World of
Vaccinology 2024

World of Vaccinology 2024

Editors

MI Sahadulla
MD FRCP (Ire) FRCP (Lon) MBA
Chairman and Managing Director
KIMS Healthcare Management Ltd.
Thiruvananthapuram, Kerala, India

Sayenna A Uduman
MD FAAP
Professor Emeritus of Pediatrics and
Pediatric Infectious Diseases (Clinical Virologist)
UAE University
Emeritus Fellow and Senior Member
American Academy of Pediatrics
Visiting Professor of Infectious Diseases
KIMS Healthcare Management Ltd.
Thiruvananthapuram, Kerala, India

Forewords

G Vijayaraghavan
TK Parthasarathy

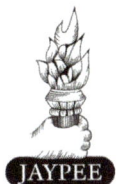

JAYPEE BROTHERS MEDICAL PUBLISHERS
The Health Sciences Publisher
New Delhi | London

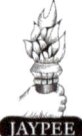 **Jaypee Brothers Medical Publishers (P) Ltd**

Headquarters
Jaypee Brothers Medical Publishers (P) Ltd
EMCA House, 23/23-B
Ansari Road, Daryaganj
New Delhi 110 002, India
Landline: +91-11-23272143, +91-11-23272703
+91-11-23282021, +91-11-23245672
Email: jaypee@jaypeebrothers.com

Overseas Office
JP Medical Ltd.
83, Victoria Street, London
SW1H 0HW (UK)
Phone: +44 20 3170 8910
Email: info@jpmedpub.com

Corporate Office
Jaypee Brothers Medical Publishers (P) Ltd
4838/24, Ansari Road, Daryaganj
New Delhi 110 002, India
Phone: +91-11-43574357
Fax: +91-11-43574314
Email: jaypee@jaypeebrothers.com

EU GPSR Authorised Representative
Logos Europe, 9 rue Nicolas Poussin
17000, La Rochelle, France
Phone: +33 (0) 6 67 93 73 78
E-mail: Contact@logoseurope.eu

Website: www.jaypeebrothers.com
Website: www.jaypeedigital.com

© 2024, Jaypee Brothers Medical Publishers

The views and opinions expressed in this book are solely those of the original contributor(s)/author(s) and do not necessarily represent those of editor(s) or publisher of the book.

All rights reserved. No part of this publication may be reproduced, stored or transmitted in any form or by any means, electronic, mechanical, photocopying, recording or otherwise, without the prior permission in writing of the publishers.

All brand names and product names used in this book are trade names, service marks, trademarks or registered trademarks of their respective owners. The publisher is not associated with any product or vendor mentioned in this book.

Medical knowledge and practice change constantly. This book is designed to provide accurate, authoritative information about the subject matter in question. However, readers are advised to check the most current information available on procedures included and check information from the manufacturer of each product to be administered, to verify the recommended dose, formula, method and duration of administration, adverse effects and contra indications. It is the responsibility of the practitioner to take all appropriate safety precautions. Neither the publisher nor the author(s)/editor(s) assume any liability for any injury and/or damage to persons or property arising from or related to use of material in this book.

This book is sold on the understanding that the publisher is not engaged in providing professional medical services. If such advice or services are required, the services of a competent medical professional should be sought.

Every effort has been made where necessary to contact holders of copyright to obtain permission to reproduce copyright material. If any have been inadvertently overlooked, the publisher will be pleased to make the necessary arrangements at the first opportunity.

Inquiries for bulk sales may be solicited at: jaypee@jaypeebrothers.com

World of Vaccinology 2024

First Edition: **2024**

ISBN: 978-93-5696-744-1

Dedication and Devotions

This book on vaccinology and evolving immunotherapies is dedicated to:
- All medical professionals and researchers who tirelessly advance medical science and enhance patient care.
- My mentors and colleagues in the USA, whose invaluable guidance and collaboration have shaped this work.
- My family and friends, who provide unwavering support and encouragement, serving as my constant source of strength.
- Dr MI Sahadulla, Chief Medical Director at KIMSHEALTH, Thiruvananthapuram, Kerala, whose endless support and patience have been pivotal throughout our journey in infectious diseases prevention.
- My beloved wife Sainambu, my children, and grandchildren, whose enduring strength and support have been my pillars throughout this journey.
- Patients, whose experiences and resilience continually inspire to push the boundaries of medical innovation.

With gratitude, I thank all colleagues and friends in the USA including the Director and Lead Scientist of Bioinformatics and Data Sciences at Cell Signaling Technology Inc. and the Former Director of Immuno-oncology Computational Biology at the Center for Immuno-oncology, Dana-Farber Cancer Institute, Harvard Medical School, Boston, MA and the Detroit healthcare experts in transplant and cancer.

Also, I extend my heartfelt thanks to the department heads and leaders in Laboratory Medicine and Microbiology at KIMSHEALTH for their contributions, inspiration, and belief in a healthier future.

And once again, thanks go to all patients, whose courage and resilience drive us to expand the frontiers of medical innovation.

Contributors

- **Mohd Uduman** BS MS (Bioinfo) MS (Compu Biologist) PhD (Yale University in Bioinformatics and Computational Biology)
  Director and Lead Scientist, Bioinformatics and Data Sciences, Cell Signaling Technology Inc.
  Former Director, Immuno-oncology Computational Biology
  Center for Immuno-Oncology, Dana-Farber Cancer Institute
  Harvard Medical School, Boston MA, USA

- **Jr Uduman** MD MS (Clinical Research)
  Medical Director (Inpatient Dialysis and CRRT), Division of Nephrology and Hypertension and
  Clinical Associate Professor, Michigan State University, Henry Ford Hospital, Detroit, MI, USA

- **AK Uduman** MD (USA Board Certified in Internal Medicine, Respiratory Medicine, Critical Care Medicine, and Sleep Medicine)
  Clinical Assistant Professor, College of Human Medicine, Michigan State University, Detroit, MI, USA

- **Afreen Allam** MBA
  Founder and CEO, SiNON Nano Sciences, Durham, NC, USA

- **Ajeeba Assan AKU** MSc
  Microbiologist, Detroit, USA

KIMSHEALTH Thiruvananthapuram Colleagues for their enthusiasm and support under Dr Sahadulla, CMD Leadership namely:
- *Zuhara PM*, Director, Emergency Department and Coordinator, Family Medicine, KIMSHEALTH.
- **Rajan B**, Director, Clinical Services, KIMSHEALTH
- **Samitha Nair**, Director, Lab Services, and her colleagues for their enthusiasm
- **Mani Varghese**, Senior Consultant, Department of Pediatrics, KIMSHEALTH
- **Arjun P**, Respiratory Medicine, KIMSHEALTH
- *Viji Mohan*, Microbiology, KIMSHEALTH
- **Sreerenjinii L**, General Manager, Pharmacy, KIMSHEALTH
- **Sister Aisha Mubarak and Staff**, Hospital Infection Control Committees, under Leads ID Consultant Dr Rajalakshmi, Dr Mohammed Niyas, Department of Infectious Diseases, KIMSHEALTH.
- *HODs, High-risk Obstetrician and Gynecologist and Fatal Medicine, Obstetrics and Gynecology, Pediatrics, and Internal Medicine.*

Finally, sincere thanks to all those who contributed their experience and knowledge developed by the Essential Program on Immunization (EPI), Department of Immunization, Vaccines and Biologicals of the World Health Organization (WHO), with extensive review and inputs from the US-CDC and P. Also, numerous colleagues in headquarters and regional offices, individuals and consultants, and partner organizations.

Foreword

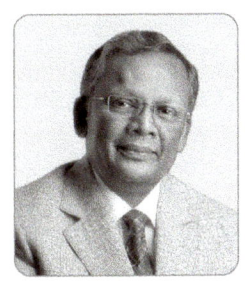

The basis for vaccination began in 1796 when the English Doctor Edward Jenner noticed that milkmaids who had gotten cowpox were protected from smallpox. Jenner also knew about variolation and guessed that exposure to cowpox could be used to protect against smallpox. The *smallpox vaccine*, introduced by *Edward Jenner* in 1796, was the first successful *vaccine* to be developed. The world and all its people have won freedom from smallpox, which was the most devastating disease. In 1980, the World Health Assembly declared smallpox eradicated (eliminated), and no cases of naturally occurring smallpox have happened since. Widespread immunization and surveillance were conducted around the world for several years. The last known natural case was in Somalia in 1977. In 1980, WHO declared smallpox eradicated—the only infectious disease to achieve this distinction. Allen does not ignore the history of vaccine disasters. He includes the fiasco in the US military in 1942, when yellow fever vaccine contaminated with hepatitis B caused 100 deaths, and the mass vaccination against smallpox in New York in 1947 that caused six deaths (four more than the outbreak itself). In the Cutter incident in the 1950s, inadequately inactivated polio vaccine caused 164 cases of paralysis and 10 deaths. While acknowledging these failures, Allen pays tribute to immunization authorities—such as Henry Kempe and Bob Chen—who have campaigned to improve vaccine safety. Allen does not ignore the history of vaccine disasters.

In 2021 when the world was threatened by the COVID-19 pandemic, there was a resurgence in vaccinology when newer vaccines were treated, and efficacy was critically analyzed. The mRNA vaccines entered the field with varying results. The first mRNA vaccines approved for use in humans—the *Pfizer/BioNTech and Moderna COVID-19 vaccines*—are being rolled out around the world.

These vaccines deliver *mRNA*, coated in lipid (fat), into cells. Once inside, your body uses instructions in the mRNA to make SARS-CoV-2 spike proteins. The immune response protects around 95% of people vaccinated with either vaccine from developing COVID-19.

Such mRNA vaccines have many benefits. They are quick to design, so once the manufacturing platform is set up, mRNA vaccines can be designed to target different viruses, or variants, very quickly. The vaccine manufacturing is also fully synthetic and does not rely on living cells like chicken eggs or cultured cell lines. So this technology *is here to stay*.

G Vijayaraghavan (Padmashri Awardee)
MD DM (Cardio) FRSM FRCP (Edin & Lond) FACC FHA
Vice Chairman and Founder Director
KIMSHEALTH
Thiruvananthapuram, Kerala, India
Dean, Postgraduate Medical Education
Advisor Emirates Royal College of Edinburg
Senior Consultant and Cardiologist

Foreword

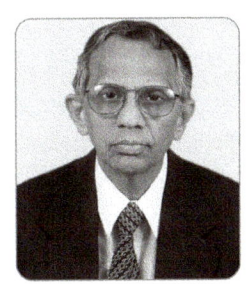

This book is designed to provide straightforward, basic information about immunizations for medical providers looking to enhance their skills. Authored by expert medical educators specializing in infectious diseases, medical microbiology, and pediatrics, it serves as a valuable resource for all healthcare professionals.

The book begins by detailing the fundamentals of vaccines, including their composition, manufacturing processes, and the methods used to test their safety and efficacy. It highlights the rapid development of mRNA vaccines for COVID-19, which was propelled by years of prior research and the urgent need to combat the global pandemic.

Furthermore, the authors have updated the current vaccine recommendations, organizing them alphabetically by infection. The Section 1 of the vaccinology section addresses practical issues that vaccinating clinicians face, such as vaccine confidence and hesitancy, common misconceptions, and strategies for effective patient communication. These topics are developed and presented in a manner accessible to healthcare providers at all levels, from medical students to seasoned practitioners.

Dr Uduman's work on vaccinology is presented as a practical guide and an excellent learning tool for students and providers involved in vaccine administration. This includes infectious disease specialists, other internal medicine subspecialists, pediatricians, geriatricians, and all primary care physicians, as well as nurse practitioners, physician assistants, and nurses.

The Section 2 delves into the use of vaccines beyond infectious diseases, exploring their application in combating cancer and noncommunicable diseases (NCDs). This section describes the innovative and evolving high-tech vaccines that are not only preventive but also therapeutic, offering potential cures for various cancers and NCDs.

Immunotherapy is highlighted as a versatile treatment for many types of cancer and NCDs, including neurodegenerative and inherited genetic disorders such as Alzheimer's disease. I congratulate the authors for their important and thought-provoking contributions to the field of vaccinology, which enhance our understanding and application of these sciences in clinical practice.

TK Parthasarathy
AB FRCSC FACS
Director of International Relations
Former Vice-Chancellor and Pro-Chancellor
Sri Ramachandra Institute of Higher
Education and Research (Deemed University)
Chennai, Tamil Nadu, India

Preface

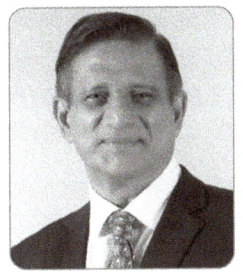

The science of vaccine development, production and application is called vaccinology. Edward Jenner is often credited as the originator of vaccinology. On May 14, 1796, he performed a smallpox vaccine experiment using material from lesions of cowpox on the hands of a dairymaid. This is probably one of the most significant scientific developments that has positively affected humanity by controlling several communicable diseases and epidemics.

World of Vaccinology 2024 is a multi-disciplinary scientific initiative dedicated to understanding the evolving cellular and molecular biology of vaccines within the field of biomedicine.

When I discussed vaccinology and immune therapeutics with my good friend, Professor Sayenna A Uduman, who is a Clinical Virologist and Epidemiologist, we realized that there is a significant need for greater public awareness in this field. This consists of two aspects:

1. Scientific basis—understanding the basic biology of vaccine development.
2. Social and public health issues—addressing the complex social, healthcare, legal, and ethical issues related to vaccination and immune therapeutics.

Interestingly, even in developing countries, vaccines are well maintained during childhood and adolescence. However, they do not receive enough attention among the adult and elderly populations, which is a major public health concern. Therefore, we decided to focus our efforts on promoting vaccinology in a way that is useful for practicing clinicians and infectious disease specialists.

I want to congratulate my dearest colleague Professor Sayenna A Uduman for all the efforts put into making this a reality. I sincerely hope that this will become a reference book and will be used as a guide by clinicians around the world.

MI Sahadulla

Preface

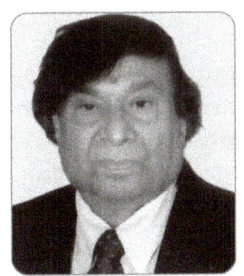

Unlike other science books, this definitive guide to immunotherapies including vaccines and vaccinology is expressed in an open-minded, persuasive narrative style. The book chapters start with a historical overview of vaccination, highlighting key milestones and breakthroughs in the field. The book opens with a historical account, tracing the advancements in vaccination and introducing the pioneers of vaccine discovery. It aims to give readers a clear understanding of the progression of immunization practices and to spark thoughts on the future directions in this vital area of science. This *World of Vaccinology 2024*, with its colorful text and illustrations, explains the immunization history and benefits of saving humans from the world's pandemics.

There are fascinating stories about vaccine discovery and vaccinologists, combined with fresh design elements, which will help the readers to understand future immunization direction and get them thinking about where human ingenuity will take us next. In the archives of human history, few scientific advancements have matched the transformative power of vaccines and immunotherapy. From the eradication of once-rampant diseases to the prospect of personalized cancer treatments, the fields of medical vaccinology and immunotherapy stand as beacons of hope, resilience, and innovation.

Vaccines have evolved significantly over the years, incorporating both traditional methods and high-tech innovations to prevent infectious diseases. We discuss the various types of these traditional and advancing vaccines, and their safety including subunit, recombinant, polysaccharide, conjugate, DNA, and viral vector vaccines, explaining the mechanisms of action and examples of each type of vaccine formulation. These vaccines use pieces of the germ like its protein, sugar, or capsid to stimulate an immune response. Examples include the human papillomavirus (HPV) vaccine and the Hib vaccine.

This book provides information on vaccine administration schedules and considerations for different populations, such as infants, pregnant mothers, elderly individuals, and immunocompromised patients. Also, it addresses issues related to vaccine development and distribution, including vaccine mandates, public health strategies, vaccine hesitancy, and surrounding ethical considerations.

Parallelly, immunotherapy represents a revolutionary approach to treating diseases, particularly cancer, by harnessing and enhancing the innate powers of the immune system. From monoclonal antibodies and checkpoint inhibitors to cancer vaccines and adoptive cell transfer, immunotherapeutic strategies have transformed the landscape of cancer treatment. This book will provide insights into the mechanisms by which these therapies modulate the immune system to recognize and combat cancer cells, offering hope to patients for whom traditional treatments have fallen short.

This book delivers and is substantially assembled, illustrious, and well researched. It is a collated evolving scientific piece of information. Vaccines and immunotherapies can change the world and breakdown big science concepts into easy understandings. There is an exceptional level of care paid to the people in these stories, so much so that connecting with the evolving science is also fantastic, going into great detail with laboratory expertise all around, globally.

Authors periodically have updated and rationalized with the new evolving pieces of knowledge in the infectious diseases specialty books that have been released in recent years including:

- *2014*: UAE University's "*Uduman's Pediatrics Handbook of Antimicrobial*" periodically updated and released by the UAE University Press
- *2016 and 2019*: KIMSHEALTH Trivandrum, India, Released Compendium *Textbook of Infectious Diseases* (book published by Jaypee Brothers Medical Publishers (P) Ltd, New Delhi, India)

- *2022*: SARS-2 CoV-19 Virology and the Pandemic Era Book released by DC Book Publishers.
- *2024*: "*Uduman's World of Vaccinology*" on vaccines, immunization, and evolving immunotherapies of this current science status. Hopefully authors desire this book to be periodically updated by KIMS Health Global specialty experts in oncology and by transplant-related infectious disease researchers on a periodical continuum basis.

This sets the stage for the exploration of the intricate and vital aspects of medical vaccinology and immunotherapy, highlighting the significance of these fields and the collective effort required to advance them.

Furthermore, the book will address the challenges that lie at the intersection of vaccinology and immunotherapy, including vaccine hesitancy, the complexities of developing vaccines for rapidly mutating pathogens, and the ongoing quest for effective cancer vaccines. It will also highlight the cutting-edge research and technological innovations driving the future of these fields, such as novel vaccine platforms and the potential of combination therapies in cancer treatment.

As we stand on the crossover of a new era in medical science, the authors of this book aim to provide healthcare professionals, researchers, and students with a comprehensive understanding of the principles and practices of vaccinology and immunotherapy. Through a multidisciplinary lens, we will explore how these fields continue to shape our approach to preventing and treating diseases, ultimately paving the way for a healthier future for all.

Power of Collaboration

Our book, the *World of Vaccinology 2024*, is a multidisciplinary scientific initiative dedicated to understanding the evolving cellular and molecular biology of vaccines within Regenerative Medicine.

This book is founded on the principles of collaboration and teamwork, encouraging contributions from experts across various disciplines, both nationally and internationally.

As genomics advances and new sophisticated technologies emerge, requiring expertise from multiple medical domains, the authors have endeavored to enhance the impact of preventive medicine.

Our goal is to elevate role models in this field and underscore the benefits of these advancements to human health and scientific innovation.

Recent breakthroughs in vaccination and immunization have shed light on the therapeutic applications of vaccines for a more comprehensive array of cancers and immunologically- mediated diseases, revealing new possibilities in disease prevention and treatment.

This version maintains the original message but enhances clarity and flow, emphasizing the collaborative nature and innovative aspirations of Uduman's *World of Vaccinology 2024*.

Sayenna A Uduman

Acknowledgments

- I would like to express my deepest gratitude to everyone who contributed to the development and publication of this book. Your support, guidance, and encouragement were invaluable throughout this journey.
- I am profoundly grateful to Dr Sahadulla whose expertise and insights in medical innovation were crucial to the foundation of this book. His mentorship has been instrumental in shaping my understanding and approach to this complex subject.
- Our appreciation to the Department of Family Medicine—Dr Zuhara PM, Director of Pharmacy and Emergency Medicine; Sree Ranjinii, Pharmacy Head; Dr Samitha, Laboratory Medicine; and her colleagues for their enthusiasm and support under Dr Sahadulla, CMD Lead.
- Afreen Allam, Nano-Scientists (Founder and CEO President, SiNON Therapeutic, Boston, USA) and Ajeeba Assan AKU, MSc Microbiologist, Detroit, USA
- Dr Rajan B, Director, Clinical Services (Reviewed chapters 9 and 11—Cancer-related Chapters)
- We extend our deepest gratitude to all the Heads of Departments (HODs) at KIMSHEALTH, particularly in Infectious Diseases (Dr Rajalakshmi, Dr Mohammed Niyas), Pediatrics, Obstetrics and Gynecology, and the Medicine Department.
- Our special appreciation is extended to Dr Mani Varghese, Senior Pediatric Consultant and Dr Arjun, Chief of Pulmonary Medicine.
- Ms Reshmi Aysha, CEO, KCC, and CSR.
- We also express our appreciation to the KIMSHEALTH Hospital Infection Control Committee, led by Sister Aisha Mubarak and her team.
- Mr Vamadevan C, Executive Secretary, with his never-failing confidence and enthusiasm, for this Uduman's World of Vaccinology 2024 that is in your hand with an impactful message that readers can quickly understand and appreciate. Uduman wishes to extend our deepest gratitude to Vamadevan, for his exceptional work on the publication of this medical book on vaccination. Vamadevan's meticulous attention to detail, unwavering dedication and hard work, and communication with the publishers have been instrumental in bringing this historical vaccinology and immunotherapy book to fruition.
- Ms Jessy Ajith, General Manager, CMD Office and Administrator, IMT, KIMSHEALTH, Thiruvananthapuram, Kerala, India.
- Ms Divya Ravidas, Manager, Corporate HR, KIMSHEALTH, Thiruvananthapuram, Kerala, India.
- Mr Ashok Kumar S, Assistant General Manager, Audiovisual, KIMSHEALTH, Thiruvananthapuram, Kerala, India.

Contents

SECTION 1 — ESSENTIAL AND CUTTING-EDGE IN VACCINOLOGY
Uduman SA, Sahadullah MIS

1. Introduction 3
2. Vaccines Evolution: Historical Background and Breakthroughs 7
3. Success Stories and Ongoing Challenges 24
4. Vaccine Components—Highpoints 36
5. Pediatric Immunizations 68
6. Adult Immunizations for Ages 19 Years or Older 84
7. Pregnancy and Lactation Periods' Vaccinations 97
8. Vaccines for the Elderly (Older Adults) (Senior Care Vaccinations) 119

SECTION 2 — IMMUNOTHERAPIES: PREVENTIVE AND THERAPEUTIC ADVANCEMENTS
Mohd Uduman, Jr Uduman, AK Uduman

9. Immunotherapy and Gene Therapy Approaches in Disease Prevention and Treatments 129
   Mohd Uduman
10. Immunization in Special Clinical Circumstances Including Solid Organ Transplant (Immunocompromised and Immunosuppressed SOT and HSCT Recipients) 173
    Jr Uduman, AK Uduman
11. Cancer Vaccines: Preventive and Therapeutics 189
    Mohd Uduman, Jr Uduman, AK Uduman
12. Vaccines and Immunotherapies against Noncommunicable Diseases 225
    Jr Uduman, AK Uduman
13. Innovative Infectious Diseases Vaccines (The Future of Vaccines) 256
    Mohd Uduman

SECTION 3 — VACCINES FOR TRAVELERS, SCHOOL CHILDREN, AND HEALTHCARE STAFF: DISPELLING MYTHS WITH MEDICAL AI AND ENSURING VACCINE SAFETY
Sahadulla MIS, Zuhara PM, Reshmi Aysha, Uduman SA

14. Travel Vaccine (Travel Immunizations) 301
15. Vaccine Safety and Efficacy 308

16. Artificial Intelligence and Machine Learning in Vaccinology 312
17. Catch-up Vaccinations in Childhood Immunizations 316
18. Combination Vaccines (Combos) 319
19. School Health Immunization.. 322
20. Healthcare Personnel Vaccine Needs 325
21. Vaccine Hesitancy and Providing Confidence in Vaccinations 330
22. Some Facts, Myths, and Misconceptions.. 334

Index 343

SECTION 1: Essential and Cutting-edge in Vaccinology

Uduman SA, Sahadullah MIS

1. Introduction
2. Vaccines Evolution: Historical Background and Breakthroughs
3. Success Stories and Ongoing Challenges
4. Vaccine Components—Highpoints
5. Pediatric Immunizations
6. Adult Immunizations for Ages 19 Years or Older
7. Pregnancy and Lactation Periods' Vaccinations
8. Vaccines for the Elderly (Older Adults) (Senior Care Vaccinations)

CHAPTER 1

Introduction

Vaccination is a powerful method of disease prevention for people of all ages worldwide as evidenced by its impact during the coronavirus disease 2019 (COVID-19) pandemic. It is a common misconception that the importance of immunizations wanes after childhood. Vaccines continue to play a critical role throughout adolescence and adulthood, bolstering the defenses established in early years and safeguarding against diseases that can emerge when immunity fades. The importance of vaccination in adult populations, particularly those aged over 60 years, is frequently overlooked, despite their continued critical role in maintaining health.

Immunization currently prevents 3.5–5 million deaths every year from diseases such as diphtheria, tetanus, pertussis, influenza, and measles. India's strides in child health over the last two decades are commendable, with the country achieving polio-free status in 2014 and eliminating maternal and neonatal tetanus a year later. Yet challenges persist as evidenced by the 1.6 million children who were unvaccinated or undervaccinated in 2022, despite high national coverage rates of 93%.

India's Universal Immunization Program (UIP) provides free vaccinations to combat 12 vaccine-preventable diseases (VPDs). These include diphtheria, pertussis (whooping cough), tetanus, polio, measles, rubella, a severe form of childhood tuberculosis, rotavirus diarrhea, hepatitis B, as well as meningitis and pneumonia caused by Haemophilus influenzae type b (Hib), among others. On the flip side, many medical students and young physicians today have limited firsthand experience with these diseases due to the success of the vaccines. This detachment from the real impact of VPDs underscores the hidden burden of these illnesses, especially among adults, where vaccination rates are dismally low. Without national guidelines, the adult immunization strategy in India remains fragmented and unclear.

The true burden of VPDs among Indian adults is unknown, with coverage for adult vaccination remaining critically low. Adults are particularly vulnerable during outbreaks due to a lack of immunization, waning immunity, age-related factors (e.g., chronic conditions and immunosenescence), and epidemiological shifts; the adult population beyond 18 years of age is particularly vulnerable during outbreaks.

There are no national adult immunization guidelines in India and although several medical societies have published adult immunization guidelines, these vary, making it unclear who should receive which vaccines (based on age, underlying conditions, etc.). *Other barriers to adult immunization* include vaccine hesitancy, missed opportunities, and cost. Steps to improve adult vaccination could include the adoption of national guidelines, education of the public, and promotion of courses on vaccinology and immunization. Improving adult vaccine coverage could help reduce the burden of VPDs, particularly among older adults.

Vaccines stand as one of the most monumental achievements in medical history. They not only confer individual protection against bacterial and viral diseases but also safeguard the broader community by fostering herd immunity. This communal protection is vital for those with health complications and for all age groups within a society.

Increased vaccination rates promote herd immunity which not only protects individuals with serious conditions but also protects all children and adults in a community. Unlike the Pediatric Immunization Guidelines, given by the Indian Academy of Pediatrics (IAP) and the National Immunization Programs (NIP), the strategies for vaccination in healthy adults are not mandatory and may vary from region to region. Usually, parents are particular and regular when it comes to vaccinating their children, but they fail to realize that adult vaccination is just as important as getting their children vaccinated. Also, any adults above the age of 65 years or any age with chronic conditions such as diabetes, heart conditions, chronic lung disease, chronic liver disease, and cancer are also at high risk and must take age-appropriate vaccination protections.

This "World of Vaccinology Tablet" is a brochure that attempts to synthesize the evolving evidence for current immunization and immunotherapies beyond pediatrics.

Recent global outbreaks of VPDs have predominantly affected unvaccinated individuals. This lack of vaccination often stems from eligibility issues, such as age constraints or preexisting medical conditions. However, there is also a notable portion of the unvaccinated population who opt out due to personal belief or religious exemptions.

Unvaccinated children drive surge in deadly outbreaks: The world is witnessing significant outbreaks of diseases that are particularly lethal to children. This concerning trend is a direct consequence of health system disruptions during the COVID-19 pandemic. As a result, over 60 million children globally have missed out on standard childhood vaccinations.

Many of the children who missed their shots have now aged out of routine immunization programs. So-called "zero-dose children" account for nearly half of all child deaths from VPDs, according to the Global Alliance for Vaccines and Immunization (GAVI), the organization that helps fund vaccination in low- and middle-income countries.

Furthermore, many of the large outbreaks of VPDs occur among religious groups and the major concerns are over the vaccine safety which drives them to avoid vaccines not based on any real religious doctrine. The main problem is that these groups of unvaccinated people become clustered together in religious activities, helping to fuel large outbreaks of VPDs.

FUTURE OF IMMUNIZATION/ IMMUNOTHERAPIES

The future of immunization hinges on the ongoing progress in medical research aimed at developing innovative vaccines. Future vaccines are anticipated to offer broader protection against variants, longer-lasting effects, and superior capabilities in preventing infection and transmission, including mucosal vaccines, compared to the vaccines currently available. Although predicting the specific characteristics of future vaccines is challenging, numerous promising research and development areas are shaping the future of immunization.

Ideally, vaccines of the future will not only be quick to develop but can offer:

- *Long-term stability at warm temperatures:* This addresses a crucial challenge in vaccine distribution, particularly in regions where maintaining cold chains is difficult, thereby facilitating global accessibility.
- *High efficacy in immune-compromised and elderly populations:* This is an important goal, as these groups are often more vulnerable to diseases yet may respond less effectively to current vaccines.
- *Durable immunity with minimal dosing and self-administration capability:* This would enhance vaccine uptake and compliance, making immunization more convenient and accessible to a broader population.

For the first time, the COVID-19 pandemic brought messenger ribonucleic acid (mRNA) vaccines to the forefront, demonstrating their potential of providing a more rapid response to emerging infectious diseases (IDs) compared to traditional vaccines.

The *mRNA technology* has emerged as a revolutionary breakthrough in vaccine development, highlighting its potential and leading to the rapid deployment of mRNA-based vaccines. This technology provides a platform for quicker and adaptable vaccine production, offering hope in the fight against emerging IDs.

Current vaccines are typically designed to target specific strains or variants of a pathogen. However, the development of universal vaccines aims to create vaccines that provide broad protection against multiple strains or even entire families of pathogens. Universal influenza vaccines, for example, would eliminate the need for annual vaccine updates and provide long-lasting immunity against multiple influenza strains.

Also, there are many "personalized vaccines" that involve tailoring vaccines to an individual's specific immune profile or genetic makeup. This approach has the potential to improve vaccine responses in individuals with weakened immune systems or to target specific cancer cells in cancer immunotherapy.

It is important to note that these futuristic vaccine/immunotherapy technologies are still in various stages of research and development. While they hold great promise, it may take time before they become widely available for clinical use. Omalizumab (Xolair), recently approved by the United States (US) Food and Drug Administration (FDA) as monotherapy for the treatment of food allergies, may now bring peace of mind to these patients and their families by reducing their risk of dangerous allergic reactions to accidental exposure.

In recent years, the pace of innovation in the field of immunizations has accelerated like never before. Pioneering technologies, from mRNA and deoxyribonucleic acid (DNA) platforms to artificial intelligence (AI), are reshaping the landscape of vaccine development, distribution, and administration. These innovations hold the promise of not only enhancing the efficacy and safety of vaccines but also addressing critical challenges such as accessibility and affordability, bequeathing a future where preventable diseases are minimized or eradicated.

mRNA-based Vaccines and mRNA Therapeutics—What is Beyond COVID-19?

The COVID-19 mRNA vaccines were developed and approved at unprecedented speed and have demonstrated significant effectiveness against infections and acute COVID-19 in the real world. The knowledge of using mRNA as a simple and promising way to deliver vaccines or therapeutic drugs had been around for decades before the onset of the recent global pandemic. The success of mRNA vaccines against COVID-19 has created huge enthusiasm around this concept and significantly boosted the applications of this class of medicines in other areas. As the pandemic gradually fades, we cannot stop thinking about what the world has gained in this chaos—the realization and authentication of the power of mRNA in modern medicine.

As the recent global pandemic gradually fades, a significant amount of research has now been concentrated on developing mRNA vaccines, mRNA therapeutic drugs, and delivery systems against infectious and immune diseases, cancer, and other debilitating noncommunicable diseases (NCDs) and has demonstrated encouraging results. *RNA therapeutics are the medicines of the future.*

At this crucial juncture of the pandemic, what we need is an "infection-blocking vaccine" and not vaccines that only protect you against severe disease. While these vaccines have saved countless lives, it is unlikely that they will, on their own, stop viral transmission and prevent the emergence of new viral variants.

Intramuscular injections generate systemic immunity but little or no immune response in the nose, where respiratory viruses such as SARS-CoV-2 (severe acute respiratory syndrome coronavirus 2) typically enter the body. In contrast, *intranasal vaccines*, which can elicit both mucosal and systemic immune responses, are targeting SARS-CoV-2 and are in development. Could they pave the way for widespread nasal vaccination in the future?

Noncommunicable Diseases' Vaccines and Immunotherapies

As life expectancy has increased, the burden of NCDs such as cancer, hypertension, atherosclerosis, and diabetes has increased. Therefore, scientists hope a new type of vaccine could treat and prevent NCDs; this could include autoimmune diseases, such as multiple sclerosis (MS), type 1 diabetes, allergic asthma, Alzheimer's, myasthenia gravis, and Crohn's disease, among others. The NCD vaccines present an interesting challenge for the US FDA which is tasked with approving new treatments on the basis of efficacy and safety.

Like traditional vaccines, NCD vaccines work by modulating the human immune system, but target cells, proteins, or other molecules that are associated with the NCD in question rather than pathogens or pathogen-infected cells. These vaccines are still in development and have not been systematically tested on humans.

- Effective vaccination will have a significant impact on the disease burden of both VPDs and NCDs and beyond.
- Immunotherapies, for example, monoclonal antibodies (mAbs) and T-cell therapies in cancer treatment approach based on the concept of harnessing the patient's immune system to fight tumor cells. Newly evolving tumor cell-specific mAbs have redefined cancer treatment and identify how human gut microbiomes alter the body's response to a common form of cancer immunotherapy.
- Over the past two decades, the immune system has attracted increasing attention for its role in fighting cancer. As researchers have learned more and more about the cancer-immune system interplay, several antitumor immunotherapies have become FDA-approved and are now regularly used to treat multiple cancer types.

Yet despite these advances, much remains unknown about how the immune system fights cancer and about immunity in general. CRISPR-based gene editing, in which scientists modify the genome using a tool developed just over a decade ago, has become a mainstay of biological discovery, providing relatively quick insight into the function of individual genes and targets for new therapies.

Gene and cell therapies have seen a massive transformation over the past decade from promising experimental treatments to approved medicines for a wide range of patients with genetic or acquired diseases.

Vaccine hesitancy and vaccine refusal (anti-vaxxers)—growing public health concerns:
Multiple factors are associated with vaccine hesitancy, and this has been increasingly identified as a global

health worry. This may upset the success of vaccination programs against IDs.

There are many likely contributing factors for vaccine refusal, such as unfamiliarity with VPDs, cultural–social differences, religious beliefs, and media information. Most major religions like Christianity, Judaism, Islam, and Hinduism do not oppose the idea of vaccinations, however, for certain sociocultural reasons oppose the immunization benefits. Notably, religious affiliations have been linked with lower vaccination coverage, especially in more conservative religious communities globally. Therefore, engaging religious leaders in immunization programs is crucial for enhancing the vaccine's uptakes significantly.

The government of India is set to launch a "U-Win" portal, designed on the lines of "Co-Win" that was launched during the COVID-19 pandemic. The U-Win program has been designed to digitize the UIP and it is presently being run in a pilot mode in certain districts of each state and Union Territory Official sources claim. It is expected that this U-Win platform will be used to register and vaccinate every pregnant woman, record her delivery outcome, register every newborn delivery, administer birth doses, and all vaccination events thereafter.

■ CONCLUSION

This introductory paragraphs of this World of Vaccinology book offers a comprehensive overview of the current and future state of vaccines. It serves as an essential resource for students, public health professionals, researchers, and anyone keen to deepen their knowledge of vaccines, vaccinations, and vaccinology. It addresses prevalent queries about vaccine usage in an era increasingly influenced by antivaccine sentiments and it deliberates on the societal versus individual benefits of vaccines.

Furthermore, it is important to acknowledge and appreciate the remarkable contributions of ID scientists and healthcare professionals. Their unwavering commitment to research and innovation plays a pivotal role in guiding us toward a healthier, disease-free future. Immunization transcends personal choice; it represents a shared duty to uphold global health and well-being.

Compilation of immunotherapies against diseases prevention including human vaccinology has been complex with substantial challenges, but we have attempted to bring together recent knowledge about the immune system including the immune-mediated illnesses and types of immunotherapies. The development of new specialized equipment and immunological techniques, genetic approaches, animal models, and a long list of mAbs, among many other factors, are improving our knowledge of this sophisticated human systems.

This knowledge is filling many of the gaps through immunotherapies, i.e., on the different types of cell subsets, cytokines soluble factors, membrane molecules, and cell functionalities are some aspects that we are starting to understand, together with their roles in health, aging, illness, and immunization. With significant advances in protein nanoparticle science, mRNA technology, adjuvant development, and B-cell and antibody analyses, a new wave of clinical trials are on the way.

As we delve into these above chapters, we embark on an exploratory journey of these transformative innovations in immunization. This journey is not only about scientific discovery but also about instilling hope and securing the health of humanity for generations to come.

■ SUGGESTED READING

1. Human Vaccines & Immunotherapeutics, Volume 20, Issue 1 (2024). https://www.tandfonline.com/toc/khvi20/current
2. Thomas A. Waldmann, Immunotherapy: past, present and future. Nature Medicine. 2003;9:269-77
3. Vaccines and Immunizations (Basics and Common Questions). Centers for Disease Control and Prevention (CDC and P) 24/7. https://www.cdc.gov/vaccines/vac-gen/imz-basics.htm
4. Zeng Z, Fu J, Cibulskis C, Jhaveri A, Gumbs C, Das B, et al. Cross-site concordance evaluation of tumor DNA and RNA sequencing platforms for the CIMAC-CIDC network. Clin Cancer Res. 2021;27(18):5049-61.

CHAPTER 2

Vaccines Evolution: Historical Background and Breakthroughs

◼ INTRODUCTION

The evolution of vaccination: Vaccination, a practice dating back to the 10th century, has evolved drastically since its inception. The advent of the smallpox vaccine in the 18th century laid the foundation for modern immunization. From the humble beginnings of variolation against smallpox to the sophisticated messenger ribonucleic acid-(mRNA)-based coronavirus disease 2019 (COVID-19) vaccines, the journey has been awe-inspiring. This progress has been driven by a continuous quest for safer, more effective vaccines and vaccination strategies.

This chapter on historical aspects of vaccines and vaccine developments is briefed despite its many-sided complexity. Here are some key points that readers will be looking at:

- *Growth and developments of selective vaccines such as* Bacille Calmette–Guérin (BCG), hepatitis B (HepB) virus, polioviruses, diphtheria–tetanus–pertussis (DTP) combination formulations, first conjugated *Haemophilus influenzae* type b (Hib) for children, pneumococcus journey from polysaccharide component, rotaviruses (RVs) for kids under 8 months of age, *Neisseria meningitis* including type B in one shot, measles, mumps, and rubella (MMR) and varicella (MMR-V) combination, zoster protection for elderlies, annual seasonal flu shot still, hepatitis A (HepA) virus (HAV) shot, dengue vaccine still not perfected, COVID-19 to all, human papillomavirus (HPV) three doses to single dose, toward human immunodeficiency virus (HIV) vaccine, malaria vaccine, and at last, the respiratory syncytial virus (RSV) and group B streptococcus (GBS) arrived for prevention.
- Artificial intelligence (AI) and machine learning (ML) in vaccine design.
- Global politics of vaccines and vaccinations.

Vaccinology, the study of vaccines and vaccination, has a rich history that spans several centuries. Vaccines have had a profound impact on public health, saving millions of lives and preventing the spread of infectious diseases. For over two centuries, people have been vaccinated against deadly diseases ever since the world's first vaccine was devised against smallpox.

Vaccines represent one of the greatest successes of medicine, histrionically reducing the incidence of serious or life-threatening infectious diseases and allowing people to live longer healthier lives. Diseases that once caused significant morbidity and mortality in children are at all-time nadirs in many parts of the world.

Vaccinations continue to evolve with ongoing research and development (R&D) of new vaccines, improvements in vaccine delivery systems, and efforts to address vaccine hesitancy and access barriers. The COVID-19 pandemic has revealed how devastating a disease outbreak can be in our societies.

The history of vaccinology begins with smallpox, one of the deadliest diseases in human history. In the late 18th century, *Edward Jenner,* an English physician, observed that milkmaids who had contracted cowpox, a less severe disease, seemed to be immune to smallpox. In 1796, Jenner conducted an experiment where he inoculated a young boy with material from a cowpox sore and then exposed him to smallpox. The boy did not develop smallpox, demonstrating the concept of vaccination. Following Jenner's discovery, other scientists and researchers began developing vaccines for various diseases. Edward Jenner was the first to test a method to protect against smallpox scientifically, and he is often considered the *"father of vaccines"* because of his scientific approach that proved the method worked.

Louis Pasteur, a French scientist, is credited with developing the first attenuated vaccine for chicken cholera in 1879. He later went on to develop vaccines for anthrax and rabies.

In the 20th century, significant advancements were made in vaccinology.

- In the 1920s, Albert Calmette and Camille Guérin developed the BCG vaccine for tuberculosis (TB).
- In the 1950s, Jonas Salk and Albert Sabin independently developed vaccines for polio, leading to the near eradication of the disease.

In the latter half of the 20th century, vaccination programs expanded globally. The World Health Organization (WHO) launched the Expanded Program on Immunization (EPI) in 1974, aiming to provide vaccines for diseases such as DTP, polio, and measles to children worldwide.

In recent decades, there have been significant advancements in vaccine technology. This includes the development of new vaccine platforms, such as recombinant deoxyribonucleic acid (DNA) technology, viral vectors, and mRNA-based vaccines. These advancements have enabled the rapid development of vaccines for emerging infectious diseases, such as COVID-19.

Global vaccination efforts: Vaccination campaigns have played a crucial role in reducing the burden of many infectious diseases worldwide. Global initiatives, such as the Global Vaccine Action Plan (GVAP) and Global Alliance for Vaccines and Immunization (GAVI), the vaccine alliance, have focused on increasing access to vaccines in low-income countries and improving immunization coverage.

Scientific evidence from the fights against smallpox measles, rubella, polio, and now COVID-19 has demonstrated that vaccines are among the most effective and safest means to prevent individual illness and protect public health. We now have more than 30 vaccines that have been approved for general or emergency use in countries around the world. However, the number of approved vaccines and their specific recommendations can change over time as new vaccines are developed and existing ones are periodically updated.

Vaccination schedules may vary from country to country and can also depend on factors such as the baby's health, maternal immunity, and local disease prevalence. The WHO regularly updates its recommendations and provides information on vaccines for different age groups and regions. Vaccination is one of the most beneficial and cost-effective measures that we can adopt to protect ourselves from potentially fatal illnesses.

Good vaccination practices begin shortly after birth and during early infancy. Vaccines are tested to ensure that they are safe and effective for children to receive at the recommended ages. Most of the recommended childhood immunizations are 90–100% effective. However, for reasons that are not completely understood, sometimes a child will not become fully immunized against a disease after receiving a vaccine.

The basic bacterial and viral components typically start in early infancy and childhood immunization practices are:

■ BACILLE CALMETTE–GUÉRIN HISTORY

In many countries, the BCG vaccine is given shortly after birth to protect against TB which is the only currently available preventive vaccine for TB. The newborns at birth are routinely vaccinated in many parts of the world, particularly in areas with a high prevalence of TB. However, not all countries include BCG immunization in their routine vaccination schedules.

The BCG vaccine is an attenuated strain of *Mycobacterium bovis*, a bacterium related to *Mycobacterium tuberculosis* (MTB), which causes TB in humans. The first human to receive the BCG vaccine was a newborn infant named Albert, who was vaccinated on July 18, 1921, marking the beginning of human BCG vaccination.

Bacille Calmette–Guérin's effectiveness in preventing TB varies and is generally higher in protecting against severe forms of childhood TB, such as TB meningitis and miliary TB. The BCG's effectiveness in preventing adult pulmonary TB, which is the most common form of TB, however, is limited. It provides partial protection and is less effective in adults than in children.

Despite its limitations, BCG remains the only available TB vaccine. Efforts to develop a more effective TB vaccine have been ongoing for many years that could provide better protection against TB infection and diseases. An effective vaccine would revolutionize TB control (Refer to Chapter 13: Innovative Infectious Diseases Futuristic TB vaccines).

Over the years, efforts have been made to develop new and more effective TB vaccines. Several vaccine candidates are currently in various stages of clinical trials, aiming to provide better protection against TB, including in adults and individuals with HIV.

■ HEPATITIS B VIRUS VACCINE DEVELOPMENTS

The development history of the HepB virus (HBV) vaccine is a significant milestone in the field of immunization and public health, the science of protecting and improving the health of populations. In the 1960s, the HBV vaccine development journey began in the United States of America (USA). *Dr Baruch Blumberg* was awarded the Nobel Prize in 1976 for his discovery of HBV and the development of the developing diagnostic tests.

In the 1970s, *Dr Saul Krugman*, the longest term served as head of pediatrics, at New York (NY) University discovered that heat-treated serum from a chronic carrier of HepB could elicit protective antibodies in a susceptible person without causing the disease. This brilliantly simple discovery paved the way for the development of various HBV vaccines now licensed worldwide.

Development of the First-Generation Vaccine (Recombinant Protein Vaccine)

In the early 1980s, researchers made a significant breakthrough in HBV vaccine development. Dr Maurice Hilleman and his team at Merck developed the first-generation vaccine, known as the "recombinant protein vaccine". This vaccine was based on using a part of the HBV surface antigen (HBsAg) produced through recombinant DNA technology. In 1982, the vaccine was licensed for use in the United States (US) by the Food and Drug Administration (FDA). Other countries followed suit in approving the vaccine.

In summary, the development of the HepB vaccine is a remarkable achievement in the history of medicine and public health. The first dose of this vaccine is often given shortly after birth, usually within the first 24 hours. This vaccine requires a series of shots for full protection. It has saved countless lives and contributed to the prevention of HBV-related diseases and disorders worldwide.
- The HepB vaccine is also known as the first "anti-cancer" vaccine because it prevents HBV, the leading cause of liver cancer worldwide.

POLIO VIRUS VACCINE BACKGROUND HISTORY

The history of the polio virus vaccine is a significant chapter in the field of public health and medicine. Polio, short for poliomyelitis, is a highly contagious viral disease that can lead to paralysis and, in severe cases, death. Before the first vaccine for polio was developed in the 1950s, it was a terrifying disease.

A breakthrough occurred in 1949 when poliovirus was successfully cultivated in human tissue at Boston Children's Hospital by *John Enders*, Thomas Weller, and Frederick Robbins. Their pioneering work was recognized with the 1954 Nobel Prize.

Polio has been known since ancient times, but large-scale outbreaks began occurring in the late 19th and early 20th centuries. These outbreaks led to increasing concern and research into finding a vaccine.

In the early 1950s, one of the most pivotal moments in the history of the polio vaccine was the development of the inactivated polio vaccine (IPV) by *Dr Jonas Salk*, in the USA. In 1954, Salk and his team conducted extensive clinical trials, culminating in a successful field trial involving over 1.8 million children. The vaccine was announced as safe and effective in 1955, marking a major breakthrough. On April 12, 1955, the US physician Jonas Salk's IPV was licensed. Six pharmaceutical companies were licensed to produce IPV and Salk did not profit from sharing the formulation or production processes. In an interview, when asked who owned the patent for IPV, Salk replied: "Well, the people, I would say. There is no patent. Could you patent the sun?"

Around the same time as Salk's work, *Dr Albert Sabin* was developing an oral polio vaccine (OPV) using *attenuated live poliovirus strain*, in NY, USA. Sabin first used an experimental OPV vaccine on himself and his family, but he had to go further afield for larger-scale trials. The OPV was easier to administer and played a crucial role in the global effort to eradicate polio. It was licensed for use in the 1960s. The Global Polio Eradication Initiative (GPEI), launched in 1988, has reduced polio cases by over 99%. Wild poliovirus transmission remains in just a few countries, highlighting the effectiveness of vaccines in controlling the disease.

In 1988, the World Health Assembly launched the GPEI to eradicate polio worldwide. This initiative, led by organizations such as the WHO, United Nations International Children's Emergency Fund (UNICEF), Rotary International, and the Bill and Melinda Gates Foundation, has made significant progress and many countries have been declared polio free.

Switch to IPV: In some countries, including the US, the use of OPV was phased out in favor of IPV due to rare cases of vaccine-derived poliovirus. The role of philanthropic organizations such as the Bill and Melinda Gates Foundation have played a significant role in supporting polio eradication efforts by providing funding and resources.
- The first dose of the OPV or the IPV is often given at 2 months of age (can be given at 6 weeks of age) followed by three more doses for full primary protection.

Historical Aspects of 1952 Polio Survivor in the USA who died on March 15, 2024:
Paul Alexander, world record holder and polio survivor, popularly known as "Man in the iron lung" died at 78, on

March 15, 2024 (WJW-TV Cleveland). Paul was a polio survivor and was dependent on an artificial respiratory system to breathe. Paul contracted polio in 1952, at the age of 6 years, which left him paralyzed from the neck down and reliant on a mechanical respirator to breathe for much of the time. This was before the first poliovirus vaccine in 1955, children affected by polio were dependent on iron lungs for their survival. Paul hailed from Dallas, Texas.

Though often confined to his submarine-like cylinder, the so-called iron lung helped him breathe and he could leave the cylinder for short periods (**Fig. 1** "The Iron Lung and Polio" under Vaccine-Preventable Diseases Photo Gallery). He even learned to breathe by himself. Paul excelled in his studies, earned a law degree, practiced law, and even published a memoir book. He held the official Guinness World Record for time spent in a lung. According to his Guinness page, he was able to leave the device for periods after he learned to "frog breathe" with the help of a physical therapist.

DIPHTHERIA, TETANUS, AND PERTUSSIS VACCINE FORMULATION BACKGROUNDS

The DTP vaccine is a combination vaccine used to immunize against three serious bacterial diseases: diphtheria, tetanus, and pertussis. Diphtheria and tetanus vaccines were developed in the early 20th century, while the pertussis vaccine was developed in the 1930s.

The individual vaccines were initially administered separately. The idea of combining these (combo) vaccines into a single shot, the DTP vaccine, was proposed to simplify immunization schedules and improve vaccination coverage.

The DTP vaccine was first introduced in the US in the 1940s and was widely adopted for routine childhood immunization. It has become a critical component of childhood vaccination programs in many countries. In India, the DTP vaccine was introduced in routine immunization in 1978, resulting in a substantial decline in incidence in the pediatric populations. The effect was a shift of the infection to the older age groups. In 1998, around 65% of cases occurred above 3 years of age.

In the 1970s and 1980s, concerns were raised about the safety of the DTP vaccine, particularly regarding rare but serious adverse reactions. These concerns led to changes in vaccine formulations and recommendations.

DTP transition to DTaP annotations for diphtheria, tetanus toxoids, and acellular pertussis antigens—to address safety concerns, acellular pertussis vaccines were developed, leading to the transition from DTP to DTaP vaccines in many countries. DTaP vaccines contain purified components of the pertussis bacterium, which are thought to have a lower risk of side effects compared to whole-cell pertussis vaccines used in DTP. In some countries, the DTaP vaccine is given to children at specific ages, followed by booster doses in later childhood. The immunization schedule can vary by country and region.

- Tdap contains a lower concentration of diphtheria and pertussis toxoids than DTaP.

The DTP or DTaP vaccines are included in the routine childhood vaccination schedules of most countries around the world. They are part of the WHO's EPI, which aims to protect children from vaccine-preventable diseases.

The first dose of the vaccine is typically given at 2 months of age (can be given at 6 weeks of age)*, with booster doses scheduled at intervals. Vaccination programs are essential for maintaining immunity and preventing outbreaks of these serious diseases.

It is important to note that the specific vaccines, recommendations, and schedules may vary by country and over time. The DTP/DTaP vaccine has been a crucial tool in preventing DTP, contributing to public health efforts to reduce the burden of these diseases.

Just to lessen the confusions on the abbreviated, for example, DTaP/Tdap/DTP (DPT)/tetanus-diphtheria (Td), and the best utility of these acronyms about what vaccine children and adults need, one should follow these general guidelines:

- 6 weeks through 6 years—DTaP
- 7-9 years of age—Td
- 10 years through 64 years—Tdap (especially if you have close contact with an infant) or Td
- 65 years or older—Td (or talk to your doctor if you have close contact with an infant).

Sources:
1. Centers for Disease Control and Prevention (CDC). (2021). Epidemiology and Prevention of Vaccine-Preventable Diseases: Chapters. Available from: https://www.cdc.gov/vaccines/pubs/pinkbook/chapters.html [Last accessed May, 2024].

HAEMOPHILUS INFLUENZAE TYPE B VACCINE SUCCESS

Prior to the introduction of the Hib vaccine, Hib infections were a major cause of morbidity and mortality among children worldwide. In the early 20th century, the Hib bacterium was responsible for a range of illnesses, including sepsis, meningitis, pneumonia, and other serious infections, primarily affecting young children.

In the early 1980s, historical breakthroughs occurred with the development of a safe and effective vaccine against Hib. Both Dr David Smith and Dr Porter Anderson are credited with developing the first successful Hib vaccine. The Hib vaccine was introduced for routine childhood immunization in the US in the late 1980s and early 1990s. This marked the beginning of a significant reduction in Hib-related diseases. Importantly, the Indian Academy of Pediatrics (IAP) had already recommended in 2006 the use of Hib vaccine for all children. The use of Hib vaccines in the private sector has been widespread in India for almost a decade.

The success of the Hib vaccine in reducing disease burden led to global efforts to make it accessible to children worldwide through vaccination programs. International organizations such as the WHO have promoted the inclusion of the Hib vaccine in routine immunization schedules. The Hib-associated diseases affect around 337,000 Indian children every year and the vaccination against Hib was introduced in 2011 as part of the pentavalent vaccine and scaled up nationwide.

The development and successful implementation of the Hib vaccine serve as a model for the development and deployment of vaccines against other infectious diseases. It demonstrates how vaccines can have a profound impact on public health by preventing serious illnesses and saving children's lives.

Childhood Hib immunization usually starts at 2 months of age (can be given at 6 weeks of age) followed by three more doses to complete the series before 15 months of age. It can be administered as a single antigen or in combination shots.

Children over 5 years and adults usually do not receive the Hib vaccine, but it might be recommended for older children or adults with asplenia or sickle cell disease, before surgery to remove the spleen or following a bone marrow transplant. Hib vaccine may also be recommended for people 5–18 years old with HIV.

PNEUMOCOCCAL BACTERIUM VACCINE DEVELOPMENT

The pneumococcal bacterium, *Streptococcus pneumoniae*, was first identified by the Austrian microbiologist Anton Weichselbaum in 1881. He isolated it from the lungs of patients who had died of pneumonia. The first pneumococcal vaccine was developed in the 1940s and it was a pneumococcal *polysaccharide vaccine* that protected against some of the most common strains of the bacterium. This vaccine was effective but had limitations in its coverage.

The breakthrough in pneumococcal vaccination came with the development of *pneumococcal conjugate vaccines (PCV)*. In the late 20th and early 21st centuries, scientists created vaccines that conjugated pneumococcal polysaccharides to carrier proteins, making them more effective, especially in children.

The first PCV, known as PCV7, was introduced in the US in 2000. Over time, more PCVs were developed, with increasing coverage against various strains of *Streptococcus pneumoniae* (→PCV10, →PCV13, →PCV15, →PCV20). These vaccines have been instrumental in reducing the incidence of invasive pneumococcal diseases, sepsis, pneumonia, and other serious infections caused by this bacterium.

Global vaccination efforts: Pneumococcal vaccines have been included in the routine childhood immunization schedules of many countries, contributing to the decline in pneumococcal disease worldwide. Organizations such as the WHO and GAVI, the Vaccine Alliance, have supported efforts to make these vaccines accessible to children in low- and middle-income countries.

India began the phased roll out of PCV with support from GAVI in June 2017. The Serum Institute of India's (SII's) pneumococcal vaccine, *Pneumosil*, was developed through a collaboration spanning over a decade with the health organizations PATH and the Bill and Melinda Gates Foundation. The vaccine was launched by the Union Health Ministry on December 29, 2020. In 2021, the Vaccine Alliance provided new funding to procure more than 9 million PCV doses, which supported an additional expansion to all Indian states.

A historic challenge with pneumococcal vaccination has been serotype replacement. As some serotypes are targeted and reduced through vaccination, other non-vaccine serotypes can become more prevalent. This emphasizes the importance of ongoing research and vaccine development to address evolving strains. These vaccines have played a crucial role in reducing the burden of pneumococcal disease and saving countless lives, especially among children.

The Centers for Disease Control and Prevention (CDC) recommends that all children under 5 years of age receive the pneumococcal vaccine. The first dose is often given at 2 months of age. The vaccine is given in a series of four doses.

ROTAVIRUS VACCINE DEVELOPMENT

The RV vaccine, which protects against severe diarrhea, is usually given starting at 2 months of age.

The development of the RV vaccine is a significant advancement in public health, as RV is a leading cause of severe diarrhea in infants and young children worldwide.

Rotaviruses were first discovered in the 1960s and research began to understand their role in causing gastroenteritis, especially in children. Initial attempts to develop a vaccine focused on using live, attenuated RV strains, similar to the approach used for other viral vaccines such as the measles and polio vaccines. However, these early attempts were not successful due to safety concerns. Dr Timo Vesikari's (Finland University) research work has significantly contributed to the introduction of the rotavirus vaccine into childhood vaccination programs worldwide. Timo Vesikari has worked with the WHO from 1988 to 1990 and has been a member of many WHO committees over the years.

In 1998, an RV vaccine (Rota Shield, by Wyeth now part of Pfizer) was first licensed and approved for use in the US. The first RV vaccine to be licensed and approved for use in the US. In 1999, Rota Shield was withdrawn from the market, just a year after its introduction, due to concerns about an increased risk of intussusception, in vaccinated infants.

In 2006, RotaTeq, developed by Dr Paul Offit and his colleagues, was licensed by Merck & Co., Inc. It is an oral vaccine containing a mixture of five human–bovine reassortant strains of RV. RotaTeq has been highly effective in preventing severe RV infections and has been widely used in many countries.

In 2008 Rotarix, developed by GlaxoSmithKline (GSK), was licensed. It is an oral vaccine based on a single human RV strain (G1P). Rotarix has also been effective in preventing RV gastroenteritis and has been used globally. Both RotaTeq and Rotarix have been included in national immunization programs in many countries, significantly reducing the burden of rotavirus-related hospitalizations and deaths among children.

India introduced the RV vaccine on March 26, 2016. It was the first country in the WHO's Southeast Asia region to do so. Currently, three live oral vaccines are licensed and marketed in India. They include a human monovalent live vaccine (Rotarix), a human–bovine pentavalent live vaccine (RotaTeq), and a vaccine based on Indian neonatal strains, 116E (ROTAVAC).

Rotavirus gastroenteritis disease burden in India 2011–2013 estimated 11.37 million episodes of RV gastroenteritis requiring 3.27 million outpatient visits, 872,000 inpatient admissions, and 78,000 deaths annually in India. With the RV immunization coverage and the potential impact of vaccine efficacy, i.e., 686,277 outpatient visits, 291,756 hospitalizations, and 26,985 deaths were prevented annually in India.

NEISSERIA MENINGITIDIS VACCINES

Meningococcal disease has been recognized for centuries, with outbreaks recorded as far back as the 1800s. However, it was not until the 20th century that the bacteria responsible for the disease, *Neisseria meningitides*, was identified.

Meningococcal vaccines have played a crucial role in preventing and controlling meningococcal disease, serious and potentially life-threatening meningitis, and sepsis. The vaccines are serogroup specific, as *Neisseria meningitidis* can be classified into different serogroups based on the composition of their capsules. The most common serogroups associated with disease are A, B, C, W, X, and Y. Different vaccines have been developed to target-specific serogroups.

Before the introduction of vaccines in 2010, a revolutionary vaccine—Neisseria meningitidis serogroup A (NmA) accounted for 80–85% of meningitis epidemics in the African meningitis belt.

The first successful vaccine against meningococcal serogroup A was introduced in the 1960s. This vaccine was based on a purified polysaccharide antigen that provided short-term protection and was not effective in young children.

There are two types of conjugated meningococcal vaccines available in the US:

- Meningococcal conjugate or meningitis ACWY (MenACWY) vaccines (Menactra®, Menveo®, and MenQuadfi®)
- Serogroup B meningococcal or MenB vaccines (Bexsero® and Trumenba®).

These conjugated vaccines combined the polysaccharide antigen with a carrier protein, improving their effectiveness and extending protection to infants and young children.

Meningococcal vaccines have been instrumental in preventing epidemics and reducing the burden of meningococcal disease in various parts of the world. Mass vaccination campaigns have been conducted in response to outbreaks and in high-risk populations. In sub-Saharan Africa, a region known as the "Meningitis Belt", large-scale vaccination campaigns have been conducted to combat the high incidence of meningococcal meningitis, particularly caused by serogroup A.

Over time, new meningococcal vaccines have been developed and approved, including vaccines targeting serogroup B, which has been a challenge due to the unique characteristics of the serogroup B capsule. These newer vaccines have expanded the options for preventing meningococcal disease. These vaccines have played a crucial role in preventing outbreaks and protecting vulnerable populations.

With the conjugated quadrivalent vaccine availability, the WHO and CDC now routinely recommend all 11–12 year olds should get a MenACWY vaccine, with a booster dose at 16 years of age. Teens and young adults (16 through 23 years old) also may get a MenB vaccine. The CDC also recommends meningococcal vaccination for other children and adults who are at increased risk for meningococcal diseases.

"A new era for equity in meningococcal disease prevention": October, 2023 marks an important development of the *pentavalent* vaccine against the five most virulent strains with one shot in the prevention of meningococcal disease. The US FDA approved a single vaccine PENBRAYA that has the potential for the prevention of the five most common serogroups causing meningococcal disease in adolescents.

Ongoing challenges: Despite significant progress in meningococcal vaccine development, challenges remain, including the need for broader protection against multiple serogroups and addressing vaccine hesitancy and accessibility issues in some regions.

MEASLES, MUMPS, AND RUBELLA AND VARICELLA VACCINE

Measles is one of the most contagious diseases humans have ever faced. An ancient disease, it was described as early as the 9th century by Persian physician and scholar Abū Bakr Muhammad Zakariya Rāzī, also known by the Europeanized name Rhazes **(Fig. 1)**. It became more widespread as global exploration increased. In 1757, Scottish doctor Francis Home discovered that measles was caused by a pathogen—he transmitted the disease to healthy individuals using the blood of infected patients and demonstrated that it was caused by an infectious agent.

Before the advent of vaccination, measles had long been endemic around the world and it remains a worldwide epidemic disease. Globally, mortality rates remained high, with approximately 30 million cases and over 2 million deaths occurring each year.

In 1954, a measles outbreak at a boarding school just outside Boston, Massachusetts, provided an opportunity for doctors at Boston Children's Hospital to try and isolate the measles virus, taking throat swabs and blood samples from infected students. The culture that Thomas Peebles, MD, obtained from 11-year-old schoolboy *David Edmonston* successfully led to the virus' cultivation and enabled doctors to create the first vaccine against measles. *John Franklin Enders*, Peebles' boss, often called *"the father of modern vaccines"*, developed the measles vaccine from the "Edmonston-B" strain, named after David and used as the basis for most live, attenuated

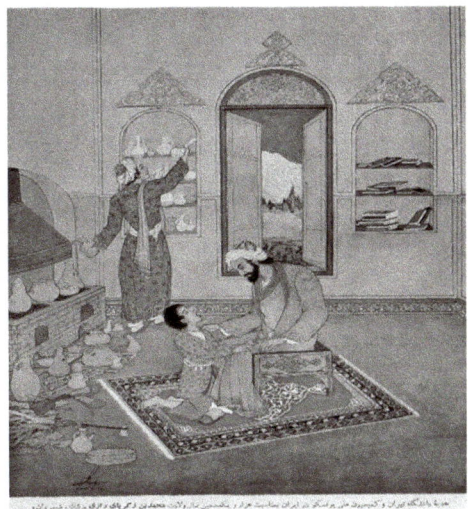

Fig. 1: Persian physician.

vaccines to this day. In 1961, it was hailed as 100% effective and the first measles vaccine was licensed for public use in 1963.

Despite challenges such as the difficulty of maintaining the cold chain when transporting and storing the heat-sensitive vaccine, an improved version of the measles vaccine was created in 1968 when *Dr Maurice Hilleman*, a pioneer in vaccine development, passed the virus through chick embryo cells 40 times (high passage) to weaken it, producing a vaccine that did not cause such severe side effects. This attenuated, weaker version, known as *the Edmonston–Ender's strain*, was developed into some of the strains still used in measles vaccines today.

Dr Maurice Hilleman, the chief virologist at Merck Research Laboratories, suspected he needed to start anew with a different strain of the mumps virus—and he got his chance when his daughter Jeryl Lynn awoke him one night to show him her swollen cheeks **(Fig. 2)**. That night Hilleman swabbed her throat to collect a sample of the virus and then drove the sample to his laboratory.

Human testing of Hilleman's officially designated "Jeryl Lynn Strain" vaccine proved that it achieved that delicate balance of producing strong immunity without causing the disease in vaccinated children. Although Jeryl Lynn could not benefit directly from the vaccine that bears her name, her younger sister did. In 1966, Kirsten Jeanne Hilleman was immunized with the investigational vaccine. In early 1968, doctors began administering the Jeryl Lynn Strain mumps vaccine to the American public.

In 1971, Hilleman combined the recently developed vaccines against measles, mumps, and rubella into the MMR vaccine, administered as a single shot, with one booster dose following—and in 2005, the varicella vaccine was added, to make the combined MMR-V vaccine a combination vaccine that protects against four different infectious diseases—measles, mumps, rubella, and varicella (chickenpox). The first dose is typically administered around the age of 1 year. Before the development of the MMR-V vaccine, these four diseases were typically prevented through separate vaccines.

In essence, the measles vaccine was developed in 1963 and by the late 1960s, vaccines were also available to protect against mumps (1967) and rubella (1969). These three vaccines were combined into the MMR vaccine by Dr Maurice Hilleman in 1971, administered as a single shot, with one booster dose following—and in 2005, the varicella vaccine was added as MMR-V.

Rubella Vaccine Development

The development of the rubella vaccine was prompted by rubella epidemics that swept Europe in 1962–1963 and the US in 1964–1965. In 1964, working in his Wistar Institute laboratory, Stanley Plotkin invented the rubella vaccine. They are prepared through a process of long-term cell culture passage, which leads to attenuating mutations in wild-type sequences. Before the first rubella vaccine was licensed in 1969, rubella was cyclical, coming in outbreaks every 4–6 years.

In 1969, Dr Saul Krugman and Dr Louis Cooper of the NY University Medical School revolutionized through their "Rubella Projects" clinical trial of live attenuated rubella virus vaccine, HPV-77 strain. This strain, designated HPV-77, exhibited desirable qualities of immunogenicity and obvious attenuation in men.

In 1971, the combined MMR vaccine was licensed for use in the US. In 2005, a combination of MMR-V vaccine was licensed.

After two decades, India introduced the measles vaccine in 1985. In 2017, India introduced RCV and the measles- and rubella-containing vaccine (MRCV) replaced measles-containing vaccine dose 1 (MCV1) and MCV2 in the routine immunization schedule.

Vaccine safety concerns: The MMR vaccine has been a subject of controversy and vaccine safety concerns, particularly in the late 1990s due to a now discredited study that suggested a link between the MMR vaccine

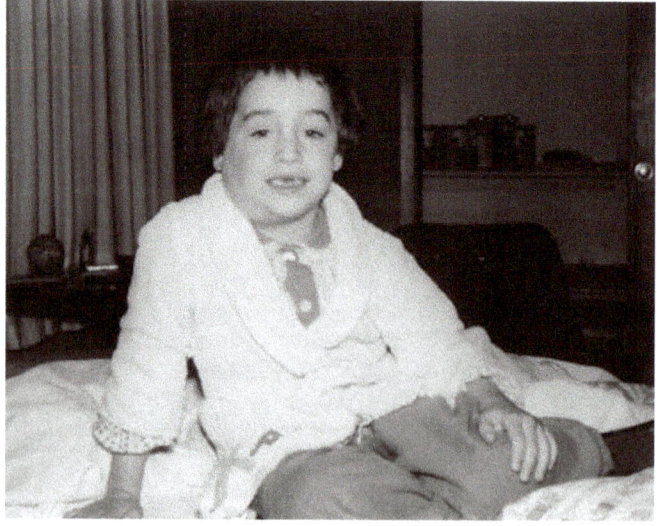

Fig. 2: Jeryl Lynn Hilleman displays mumps cheeks in 1963.

and autism. Extensive scientific research has since debunked this claim and the MMR vaccine is considered safe and effective.

Over the years, MMR-V vaccines have been included in vaccination schedules in many countries around the world as part of routine childhood immunization programs.

The development of the varicella vaccine began in the mid-20th century and *Japan was among the first countries to vaccinate for chickenpox in 1974*. The vaccine virus was developed from a cell culture virus isolated (Oka strain) from an otherwise healthy child with varicella disease. A live attenuated varicella Oka strain vaccine, the Oka strain, was developed by Takahashi and his colleagues in Japan in the early 1970s (Takahashi et al., 1974).

In contrast, the varicella vaccine developed by Hilleman was first licensed in the US in 1995 when Dr Philip Brunel and Anne Gershon (NY University, USA) started researching ways to prevent chickenpox and zoster between 1965 through 1975. The first varicella vaccine, Varivax, was developed by Merck and approved for use in the USA by the FDA in 1995. Another varicella vaccine, ProQuad, which combines the varicella vaccine with the MMR vaccine, was also developed and approved later.

▪ ZOSTER VACCINATION

The herpes zoster (HZ) vaccine, also known as the shingles vaccine, has an interesting historical aspect. The story of the zoster vaccine begins with the development of the varicella (chickenpox) vaccine. In the 1970s and 1980s, researchers (Dr P Brunel et al.) worked on creating a vaccine to prevent chickenpox, which is also caused by the VZV. The zoster vaccine, specifically designed to prevent shingles, was developed based on the knowledge that VZV can reactivate.

The first shingles vaccine, called *Zostavax*, was developed by Merck and approved by the US FDA in 2006. It was a live attenuated vaccine form of the varicella zoster virus (VZV), which causes both chickenpox and shingles. Despite its effectiveness, Zostavax had some limitations, such as a lower efficacy in older adults which waned over time, leading to a decreased protection against shingles and postherpetic neuralgia (PHN). Additionally, it was a live vaccine and was not recommended for individuals with weakened immune systems.

In 2017, a new shingles vaccine called *Shingrix* was approved by the FDA. Shingrix is a nonlive recombinant vaccine that contains a protein component of the VZV subunit vaccine (HZ/su) (Shingrix®). It is administered in two doses and has shown higher efficacy and longer-lasting protection compared to Zostavax. Clinical trials have demonstrated that Shingrix is more than 90% effective in preventing shingles and PHN in adults aged 50 years and older.

Due to its improved efficacy and safety profile, the CDC now recommends Shingrix as the preferred shingles vaccine for adults aged 50 years and older, including those who previously received Zostavax. The higher efficacy and broader age recommendation have led to increased vaccination rates and a greater reduction in the incidence of shingles and its complications.

The historical aspect of the HZ vaccine highlights the continuous efforts to develop more effective and safer vaccines to prevent shingles. The transition from Zostavax to Shingrix has brought about significant advancements in shingles prevention, providing better protection for individuals at risk of developing this painful condition.

▪ INFLUENZA VACCINE

The CDC recommends annual flu shots for everyone 6 months and older each flu season. September and October are the best times for most people to get vaccinated each year.

The influenza virus (IFV) was first isolated and identified in the 1930s. Influenza vaccine development is an ongoing process and evolving history that aims to create effective vaccines to prevent influenza infections. Scientists realized that there were different strains of the virus, which made vaccine development challenging.

Surveillance systems are in place to monitor the circulating strains of IFV. Based on these data, the recent circulating virus strains should be included in the renewed annual vaccination.

There are different types of influenza vaccines, including inactivated, live attenuated, and recombinant vaccines. Each type has its own production methods.

- In the 1940s,- the first inactivated vaccine was developed by growing the IFV in chicken eggs and then inactivating it with heat. It was first used in the military.
- In the 1950s, a trivalent vaccine was introduced, targeting three different IFV strains. This marked a significant advancement in vaccine development.

- In 1970s,- shift from "egg-based" to "cell-based" vaccines—the traditional method of growing IFV in chicken eggs remained the primary method for vaccine production for many years. However, research in the 1970s explored cell-based vaccine production methods, which offered advantages in terms of scalability and speed.
- In the 2000s, a quadrivalent influenza vaccine was developed, targeting four different influenza strains (two influenza A strains and two influenza B strains). This provided broader protection against circulating strains.
- The H1N1 pandemic in 2009 was the first major influenza outbreak in the 21st century. The official death toll of 18,500 was later revised upward by The Lancet Medical Journal to between 151,700 and 575,400 dead.
- The 2010s saw the emergence of new vaccine technologies, including recombinant DNA technology and the development of influenza vaccines that did not rely on growing the virus in eggs. These innovations increased vaccine production efficiency.
- In 2020s,- ongoing R&D is focused on developing universal influenza vaccines that offer long-lasting protection against multiple strains of the virus, potentially eliminating the need for annual updates.

Throughout its history, the influenza vaccine has gone through various improvements and adaptations to address the challenges posed by the ever-changing nature of the IFV. The goal of these developments is to provide better protection against seasonal flu strains and prepare for potential pandemics.

It is important to note that IFV can change over time and new strains may emerge. Therefore, ongoing R&D efforts are necessary to ensure that influenza vaccines remain effective against the circulating strain.

In India, the flu vaccine is only recommended for certain high-risk individuals. The IAP has not yet recommended the introduction of the influenza vaccine into the Universal Immunization Program (UIP) for several reasons, including limited data on the morbidity and mortality of influenza in India.

HEPATITIS A VIRUS VACCINE

The HAV was first identified and characterized in the 1970s. Based on the knowledge of the virus, researchers began to explore the development of an inactivated vaccine to prevent HAV infection.

After successful clinical trials and safety assessments, the vaccine went through the regulatory approval process in various countries. The first HepA vaccine was approved in Europe in 1991 and in the US in 1995. The WHO recommends universal vaccination in areas where the disease is moderately common. Single-antigen HepA vaccines were licensed for use in the US in 1995 (Havrix) and 1996 (Vaqta). Vaccination recommendations vary by country and region.

The HAV vaccine has had a significant impact on reducing the incidence of HAV infection. In India, HepA vaccines have been included in routine childhood immunization schedules and is also recommended for travelers to areas with higher HAV risk.

The HAV vaccine is typically administered in two doses, with the second dose given 6–18 months after the first. All children should receive two doses of the HepA vaccine beginning at age of 1 year (i.e., 12–23 months). It is highly effective in preventing infection and its associated complications. As a result of vaccination efforts, the incidence of HAV has significantly decreased in many parts of the world, contributing to improved public health.

All HAV vaccines are licensed for use in children aged 1 year or older. However, in the Indian scenario, it is preferable to administer the vaccines at the age of 18 months or more when maternal antibodies have completely declined. Two doses 6 months apart are recommended for all HAV vaccines.

It is important to note that ongoing R&D efforts may lead to improvements in HAV vaccines and potentially the development of combination vaccines that protect against multiple hepatitis viruses (e.g., HAV and HBV). Additionally, vaccine recommendations and availability may vary by region and over time, so it is advisable to consult with public health authorities for the most up-to-date information on HAV vaccination.

DENGUE VIRUS VACCINES HISTORICAL PERSPECTIVE

The WHO considers the dengue virus (DENV) to be one of the fastest-spreading arboviral diseases caused by any of four antigenically and genetically distinct *mosquito-borne DENV serotypes* (1, 2, 3, and 4). The majority of DENV infections are silent, but approximately 25% of these result in clinically apparent disease, which may manifest as dengue fever, a self-limiting febrile illness, or more severe dengue hemorrhagic fever and dengue shock syndrome.

India is home to nearly a third of the global population at risk of dengue. Approximately, 390 million DENV infections occur annually worldwide, of which 96 million have clinical manifestations, including 500,000 hospitalizations and 20,000 deaths every year (CDC, USA, 2023).

In recent years, DENV activities have been much more than the sum of all dengue cases reported over a decade in India and it is endemic. DENV is a major global public health problem requiring a safe and efficacious vaccine. For more than 75 years, scientists and product developers have attempted to design safe DENV vaccine candidates, but the challenges have been substantial and formidable.

The development of DENV vaccines began in 1929. The first dengue vaccine was developed in 1997 by Thomas Chambers, an associate professor of molecular microbiology and immunology at Saint Louis University. The vaccine was developed using a virus inactivated with phenol, formalin, or bile. Dengue vaccine development has been a complex and ongoing process.

The development of a DENV vaccine has faced challenges due to the unique characteristics of the virus and the need to provide protection against all four serotypes.

In the early 2000s, the National Institutes of Health (NIH), the University of St Louis, and Acambis Inc. developed the Dengvaxia vaccine. Sanofi Pasteur licensed the vaccine, which uses ChimeriVax™ technology. Dengvaxia is approved for use in individuals 6 through 16 years of age with laboratory-confirmed previous dengue infection and living in endemic areas.

- Dengvaxia [chimeric yellow fever virus–tetravalent dengue vaccine (CYD-TDV)]: A live attenuated tetravalent vaccine developed by Sanofi Pasteur, it was one of the first dengue vaccines to be licensed for use and administered in multiple doses. Designed to provide protection against all four serotypes of the DENV. It was approved in several countries, including the Philippines, Brazil, Mexico, and some other dengue-endemic regions. However, *its use is limited to individuals who have had a prior dengue infection.* This is because the vaccine can increase the risk of severe dengue in individuals who have not been previously infected.

There is another tetravalent DENV vaccine, TAK-003 (Takeda), also known as TAK-875, developed by Takeda Pharmaceuticals. TAK-003, also known as TAK-875, has shown promising results in clinical trials, demonstrating efficacy against all four dengue serotypes. It is important to note that the effectiveness of dengue vaccines can vary depending on factors, such as age, prior dengue infection status, and the specific serotype circulating in a particular region.

Other Candidate Dengue Virus Vaccines

- *TV003/TV005 vaccine:* Developed by the NIH in the US. These vaccines are based on a live attenuated virus and were being evaluated in clinical trials to assess their safety and efficacy.

Several other dengue vaccine candidates were in different stages of development by various pharmaceutical companies and research institutions. These candidates used various approaches, including live attenuated vaccines, subunit vaccines, and DNA-based vaccines. Each candidate utilizes different strategies to stimulate an immune response against the DENV.

- The availability and recommendations for dengue vaccines may vary by country and region, depending on the prevalence of dengue and the specific vaccines that have been approved for use.

The development of a safe and effective dengue vaccine remains a priority, as dengue continues to be a significant global health concern. Efforts are focused on improving vaccine efficacy, safety, and the ability to provide long-lasting protection against all four dengue serotypes. Continued research and collaboration among scientists, public health agencies, and vaccine manufacturers are crucial in advancing dengue vaccine development.

In recent years, the development of dengue vaccines has accelerated. India's first DNA vaccine candidate for dengue has shown promising results in preliminary trials on mice. The candidate generated a robust immune response and improved survival rates after exposure to the disease.

SARS-COV-2 (COVID-19) VACCINATION

Coronavirus disease 2019 has rapidly evolved and is an ongoing story, caused by the novel coronavirus SARS-CoV-2 (severe acute respiratory syndrome coronavirus 2), which was first identified in Wuhan, China, in late 2019. As the virus spread globally, researchers and pharmaceutical companies began efforts to develop vaccines to combat the pandemic. COVID-19 vaccines were distributed worldwide as part of a massive global vaccination effort. Many countries-initiated vaccination campaigns to inoculate their populations against the virus.

Messenger RNA vaccines: One of the newest and most exciting areas in vaccine technology is the use of mRNA vaccines, unlike conventional vaccines which can take many months or even years to cultivate. In contrast, mRNA vaccines can be developed quickly using the pathogen's genetic code. It is now proven and widely accepted that the *spike (S) glycoprotein* [receptor-binding domain (RBD)] is responsible for virus binding and entry into the host cell. The S protein is used by the virus to attach to human cells and hence gain cell entry to the human body system **(Fig. 3)**.

The S protein is most promising immunogenic for producing protective immunity. However, it is likely that the S protein has evolved to perform its functions while evading host-neutralizing antibody responses and thus should be engineered to ensure an optimal immune response.

Two of the most notable vaccines developed are the Pfizer-BioNTech and Moderna vaccines. Both of these vaccines are based on mRNA technology, a relatively new approach to vaccination. They were developed and authorized for emergency use in late 2020.

The AstraZeneca–Oxford vaccine is a *viral vector vaccine*. It uses a harmless adenovirus to deliver a piece of the SARS-CoV-2 virus' genetic material, triggering an immune response. It was authorized for emergency use in various countries in late 2020 and early 2021.

Another viral vector vaccine, developed by Johnson & Johnson's Janssen Pharmaceuticals, received emergency use authorization in early 2021. *It has the advantage of requiring only a single dose.*

Chinese and Russian vaccines: China and Russia developed several COVID-19 vaccines, such as Sinopharm, Sinovac, and the Russians Sputnik V. These vaccines were used in various countries and authorized for emergency use.

Challenges and variants: The development and distribution of vaccines faced challenges such as vaccine hesitancy, distribution logistics, and concerns about the emergence of new virus variants that might affect vaccine effectiveness. Some vaccines required updates to address variant strains.

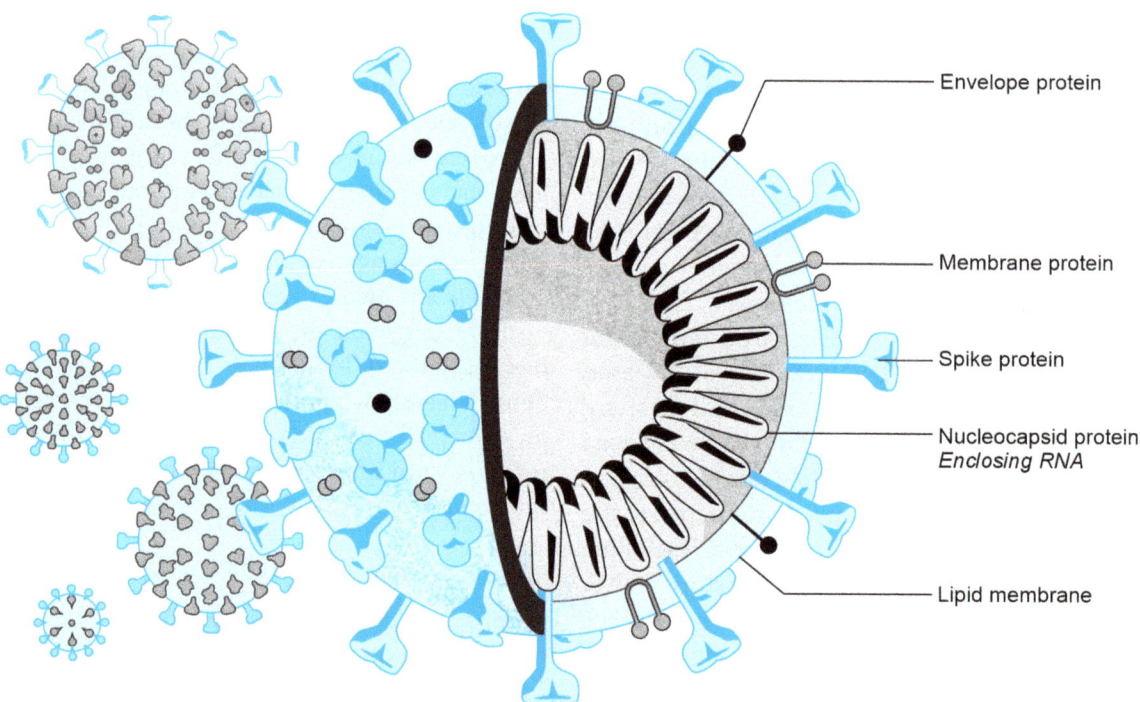

Fig. 3: Schematic representation of severe acute respiratory syndrome coronavirus-2 (SARS-CoV-2) encodes four structural proteins similar to other CoVs.

Booster shots: As the pandemic evolved, discussions about booster shots to maintain immunity levels among vaccinated individuals emerged. Some countries began administering booster shots in 2021 to enhance and prolong immunity.

Prime-boost vaccinations can enhance immune responses, whereas chronic antigen exposure (repeated booster doses) can cause immune tolerance. In humans, the benefits, limitations, and risks of repetitive vaccination remain poorly understood. An anecdotal report shows that SARS-CoV-2 hypervaccination did not lead to adverse events and increased the quantity of spike-specific antibodies and T-cells without having a strong positive or negative effect on the intrinsic quality of adaptive immune responses. It does not endorse hypervaccination as a strategy to enhance adaptive immunity.

Global efforts: Organizations like COVID-19 Vaccine Global Access (COVAX) is a worldwide initiative working to ensure fair, equitable access to the vaccines for every country that participates were established to ensure equitable vaccine distribution to low- and middle-income countries, aiming to combat the global pandemic on a larger scale.

Please keep in mind that the COVID-19 situation is highly dynamic and constantly evolving. Therefore, it is essential to consult up-to-date sources and follow the guidance of health authorities for the most current information on COVID-19 vaccines and their history.

A recent long-COVID study found Epstein–Barr virus (EBV) infection to be one of four major risk factors, suggesting that some long-COVID symptoms might be caused by reactivation of EBV when the body is weakened from fighting the coronavirus. This association is perhaps not surprising. The good message is SARS-CoV-2 vaccination clearly reduces the severity and the frequency of long-term COVID-19. The only debate is to what extent the vaccination reduces the long-haul symptoms and the experts have estimated that to have ranged from 15% to 50%. Further Spanish researchers have tested a newly developed vaccine that prevents COVID infections from impacting patients' neurological function. They claim that their work is "the first study of a vaccine that is 100% effective against brain damage caused by SARS-CoV-2 in a susceptible mouse and the results obtained strongly suggest that the vaccine could prevent persistent COVID observed in several people infected with SARS-CoV-2".

On October 2, 2023, nearly 3 years after the rollout of mRNA vaccines across the world, Katalin Karikó, an adjunct professor of neurosurgery at Penn's Perelman School of Medicine and Drew Weissman, the Roberts Family Professor of Vaccine Research in the Perelman School of Medicine *won the 2023 Nobel Prize in Physiology or Medicine* for discoveries enabling the development of novel COVID-19 vaccines and for their groundbreaking work on nucleoside base modification of mRNA.

■ HUMAN PAPILLOMAVIRUS VACCINES

Human papillomavirus vaccines were first introduced in the early 2000s and it is a preventive cancer vaccines such as the HepB vaccines. The two most well-known HPV vaccines are Gardasil (*made by Merck*) and Cervarix (*made by GSK*). These vaccines target several strains of HPV that are known to cause various cancers, including cervical cancer.

Initially, these vaccines were primarily targeted at adolescent girls, but vaccination programs have often been extended to include boys as well to reduce transmission and protect against related cancers such as oropharyngeal cancer. Over the years, many countries expanded their HPV vaccination programs to include a wider age range and population.

These vaccines have been shown to be highly effective in preventing HPV infection and related cancers. Despite the benefits of HPV vaccines, there have been challenges and controversies, including concerns about vaccine safety, hesitancy, and misinformation. In many countries, the dosing schedule for HPV vaccines has been simplified from three doses to two doses for adolescents, which may improve vaccine uptake.

Apart from these preventive vaccines, there is ongoing research into therapeutic HPV vaccines that could potentially help treat existing HPV infections and related cancers. In addition to vaccination, efforts to improve screening and early detection of HPV-related cancers, particularly cervical cancer, continue to be a focus of healthcare systems worldwide.

In India, bivalent and quadrivalent HPV vaccines were licensed in the country in 2008 and a monovalent vaccine was licensed in 2018. The HPV vaccine has also faced pushback in India. It was, without evidence, that vaccination will lead to riskier sexual behavior among young people. There is also lingering public mistrust due to a controversial HPV vaccine study more than a decade ago.

Apart from the vaccine cost, there has also been in short supply. Demand shot up in recent years after the WHO recommended vaccinating not just 9–14-year-old girls but also older teens. Several countries debuted the vaccine and some began inoculating boys too, causing global demand to double between 2017 and 2018. But pharmaceutical companies were not able to catch up, resulting in "a crisis of supply". Low-income countries were left without HPV vaccines as most of the limited supply was taken by high-income countries.

Experts say that even though vaccine hesitancy is relatively low in India compared to several western nations, including the US, the HPV vaccine's sexual connotation complicates things.

HUMAN IMMUNODEFICIENCY VIRUS VACCINES DEVELOPMENTS

It has been more than four decades since HIV emerged, causing a pandemic that has left more than 40 million people dead and more than 38 million currently living with the infection worldwide.

There is currently no vaccine available that will prevent HIV infection or treat those who have it. However, scientists are working to develop one. NIH is investing in multiple approaches to prevent HIV, including a safe and effective preventive HIV vaccine.

The development of an HIV vaccine has been a complex and challenging process due to its high genetic variability and the ability to evade the immune system. Developing a vaccine that can provide broad protection against the diverse strains of HIV remains a significant encounter. Ongoing research focuses on identifying conserved regions of the virus, optimizing vaccine regimens, and exploring novel strategies such as mosaic vaccines and gene-editing technologies.

Following the identification of HIV as the causative agent of acquired immunodeficiency syndrome (AIDS) in the early 1980s, researchers began working toward developing a vaccine. Initial efforts focused on using inactivated or attenuated forms of the virus, similar to traditional vaccine approaches. However, these early attempts did not yield successful results.

One of the most significant milestones in HIV vaccine research was the RV144 trial conducted in Thailand (2009). That trial showed a modest level of efficacy, with a 31% reduction in HIV infection rates among vaccinated individuals compared to those who received a placebo. The RV144 trial provided valuable insights into the immune responses that may confer protection against HIV. It highlighted the importance of inducing both antibody and cellular immune responses for an effective vaccine. The trial findings have since guided further R&D efforts.

In recent years, broadly neutralizing antibodies (bNAbs) against HIV have sparked new hope for vaccine development. These antibodies can neutralize a wide range of HIV strains. Researchers are studying these bNAbs to understand their mechanisms of action and exploring ways to elicit similar responses through vaccination.

The "beauty of mRNA" technology: With the success of safe and highly effective COVID-19 vaccines, scientists now have an exciting opportunity to learn whether mRNA technology can achieve similar results against HIV infection.

The International AIDS Vaccine Initiative (IAVI) and Moderna, the companies to develop a COVID-19 mRNA vaccine, have also launched a trial of an mRNA HIV vaccine, to be conducted at the Center for Family Health Research in Kigali, Rwanda, and The Aurum Institute in Tembisa, South Africa. Although mRNA technology could accelerate the testing of HIV vaccines, it "will not solve the primary challenge facing HIV vaccines that involve immunogen design".

Other various vaccine approaches are being explored, including viral vector-based vaccines, protein subunit vaccines, DNA vaccines, and mRNA vaccines. These approaches aim to stimulate both humoral (antibody) and cellular immune responses to prevent HIV infection or control the virus in individuals who become infected.

MALARIAL VACCINES' DEVELOPMENT

Malarial vaccines' development began in the 1960s when rodents, primates, and human volunteers were immunized with irradiated sporozoites. In 1967, mice were immunized with radiation-attenuated *Plasmodium berghei* sporozoites.

Malaria is a life-threatening mosquito-borne disease caused by a diversity of *Plasmodium* species. The development of the malaria vaccine was difficult because the *Plasmodium* parasite that causes malaria has a multistage life cycle, which presents different antigens at different stages. There have been several challenges in developing a malaria vaccine, but there has been significant progress in recent years. Even with successful vaccination, the immune response may not completely eliminate the parasite, leading to breakthrough infections.

In 2021, the WHO approved the first malaria vaccine, *RTS, S/AS01 vaccine (Mosquirix™)* for widespread use and is designed to target the *Plasmodium falciparum* parasite, which is the most lethal species.

Additional malaria vaccine candidates are in various stages of development, including those targeting different stages of the parasite's life cycle, aiming for better efficacy and broader coverage. While progress has been made, continued investment in malaria vaccine research and distribution infrastructure is crucial to achieving further success in the fight against this deadly disease.

The WHO recommends second malaria vaccine, R21, an easier to manufacture and cheaper than RTS, S, while demonstrating similar effectiveness. These two vaccines can help bolster malaria prevention and control efforts and save hundreds of thousands of young lives globally.

Malaria vaccines have been in development for almost 60 years. The RTS, S/AS01 vaccine has now been approved but cannot be a stand-alone solution. Development should further continue on promising candidates such as R21 and also for a vaccine against *Plasmodium vivax (P. vivax)* infections.

- Multicomponent vaccines may be a useful addition to other malaria control techniques in achieving eradication of malaria.

BACKGROUND OF GROUP B STREPTOCOCCUS AND RESPIRATORY SYNCYTIAL VIRUS VACCINES' DEVELOPMENTS

Maternal immunization and maternal immunity— exemplified by these GBS and RSV vaccines development for infant protections

- Vaccines given to pregnant women (maternal immunization) that are intended to prevent illness in young infants rely on this process of transplacental antibody transfer.
- When a pregnant woman is vaccinated, her immune response produces vaccine-specific antibodies, which can then be transferred to the fetus.
- This protection from the mother is called "maternal immunity" and is critical for helping infants fight off potential infections during the most vulnerable first months of life when their immune system is still developing.

Group B streptococcus vaccines: In August 2022, the GBS6 vaccine received breakthrough therapy designation from the US FDA for the prevention of invasive GBS disease due to the vaccine serotypes in newborns and young infants by active immunization of their mothers during pregnancy.

Group B streptococcus 6 is designed to offer protection against the six most prominent GBS serotypes, which account for 98% of GBS disease worldwide.

Respiratory syncytial virus vaccines: They are finally here after decades of failed attempts and have given way to several successful vaccines and treatments for the respiratory disease RSV. Scientists began developing a vaccine for RSV shortly after the virus was discovered in 1956.

Respiratory syncytial virus vaccine development began in the 1960s with an unsuccessful formalin-inactivated RSV vaccine that induced a severe and in two cases lethal lung inflammatory response during the first natural RSV infection after vaccination of RSV-naïve infants.

The problem with RSV was that scientists did not know what caused its antibody-dependent enhancement. For the next two decades, RSV vaccine progress stagnated. Researchers developed multiple live attenuated vaccines using a virus that was weakened instead of neutralized or deactivated.

Now, at last, *the US FDA has approved ABRYSVO™ (Pfizer), a bivalent RSV prefusion F (RSVpreF) vaccine*, for the prevention of lower respiratory tract diseases (LRTD)—primarily targeting against RSV—severe LRTD in infants from birth up to 6 months of age by active immunization of pregnant individuals at 32 through 36 weeks' gestational age.

There are also phase 1 clinical trials planned or under way to evaluate mRNA RSV vaccines in pregnant persons and in children, which may provide more tools for preventing RSV infection in the future.

ROLE OF ARTIFICIAL INTELLIGENCE AND MACHINE LEARNING IN VACCINE DESIGN

The axiom and origins of the phrase "artificial intelligence" in healthcare was first coined in a Dartmouth College conference proposal in 1955. But the AI applications did not enter the healthcare field until the early 1970s, when research produced MYCIN, an AI program that helped identify blood infection treatments. In recent years, scientists have leveraged ML and AI to search the scientific literature for knowledge on how to build effective vaccines against new infectious viruses and bacteria.

- The application of AI and ML in the field of vaccine evolution has become ubiquitous due to the advent of new and fatal diseases.
- These technologies assist in predicting how a virus may mutate, enabling faster adjustments to existing vaccines or the creation of new ones.

Artificial Intelligence and Machine Learning in Vaccine Progress

Artificial intelligence is a young discipline of 60 years, which is a set of sciences, theories, and techniques including mathematical logic, statistics, probabilities, computational neurobiology, and computer science that aims to imitate the cognitive abilities of a human being. Basically, it is a computer-controlled robot or a software think intelligently like the human mind, accomplished by studying the patterns of the human brain and by analyzing the cognitive process. The outcome of these studies develops intelligent software and systems.

The AI refers to the simulation or approximation of human intelligence in machines. The objectives include computer-enhanced learning, reasoning, and perception, and are being used today across different industries from finance to healthcare systems. An AI system can sort through thousands of components in a complicated structure to find the ones most likely to elicit a strong immunological response. Studying the proteins that make up the virus, such as the spike protein-S of the SARS-CoV-2, is one of the roles and functions of AI in vaccine development.

Historically, vaccine development is a lengthy and expensive process. Very often, it takes multiple years and millions of dollars to complete. Vaccines are typically made using one of several different strategies or "platforms". However, different strategies can generate different immune responses. Through the Rapid Assessment of Platform Technologies to Expedite Response (RAPTER) project, the scientists leverage ML and AI to search the scientific literature for knowledge on how to build effective vaccines against new infectious viruses and bacteria. With RAPTER, researchers figure out which strategy would work best for a specific virus or bacteria to maximize the value of immune responses from the host. The tool aims to help produce new vaccines more rapidly and with a reduced timeline and cost.

Today, the field of vaccine development has rapidly evolved. AI is one of the predominant technologies that can help, analyze, and interpret crucial and viable genetic information. Furthermore, AI can aid in predicting the reaction and behavior of the target molecules in cells. One such tool is artificial neural networks (ANNs). They work like biological neurons and carefully interact with the body. These ANNs can be trained by continuously feeding data and adjusting their connections. ANNs can help in the development of treatment strategies, prognosis of a disease, and treatment outcomes. Automated systems can also be developed to analyze large amounts of data.

Thus, AI is a powerful tool that can advance and revolutionize the development of vaccines. Implementation of AI-based algorithms and networks in the R&D sector can assist in pharmaceutical applications.

POLITICS OF VACCINATION: A GLOBAL HISTORY

The topic of vaccines and vaccinations is a complex and many-sided topic that can sometimes become politicized, with various political and philosophical viewpoints influencing public discourse and policy decisions.

Here are some key points to consider regarding the politics of vaccines and vaccinations:

Vaccine policy decisions, such as the inclusion of specific vaccines in national immunization schedules or the allocation of resources for vaccine R&D, can be influenced by political considerations. Government bodies, at the local, national, and international levels, play a crucial role in shaping vaccination policies. Policymakers must balance healthcare interests, scientific evidence, fiscal factors, and public opinion when making decisions related to vaccines and vaccinations. These policies are often influenced by expert recommendations from health organizations such as the WHO and the CDC.

Mandatory and disciplinary vaccination policies, such as requiring vaccination certificates for public activities and firing employees who refuse vaccination, have raised considerable hostilities. These mandates are often subject to political debate, with some arguing for individual freedom and others emphasizing the importance of free and transparent public health.

Vaccine distribution: The equitable distribution of vaccines, both domestically and internationally, can be a contentious issue. Global politics can influence the allocation of vaccines to countries and regions and there are ongoing debates about how to ensure that vaccines reach underserved populations.

Public opinion and misinformation: The politics of vaccines are also influenced by public opinion and the spread of vaccine-related misinformation. Vaccine hesitancy and refusal can be driven by a variety of factors, including mistrust of government, concerns about vaccine safety, and the influence of antivaccine movements.

During COVID-19, India faced low rates of vaccine administration during the initial stages of the vaccination campaign, likely because of vaccine hesitancy and misinformation propagated by social media.

It is essential to approach discussions about vaccines and vaccinations with evidence-based information, respect for diverse perspectives, and a focus on public health outcomes. Healthcare professionals and public health experts play a crucial role in providing accurate information, addressing concerns, and promoting vaccination as a vital public health intervention.

The pharmaceutical industry plays a significant role in vaccine development and production. The relationship between governments and vaccine manufacturers can influence pricing, patents, and vaccine availability. Political decisions about allocating resources to vaccine development can have a significant impact on the availability and accessibility of vaccines.

CONCLUSION

This historical aspect of vaccine history offers valuable lessons that can inform our understanding of vaccines and their preventive role in medical practices. These lessons provide insights into the impact of vaccination on public health and the challenges associated with vaccine development, distribution, and acceptance at the global level. These historical lessons can guide policymakers, healthcare professionals, and the public in making informed decisions about vaccines and their role in preventing both infectious diseases and controlling noncommunicable diseases.

SUGGESTED READING

1. Cooper LZ, Giles JP, Krugman S. Clinical trial of live attenuated rubella virus vaccine, HPV-77 strain. Am J Dis Child. 1968;115(6):655-7.
2. Haelle T. (2023). RSV Vaccines Are Finally Here after Decades of False Starts. Available from: https://www.scientificamerican.com/article/rsv-vaccines-are-finally-here-after-decades-of-false-starts/ [Last accessed May, 2024].
3. John J, Sarkar R, Muliyil J, Bhandari N, Bhan MK, Kang G. Rotavirus gastroenteritis in India, 2011-2013: revised estimates of disease burden and potential impact of vaccines. Vaccine. 2014;32(Suppl 1):A5-9.
4. Kocher K, Moosmann C, Drost F, Schülein C, Irrgang P, Steininger P, et al. Adaptive immune responses are larger and functionally preserved in a hypervaccinated individual. Lancet Infect Dis. 2024;24(5):e272-4.
5. Medical Forum. (2023). New vaccine for long-COVID. Available from: https://mforum.com.au/long-covid-vaccine/ [Last accessed May, 2024].
6. PATH. (2024). RSV vaccine and mAb snapshot. Available from: https://www.path.org/resources/rsv-vaccine-and-mab-snapshot/ [Last accessed May, 2024].
7. Pfizer. (2023). Pfizer Announces New England Journal of Medicine Publication on Group B Streptococcus (GBS) Maternal Vaccine Candidate. Available from: https://www.pfizer.com/news/press-release/press-release-detail/Pfizer-announces-new-england-journal-medicine-publication [Last accessed May, 2024].
8. Power LE. The Politics of Vaccination: A Global History. Emerg Infect Dis. 2018;24(11):2135.
9. Ramsey L. (2023). Scientists leverage machine learning and AI to guide vaccine development. Available from: https://www.news-medical.net/news/20230811/Scientists-leverage-machine-learning-and-AI-to-guide-vaccine-development.aspx#:~:text=Through%20the%20Rapid%20Assessment%20of,new%20infectious%20viruses%20and%20bacteria [Last accessed May, 2024].
10. Swaminathan S, Khanna N. Dengue vaccine development: Global and Indian scenarios. Int J Infect Dis. 2019;84S:S80-6.
11. Vesikari T. From rubella to rotavirus, and beyond. Hum Vaccin Immunother. 2015;11(6):1302-5.

CHAPTER 3

Success Stories and Ongoing Challenges

VACCINE SUCCESS STORIES AND CHALLENGES

- Smallpox eradication, bacillus Calmette-Guérin's (BCG's) success, and child *Haemophilus influenzae* type b (Hib) toward elimination
- Rubella, measles, and mumps control, polio eradication, and rotavirus (RV) control
- Tetanus and diphtheria (TD) control, pertussis success and challenges
- Hepatitis A virus (HAV) control and hepatitis B virus (HBV) vaccine success stories, pneumococcus (PCV) benefits
- Human papillomavirus (HPV) toward control of cancers, severe acute respiratory syndrome coronavirus 2 (SARS-CoV-2) vaccines efficacy and challenges
- Meningococcus control.

Vaccination currently saves an estimated 3–4 million lives per year throughout the world and so topped the list in terms of lives saved, making it one of the most cost-effective health interventions available in modern times. India has a long history of successful vaccination with historical accounts of inoculation dating back to the 18th century. The World Health Organization (WHO), working in partnership with both public and private sectors, has a proud history of vaccinology.

Vaccines and immunizations have been one of the most successful public health interventions in modern medical history. The main challenge faced by developing countries is the *affordability* of vaccines and for the developed countries has been with the *vaccine acceptability*. Despite multiple challenges, developing countries like India have achieved remarkable feats with childhood immunizations and continue to do so with COVID-19 preventive measures including vaccinations. These vaccine's success story gives us hope to defeat any such emerging pandemic, as we look back to all that vaccines have achieved for humanity.

Apart from well-known smallpox eradication at the global level in 1980, the late Dr Saul Krugman, a long-time (47 years) Head of Pediatrics at the New York University School of Medicine (renamed now as NYU Grossman School of Medicine) has done "more to eliminate pediatric infectious diseases than any other person ever".

Dr Krugman has been the leader in the development of vaccines against childhood measles and unraveled the mysteries of viral hepatitis field clinical trials during the 1070s. Also proved the effectiveness of the first vaccine against rubella in 1969. Similarly, he led the way with tests to gain the approval and wide use of the first vaccine against measles, once a threat to all children.

The COVID-19 vaccine's success is a springboard for further vaccine research. Despite the staggering amount of suffering and deaths during the pandemic of COVID-19, a remarkable success story has emerged. The development of several highly efficacious vaccines against a previously unknown viral pathogen, SARS-CoV-2, which emerged in <1 year after the identification of the virus, is unprecedented in the history of vaccinology.

Development of successful vaccines is typically easier when there is:

- A single serotype and the pathogen are antigenically stable, the best examples are the smallpox virus, HBV, gram-negative Hib, etc.
- The pathogen is antigenically stable.
- Diagnostic tests/clinical measures for measuring disease burden are available.
- The vaccine is both safe and effective.

In addition to examples of successful vaccines, there are also a large number of partially successful vaccines that are near or substantially toward elimination. Challenging pathogens, such as those with multiple serotypes, complex lifecycles, or high antigenic variability are the ones that are most likely to have a partially successful vaccine.

Partially successful vaccine histories in immunizations refer to cases where vaccines provide some level of protection against disease but may not provide complete lasting immunity or may have limited effectiveness. It is important to note that partial protection from vaccines can still significantly impact public health by reducing the severity of diseases, decreasing transmission rates, and preventing complications. There are several examples of vaccines that have demonstrated partial success in human immunization for various reasons:

- The *BCG* immunizations provide partial protection against tuberculosis (TB), particularly in children. However, its effectiveness varies and may wane over time, making it less effective in adults.
- Diphtheria, pertussis (whooping cough), and tetanus (DPT) is a class of combination vaccines against three infectious diseases in humans—DPT with the good success of disease control at a global level. However, pertussis vaccine effectiveness can decrease over time, leading to a resurgence of the disease in some areas.
- In 1995, following the *Global Polio Eradication* Initiative (GPEI) of the WHO (1988), India launched "Pulse Polio" with the Universal Immunization Program (UIP) which aimed at 100% vaccination coverage. The last reported cases of wild polio in India were in West Bengal and Gujarat on 13 January 2011. On 27 March 2014, the WHO declared India a polio-free country, since no cases of wild polio had been reported in 5 years.
  - *The challenges are* the nonpolio acute flaccid paralysis (AFP) rates with pulse polio frequency in India. The WHO is attempting to phase out the use of oral polio vaccine (OPV) to eliminate the risk that the active virus in the vaccine could mutate into a form that can harm unvaccinated children.
- *Measles, mumps, rubella (MMR):* India had set a target to eliminate measles and rubella (MR) by 2023, having missed the earlier deadline of 2020, due to various reasons, exacerbated by disruptions due to the pandemic. In India, rubella is still a common cause of febrile rash in children and is also a public health problem because of the teratogenic effects of rubella infection in pregnant women [congenital rubella syndrome (CRS)].
- *The RV vaccine* is highly effective in preventing severe cases of RV gastroenteritis in infants and young children. However, it may not provide complete protection against all strains of the virus.
- *The influenza vaccine* is updated annually to target the most prevalent strains of the virus. While it can significantly reduce the risk of getting the flu and its severity, it does not guarantee complete protection due to the ever-changing nature of the influenza virus.
- *Dengue fever vaccine, DENV (Dengvaxia):* Vaccines provide partial protection against dengue fever but are less effective against certain strains of the virus. DENV with its four inter-related serotypes, has also raised safety concerns in some populations.
- *Malaria vaccine* (RTS, S/AS01) has shown partial success in reducing the risk of malaria infection, but it does not offer complete protection. Plasmodium is a parasite with a complex multistage lifecycle that causes malaria, and its effectiveness can vary depending on factors such as age and location.
- Developing an *effective HIV vaccine* has proven challenging due to the virus's ability to mutate rapidly and evade the immune system. Several experimental HIV vaccines have shown partial success in early-stage trials but have not yet provided full protection.

Vaccines are continually researched and improved to enhance their effectiveness, and new vaccines are developed to address diseases for which no vaccines currently exist.

Childhood vaccination is critical and routine childhood immunization programs have significantly reduced the incidence of various diseases, including DTP, polio, MMR, and varicella. These vaccines have prevented countless cases and deaths, allowing children to grow up healthier. Vaccines are a critical part of public health efforts, and their continued use and promotion are essential for preventing these and other vaccine-preventable diseases (VPDs). Additionally, vaccine recommendations and schedules may vary by country and region, so individuals should consult with their healthcare providers to ensure they are up to date on their vaccinations.

SMALLPOX (VARIOLA) SUCCESS STORY

Vaccination with the vaccinia (cowpox) virus is not only the first vaccine ever developed by Jennifer, but it is the most well-known example of a highly effective vaccine at the time when people were faced with deadly smallpox outbreaks.

In May 1796 English physician Dr Edward Jenner created the first successful vaccine. He found that people infected with cowpox were immune to smallpox.

In 1806, French emperor Napolean Bonaparte and American President Thomas Jefferson acknowledged Dr E Jenner's work and endorsed the smallpox vaccine. Other members of this genus that can infect humans include monkeypox virus, cowpox virus, vaccinia virus, and several putative novel species. The cowpox virus is believed to have been used by Jenner as material for the first smallpox vaccine. Later, the cowpox virus was replaced with the vaccinia virus.

Variola major, the causative agent of smallpox no longer exists in nature. This represents the best example in which a vaccine was decisively used to drive a species to extinction. Through a global vaccination campaign led by the WHO, smallpox was declared eradicated in 1980. This success demonstrated the power of vaccines and international cooperation. It has been 44 years since the WHO declared the complete eradication of smallpox in the world—a tremendous victory attributed entirely to the intensified, large-scale vaccination programs across the world.

The last known smallpox case, anywhere in the world, was reported in the late 1970s. Since no animals other than humans are known to carry or transmit smallpox, the risk of getting the illness has effectively been reduced to zero.

An emerging global threat is the appearance of mpox (formerly known as monkeypox) during the COVID-19 pandemic. Mpox is a rare disease that leads to rash and flu-like symptoms. A live, nonreplicating vaccinia vaccine (Jynneos-BN) was approved by the FDA in 2019 for the prevention of smallpox and monkeypox in people 18 years and older who are at high risk for smallpox or monkeypox.

BACILLUS CALMETTE-GUÉRIN USEFULNESS IN CONTROLLING TUBERCULOSIS

The only licensed TB vaccine to date, known as the BCG vaccine, was developed over a century ago. First administered to a human subject as a TB vaccine on July 18, 1921, BCG has a long history of use for the prevention of TB and later the immunotherapy of bladder cancer. For TB prevention, BCG is given to infants born globally across over 180 countries and has been in use since the late 1920s.

The BCG vaccine saves thousands of lives every year by protecting young children from severe forms of tuberculosis, but it does not adequately protect adolescents and adults, who account for most TB transmission. With about 352 million BCG doses procured annually and tens of billions of doses having been administered over the past century, it is estimated to be the most widely used vaccine in human history.

In India: A recent modeling analysis on the potential impact of neonatal BCG highlights how even a vaccine with moderate effectiveness (50%) could achieve substantial reductions in TB.

Challenges are the Adult Onset of Contagious Pulmonary Tuberculosis

India, Indonesia, and the Philippines hold a majority (60%) of the global case reductions and India recorded 27% of the world's TB cases in 2022. An estimated 10.6 million people have developed TB in 2022, in India. A majority of those 7.5 million people were diagnosed with airborne lung disease for the first time. This is significant because of *Mycobacterium tuberculosis* (M. tb) disease reactivations.

In its Global Tuberculosis Report 2023, the WHO says this has been the highest annual record of new cases of TB since it started monitoring the disease in 1995, and this sharp rise may be linked to delays in treatment caused by the COVID-19 pandemic.

Novel TB vaccines effective in adolescents and adults could reduce this burden. M72/AS01E and BCG revaccination have recently completed phase IIb trials and estimates of their population-level impact are needed.

HAEMOPHILUS INFLUENZAE TYPE B DISEASE ELIMINATIONS

The Hib immunization success has served as a model for the development and implementation of other vaccines.

The first conjugate vaccine used in humans became available in 1987. This was the (Hib) conjugate, which protects against meningitis. The vaccine was soon incorporated into the schedule for infant immunization in the United States demonstrating the importance of vaccination in preventing infectious diseases.

The success story of the Hib vaccine is a testament to the power of vaccination in preventing devastating diseases, particularly among children. This vaccine is typically administered in multiple doses during infancy. In many countries, the Hib vaccine is now a routine part of childhood immunization schedules, given along with other vaccines such as DTP/DTap, polio, MMR, and varicella.

The success of Hib vaccination is not limited to a single country. It has had a global impact, saved countless lives, and prevented lifelong disabilities. In countries with high vaccination coverage, Hib infections have become rare, and many children have grown up without experiencing these life-threatening illnesses.

In India, 445 (48%) pediatricians ranked the universal use of the Hib vaccine in the national immunization program as the most important strategy to prevent and control Hib disease in India (ICMR, 2020).

Despite the fact that the success of Hib vaccination is evident, it is essential to maintain high vaccination coverage to prevent the resurgence of the disease. Health authorities should continually monitor Hib and vaccination rates to ensure protection.

RUBELLA ELIMINATION–MEASLES–MUMPS DISEASES CONTROL

The world was immersed in the rubella pandemic of 1964–65. In the United States alone, an estimated 12.5 million people were infected with rubella, 11,000 pregnant women lost their babies, 2,100 newborn infants died, and 20,000 infants were born with congenital rubella birth defects, called congenital rubella syndrome. The rubella virus was first isolated in 1962, and rubella vaccines became available by the end of the same decade (1969).

- Systematic vaccination against rubella, usually in combination with measles, has eliminated both the congenital and acquired infection from some developed countries including the USA.
- In developing countries, specifically in India, rubella has been observed that around 40–45% of women of childbearing age are susceptible to rubella. Moreover, it is surprising to know that over two lakh babies are born with birth defects because of rubella infection during pregnancy in the Indian subcontinent.

It is worth recalling the historical aspects of the rubella vaccine invention by Stanley Plotkin in his Wistar Institute laboratory, and the "R" in MMR combo vaccines that are now used worldwide. Further, rubella was eliminated from the United States in 2004 as the result of the dedicated and unprecedented pioneering work of the late Professor Louis Z Cooper's (LZC), Rubella Project of the Bellevue Hospital, NY University, USA, for the elimination of both rubella pandemic devasted CRS and measles virus circulation in many parts of the world.

Literally moving from the bench to the bedside, LZC isolated the rubella virus and measured antibody responses in the laboratory while also evaluating hundreds of mothers and infants with CRS. Through these efforts, LZC established the clinical definition, features, and health impacts of CRS. Realizing that defining the disease and diagnosing the infection were only a part of what was needed to control any future pandemic diseases.

As rightly worded in the "2021 Red Book Dedication for LZC": Quote "he 'would say that nothing is unprecedented (in this COVID pandemic),' we just need to know where to look to find the guidance from the past to lead us through the challenges of the present". Unquote. Yes, when Dr LZC entered Saul Krugman's laboratory (NYU), the rubella pandemic had not yet flared, but he was in the right place at the right time, and this, coupled with his passions and energies, changed the course of that pandemic—a good analogy for Dr LZC's dedicated professional talents and his compassionate services.

Measles elimination is important because measles outbreaks can cause severe complications and deaths, especially among young, malnourished children. The WHO defines measles elimination as the absence of endemic measles virus transmission in a defined geographical area for at least 12 months. Experts say that a two-dose measles immunization schedule is necessary to achieve the ~95% population immunity necessary to interrupt measles virus transmission.

India had set a target to eliminate MR by 2023 but missed the earlier deadline of 2020. Four countries have eliminated measles—Bhutan, Maldives, DPR Korea, and Timor-Leste. In countries close to measles elimination, cases imported from other countries remain an important source of infection.

Measles control: In 1963, John Enders and colleagues transformed their Edmonston-B strain of measles virus into a vaccine and licensed it in the United States. In 1968, an improved and even weaker/attenuated measles vaccine, developed by *Maurice Hilleman and colleagues at Merck Research Lab*, was distributed. >500,000 cases of measles occurred each year in the US in the 20th century compared with 13 cases in 2020 and is considered eliminated in the US unvaccinated children are at risk of getting measles, but so are other people who are not able to get the vaccine or who have compromised immune systems.

Measles, a highly contagious disease, used to cause millions of deaths worldwide. One of the most common live-attenuated vaccines in use today is the MMR vaccine, which has dramatically reduced measles cases and deaths. Measles was declared eliminated in the United States in 2000, although sporadic outbreaks can still occur when vaccination rates drop. However, ongoing efforts are needed to maintain control and prevent outbreaks.

Since the beginning of 2022, Mumbai has recorded over 20 outbreaks of measles, with the D8 strain of virus found to be associated with the most recent outbreak. However, there are no structural changes found in the virus strain, and the recent outbreak is primarily due to immunization gaps. The re-emergence of measles is posing an imminent global threat owing to a decline in its vaccination rates amid the COVID-19 pandemic–a special focus on the recent outbreak in India—a call for a massive vaccination drive to be enhanced at the global level.

Mumps: According to Dr Paul Offit's book Vaccinated, during the 1960s "mumps virus infected a million people in the United States every year. Most people who contract the disease recover fully. However, beyond those chipmunk cheeks, mumps can have serious (and sometimes permanent) complications that are not so comical—inflammation of the testicles and ovaries, encephalitis, meningitis, and deafness". In early 1968, doctors began administering the Jeryl Lynn Strain mumps vaccine to the American public.

Although originally designed as three separate vaccines, attenuated strains of MMR were successfully formulated into a single combination vaccine in the US in 1971 and it continues to be used to provide protective immunity against pathogens responsible for what were once considered common childhood diseases. *Dr Maurice Hilleman at Merck* was also the first person to combine viral vaccines when he created the MMR vaccine, which has changed the entire world. On December 14, 2018, the US celebrated "50 years of mumps vaccination in America", helping to make "chipmunk cheeks and swollen testicles a thing of our nation's past". Although the MMR vaccine is not a part of the national immunization schedule of India, it was introduced in the state immunization program of Delhi in 1999 as a single dose between 15 and 18 months.

The MMR combos greatly improved vaccination coverage and reduced the incidence of these diseases. The MMR-V vaccine, which includes varicella (chickenpox) protection, was introduced in 2005 to further simplify vaccination schedules and reduce the number of shots a child needs to receive. The widespread use of MMR-V vaccines has led to significant reductions in the incidence of these diseases, preventing numerous cases of illness, hospitalizations, and deaths. Even when MMR combined with live, attenuated VZV to provide a quadrivalent vaccine, seroconversion rates remain high (measles; 97.1%, mumps; 96.0%, rubella; 98.8%, and varicella; 93.5%, respectively.

POLIO TOWARD ERADICATION

Polio is a highly infectious viral disease that largely affects children under 5 years of age. The virus is transmitted by person-to-person spread mainly through the fecal-oral route or, less frequently, by a common vehicle (e.g., contaminated water or food) and multiplies in the intestine, from where it can invade the nervous system and cause paralysis.

Thanks to vaccines polio, has seen significant progress toward eradication. The development of vaccines to prevent polio has been a major success story in the fight against infectious diseases. The polio vaccines have nearly eradicated life-threatening paralytic diseases and have prevented an estimated 29 million cases of paralysis between 1960 and 2021. The GPEI is financed by a wide range of public and private donors, who help meet the costs of the Initiative's eradication activities.

In 1955 Dr Jonas Salk's inactivated polio vaccine (IPV) was licensed in the USA. However, the OPV was easier to administer and played a crucial role in the global effort to eradicate polio which was licensed for use in the 1960s.

Mass vaccination campaigns: The introduction of polio vaccines led to mass vaccination campaigns in many countries. These efforts helped to reduce the incidence of polio dramatically in the Western world and other regions.

Progress toward eradication: Polio cases had declined dramatically worldwide by the early 21st century. The final push to eradicate the virus is challenging but remains a global health priority. By 2003, polio remained endemic in only 6 countries—and by 2006, that number had dropped to 4. As of July 2021, only two cases of wild poliovirus have been recorded globally this year to date: one each in Afghanistan and Pakistan.

Alongside the success and safety of the OPV in areas where vaccination coverage is low, comes *a disadvantage, i.e., vaccine-associated paralytic poliomyelitis (VAPP).* Continued use of the vaccine poses a risk of spreading the disease by the attenuated vaccine virus begins to circulate in undervaccinated communities. When this happens to circulate for sufficiently long enough time, it may genetically revert to a "strong" virus, able to cause paralysis, resulting in what is known as circulating vaccine-derived polioviruses (cVDPVs).

If a population is adequately immunized, it will be protected against both wild VAPP and cVDPVs.

Because of its widespread OPV use in the US, this resulted in an average of nine children each year from 1961 to 1989 who suffered VAPP paralysis due to OPV. Since polio was no longer endemic in the US, the OPV vaccine was causing more cases of paralysis than the wild-type polioviruses that it was designed to prevent. In 2000, the OPV vaccine regimen was abandoned in favor of the safer IPV series and VAPP was eliminated in the USA.

Implementation of an all IPV vaccine schedule in 2000 halted the occurrence of VAPP cases in the United States. The polio story continues with ongoing global eradication efforts striving to stop all poliovirus transmission.

Challenges and Setbacks

Since the launch of GPEI, polio cases have decreased by >99%, from an estimated 350,000 cases in >125 endemic countries to six reported cases in 2021. Of the three strains of wild poliovirus (type 1, type 2, and type 3), wild poliovirus type 2 was eradicated in 1999 and wild poliovirus type 3 was eradicated in 2020. As of 2022, endemic wild poliovirus type 1 remains in two countries—(1) Pakistan and (2) Afghanistan. Despite substantial progress, polio eradication efforts have faced challenges, including vaccine hesitancy, conflict zones, and logistical hurdles.

ROTAVIRUS GASTROENTERIC CONTROL BY ORAL VACCINES

Before the widespread use of vaccines, RV was the most common cause of community-acquired acute gastroenteritis (AGE) and healthcare-associated diarrhea in young children. In India: it is estimated that RF causes 872,000 hospitalizations, 3,270,000 outpatient visits, and an estimated 78,000 deaths annually in India. RV diarrhea presents in a similar manner to any other diarrhea but can mainly be prevented through orally administered RV vaccination.

Although RV is not amenable to eradication because of animal reservoirs, live, and attenuated oral vaccines have been the bedrock of both prevention and control programs, providing intestinal and humoral immunity.

Dr Timo Vesikari is a specialist in pediatric infectious diseases with a particular research interest in virology and viral vaccines. His research work has significantly contributed to the introduction of RV vaccine into childhood vaccination programs, worldwide.

The success story of RV vaccination is remarkable in the field of public health. It has demonstrated how vaccines, when developed, implemented, and distributed effectively, can significantly reduce the burden of a deadly and highly contagious disease, saving countless lives and improving the quality of life for children and families around the world. RV success stories are evidenced by a recent study that norovirus (NoV) has become the most prevalent pathogen among children with AGE in the post-RV vaccine era.

The global burden and the trends of RV infection-associated deaths have also decreased substantially. The epidemiology and burden of RV disease in the United States have changed dramatically following the introduction of RV vaccines in 2006 and 2008.

The Rota Shield vaccine developed against RV represents a vaccine that failed post-licensure due to an unacceptably high rate of reactogenicity in which serious adverse events (e.g., intussusception) reached 90–214 cases per million administered doses. Following licensure in 1998, it was subsequently pulled from the market by the end of 1999.

Live, attenuated RV vaccines with improved safety profiles (Rotarix® and RotaTeq®) have now entered the market to address this important clinical need. These vaccines have significantly reduced the healthcare burden associated with RV since the year 2006.

TETANUS AND DIPHTHERIA VACCINES ROLE

The DTP vaccine has been highly effective in preventing DTP. It played a significant role in reducing the incidence of these diseases and their associated morbidity and mortality.

The success of these vaccines can be attributed to their ability to provide long-lasting immunity against TD, significantly reducing the incidence of these diseases and their associated morbidity and mortality. Vaccination programs, along with proper wound care and hygiene practices, have played a crucial role in controlling tetanus, while also preventing diphtheria outbreaks.

The TD vaccine consists of formaldehyde-inactivated toxoids with the diphtheria toxoid developed in 1920 and the tetanus toxoid first described in 1924. Immunity for both diseases is achieved through antibody-mediated toxin neutralization.

For tetanus, immunity is considered 100% effective in preventing death if preexisting antibody levels are above a putative protective threshold of 0.01 IU/mL.

For diphtheria, a minimal protective serum titer has also been defined as 0.01 IU/mL.

Furthermore, protection against both diseases can be achieved with relatively low levels of toxin-specific antibodies compared to the high levels of antibodies elicited through current vaccination schedules. The tetanus vaccine, often given in combination with other vaccines such as adult dose diphtheria and acellular pertussis (DTaP or Tdap), stimulates the immune system to produce antibodies against these diseases.

Booster shots are recommended every 10 years to ensure ongoing immunity because the tetanus bacterium is widespread in the environment, and potential exposure to the bacteria through wounds is always possible.

Diphtheria vaccine is also commonly administered in combination with tetanus and pertussis vaccines (DTaP or Tdap). In countries with high vaccination rates, diphtheria has become rare. However, it is essential to maintain vaccination coverage to prevent its resurgence.

The success of these vaccines can be attributed to the development of herd immunity when a significant portion of the population is vaccinated, reducing the circulation of the bacteria in the community. Vaccination not only protects individuals but also contributes to the overall public health by preventing outbreaks of these diseases.

It is important to follow recommended vaccination schedules and receive booster shots as advised by healthcare professionals to maintain immunity against TD throughout one's life. In light of these results, the current US recommendation for adult TD booster doses to be administered every 10 years should be reconsidered.

PERTUSSIS VACCINE SUCCESS AND CHALLENGES

Following the implementation of a whole-cell inactivated pertussis (wP) vaccine in the 1940s, the disease burden dropped dramatically to a low of 0.5 cases per 100,000 persons by 1976. The wP vaccines were developed first and are suspensions of the entire *Bordetella pertussis* organism that has been inactivated, usually with formalin.

Vaccination has been the primary strategy for preventing pertussis, but there are several challenges associated with pertussis vaccination:

The wP vaccine elicited a relatively high rate of local and systemic adverse events. The most concerning adverse event was a potential link between vaccination and permanent brain damage due to encephalopathy. Nevertheless, the reappraisal of earlier studies calls into question whether any link between wP vaccination and encephalopathy truly exists.

Now in immunization practices, two forms of vaccine are in use, the wP, and the acellular vaccine (aP). Concerning the safety of the wP vaccine, several replacement subunit acellular pertussis (aP) candidate vaccines were developed. Both are generally safer and cause fewer side effects, but they may offer less long-lasting protection. *Balancing safety and effectiveness is an ongoing challenge.*

- *Waning immunity:* The pertussis vaccine can wane over time and achieving high vaccination coverage rates within a population is essential for herd immunity. This means that even individuals who have been vaccinated can become susceptible to the disease as they get older. This has led to a resurgence of pertussis in adolescents and adults, who can then transmit the infection to vulnerable infants.
- *Vaccine hesitancy:* Vaccine hesitancy and refusal are growing concerns globally. Misinformation and distrust of vaccines can lead to lower vaccination rates, reducing the overall protection against pertussis and other preventable diseases.
- *Incomplete vaccination coverage:* Some individuals may not receive the full recommended vaccine series due to various reasons, including vaccine hesitancy, access issues, or medical contraindications. This can leave pockets of susceptibility in the population.
- *Mutating bacteria: B. pertussis* bacteria can mutate over time, potentially affecting the effectiveness of vaccines. This could result in new strains that are less susceptible to immunity conferred by existing vaccines.
- *Pregnant women and infants:* Pertussis is particularly dangerous for infants, and maternal vaccination during pregnancy has been recommended to protect newborns. However, ensuring high coverage among pregnant women can be challenging, and some may have concerns about vaccine safety during pregnancy.

To address these challenges, ongoing research is focused on improving pertussis vaccines, developing new strategies for vaccination, and increasing public awareness about the importance of vaccination. Boosters for adolescents and adults, continued surveillance, and public health efforts to educate the public about the safety and efficacy of vaccines are critical components of pertussis control. Public health authorities also monitor pertussis outbreaks and may implement additional vaccination measures when needed to control the spread of the disease.

Unlike tetanus, diphtheria, and Hib, one of the major limitations with the development of subunit vaccines for pertussis was the lack of a defined correlate of immunity against a specific *B. pertussis* component for vaccine-induced immunity. The answer to this public health problem is unclear. A range of potential solutions have been proposed and although a return to the old wP vaccine is considered unlikely, new wP vaccines with high efficacy and improved safety profiles might still be a viable option.

Until researchers can find an improved approach to elicit durable immunity while retaining an acceptable safety profile, pertussis will represent a continuing problem for the foreseeable future.

HEPATITIS A VIRUS CONTROL BY VACCINATIONS

It represents a striking success for whole-virion inactivated vaccines, with incomparable efficacy. Dr Saul Krugman of the NY University was the first scientist to prove that "infectious" (type A) hepatitis, transmitted by the fecal-oral route, and the more serious "serum" (type B) hepatitis, transmitted by blood, body secretions, and sexual contact, were caused by two immunologically distinct viruses.

The HAV vaccine has been included in many national immunization programs, contributing to global efforts to reduce the burden of hepatitis A. One of the most impressive aspects of the inactivated HAV vaccines has been the durability of vaccine-induced antibody responses, often for a lifetime. After completing the recommended vaccine schedule, long-term antibody persistence was demonstrated for up to 20 years postvaccination. This has led to significant reductions in the number of cases and deaths associated with the disease.

These critical elements supported the eventual development and licensure of two inactivated whole-virion, alum-adjuvanted vaccines *(Havrix® and Vaqta®)* in the US. Efficacy for both vaccines is high, with estimates ranging from 94 to 100%. HAV-specific antibodies have been identified as the key correlate of protective immunity following vaccination, and although an absolute lower limit has not been defined, titers >10–20 mIU/mL are generally considered protective.

Outbreak Control

The vaccine has been crucial in controlling HAV outbreaks, especially in settings where the virus can easily spread, such as in communities with poor sanitation, daycare centers, and restaurants. The vaccine has also been beneficial for travelers, as it protects against HAV when visiting regions with a higher prevalence of the virus. Many countries have even made the vaccine a requirement for travelers entering areas with a high risk of HAV.

Overall, the HAV is a remarkable success story in the realm of vaccines and public health. It has not only saved innumerable lives but also reduced the economic and societal burden by preventing infections and their associated complications. Its widespread use continues to be a central component of global efforts to control and ultimately eliminate hepatitis A as a public health threat.

HEPATITIS B VIRUS VACCINATION SUCCESS STORY

The success of the HBV vaccine led to the implementation of universal vaccination programs in many countries. Over time, improved versions of the HBV were developed, including second and third-generation vaccines. These newer vaccines have further enhanced safety and efficacy profiles. The ultimate goal is to eliminate hepatitis B as a public health threat. *The success story of the HBV vaccination is a remarkable* one that has had a profound impact on public health worldwide.

The first-generation HBV vaccine, consisting of purified HBV surface antigen (HBsAg), was licensed for use in the United States in 1981. Subsequent advances led to improved vaccines, including recombinant DNA technology to produce the antigen, which greatly enhanced the safety and effectiveness of the vaccine.

In 1983, Dr Krugman, achieved the Albert Lasker Public Service Award for his courageous leadership in conceiving, developing, and testing vaccines against various viral diseases, especially hepatitis B, with vast impact on world health.

Many countries have implemented universal vaccination programs to ensure that infants receive the HBV shortly after birth. This has been particularly effective in preventing mother-to-child transmission during childbirth, which was a common mode of transmission before the vaccine. The CDC has updated its guidance for hepatitis B testing for the first time since 2008 and now recommends that all adults in the US be tested for HBV at least once in their lifetime

"Along with vaccination strategies, universal screening of adults and appropriate testing of persons at increased risk for HBV infection will improve health outcomes, reduce the prevalence of HBV infection in the US, and advance viral hepatitis elimination goals".

As a result of vaccination efforts, the incidence of hepatitis B infection has significantly declined in many parts of the world. The vaccine provides long-lasting immunity, often for a lifetime, with a high rate of protection This has led to a substantial decrease in the number of new cases of chronic hepatitis, cirrhosis, and liver cancer associated with hepatitis B.

In summary, the HBV vaccination success story is characterized by the development of an effective vaccine, widespread adoption of vaccination programs, and a significant reduction in the incidence of hepatitis B and its related health problems. The National Strategy for Viral Hepatitis B and C 2023-2030 (NSVH) focuses on strengthening existing preventive services for viral hepatitis B and C and further expand the coverage of diagnostics and treatment services to the communities.

PNEUMOCOCCAL VACCINES BENEFITS

These vaccines have had a profound impact on reducing the incidence of pneumococcal diseases, including pneumonia, meningitis, and invasive bacteremic diseases. The introduction of conjugated vaccines such as Prevnar 7 (PCV7), Prevnar 13 (PCV13), and targeted pneumococcal strains has significantly reduced the incidence of invasive pneumococcal diseases, particularly in children.

Overall the pneumococcal vaccines are 60–70% effective in preventing invasive disease caused by serotypes in the vaccine and 3 in 4 adults 65 years or older against invasive disease.

Although the PCV has been introduced into state immunization programs (SIPs) in India, many children remain unvaccinated. Recently, India's Advisory Committee on Vaccines and Immunization Practices recommended PCV on the pediatric immunization schedule nationally. Thus, currently, pneumococcal vaccines seem to be the only public health tool capable of rapidly reducing the burden of pneumococcal diseases in India. Implementing PCV SIPs throughout India, would not only prevent a substantial amount of pneumococcal disease cases and consequent deaths.

By reducing the incidence of pneumococcal diseases, vaccines also play a role in preventing the overuse of antibiotics, which can contribute to antimicrobial resistance (AMR).

Organizations like Gavi, the Vaccine Alliance, have supported the introduction of PCVs in low-income countries, further contributing to the reduction of pneumococcal diseases.

Researchers continue to monitor pneumococcal disease trends to ensure that vaccination programs are effective and to identify any emerging issues, such as changes in bacterial strains.

THE HUMAN PAPILLOMAVIRUS VACCINES ARE SO EFFECTIVE!

The HPV vaccine has been available since 2006. Of the known identified 200 types of sexually transmitted HPV, at least 12 can cause urogenital cancers. HPV vaccines have been successful in preventing cervical cancer and other HPV-related diseases.

After the introduction of HPV vaccines, real-world studies have demonstrated decreases in the prevalence of vaccine HPV types as well as reduced rates of high-grade cervical lesions and invasive cervical cancer in vaccinated populations. Accumulated safety data from large post-marketing surveillance studies and epidemiologic studies have been consistent with the safety profile in clinical trials.

In India, HPV prevalence in studies in different settings has ranged from 7 to 27% among healthy women. Vaccinating girls against HPV is a cost-effective strategy to reduce the incidence of cervical cancer and mortality due to cervical cancer.

Advances in vaccine technology and research may lead to improved vaccines and broader protection against additional HPV strains in the future.

Widespread use of HPV vaccines represents a significant success story and has the potential to greatly reduce the incidence of these cancers in the future.

Expanding vaccination programs to include boys and young men may reduce HPV prevalence. Therefore, it is essential to continue efforts in vaccination and education to further reduce HPV-related diseases and cancers, with a particular focus on reaching underserved populations and increasing vaccine access globally.

Additionally, regular screenings, such as Pap tests and HPV testing, remain crucial for early detection and management of HPV-related diseases.

SARS-CoV-2 (COVID-19) VACCINES EFFICACY AND CHALLENGES

Good of COVID-19 Vaccines and Vaccinations

COVID-19, caused by SARS-CoV-2, has led to a global pandemic (2022–2023). Several highly efficacious vaccines including new RNA technology have been developed to control the spread of a previously unknown viral pathogen at a speed that never happened in vaccine development history. This is indeed a scientific miracle empowered by technological advancements and forms a platform for future vaccine manufacturing against human diseases and disorders including cancer vaccine progress.

Early in January 2020, SARS-CoV-2 culturing and genomic analysis happened at a record pace. Before learning and mapping out the catastrophic effects of COVID-19 on our human system and with no specific antiviral drugs identified, countries such as China, the USA, and the UK started the race for vaccine design and manufacturing. All these efforts resulted in the first mRNA SARS-CoV-2 vaccines against COVID-19 when it was rolled out in mid-Dec 2020.

It is an unprecedented event in the history of vaccinology in less than a year! from the identification of the virus until the EUA in less than a year!

The rapid development of multiple COVID-19 vaccines distributed with speed, worldwide in a record time; has been a testament to the effectiveness of scientific innovation and international collaboration. Some key vaccines that were widely used or in development at that time:

- *Pfizer-BioNTech* mRNA vaccine was one of the first COVID-19 vaccines to receive emergency use authorization (EUA) in many countries. It is highly effective in preventing COVID-19. Similar to the Pfizer-BioNTech vaccine, the Moderna COVID-19 vaccine is also an mRNA-based vaccine and has shown high efficacy against the virus.
- *Johnson & Johnson (Janssen):* Vaccine is a viral vector vaccine that uses a harmless adenovirus to deliver a piece of the SARS-CoV-2 spike protein. It has the advantage of requiring only one dose.
- *AstraZeneca-Oxford, UK:* Developed by the University of Oxford vaccine was widely used in many countries. CoviShield is a vaccine made by the Serum Institutes of India (SII), Pune in collaboration with AstraZeneca known as "ChAdOx1 nCoV-19 or AZD1222" (chimpanzee adenovirus-vectored vaccine) against severe SARS-CoV-2.

Because of some uncertainty over earlier clinical trial results clouded its prospects until Dec 31, 2020, and India approved this Pune-made vaccine on January 1, 2021; However, it faced some concerns about rare blood clotting issues, leading to temporary suspensions and changes in recommendations in some regions, many Indian hospitals are inoculating healthcare workers with this AstraZeneca strain vaccine.

- *Sinopharm and Sinovac:* Threse are Vero-cell inactivated vaccines developed in China. They have been used in several countries, including in the UAE, India, etc., and have shown efficacy in preventing COVID-19.
- *Sputnik V:* Developed in Russia, this vaccine is also a viral vector vaccine and has been authorized for use in multiple countries.
- *Novavax:* This protein subunit vaccine was in late-stage clinical trials and showed promising results in preventing COVID-19. It received authorization in some countries.
- *Bharat Biotech's Covaxin:* It is another home-grown vaccine manufactured in Hyderabad by Bharat Biotech, is an "inactivated SARS-CoV-2" prepared from India India-derived virus–strain received EUA in India and was widely used there.
- *The Covaxin vaccine:* It is similar to the Chinese manufactured virus strains called "Sinopharm" (Govt) and "Sinovac" inactivated vaccines that are used in the far East and many Mid-East countries now. But hospitals that have been administering Covaxin have seen many doctors hesitate to get the shot. Both these two vaccines may have certain immediate transient adverse reactions like any other immunizations, but the long-term adversarial effects, are probably of a rarity. Also, the vaccine-induced lasting immunity for all the approved vaccines remains to be followed prospectively.

It is important to note that COVID-19 vaccines may have further evolved since were approved and updated to address emerging variants of the virus. The effectiveness, safety, and availability of vaccines can vary by region, so it is essential to refer to local health authorities and stay informed about the latest developments related to COVID-19 vaccines in your area.

Also, vaccination cuts long COVID risk:
- Individuals who received one or more doses of the COVID-19 vaccine before their initial infection were found to be 58% less likely to receive a diagnosis of post-COVID conditions than their unvaccinated counterparts. Furthermore, the study revealed a dose-response effect, increasing vaccine effectiveness with each successive dose administered before infection.
- In the latest (Nov 28, 2023), WHO epidemiological update on COVID-19 showed—"over half a million

new cases and over 2,400 deaths were reported during the last 28-day period from October 23 to November 19, 2023—a decrease of 13% and 72%, respectively, compared with the previous 28 days".
- The public can be assured that these updated vaccines have met the agency's rigorous scientific standards for safety, effectiveness, and manufacturing quality. "Vaccination remains critical to public health and continued protection against serious consequences of COVID-19, including hospitalization and death".

MENINGOCOCCAL OUTBREAK CONTROLS

Meningococcal vaccines have been instrumental in preventing and controlling meningococcal outbreak diseases, especially in crowded settings like college campuses. The availability of vaccines has been crucial in controlling these outbreaks, preventing further spread of the disease, and protecting at-risk populations.

Meningococcal vaccines have been developed over several decades, with the first polysaccharide-based vaccine introduced in the 1970s. These early vaccines targeted different serogroups of the *Neisseria meningitidis*. The most common serogroups associated with disease are A, B, C, W, and Y and vaccines were developed to protect against these serogroups.

Over time, advancements in vaccine technology led to the development of conjugate vaccines, which were more effective and provided longer-lasting immunity. The introduction of conjugate meningococcal vaccines has led to a significant reduction in the incidence of meningococcal disease, particularly in high-risk populations such as infants, adolescents, and college students.

Mass vaccination campaigns during outbreaks have helped to rapidly contain the spread of the disease and save lives. Adolescents and young adults are among the groups most susceptible to meningococcal disease. Vaccination efforts have targeted this age group to provide protection during a period of increased risk. In several countries, widespread vaccination campaigns have successfully eliminated meningococcal serogroup C as a public health threat. This achievement demonstrates the effectiveness of vaccination programs in reducing the incidence of meningococcal disease.

Research and Development for serogroup B has been challenging to vaccinate against because of its unique properties. However, ongoing research has led to the development of vaccines targeting serogroup B, which are now available in some regions. The introduction of new multivalent meningococcal conjugate vaccines (*MenFive*®), is a critical addition to the toolbox that will save thousands of lives every year.

Meningococcal vaccines have had a global impact, reducing the burden of meningococcal disease in various countries. Organizations like the WHO have supported vaccination campaigns in regions with high disease prevalence.

In summary, meningococcal vaccines have been a success story in the field of vaccinology. They have substantially reduced the burden of a potentially devastating and life-threatening disease, prevented outbreaks, and saved lives worldwide. Through vaccination campaigns and research efforts, many regions have seen a significant reduction in meningococcal disease-associated morbidity and mortality.

CONCLUSION

Successful vaccines have been developed against many of the most common human pathogens and this success has not been dependent upon any one specific class of vaccine since subunit vaccines, nonreplicating whole-virus or whole-bacteria vaccines, and attenuated live vaccines have all been effective for particular vaccine targets.

After completing the initial vaccination series, one common aspect of successful vaccines is that they induce long-term protective immunity. In contrast, several partially successful vaccines appear to induce relatively short-lived protection, and long-term protective immunity will likely be critical for making effective vaccines against our most challenging diseases such as acquired immunodeficiency syndrome (AIDS) and malaria.

Although nearly all vaccines require at least one booster dose to maintain long-term protective immunity, many of our most successful vaccines have achieved the appropriate balance of both safety and efficacy.

SUGGESTED READING

1. Amanna IJ, Slifka MK. Successful Vaccines. Curr Top Microbiol Immunol. 2020;428:1-30.
2. American Academy of Pediatrics. (2021). 2021 Red Book Dedication for Louis Z. Cooper, MD, FAAP. Available from: https://publications.aap.org/redbook/book/347/chapter/5748898/2021-Red-Book-Dedication-for-Louis-Z-Cooper-MD [Last accessed April, 2024].
3. Arinaminpathy N, Rade K, Kumar R, Joshi RP, Rao R. The potential impact of vaccination on tuberculosis burden

in India: A modelling analysis. Indian J Med Res. 2023; 157(2&3):119-26.
4. Ghia CJ, Horn EK, Rambhad G, Perdrizet J, Chitale R, Wasserman MD. Estimating the Public Health and Economic Impact of Introducing the 13-Valent Pneumococcal Conjugate Vaccine or 10-Valent Pneumococcal Conjugate Vaccines into State Immunization Programs in India. Infect Dis Ther. 2021:10:2271-88.
5. Lee BR, Harrison CJ, Hassan F, Sasidharan A, Moffatt ME, Weltmer K, et al. A Comparison of Pathogen Detection and Risk Factors among Symptomatic Children with Gastroenteritis Compared with Asymptomatic Children in the Post-rotavirus Vaccine Era. J Pediatr. 2023;261: 113551.
6. National Museum of American History. (2018). Happy 50th anniversary of no mumps. Available from: https://americanhistory.si.edu/blog/mumps-vaccine [Last accessed April, 2024].
7. Sabin AB. The 1981 International Symposium on Viral Hepatitis. Available from: https://drc.libraries.uc.edu/server/api/core/bitstreams/d0b20cc3-ba11-42eb-8599-873246173d12/content [Last accessed November, 2024].
8. Saxon W. (1995). Saul Krugman, 84; Led Fight to Vanquish Childhood Diseases. Available from: https://www.nytimes.com/1995/10/28/nyregion/saul-krugman-84-led-fight-to-vanquish-childhood-diseases.html [Last accessed April, 2024].
9. Suvvari TK, Kandi V, Mohapatra RK, Chopra H, Islam MA, Dhama K. The re-emergence of measles is posing an imminent global threat owing to decline in its vaccination rates amid COVID-19 pandemic: a special focus on recent outbreak in India—a call for massive vaccination drive to be enhanced at global level. Int J Surg. 2023;109(2): 198-200.
10. Vesikari T, Karvonen A, Ferrante SA, Ciarlet M. Efficacy of the pentavalent rotavirus vaccine, RotaTeq®, in Finnish infants up to 3 years of age: the Finnish Extension Study. Eur J Pediatr. 2010;169(11):1379-86.
11. Weng MK, Doshani M, Khan MA, Frey S, Ault K, Moore KL, et al. Universal Hepatitis B Vaccination in Adults Aged 19-59 Years: Updated Recommendations of the Advisory Committee on Immunization Practices—United States, 2022. MMWR Morb Mortal Wkly Rep. 2022; 71(13):477-83.
12. World Health Organization. Learn the story of these life-saving jabs. Available from: https://www.who.int/news-room/spotlight/history-of-vaccination/a-brief-history-of-vaccination [Last accessed April, 2024].

CHAPTER 4

Vaccine Components—Highpoints

■ INTRODUCTION

This chapter's contents highlight immunogenic components of commonly approved and added vaccines for use in clinical practices. Safety, efficacy, and promising approaches for vaccine delivery are discussed in comprehensive.

Fundamentally, all the approved vaccines are either one of the following:
- Toxoid vaccines
- Inactivated vaccines
- Live-attenuated vaccines (LAVs)
- Polysaccharide and conjugate vaccines
- Recombinant and subunit vaccines
- Messenger ribonucleic acid (mRNA) vaccines
- Viral vector vaccines

There are around 25 plus vaccines, e.g., compositions, doses, interactions, adverse reactions, and management are provided.

■ LANDSCAPE AND PROGRESS OF VACCINE DEVELOPMENT

A vaccine generally contains an agent that resembles a disease-causing microorganism and is usually made of the microbe, its toxins, or one of its surface proteins. Vaccines were initially developed on an experimental basis, depending mostly on live attenuation or inactivation of pathogens.

The live-attenuated viral vaccines currently available and routinely recommended are measles, mumps, rubella, varicella (MMRV), rotavirus, and influenza (intranasal). Other nonroutinely recommended live vaccines include the adenovirus vaccine (used by the military), typhoid vaccine (Ty21a), and bacille Calmette-Guérin (BCG).

Advances in immunology, molecular biology, biochemistry, genomics, and proteomics have added new outlook to the vaccinology field. Live recombinant bacterial and viral vectors effectively stimulate the immune system as in natural long-term cellular immune responses that are needed for disease protection. In general, all these methods have shown advantages and disadvantages.

The mRNA vaccine technology has provided a platform for quicker and adaptable vaccine production, offering hope in the fight against emerging infectious diseases.

Messenger Ribonucleic Acid Vaccines—A New Era in Vaccinology

Until recently most people had never even heard of mRNA vaccines; thanks to decades of mRNA research and innovation. As scientists put it, "The whole field of mRNA is just exploding. It is a game-changer in medicine. Now scientists believe that the mRNA vaccine technology may be the key to solving a wealth of health problems and even gave this new era a name: "the RNAissance" (Rebirth)".

Role of Nanotechnology Behind the Success of mRNA Vaccines for COVID-19

Instead, the mRNA vaccines use the synthetic genetic sequence or "code" of the antigen translated into mRNA. It is a ghost of the real thing, fooling the body into creating very real antibodies. The artificial mRNA itself then disappears, degraded by the body's natural defenses including enzymes that break it down, leaving us with only the antibodies.

Nanotech Offers a Promising Approach to Vaccine Delivery

Nanoparticles can encapsulate antigens, protecting them and facilitating controlled release, potentially leading to improved vaccine stability and enhanced immune responses. This innovation holds the potential for developing next-generation, highly effective vaccines.

Various Other Approaches for Vaccine Development

Recombinant vaccine, i.e., mixing of two deoxyribonucleic acid (DNA) from different sources is called a recombinant vaccine technology, in which the DNA encoding the genetic determinant of the bacteria, insect, yeast, and mammalian cells can be inserted and expressed. This technology is gaining traction due to its potential for rapid vaccine development and the ability to induce robust and long-lasting immune responses. Examples are hepatitis B virus (HBV) vaccines, flu vaccines, and rabies.

The recombinant vaccines can be broadly classified into three groups:
1. Attenuated recombinant, e.g., cholera and *Salmonella* spp.
2. Subunit recombinant vaccines are proteins, peptides, and DNA extraction methods, HBV, human papillomavirus (HPV), and hand-foot-mouth disease (HFMD)
3. Vector recombinant uses an attenuated virus or bacterium to introduce microbial DNA to cells of the body, e.g., influenza, vesicular stomatitis virus (VSV), measles virus, and adenovirus.

Several recombinant vaccines are available commercially, and many more are projected to be available soon, so the future of recombinant vaccines is bright. It is important to understand the immune response of the host to ensure that the vaccine induces the appropriate immunological reaction. In addition to using conventional delivery routes such as oral, intranasal, intradermal (ID), transcutaneous, intramuscular (IM), and intraperitoneal (IP,) scientists are experimenting with needle-free systems and vaccine strategies that allow mass vaccination of many individuals simultaneously.

Peptide vaccines are synthetic proteins that mimic naturally occurring proteins from viruses, causing an immune response. Peptide vaccines have shown great potential in cancer immunotherapy by targeting tumor antigens and activating the patient's immune system to mount a specific response against cancer cells without affecting healthy cells.

Adjuvant Technologies for Vaccine Safety and Efficacy

Adjuvants are substances that are primarily added to usual vaccines to promote the body's immune response. Innovative adjuvant technologies are being developed to improve vaccine efficacy and reduce the amount of antigen needed per dose. This not only amplifies the protective response, but also allows for more competent vaccine production and distribution.

Thermostable Vaccines

Maintaining the cold chain for vaccine distribution can be challenging, especially in remote or resource-constrained areas. Innovations in thermostable vaccines that withstand a broader range of temperatures are addressing this issue, ensuring vaccine effectiveness and accessibility, even in challenging environments.

Virus-like Particle Vaccines

Mimic the structure of viruses without containing the genetic material to cause disease. They are safe and highly effective in inducing strong immune responses, making them a promising innovation in vaccine development. Examples are HBV vaccines and HPV vaccines.

Future Prospective of Nasal and Oral mRNA Vaccines or Microarray Patches Administrations

Vaccines administered through the parenteral route, especially mRNAs provide robust protection against severe disease and death. However, they do not completely prevent the spread of severe acute respiratory syndrome coronavirus 2 (SARS-CoV-2), and intranasal vaccines delivered through the nasal cavity which can elicit both mucosal and systemic immune responses. More than a dozen nasal sprays or drops are now being tested against coronavirus disease-2019 (COVID-19) in humans, either as a primary immunization or as a booster.

Around the world, more than a dozen intranasally delivered COVID-19 vaccines have entered clinical trials, and they run the gamut from adenovirus-vectored genes for viral antigens to recombinant protein-based formulations to live attenuated SARS-CoV-2. Administered, most commonly by an aerosolized spray, although nasally administered drops, powders, and gels have also been considered *(Discussed under COVID-19 Vaccine highlights with illustrious pictures in this chapter).*

Future Oral Route Administrations of DNA and RNA Vaccines

In addition to make vaccines easier to tolerate, the oral capsule-form approach could also be used to deliver other kinds of therapeutic RNA or DNA directly to the digestive tract, which could make it easier to treat gastrointestinal disorders such as ulcers. There are many immune cells in the gastrointestinal tract, and orally administered vaccines are a known way of creating an immune response and stimulating the immune system.

Like most vaccines, RNA vaccines have to be injected, which can be an obstacle for people who fear needles. Now, a team of the researchers has developed a way to deliver RNA in a capsule that can be swallowed, which they hope could help make people more receptive to them.

Microarray patches (MAPs), are coin-sized patches covered either with tiny needles coated in the dry vaccine that painlessly penetrate the skin or a formula that dissolves when the patch is pressed onto the skin for 2–5 minutes. These patches do not require cold temperatures, weight significantly less than vials requiring needles and syringes, do not require any mixing, and can be given by untrained community health workers in almost any condition. Plus, there is a needle-free advantage of painless delivery, upping the odds that people will get all of the vaccinations they need.

Microarray patches have the potential to change the way vaccines are delivered and could transform immunization coverage in lower-income countries, e.g., deliver vaccines without syringes, making them easier to distribute and administer. The simplicity, versatility, safety, and thermostability advantages make MAPs a promising alternative, allowing for the expansion and improvement of immunization programs.

There are currently two MAPs in the market pipeline; one for measles and one for rubella. Two important next steps are to evaluate where and in what circumstances MAPs would most likely be used, i.e., for routine, seasonal, or other kinds of immunizations, and in what countries or settings. Unfortunately, some challenges are standing in the way of MAPs becoming widely used. The largest roadblock at the moment is the lack of large production facilities for MAP! *(UNICEF, 2022).*

Nasal Vaccines and Mucosal Immunity

Unlike conventional vaccines, nasal vaccines are needle-free, thus simplifying immunization procedures and reducing apprehension among vaccinees. Nasal vaccines induce protective immunity that prevents the invasion of pathogens from mucosal surfaces and inhibits severe disease. Nasal vaccines are particularly appropriate for respiratory infectious diseases because of their specialized induction of effective immunity in the upper and lower respiratory tracts.

Unfortunately, we don't have an approved mucosal booster vaccine yet, and our research has shown that as simple as a spray of recombinant spike protein without any adjuvants can restimulate immune response and then establish mucosal immunity in the nasal cavity, which goes a long way in preventing infection as well as transmission. Many types of nasal vaccines and delivery systems have been developed worldwide, with those to combat COVID-19 at the top of the list.

Single-dose Vaccines

Efforts are being made to develop single-dose vaccines that provide complete immunization against certain diseases. This innovation simplifies vaccination schedules, increases compliance, and improves vaccine coverage, especially in challenging or hard-to-reach populations.

Inverse Vaccines

As of this day, February 2024, this vaccine is still in development and has not been tested on humans. Conventional vaccines train the immune system to spot infectious diseases and stop them from multiplying and spreading. An inverse vaccine, on the other hand, stops the immune system from attacking cells specifically, good and healthy cells. Instead, it retrains the immune system to save healthy cells, essentially by adding a "do not attack" flag.

Autoimmune diseases are usually treated with drugs that suppress the immune system to stop the immune cells from attacking any cells, including healthy ones. They can be effective, but have their disadvantages, too. Scientists hope the inverse vaccine could treat autoimmune diseases, such as multiple sclerosis (MS), type 1 diabetes, allergic asthma, or Crohn's disease. In autoimmune diseases, the body's immune system (our defense against illness) cannot tells the difference between good cells and bad cells and ends up attacking them all. So, you get sick either way.

The inverse vaccine is not yet ready for testing in human trials, and no other inverse vaccines have been clinically approved, either. However, early safety trials are underway, including for their use with celiac disease, and phase 1 safety trials for MS.

Adenoviruses Vaccine

Adenoviruses are nonenveloped, double-stranded DNA viruses, first discovered in the human adenoid tissue in 1953 by Rowe and his colleagues. In humans, adenoviruses generally cause mild respiratory and gastrointestinal tract infections; however, adenovirus-induced infections can be life-threatening in immunocompromised people, or people with preexisting respiratory or cardiac disorders.

These viruses are isolated from a wide variety of mammalian species, ranging from simians to chimpanzees to human beings. In humans, >80 recognized types and multiple genetic variants are divided into seven species (A–G) that infect humans.

Human adenoviruses (AdHu) are common and can cause a range of illnesses, and are associated primarily with:
- Respiratory tract disease (types 1–5, 7, 14, and 21)
- Epidemic keratoconjunctivitis (EKC)—"Madras Eye" (types 8, 19, and 37)
- Gastroenteritis (types 40 and 41)

They are typically spread through close personal contact, such as touching or shaking hands, through the air by coughing and sneezing, or by touching an object or surface with adenoviruses on it, then touching your mouth, nose, or eyes.

There is currently an adenovirus vaccine available, but it is not for general use. The adenovirus vaccine (live and oral) is a vaccine used to control disease caused by AdHu serotypes 4 and 7. It is given in a two-tablet form (one tablet for each adenovirus type) and is currently approved for military personnel aged 17 through 50 years.

"Madras Eye", also known as EKC, is a highly contagious eye infection typically caused by adenoviruses. At present, there is no specific vaccine available to prevent "Madras Eye" or EKC.

Adenoviruses have also been used as vectors in the development of other vaccines.

Adenoviruses are considered excellent vectors for delivering target antigens to mammalian hosts because of their capability to induce both innate and adaptive immune responses. Currently, adenovirus-based vaccines are used against a wide variety of pathogens, including *Mycobacterium tuberculosis*, human immunodeficiency virus (HIV), and *Plasmodium falciparum*.

Viral vector-based vaccines use a harmless virus to smuggle the instructions for making antigens from the disease-causing virus into cells, triggering protective immunity against it. Unlike other viral vectors, such as lentivirus and retrovirus, the risk of insertion mutagenesis is much less in the case of adenoviruses as they do not integrate the viral genome with the host genome. The relatively large-sized and well-characterized genome, adenoviruses are easy to manipulate genetically. Because adenoviruses cause mild infections in humans and their viral replication can be inhibited by genetic modifications, adenovirus-based vaccines are mostly safe and come with very few side effects.

To date, several adenovirus-based vaccines are in clinical and preclinical trials.

The COVID-19 vaccines use an adenovirus vector to deliver a piece of the SARS-CoV-2 virus's genetic material into cells to stimulate an immune response. This has been authorized for emergency use (AEU) amidst the COVID-19 pandemic.

Vaccines developed against HIV, Ebola virus, influenza virus, *M. tuberculosis*, and *Plasmodium falciparum* are currently under human clinical trials. There are also vaccines under preclinical trials developed against rabies virus, dengue virus (DENV), and Middle East respiratory syndrome coronavirus (CoV). The advantage of using adenovirus vectors is that they are good at entering human cells and delivering the genetic material, which can lead to a strong immune response.

Vector Design

Scientists modify the adenovirus genome by removing certain genes necessary for replication and inserting genes that encode antigens from the target pathogen. The modified adenovirus, now serving as a vector, is administered to the individual through injection, nasal spray, or another route. There are four main types of viral vectors (e.g., adeno-associated viral, adenoviral, lentiviral, and retroviral), each with its unique characteristics uses and limitations.

Antigen Presentation

Once inside the body, the modified adenovirus infects cells and releases the genetic material encoding the antigen. The cells then produce the antigen, which is recognized by the immune system as foreign. The immune system mounts a response against the antigen, producing antibodies and activating T-cells specific to that antigen.

Immune memory: After the initial immune response, memory cells are generated, providing long-term immunity against the target pathogen.

Adenovirus vector vaccines may have limitations and potential side effects, like any medical intervention. These can include mild to moderate reactions such as fever, fatigue, headache, muscle pain, and injection site reactions. Additionally, there have been rare reports of serious adverse events, such as blood clotting disorders, associated with some adenovirus vector COVID-19 vaccines.

Overall, the benefits of adenovirus vaccines generally outweigh the risks, but continued monitoring and research are essential to ensure their safety and effectiveness.

Anthrax Vaccine

Anthrax is relatively rare in most parts of the world, including India. It can have severe consequences if not treated promptly. Anthrax is one of the top 10 diseases reported in India and one of the major causes of death in livestock, with a high fatality. The anthrax resulting from natural infection or secondary to a bioterror event can occur in multiple forms, depending on the route of infection: cutaneous, inhalation, ingestion, or injection.

Human anthrax is difficult to contain. This is primarily because it is a zoonotic disease, and the disease has never been contained in the livestock of India due to lack of adequate vaccination facilities. Animal anthrax is very common in many parts of India. Human anthrax outbreaks in India were clustered around the eastern coastal regions. The states of Odisha, West Bengal, Andhra Pradesh, and Jharkhand reported a maximum number of outbreaks.

Clinicians should order the vaccine in conjunction with recommended antibiotic treatment. If not treated promptly, anthrax is often fatal, especially when a person develops the inhalation form of the disease after breathing in anthrax spores.

The anthrax vaccine is primarily recommended for adults 18 through 65 years of age who are at risk of exposure to anthrax bacteria, including certain laboratory workers who work with Bacillus anthracis and those who handle potentially infected animals or their carcasses.

BioThrax [anthrax vaccine adsorbed (AVA)], the only anthrax vaccine currently licensed in the United States for use in humans, is prepared from a cell-free culture filtrate. The vaccine's efficacy for the prevention of anthrax is based on animal studies and has proven to be effective in preventing the disease. AVA demonstrated 93% efficacy for preventing cutaneous and inhalation anthrax. Multiple reviews and publications evaluating AVA safety have found adverse events usually are local injection site reactions, with rare systemic symptoms, including fever, chills, muscle aches, and hypersensitivity.

Pre-exposure prophylaxis is only recommended for select groups of workers at continued risk of infection. Post-exposure prophylaxis (PEP) for previously unvaccinated people older than 18 years who have been exposed to aerosolized B anthracis spores consists of up to 60 days of appropriate antimicrobial prophylaxis combined with three subcutaneous (SC) doses of AVA (administered at 0, 2, and 4 weeks postexposure). AVA is not licensed for use in pregnant women. Use in pediatric populations has not been studied.

There is a vaccine in India that can help prevent anthrax, a serious infection caused by the bacterium *Bacillus anthracis*. However, this vaccine is not typically available for the general public. It is only recommended for people who are at an increased risk of coming into contact with or have already been exposed to anthracis.

Bacille Calmette–Guérin Vaccines

Bacille Calmette–Guérin vaccine is a live vaccine originally prepared from attenuated strains of *Mycobacterium bovis*. An isolate of BCG can be distinguished from wildtype *M. bovis* only in a reference laboratory. The BCG is one of the most widely used vaccines in the world. The use of BCG is recommended by the Expanded Program on Immunization (EPI) of the World Health Organization (WHO) for administration at birth.

The BCG vaccine has relatively high protective efficacy (approximately 80%) against meningeal and miliary TB in children.

In countries with a significant number of tuberculosis (TB) patients in the community, children are vulnerable to getting TB infection early in life [Centers for Disease Control and Prevention (CDC) and WHO]. Therefore, the practice of giving birth dose should be continued and highly beneficial for developing nations. It has its greatest effect in preventing miliary TB or TB meningitis. No booster dose is needed. Infants not vaccinated at birth may require tuberculin skin testing (TST) before giving BCG to children beyond 3 months of age.

Dose and Route of Administration

- An ID dose was given before the baby was discharged home with their mother.
- The usual reaction to successful BCG vaccination is induration at the injection site, followed by a local

lesion which starts as a papule two or more weeks after vaccination. It may ulcerate and then slowly subside over several weeks or months to heal, leaving a small, flat, or pitted scar.

- Neonatal BCG vaccination given intradermally at the left deltoid region leaves a pitted scar at the end of 12–14 weeks, considered proof of successful BCG immunization in the majority of infants.
- If BCG was given subcutaneously, it may induce local infection and abscess.

In successfully BCG-vaccinated children, there is a lack of evidence supporting the use of additional and/or booster doses. Infants not vaccinated at birth may require TST before giving BCG to children aged 3 months and above (WHO and CDC).

Adverse reactions are rare and uncommon (1–2% of immunizations) such as subcutaneous abscess, regional lymphadenopathy, and osteitis which generally are not serious. Disseminated fatal infection occurs rarely (approximately 2 per 1 million people), primarily in people who are severely immunocompromised, such as children with poorly controlled HIV infection or severe combined immunodeficiency. Antituberculosis therapy is recommended to treat osteitis and disseminated disease caused by BCG vaccine. Pyrazinamide is not believed to be effective against BCG and should not be included in treatment regimens.

Bacille Calmette–Guérin is not generally recommended for routine use in the USA, UK, and Australia because of the low risk of infection with *M. tuberculosis* because of the vaccine's potential interference with TST skin test reactivity. For individuals, BCG immunization should be considered only for those who have a negative TST result and who do not have contraindications in the following circumstances:

- It is offered to those who are at higher risk of acquiring TB, especially to those children visiting and/or living for three months or more in a country where there is a high rate of TB.
- The child is exposed continually to a person or people with contagious pulmonary TB resistant to isoniazid and rifampin and the child cannot be removed from this exposure.

Careful assessment of the potential risks and benefits of the BCG vaccine and consultation with personnel in local TB control programs are strongly recommended before the use of the BCG vaccine.

Bacille Calmette–Guérin vaccine has a documented protective effect against meningitis and disseminated TB in children. However, BCG immunization does not prevent primary infection and, more importantly, does not prevent reactivation of latent pulmonary infection, the principal source of bacillary spread in the community.

Adverse reactions are rare (1–2% of immunizations), e.g., local at the vaccination site reactions, such as subcutaneous abscess, regional epiphyseal, osteitis, or lymphadenopathy, which generally are not serious. Disseminated fatal infection occurs rarely (approximately 2 per 1 million vaccinated people), primarily in people who are severely immunocompromised, such as children with poorly controlled HIV infection or severe combined immunodeficiency. Antituberculosis therapy is recommended to treat osteitis and disseminated disease caused by BCG vaccine. Pyrazinamide is not believed to be effective against BCG and should not be included in treatment regimens.

The use of the BCG vaccine is contraindicated for people receiving immunosuppressive medications including high-dose corticosteroids. Although no untoward effects of the BCG vaccine on the fetus have been observed, immunization of women during pregnancy is not recommended.

Bacille Calmette–Guérin vaccine also offers protection against nontuberculous mycobacterial infections such as leprosy and Buruli ulcer. It is also used in the treatment of superficial carcinoma of the bladder. While its roles for TB prevention and bladder cancer immunotherapy are widely appreciated, over the past century, BCG has been also studied for nontraditional purposes, which include (1) prevention of viral infections and nontuberculous mycobacterial infections, (2) cancer immunotherapy aside from bladder cancer, and (3) immunologic diseases, including MS, type 1 diabetes, and atopic diseases.

Bacille Calmette–Guérin Vaccination for COVID-19

During the past year, BCG emerged as a candidate vaccine for the prevention of infection with SARS-CoV-2. Initial studies found that countries currently using BCG vaccination have lower SARS-CoV-2 incidence and death rates. A study performed in Israeli population cohorts before and after the discontinuation of BCG vaccination in the 1980s also failed to identify differences in COVID-19 incidence, arguing that BCG-induced protection is unlikely to be durable.

In contrast, in addition to these correlative studies, a retrospective observational study of a diverse cohort of 6,679 healthcare workers in Los Angeles, California, demonstrated that a history of BCG vaccination was associated with reduced COVID-19-related clinical symptoms ($p = 0.017$), as well as decreased seroprevalence of anti-SARS-CoV-2 immunoglobulin G (IgG) with an odds ratio (OR) of 0.76 [95% confidence interval (CI) 0.57–0.99; $p = 0.048$]. Importantly, no association was found with meningococcal, pneumococcal, or influenza vaccination. While preliminary, these findings strengthen the argument that BCG may exert preventive efficacy and reduction in morbidity/mortality against SARS-CoV-2.

As of this writing, there is no evidence that the BCB protects people against infection with the COVID-19 virus. Importantly, prospective randomized clinical trials are necessary to make definitive conclusions regarding the potential effect of BCG vaccination against COVID-19.

New Tuberculosis Vaccine for Adolescent/Adult Vaccination with M72/AS01

Currently, 16 candidates for TB vaccines are in various phases of clinical trials in adolescents and adults infected with *M. tuberculosis* demonstrating a prevention of disease efficacy of 49.7% (95% CI: 2.1–74.2) after 3 years of follow-up. However, M72/AS01E would need a supportive phase III trial for licensure, which is planned but likely to require years before results are available to inform policy.

COVID-19; SARS CoV-2 Vaccines

Upbringing

The authors explain COVID-19 vaccine aspects of public concerns in a recently posted query, Dated May 11, 2023.

An on-call query on the category of "infectious diseases and vaccines". *"How do we know COVID-19 vaccines are working well to protect people?. Is the COVID-19 vaccine safe to take? Which vaccine is the best one to get"?*

Author's response:
- Yes, COVID-19 vaccines are safe and effective. The US CDC continues to recommend that everyone ages 6 months and older stay up to date with all COVID-19 vaccines, including an updated vaccine when eligible.
- Vaccines continue to lower the risk for severe disease, hospitalization, and death, even against the widespread Delta, and Omicron variants.
- More than 672 million doses of COVID-19 vaccine have been given in the US from December 14, 2020, through March 1, 2023. Serious side effects that could cause long-term health problems are infrequent following any vaccination, including COVID-19 vaccination.
- A cohort study of >1.5 million hospital admissions in Canada through the first 2 years of the COVID-19 pandemic has quantified the benefit of vaccinations. Unvaccinated patients were found to be up to 15 times more likely to die from COVID-19 than fully vaccinated patients.
- The initial focus of SARS-CoV-2 vaccines was on preventing symptomatic, often severe illnesses. Most COVID-19 vaccines were two-dose vaccines, like the mRNA or adenovirus-vectored like the UK AstraZeneca's or the Indian Covishield vaccines.
- All current vaccines hinge on that important spike protein in the SARS-CoV-2 virus, which delivers instructions to the body's cells to produce the protein, but vaccines like the Novavax, USA (i.e., *Europe-made Nuvaxovid and Indian SII Covovax*) delivers the proteins directly.
- The immunity from the vaccines has been found to wane over time, requiring people to get booster doses of the vaccine to maintain protection against COVID-19. But each is slightly different!

Covidology—Vaccines Preventing Aspects

Coronavirus disease-2019 is officially the worst pandemic in modern medical history, surpassing the death toll from the 1918 Spanish Flu. The SARS-CoV-2 vaccines are a critical tool in the fight against the COVID-19 pandemic.

Messenger RNA technology has emerged as a revolutionary breakthrough in vaccine development. The COVID-19 pandemic highlighted its potential, leading to the rapid deployment of mRNA-based vaccines. This technology provides a platform for quicker and adaptable vaccine production, offering hope in the fight against emerging infectious diseases. Several kinds and spectrum COVID-19 vaccines have been developed and AEU or approved for widespread distribution in many countries.

These various technologies include mRNA, viral vectors, inactivated virus methods, protein subunits, LAVs, and toxoid vaccines.

Racing to develop and distribute a vaccine against COVID-19 has proven to be a challenging endeavor. Not only has there been the enormous scientific-technical challenge of developing the world's first vaccines against a CoV, but the subsequent ethical issues involved in vaccine allocation have been equally complex. Based on the landscape of the COVID-19 pandemic experiences, several important healthcare handling lessons have been evolved to manage any future disease pandemics.

Some of the notable pandemic-dominant COVID-19 vaccines that are currently available include the following:

- *USA—Pfizer-BioNTech (Comirnaty):* Developed by Pfizer and BioNTech, this is an mRNA-based vaccine.
- *USA—Moderna:* Another mRNA vaccine developed by Moderna.
  In the in vivo system, the mRNA vaccine (wrapped in a coating) mimics a viral infection by employing the host cell protein machinery to convert mRNA into a defined antigen and to elicit a robust humoral and cellular immune response. In fact, the mRNA in the vaccine teaches human body cells how to make copies of the spike protein. If we are exposed to the real virus later, our body will recognize it and know how to fight it off. Individuals who get an mRNA vaccine are not exposed to the virus, nor can they become infected with the virus by the vaccine.
- USA—Johnson & Johnson's COVID-19 vaccine expired as of May 6, 2023, and is no longer available in the US. Those who did get the Johnson & Johnson's shot are considered up-to-date when they get one updated (2023–2024 formula).
- *UK—Oxford AstraZeneca/Oxford*: A viral vector vaccine developed by AstraZeneca and the University of Oxford [ChAdOx1-S (recombinant) COVID-19 vaccine].
  This vaccine is safe and effective for all individuals aged 18 and above. In line with the WHO prioritization roadmap and the WHO values framework, older adults, health workers, and immunocompromised persons should be prioritized. The AstraZeneca vaccine can be offered to people who have had COVID-19 in the past. However, individuals may choose to delay vaccination for 3 months following the infection.

Serum Institute of India: Covishield (Oxford/AstraZeneca Formulation)

There is no data available when both these (India vs. Oxford) vaccines are used interchangeably. The WHO had greenlit the use of Covishield 2 years ago *for individuals aged 18 and older.*

Dr Amitav Banerjee—an epidemiologist who leads DY Patil Medical College in Pune—said that Covishield carried a "double whammy of risk". He noted that its use had been discouraged in most European countries due to blood clots. It also carries the risk of myocarditis.

A well-known British-Indian cardiologist has flagged the cardiovascular side effects of the Covishield vaccine. According to Dr Aseem Malhotra, the vaccine manufactured in India by the Serum Institute is "even worse" than mRNA COVID-19 vaccines when it comes to concerns such as heart attacks and strokes.

- *India—Bharat Biotech's Covaxin:* It is a whole inactivated virus-based COVID-19 India's first indigenous COVID-19 vaccine developed in collaboration with the Indian Council of Medical Research (ICMR).
  On April 2, 2022, WHO confirmed the suspension of supply of Covaxin (Bharat Biotech) through UN procurement agencies and recommended that countries using the vaccine take action as appropriate.
- *China—Sinopharm:* An inactivated virus vaccine developed in China.
- *China—Sinovac (CoronaVac):* Another inactivated virus vaccine developed in China.
  Both these Chinese vaccines are inactivated vaccines, which kill the SARS-CoV-2 virus. China's CoV vaccines account for almost half of the 7.3 billion doses delivered globally and have been enormously important in fighting the pandemic, particularly in less wealthy nations.
  The WHO Strategic Advisory Group of Experts on Immunization (SAGE) has thoroughly assessed the data on the quality, safety, and efficacy of the vaccine and has recommended its use for people aged 18 and above.
  Safety data is currently limited for persons above 60 years of age (due to the small number of participants in clinical trials). While no differences in the safety profile of the vaccine in older adults compared to younger age groups can be anticipated, countries considering using this vaccine in persons older than 60 years should maintain active safety monitoring.
- *Sputnik V:* Developed in Russia, this vaccine also uses a viral vector with two different adenovirus vectors (Ad26 priming and Ad5 boost).
  Efficacy of Sputnik V against COVID-19 was reported at 91.6%. The figure is based on the analysis of data on 19,866 volunteers, who received both the first and second doses of the Sputnik V vaccine or placebo at the final control point of 78 confirmed COVID-19 cases.

This vaccine was first announced as safe and effective by Russia. However, there are controversies surrounding this vaccine such as the possible decline of its immunogenicity and diminished neutralizing capacity against some COVID-19 variants.

- *Novavax vaccine:* A protein-based subunit vaccine. Sold under the brand names Nuvaxovid and Covovax, among others, is a subunit COVID-19 vaccine developed by Novavax and the Coalition for Epidemic Preparedness Innovations (CEPI).

Novavax is generally considered effective if the estimate is ≥50% with a >30% lower limit of the 95% CI. Efficacy is closely related to effectiveness, which is generally expected to slowly decrease over time.

The US Food and Drug Administration (FDA) says that what makes Novavax unique from other COVID-19 vaccines is that it is built with a much older technology for vaccine development where, instead of injecting the genetic recipe, actually inject the protein a combination of spike proteins that form what are called nanoparticles, which group together. The Novavax vaccine also has an adjuvant, an immune stimulant to get a better immune response. In some ways, this is an older technology. The protein is made outside of the human body and then injected into us, and that induces the immune response.

There are a number of widely used vaccines that inject the protein of the virus or the pathogen, like the HPV or the HBV. People will also be familiar with tetanus toxoid vaccines or diphtheria toxoid vaccines as part of a childhood vaccine series.

Mucosal Vaccines

Around the world, more than a dozen intranasally delivered COVID-19 vaccines have entered clinical trials, and they run the gamut from adenovirus-vectored genes for viral antigens to recombinant protein-based formulations to live-attenuated SARS-CoV-2.

Inhalation and Injection COVID-19 Vaccines, What is the Difference?

Different from the injection, the inhalation vaccine can not only stimulate humoral and cellular immune responses but also stimulate the production of IgA antibodies, achieving the purpose of efficiently inducing mucosal immunity and finally fulfilling triple immune protection.

A small handful of intranasal flu vaccines are commercially available, such as FluMist, which came on the US market in 2003. Other vaccines and immunizations targeting other viruses have been in development since before the COVID-19 pandemic, but none have moved to late-stage trials. Compared with IM injections, "we do not have that much experience in humans with intranasal vaccines".

Nasal vaccine inventors on patent applications related to a COVID-19 vaccine are now being tested with IM and intranasal delivery in the US and Mexico (Pfizer and other pharmaceutical companies). IM injections generate systemic immunity but little or no immune response in the nose, where respiratory viruses such as SARS-CoV-2 typically enter the body. Scientists anticipate this so-called mucosal immunity, is one of the best ways to completely inhibit infection and thereby abolish community spread **(Fig. 1)**.

Recently, "iNCOVACC(r)" is a recombinant replication-deficient adenovirus vectored vaccine with a prefusion-stabilized SARS-CoV-2 spike protein. This vaccine candidate was evaluated in phases I, II, and III clinical trials with successful results. iNCOVACC(r) has been specifically formulated to allow intranasal delivery through nasal drops. The nasal delivery system has been designed and developed to be cost-effective in low- and middle-income countries.

The vector intranasal delivery platform gives us the capability for rapid product development, scale-up, and easy and painless immunization during public health emergencies and pandemics.

COVAX

It aims to accelerate the development and manufacturing of COVID-19 vaccines and guarantee fair and equitable access for every country. It is a global effort to provide equitable access to vaccines, primarily focusing on distributing vaccines to lower-income countries.

It is important to note that the situation regarding COVID-19 and vaccines is continually evolving. New vaccines may have been developed, and recommendations for their use may have changed. Additionally, vaccine distribution, eligibility, and requirements may vary by country and region.

Vaccine Effectiveness

The COVID-19 vaccines have shown high efficacy in preventing symptomatic COVID-19 infection, severe illness, and hospitalization. However, breakthrough infections can still occur, especially with emerging variants

CHAPTER 4: Vaccine Components—Highpoints

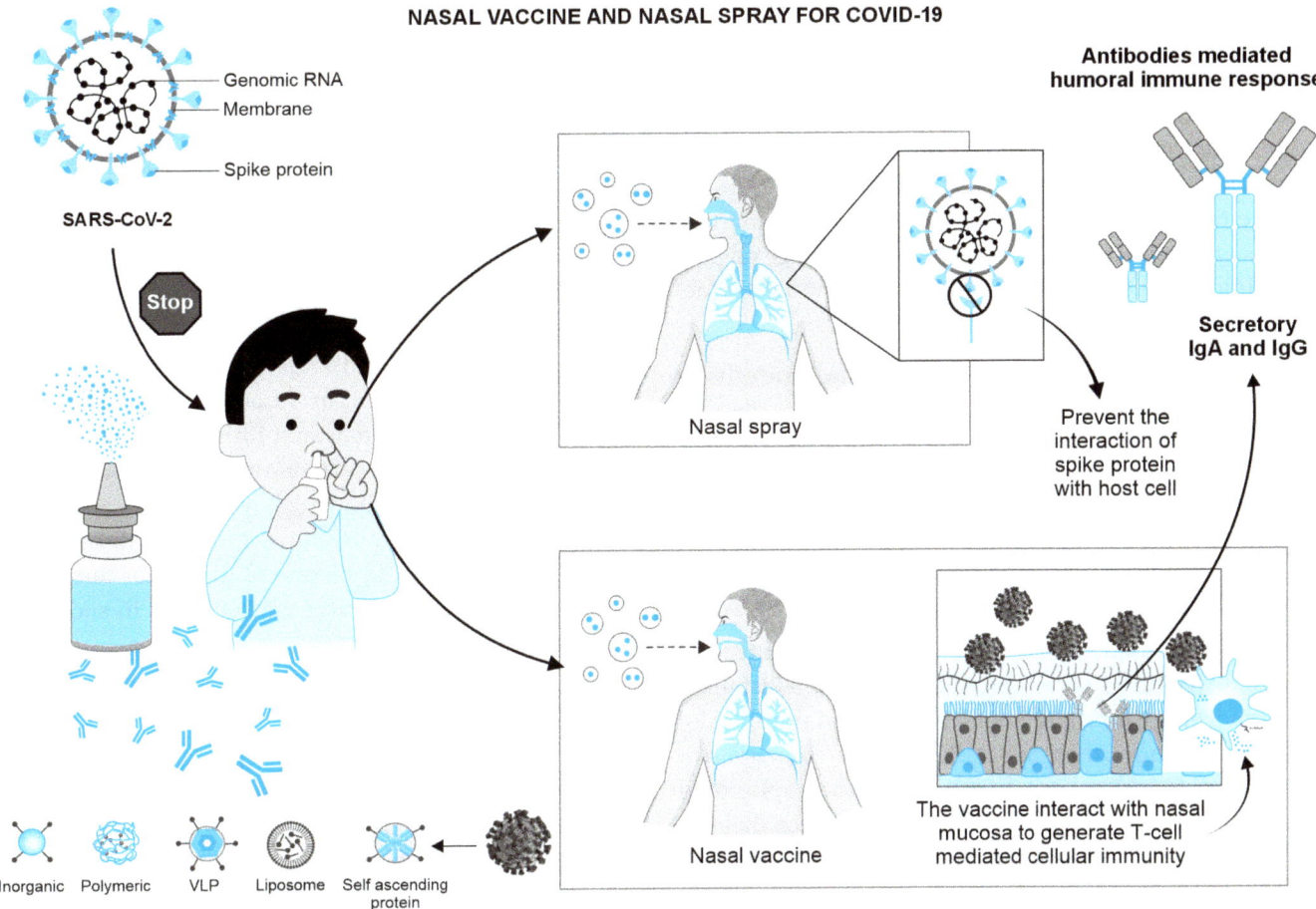

Fig. 1: Intranasal vaccine delivery platform offers several potential advantages, including the ability to induce mucosal immunity directly at the site of virus entry (the respiratory tract), ease of administration, and the possibility of reducing or eliminating the need for needles, which can improve vaccine acceptance and accessibility. There are some notable approaches and findings in the development of intranasal severe acute respiratory syndrome coronavirus-2 (SARS-CoV-2) vaccine delivery platforms: (1) Adenovirus-vector vaccine co-expressing antigens, (2) bacteriophage-based vaccine platforms, (3) virus-like particles (VLPs)-based vaccine platform, and (4) plant-derived extracellular vesicles (Evs) as a delivery platform.

of the virus. Vaccinated individuals may have milder symptoms if they do contract the virus.

Vaccine Doses

Most COVID-19 vaccines require two doses, administered a few weeks apart, to achieve optimal protection. Some vaccines, like the Johnson & Johnson vaccine, require only a single dose.

Vaccine Safety

The COVID-19 vaccines have undergone rigorous testing in clinical trials to ensure safety. Regulatory authorities closely monitor vaccine safety and investigate any reported adverse events.

- The benefits of vaccination in preventing COVID-19 outweigh the risks of potential side effects.
- The Pfizer and Moderna vaccines are strongly recommended as safe and effective at preventing serious illness or death from COVID-19.

On the safety profile, the CDC says there is a preference for the mRNA (Pfizer and Moderna) COVID-19 vaccines over the Novavax or Johnson & Johnson vaccines.

Side Effects

Common side effects of COVID-19 vaccines include pain at the injection site, fatigue, headache, muscle pain, chills, fever, and nausea. These side effects are generally mild and temporary, resolving within a few days.

Serious side effects that could cause long-term health problems are infrequent following any vaccination, including COVID-19 vaccination.

Clinicians need to stay updated with the latest guidelines and recommendations from local health authorities regarding COVID-19 vaccination. They should educate their patients about the benefits of vaccination, address any concerns or questions, and encourage eligible individuals to receive the COVID-19 vaccine to protect themselves and the community.

Note: Vaccine dosage relevant to ages and underlying disorders to FDA-approved COVID-19 vaccines.

In general, recommended vaccinations against COVID-19 were associated with reduced risk of various post-COVID thromboembolic and cardiovascular complications during acute (0–30 days) and post-acute (31–90 and 91–180 days) phases Long COVID, also known as post-acute COVID-19 sequelae or post-acute COVID-19 syndrome, is recognized as a major concern after infection with the SARS-CoV-2 virus, and will likely cause substantial global morbidity for many years. With global numbers of infections of more than 500 million and a conservative prevalence of 20–30%, more than 100 million people could be currently affected by long-term COVID-19 worldwide.

Current studies suggest that COVID-19 vaccines might have protective and therapeutic effects on long-term COVID. More robust comparative observational studies and trials are needed, however, to determine the effectiveness of vaccines in preventing and treating long COVID.

Chikungunya Vaccines

Chikungunya virus (CHIKV) causes an illness characterized by sudden high fever, severe joint pain, rash, and muscle pain. The name "chikungunya" derives from an African word meaning "to become bent and twisted", indicating the arthritic symptoms that make infected individuals appear sick in pain.

It is an RNA virus transmitted primarily by *Aedes* mosquitoes, particularly *Aedes aegypti* and *Aedes albopictus*. Although chikungunya is rarely fatal, its debilitating symptoms can persist for weeks or months, affecting a person's quality of life.

Even with the recent FDA-approved CHIKV vaccine, prevention through mosquito control measures and vaccines remains crucial in endemic regions. It has been identified in over 110 countries throughout the world.

The concerns that the main challenges of the CHIKV vaccine are the unlikely events of disease severity that was called "antibody-dependent enhancement (ADE)" effect. The AED phenomenon has been observed mainly with RNA viruses, including flaviviruses such as dengue, yellow fever, and Zika; alpha- and beta coronavirus including COVID–19; orthomyxoviruses such as influenza; retroviruses such as HIV; and orthopneumoviruses such as respiratory syncytial virus (RSV).

The ADE is a phenomenon in which the binding of a virus to suboptimal antibodies can occur from natural infection or a vaccine and or other treatment given. ADE is something researchers watch for very carefully and is extremely rare. In ADE, certain antibodies make it easier for viruses to get into cells, which would mean a virus or a vaccine makes people more at risk for severe disease. ADE in dengue is believed to be one of the major underlying mechanisms leading to increased severity in secondary DENV infection.

Cholera Vaccine

Globally, there is a shortage of cholera vaccine, with only 33 million of the 72 million requested doses delivered to countries. The International Coordinating Group, the WHO-backed organization that manages the global stockpile of oral cholera vaccines, recommended the use of a single dose, rather than the standard two-dose regimen in emergency vaccination, because of insufficient production capacity.

A single dose of EuBiologics oral cholera vaccine provided significant protection against cholera for at least 36 months.

Dengue Virus Vaccine

Dengue virus fever is among the most common mosquito-borne viral diseases worldwide. It is endemic in >100 countries and causes an estimated 390 million infections each year. While many dengue infections are asymptomatic or produce only mild illness, dengue can occasionally cause more severe disease and even death. DENV is also a leading cause of fever among travelers returning from Latin America, the Caribbean, and Southeast Asia. DENV poses a significant and growing public health burden to people living in and traveling to endemic countries.

A vaccine can help prevent dengue, which is caused by four distinct, but closely related DENVs; DENV-1,

DENV-2, DENV-3, and DENV-4. Only one dengue vaccine is currently available for use, a tetravalent, live-attenuated dengue vaccine CYD-TDV (Dengvaxia®), is safe and effective.

This vaccine must be administered as a three-shot series over a period of 6 months (at 0, 6, and 12 months) to children and adults between the ages of 9 and 45 years with a history of dengue infection or serological testing for past dengue infection. Vaccinated seropositive participants were protected against breakthrough DENV illnesses.

In 2016, the WHO recommended that countries in which dengue is highly endemic consider introducing Dengvaxia® for children over 9 years of age. A phase I trial with 60 healthy adults of 18–45 years has already been completed, showing the vaccine to be safe and well tolerated.

The vaccine is protective among those who were previously exposed but increases the risks of hospitalizations and severe illness among the unexposed. Since younger children are less likely to have been exposed to DENV, the vaccine could likely act like a primary infection in children not previously exposed to dengue, potentially contributing to a more severe illness when subsequent exposure to natural infection occurred.

One of the main challenges of introducing a dengue vaccine is "ADE", e.g., a person with low levels of antibodies against one serotype of dengue, may end up getting a more severe infection with another serotype of dengue.

QDENGA® (TAK-003) is a second dengue vaccine that is based on a live-attenuated dengue serotype 2 virus, which provides the genetic "backbone" for all four DENV serotypes and is designed to protect against any of these serotypes. This two-dose dengue vaccine, TAK-003, contains live-attenuated DENV-2 plus DENV-2 chimeras of the structural regions of DENV-1, DENV-3, and DENV-4.

QDENGA® is indicated for the prevention of dengue disease in individuals from 4 years of age and should be administered subcutaneously as a 0.5 mL dose at a two-dose (0 and 3 months) schedule under the approved dosing regimen.

Another TV005 tetravalent dengue vaccine was well-tolerated and immunogenic in young children to adults, including individuals with no previous dengue exposure. This vaccine was well-tolerated and immunogenic in a randomized, controlled trial for all TV005 four serotypes and age groups, in dengue-endemic Bangladesh.

Three Dengue Vaccines—What Now?

A single dose of Butantan-DENV prevented symptomatic DENV-1 and DENV-2, in children and adults regardless of dengue serostatus at baseline, through 2 years of follow-up. Given the realities of the dimensions of the dengue pandemic in the 20th and 21st centuries, a highly effective, one-dose, tetravalent vaccine remains in high demand. Butantan-DV clinical trials should continue and, if possible, be expanded.

Diphtheria-Tetanus-Pertussis Vaccine

There are three vaccine types in the market either whole cell pertussis component (DTwP) or acellular type (DTaP). Both are pediatric formulations of diphtheria and tetanus toxoids and acellular pertussis vaccines. The third vaccine type is the Tdap component contains tetanus toxoid, reduced adult dose diphtheria toxin, and acellular pertussis components (adolescent and adult formulations).

Purified acellular-component pertussis vaccine contains three or more immunogens derived from *Bordetella pertussis* organisms: Inactivated pertussis toxin (toxoid), filamentous hemagglutinin, fimbrial proteins (agglutinogens), and pertactin (an outer membrane protein). Acellular pertussis vaccines are adsorbed onto aluminum salts and must be administered intramuscularly. All pertussis vaccines in the United States are combined with diphtheria and tetanus toxoids; none contain thimerosal as a preservative.

A single dose of Tdap is recommended universally for people 11 years and older, including adults of any age, in place of a decennial tetanus and diphtheria vaccine (Td). The preferred schedule is to administer Tdap at the 11- or 12-year-old preventive visit, with a catch-up of older adolescents. Booster doses of Tdap are not recommended for any group of people except pregnant women.

Routine Vaccination

Administer a five-dose series of DTaP vaccine at ages 2, 4, 6, 15 through 18 months, and 4 through 6 years. The fourth dose may be administered as early as age 12 months, provided at least 6 months have elapsed since the third dose.

In contrast, the Indian Academy of Pediatrics (IAP) recommends DTwP vaccines for the primary three doses with a choice of booster doses are either the DTwP or DTaP components. It has become clear that the immunity evoked by the DTaP vaccine, which has been in wide use

since the late 1990s, is less durable than the immunity evoked by the DTwP.
- From age 11 years onward every 10 years, the Tdap is recommended.
- Administer 1 dose of Tdap vaccine to women during each pregnancy (preferred during 27 through 36 weeks of gestation) regardless of time since prior Td or Tdap vaccination.

Pertussis

A series of five pertussis shots to be given before age 7, combined with DTaP, with a booster dose (Tdap) recommended around the age of 11. The overall efficacy of the vaccine is "quite high". For 90% of people who get the recommended childhood immunization, immunity lasts longer than 10 years, and for over half, it lasts an entire lifetime.
- A recent study has shown vaccinating a parent of newborn infants against pertussis provides moderate protection against the infectious disease in young infants.
- This targeted vaccination strategy, called *cocooning*, has been recommended for more than a decade, but its uptake has been limited, absent evidence of its field effectiveness. "Cocooning" reduces whooping cough risk in Infants.
- In adolescents and adults, pertussis can be severe but is rarely life-threatening, as it can be in infants. Since children and adults can expose infants to pertussis, it is important to administer the Tdap vaccine in all persons who could be in contact with an infant; administration of the Tdap vaccine during every pregnancy, to provide transplacental antibodies, has also been recommended.

Significant advances and breakthroughs in pertussis vaccine to come soon.

Hepatotropic Viruses (HAV, HBV, HCV, HDV, HEV, etc.)

A, B, C, D, E: It is a short, menacing alphabet representing the five types of viruses causing viral hepatitis, a sickness afflicting some 400 million people around the world today. Hepatitis viruses are a set of very different pathogens that kill 1.4 million people annually and infect more than HIV and the malaria pathogen combined. Most of the deaths are from cirrhosis of the liver or hepatic cancer due to chronic infections with hepatitis viruses B or C, picked up through contact with contaminated blood.

In India, as per latest estimates, 40 million people are chronically infected with hepatitis B and 6–12 million people are chronically infected with hepatitis C. HEV is the most important cause of epidemic hepatitis, though HAV is more common among children. These sections will be devoted to the hepatitis and vaccine perspectives individually.

Hepatitis A virus (HAV) and hepatitis E virus (HEV) are enterically transmitted pathogens that produce sporadic infections as well as outbreaks of acute viral hepatitis mostly transmitted through the fecal-oral pathway. In India, HAV infection is common among children, and it generally leads to mild anicteric hepatitis. The majority of children under the age of two (85%) and nearly half of those aged 2–5 (50%) have nonspecific symptoms and are usually anicteric. HAV infection disease severity increases with the patient's age.

Chronic HEV infection is rare and, to date, has only been reported in more developed countries, mostly among organ transplant recipients with immunosuppression. Approximately 60% of recipients of solid organ transplants fail to clear the virus and develop chronic hepatitis, and 10% will develop cirrhosis.

Hepatitis B virus (HBV) and hepatitis C virus (HCV) infections are more alike, which include distribution, hepatotropic, disease transmission, and at last leading to chronic infection which may end in liver cirrhosis and hepatocellular carcinoma (HCC).

Hepatitis B virus and HCV infections do not have a standard of care due to the individual category of infected subjects so it is difficult to cure. Thus, studying the magnitude becomes a crucial component in the prevention of HBV and HCV. The current review aims to summarize and update current and evolving vaccine prevention aspects.

Over the last 50 years, researchers have identified five types of viruses that cause different forms of viral hepatitis. Each virus has its own mode of transmission and health impacts. Scientists around the world have worked to develop treatments and vaccines **(Table 1)**.

Hepatitis A Virus Vaccine (Minimum Age: 12 Months)

Several commercial injectable inactivated HAV vaccines are available internationally. All provide similar protection from the virus and have comparable side effects. No vaccine is licensed for children younger than 1 year of age. In China, a LAV is also available. In the US, Canada, and European countries, the HAV vaccines are inactivated.

CHAPTER 4: Vaccine Components—Highpoints

TABLE 1: Transmission and prevention aspects.

Hepatotropic viruses	HAV	HBV	HCV	HDV	HEV
Virus discovery year	1973	1967	1989	1977	1978
Transmission	Contaminated food and water. Contact with an infected person	Blood-contaminated syringe, sexual contact, and during birth	Blood-contaminated syringe and sexual contact	Like HBV, only occurs in those with HBV infected	Contaminated food and water. Contact with an infected person
Chronic infections?	No	Yes	Yes	Yes	No
Treatment	Supportive, no formal antivirals	Supportive, no formal antivirals	Highly effective antiviral drugs, curable	Supportive, no formal antivirals	
Preventive vaccine	Preventable	Preventable	No approved vaccines	Preventable by HBV vaccines	No approved vaccines. China uses vaccine

(HAV: hepatitis A virus; HBV: hepatitis B virus; HCV: hepatitis C virus; HDV: hepatitis D virus; HEV: hepatitis E virus)

The inactivated HAV vaccines in use are: (1) Monovalent: GSK HM175 strain, HAVRIX® (GSK US), (2) Monovalent: Merck CR326F strain, VAQTA (US), and (3) Avaxim (Sanofi Pasteur, Canada and France). These are available in children and adult formulations. Also (4) Combination: GSK HM175 strain and recombinant hepatitis B surface antigen (HBsAg), TWINRIX.

The IAP, Advisory Committee on Vaccines and Immunization Practices (ACVIP), recommends a single dose live-attenuated HAV vaccine (*Chinese viral H2 strain*) at 12 months of age based on limited published data. Near elimination of the disease was achieved in China for 14 years following the introduction of the H2 live vaccine (SC use) into the Expanded Program on Immunization (EPI). The CDC and Advisory Committee on Immunization Practices (ACIP) did not approve this oral vaccine for childhood immunization practices.

Routine vaccination: Initiate the two-dose HAV series at 12 months through 23 months; separate the two doses by 6–18 months.

- Children who have received one dose of HAV vaccine before the age of 24 months should receive a second dose 6–18 months after the first dose.
- For any person aged 2 years and older who has not already received the hepatitis A vaccine series, two doses of vaccine separated by 6–18 months may be administered if immunity against HAV infection is desired.

VAQTA is available in the following adult formulations:
- 50 U/1-mL single-dose vials
- 50 U/1-mL prefilled Luer-Lok® syringes

Dosage and administration: Adults (19 years of age and older): The vaccination schedule consists of a primary 1 mL dose administered intramuscularly and a 1 mL booster dose administered intramuscularly 6–18 months later.

Booster immunization following another manufacturer's hepatitis A vaccine: A booster dose of VAQTA may be given at 6–12 months following a primary dose of Havrix®.

Of note, HAV remains endemic in many areas of the world resulting in ongoing risks for travelers to intermediate and high endemic countries, as well as the risk for consumption of imported HAV-contaminated food from global sources.

Herd immunity does not protect against foodborne exposure.

Hepatitis B Virus Vaccine

- Hepatitis B vaccine (HepB vaccine) is highly effective in preventing HepB infection. It provides long-lasting immunity, and in most cases, a complete vaccine series confers lifelong protection.
- *Protective cut-off antibody titer:* Anti-HBs >10 mIU/mL is considered to be immune to HBV infection, either from vaccination or successful recovery from a previous HBV infection. Anti-HBs <5 mIU/mL is negative for HBV infection, but susceptible and hence requires vaccination.

There are several HepB vaccines available, but the most common one is a recombinant vaccine. These vaccines contain a small, harmless part of the HepB virus, which triggers an immune response without causing the disease itself.

First dose: Given at any time including soon after birth.
Second dose: Usually given 1–2 months after the first dose.
Third dose: Typically given 6 months after the first dose. A vaccine series can be started at any age.

- *Vaccination schedule:* The HepB vaccine is typically administered as a series of shots. The standard schedule involves three doses. There is also an accelerated schedule for adults that can be administered over a shorter period.

Hepatitis B vaccination is recommended for:
- All infants, typically given at birth
- All children and adolescents who were not vaccinated as infants
- Healthcare workers
- People with certain medical conditions
- People at increased risk due to lifestyle factors, such as those who engage in unprotected sex or use intravenous drugs
- Travelers to areas with high hepatitis B prevalence
- Close contacts of individuals with HBV and or surface antigen carriers **(Table 2)**
- Vaccination is a critical tool in preventing the spread of hepatitis B and protecting individuals from the potentially severe consequences of the infection.

Safety: These are generally safe. Common side effects include pain or redness at the injection site, mild fever, and fatigue. Severe allergic reactions are extremely rare. Existing HepB vaccines are yeast-derived recombinant DNA technology in single antigen (HBs antigen) pediatric formulations (monovalent) with an aluminum adjuvant, containing no thimerosal as a preservative. (Yeast-derived recombinant HepB vaccine produced by SmithKline Biologicals.)

Combination (Combos) vaccines: Some vaccines combine HepB with HepA or other immunizations.

Universal immunization of infants beginning at birth to prevent HBV infection and its complications. The monovalent HBV vaccine is given to all newborns before hospital discharge. The second dose should be administered at age 1 or 2 months (minimum interval of 4 weeks). Infants who did not receive a birth dose should receive three doses of an HBV vaccine on a schedule of 0, 1–2 months, and 6 months starting as soon as feasible. Administration of a total of four doses of HepB vaccine is permitted when a combination vaccine containing HBV is administered after the birth dose.

Infants born to HBsAg-positive mothers, administer HepB vaccine and 0.5 mL of hepatitis B immunoglobulin (HBIG) within 12 hours of birth. These infants should be tested for HBsAg and antibodies to HBsAg (anti-HBs) 1–2 months after completion of the HepB series at 9 through 12 months (new recommendations).

Postvaccination serologic testing for immunity is not recommended after routine vaccination of infants, children, adolescents, and adults. Postvaccination serologic testing is recommended for infants born to HBsAg-positive mothers, healthcare provider (HCP), chronic hemodialysis patients, HIV-infected and other immunocompromised persons, and sex partners of HBsAg-positive persons. Testing is recommended 1–2 months after the final dose of the vaccine series or at age 9–12 months for infants of HBsAg-positive mothers. Revaccination is recommended if anti-HBs are <10 mIU/mL.

For hemodialysis patients, the need for booster doses should be assessed by annual anti-HB testing. A booster dose should be administered when anti-HB levels decline to <10 mIU/mL.

- On February 21, 2018, the ACIP recommended HepB-CpG (HEPLISAV-B) for use in persons aged ≥18 years. The vaccine is administered in two doses, 1 month apart, and is the first new HepB vaccine in the US in >25 years and the only two-dose vaccine for adults age 18 years and older.
- HepB-CpG contains yeast-derived recombinant HBsAg and is prepared by combining purified HBsAg with small synthetic immunostimulatory cytidine-phosphate-guanosine oligodeoxynucleotide (CpG-ODN) motifs (1018 adjuvant). The 1018 adjuvant binds to toll-like receptor 9 to stimulate a directed immune response to HBsAg.
- The Heplisav-B vaccine's shorter schedule—two doses over 1 month compared with three doses over 6 months for rival products such as Engerix-B—would improve patient adherence.

Vaccine Nonresponders

HepB vaccine "nonresponder" refers to a person who does not develop protective surface antibodies after completing two full series of the HepB vaccine and for whom an acute or chronic HBV infection has been ruled out.

TABLE 2: Recommended dosages of hepatitis B vaccines.

Patients	Single-dose vaccines[a]			Combination vaccines		
	Recombivax HB[b] dose, µg (mL)	Engerix-B[c] dose, µg (mL)	Heplisav-B[d] dose, µg (mL)	Pediarix[e] dose, µg/mL	Twinrix dose, µg (mL)[f]	Vaxelis[g] dose, µg (mL)
Infants, children, and adolescents younger than 20 years (except as noted)	5 (0.5)	10 (0.5)	Not applicable	10 µg HBsAg (0.5) (ages 6 weeks through 6 years only)	Not applicable	10 µg HBsAg (0.5) (ages 6 weeks through 4 years only)
Adolescents 11–15 years of age[b]	10 (1)	Not approved for two-dose schedule	Not applicable	Not applicable	Not applicable	Not applicable
Adults 18 years or older			20 (0.5)		20 (1)	
Adults 20 years or older	10 (1)	20 (1)		Not applicable	20 (1)	
Adults undergoing dialysis	40 (1)[h,i]	40 (2)[i,j]	Not applicable	Not applicable	Not applicable	Not applicable

[a]Recombivax and Engerix-B vaccines are administered in a three-dose schedule at 0, 1, and 6 months; four doses may be administered if a combination vaccine is used (at 2, 4, and 6 months) to complete the series. Only single-Ag HepB vaccine can be used for the birth dose. Single-Ag or combo vaccine containing HepB vaccine may be used to complete the series. See text for management of infants born to HBsAg positive or HBsAg unknown mothers.
[b]Merck & Co., Inc. A two-dose schedule, administered at 0 months and then 4–6 months later, is licensed for adolescents 11 through 15 years of age using the adult formulation of Recombivax HB (10 µg).
[c]GSK Biologicals. The US FDA also has licensed this vaccine for use in an optional four-dose (0.5 mL/dose for ages birth through 10 years and 1.0 mL/dose for ages 11–19) schedule at 0, 1, 2, and 12 months for all age groups. A 0-, 12-, and 24-month schedule is licensed for children 5 through 10 years of age at a 0.5 mL dose and for children 11 through 16 years of age at a 1.0 mL dose for whom an extended administration schedule is appropriate on the basis of risk of exposure.
[d]Dynavax Technologies Corporation. A two-dose schedule administered at 0 and 1 month for use in people ≥18 years of age; safety and effectiveness of Heplisav-B have not been established in adults on hemodialysis.
[e]Combo of diphtheria and tetanus toxoids and acellular pertussis (DTaP), inactivated poliovirus (IPV), and HepB (Engerix-B 10 µg) is approved for use at 2, 4, and 6 months of age [Pediarix (GlaxoSmithKline)]. This vaccine should not be administered at birth, before 6 weeks of age, or at 7 years of age or older. For additional information, see pertussis.
[f]A combo of hepatitis B (Engerix-B, 20 µg) and hepatitis A [HAVRIX®, 720 enzyme-linked immunosorbent assay units (ELU)] vaccine; Twinrix is licensed for use in people 18 years of age and older in a three-dose schedule at 0, 1, and 6 months. Alternately, a four-dose schedule at days 0, 7, and 21 to 30, followed by a booster dose at 12 months, may be used.
[g]Combo of diphtheria and tetanus toxoids and acellular pertussis (DTaP), inactivated poliovirus (IPV), Haemophilus influenzae type b conjugate, and HepB recombinant vaccine approved for use at 2, 4, and 6 months of age to be used from 6 weeks of age through age 4. Not to be used for the birth dose or for children 5 years and older.
[h]Special formulation for adult dialysis patients administered at 0, 1, and 6 months.
[i]When administered to these populations, follow-up serologic testing is recommended 1–2 months after completion of the two-dose series.
[j]Two 1 mL doses administered in one or two injections in a four-dose schedule at 0, 1, 2, and 6 months of age.
(HBsAg: hepatitis B surface antigen)
Source: Adopted from CDC and Redbook, 2023.

Although the majority of persons vaccinated against HepB successfully respond to vaccination, an estimated 5-15% of persons may not respond due to older age, obesity, smoking, and other chronic illnesses. It is also possible that a person who does not respond to the vaccine may already be infected with HBV. Therefore, testing for the presence of the HBV infection, e.g., sAg and eAg is recommended before diagnosing a person as a "vaccine nonresponder".

The CDC recommendations for hepatitis B vaccine nonresponders:
- Persons who do not respond to the primary vaccine series (i.e., anti-HBs <10 mIU/mL) should complete a second vaccine series or be evaluated to determine if they are HBsAg-positive. For the second series, a different brand of vaccine should be administered. For adults in the US, the second series can be given using a three-dose vaccine or the two-dose vaccine.

- Persons who do not respond to an initial vaccine series have a 30–50% chance of responding to a second series. Newer vaccines might provide greater seroprotection, which can mean a greater antibody response, especially in adults who may be older, obese, or live with type 2 diabetes. If you have not responded to a primary vaccine series, talk to your doctor about whether the Heplisav-B (two-dose) or PreHevbrio (three-dose) vaccine is a better option for you.
- Revaccinated persons should be retested to check antibody response at the completion of the second vaccine series, 1–2 months following the last dose of the series.
- Persons exposed to HBsAg-positive blood or body fluids who are known not to have responded to a primary vaccine series should receive a single dose of HBIG and restart the hepatitis B vaccine series with the first dose of the HepB vaccine as soon as possible after exposure. Alternatively, they should receive two doses of HBIG, one dose as soon as possible after exposure, and the second dose 1 month later.
- The option of administering one dose of HBIG and restarting the vaccine series is preferred for nonresponders who did not complete a second three-dose vaccine series. For persons who previously completed a second vaccine series but failed to respond, two doses of HBIG are preferred.

HepB vaccine "nonresponders" who test negative for HBV infection are at risk for being infected and should be counseled regarding how to prevent HBV and to seek immediate medical care to receive a dose of HBIG if they have been exposed to potentially infected blood.

Hepatitis B vaccine "nonresponders" to vaccination who test positive for HBV should be counseled regarding how to prevent transmitting the HBV to others and the need for regular medical care and monitoring for their chronic infection.

Hepatitis C Virus Vaccine

According to the WHO, 58 million people are chronically infected with HCV globally. The majority of those infected with HCV advance to chronic infection, but 15–45% spontaneously clear viremia without treatment. There is currently no preventative or therapeutic vaccine, and treatment generally focuses on patients who are already in the chronic phase of HCV infection.

Pediatric HCV: Due to the widespread use of the HepB vaccine, HCV infection has become the most important cause of chronic hepatitis in children. There is no vaccine against HCV. Therefore, prevention efforts focus on minimizing the risk from vertical transmission and from unsafe injection of drugs.

The HCV genomic RNA was single-stranded with positive polarity, which was packaged by core protein and enveloped by a lipid bilayer containing two viral glycoproteins (E1 and E2) to form the virion. Getting tested for HCV serology is important because treatments can cure most people with HCV in 8–12 weeks.

Toward a vaccine against HCV: Recent advances aid the development of vaccines protecting against chronic liver diseases with HCV is urgently needed to address the ongoing public health crisis caused by this insidious pathogen a major cause of liver cirrhosis and cancer. Efforts toward the development of vaccines were initiated after the discovery of HCV in 1989, but to date, no vaccine has been licensed. An increased understanding of HCV protective immunity and HCV envelope glycoprotein structure and function is paving the way toward rational vaccine design and evaluation.

The HCV infections are a major global health burden. After the identification of the virus in 1989, insights into viral replication and drug development have long been hampered by the lack of efficient cell culture models. Their establishment was an important prerequisite for the development of selective antivirals.

The development of a system to propagate HCV in cell culture took more than a decade. All human hepatitis viruses are very difficult to grow in cell culture.

Hepatitis D Virus Vaccines

Yes, being vaccinated against HBV is the best way to protect against hepatitis D virus (HDV) infection. HDV, also known as hepatitis delta virus, is a defective, hepatotropic pathogenic agent among HBsAg-positive persons, approximately 5% are infected with HDV, which corresponds to approximately 12 million persons (95% CI, 8.7–18.7 million) worldwide. In three recent meta-analyses, the number of HDV-infected persons worldwide ranged from 12 to 72 million, underscoring the heterogeneity of current epidemiologic data.

In Trivandrum, KIMS Health's annual prevalence of 0.42% (2021) to 2.5% (2022) from people with

HBsAg-positive samples suggests a higher-than-expected prevalence in other parts of India. HDV requires HBsAg for virion assembly and in vivo survival. In India, the prevalence varies temporally and spatially; a recent study documents the presence of HDV with 2.1% prevalence in HepB patients treated at the tertiary care unit at Jabalpur Central India.

Individuals with chronic HBV infection are at risk of HDV superinfection. Because of the dependence of HDV on HBV, the diagnosis of hepatitis D cannot be made in the absence of markers of HBV infection. Coinfection with HDV accelerates the progression of liver disease associated with chronic hepatitis B. Bulevirtide inhibits the entry of HDV into hepatocytes.

The HDV testing should be considered for all HBsAg-positive patients with unusually severe or protracted hepatitis, especially for those emigrants from a region with endemic infection (such as Eastern European countries, Mediterranean countries, and countries in Central America), injection drug use, men who have sex with men, coinfection with HCV or HIV, or high-risk sexual practices.

Hepatitis E Virus Vaccines

Hepatitis E virus disease is more common among young adults than among children and is more severe in pregnant women, in whom mortality rates can reach 10–25% if infection occurs during the third trimester. Chronic HEV infection is rare and, to date, has only been reported in more developed countries, mostly among organ transplant recipients with immunosuppression.

Yes, there are vaccines available for HEV infections, but their availability and approval for use may vary by country. Two vaccines have been developed and are in use in some regions.

1. *Havax (Havax®):* This is an inactivated recombinant vaccine that was developed and is used in India. Administered in two doses. Hecolin was found to be safe and efficacious in a phase III trial, but WHO SAGE did not recommend it. Not US FDA-approved.
2. *Hecolin (Hecolin®):* Similar to Havax, is another inactivated recombinant vaccine that was developed and primarily used in China—administered in two or three doses. However, it is not yet prequalified by the WHO.

Available evidence suggests that 20 million people are infected annually resulting in over 70,000 deaths. Pregnant women are at the highest risk for morbidity and mortality with HEV infection. Considering the limited availability of diagnostics, insufficient surveillance, and investigation of hepatitis outbreaks, these are likely significant underestimates.

The Hecolin vaccine has been recommended by the WHO for outbreak response, since 2015. However, it is important to note that this vaccine may not be available in all countries. In the United States, there is no FDA-approved vaccine for HEV available. It is always recommended to refer to local guidelines and recommendations regarding the availability and use of HEV vaccines in specific regions. Additionally, individuals at higher risk of HEV, such as travelers to endemic regions or certain occupational groups, may benefit from vaccination.

Haemophilus Influenzae Type b Vaccines

Haemophilus influenzae type b (Hib) immunization is routinely recommended only for children under 5 years of age.

PRP-capsular antigen conjugated with CRM-197 or tetanus toxoid is used as carrier proteins. These carrier proteins are highly immunogenic after the completion of three primary doses in infants with a booster at 12–18 months. With the introduction of combination vaccine with multiple antigens (tetra, penta, and hexavalent components), there have been mix-ups among clinicians and the vaccine manufacturers have further aggravated this confusion.

- Hexavalent vaccine is composed of rHepB + DTap + Hib + IPV;
- Pentavalent is composed of rHepB + DTwP + Hib; and the
- Tetravalent vaccine is composed of DTwP or DTaP + Hib.

Administer a two- or three-dose Hib vaccine primary series and a booster dose (dose 3 or 4 depending on the vaccine used in the primary series) at age 12 through 15 months to complete a full Hib vaccine series.

Not routinely recommended for Adults. However, one dose of Hib vaccine should be administered to unimmunized persons aged 5 years or older who have anatomic or functional asplenia (including sickle cell disease) and unvaccinated persons 5 through 18 years of age with HIV infection.

- Children aged 12 through 59 months who are at increased risk for Hib disease, including chemotherapy recipients and those with anatomic or functional asplenia (including sickle cell disease), HIV infection, immunoglobulin deficiency, or early component complement deficiency, who have received either no doses or only one dose of Hib vaccine before 12 months of age, should receive two additional doses of Hib vaccine 8 weeks apart; children who received two or more doses of Hib vaccine before 12 months of age should receive one additional dose.

- For patients younger than 5 years of age undergoing chemotherapy or radiation treatment who received a Hib vaccine dose(s) within 14 days of starting therapy or during therapy, repeat the dose(s) at least 3 months following therapy completion.
- Recipients of hematopoietic stem cell transplant (HSCT) should be revaccinated with a three-dose regimen of Hib vaccine starting 6–12 months after successful transplant, regardless of vaccination history; doses should be administered at least 4 weeks apart.
- A single dose of any Hib-containing vaccine should be administered to unimmunized children and adolescents 15 months of age and older undergoing an elective splenectomy; if possible, the vaccine should be administered at least 14 days before the procedure.

Human Papillomavirus Vaccines

In the Indian context, the National Cancer Registry Programme (NCRP) of the ICMR notes the projected count of cervical cancer cases in 2023 to be above 3.4 lakhs. This alarming statistic highlights the urgent need for effective preventive measures to combat the prevalence of cervical cancer in India.

Human papillomavirus is a common sexually transmitted infection. More than 90% of sexually active men and 80% of sexually active women will be infected with HPV in their lifetime. About 50% of HPV infections involve certain high-risk types of HPV, which can cause cancer.

According to the National Center for Biotechnology Information (NCBI), about 6.6% of women in India have cervical HPV infection at any given time. HPV serotypes 16 and 18 are responsible for nearly 76.7% of cervical cancer in India. In 2025, 7.5% of all cancers in India were projected to be HPV-related. Cervical cancer (87.6%) and oropharyngeal cancer (63.2%) were the most common HPV-related cancers in India for females and males, respectively.

In most cases, the immune system can fight off an HPV infection and prevent it from developing symptoms or health conditions. Cervical lesions from noncancerous HPV infection are rare, nonharmful, and are mostly caused by HPV types 6 and 11. Meanwhile, the majority of HPV-related cancers are caused by types 16 and 18.

As of this date (February 118, 2024), there are three licensed products available for the prevention of HPV infections. These are 2vHPV (Cervarix) GSK, 4vHPV (Gardasil 4) Merck, and recently (2015) WHO approved 9vHPV (Gardasil 9) Merck **(Table 3)**.

- Gardasil 9 is the only HPV vaccine currently available in the United States and is now approved for use in males and females between the ages of 9 and 45.

TABLE 3: Background summary of licensed HPV vaccines.

Recombinant vaccines	Bivalent-HPV 2 (Cervarix) GSK	Quadrivalent HPV-4 (Gardasil 4) Merck	Gardasil-9 (HPV-9). Merck's 69 valent
Valent types	16 and 18	6, 11, 16, and 18	Covers the same HPV-4 valent as well as five additional valent types 31, 33, 45, 52, and 58
Adjuvant	ASO4	AAHS	
Licensed	Females aged 9–25 years	Females and males aged 9–26 years	To include women and men aged 27 through 45 years
Schedules	*Three doses:* 0, 1, and 6 months or two doses at 6 months to 1-year interval	*Three doses:* 0, 2, and 6 months or two doses at 6 months to 1-year interval	Three doses or two doses at 6 months to 1 year interval. For women 15 years and older, the three-dose schedule is still recommended
Immunogenicity-based neutralizing antibody	Minimal protective antibody threshold u/k	May lose detectable antibody but no loss of protection	88% effective in preventing HPV-type precancerous genital warts, vulvar and vaginal lesions, cervical precancerous and cancer lesions

Note: Revised ACIP Recommendations for HPV Vaccine
Source: Harper DM, DeMars LR. HPV vaccines: A review of the first decade. Gynecol Oncol. 2017;146(1):196-204.

Recombinant DNA technology is used to prepare HPV vaccines from the major capsid (L1) protein of HPV. The L1 proteins self-assemble into noninfectious, non-oncogenic virus-like particles (VLPs).

The number of recommended doses is based on age at administration of the first dose. Two doses are recommended for people starting the series before their 15th birthday, while three doses are recommended for those who start the series on or after their 15th birthday and for people with certain immunocompromising conditions.

Routine immunization is recommended beginning at 9 years of age. This way immunization provides optimal protection against HPV serotype 16, the most prevalent type associated with cervical cancers, as well as several other less prevalent types.

The WHO endorsed IAP-ACVIP recommendation is a two-dose regimen at 6-month to 1-year intervals for 9–14-year-old girls. However current three-dose regimen for adolescent girls aged 15 years and older will continue. For the immunocompromised individuals, including the HIV-infected, the three-dose schedule is recommended, irrespective of age.

- *Gardasil 9v* vaccine, recombinant, covers five more HPV types than its predecessor Gardasil 4v, both manufactured by the MSD. It adds protection against five additional HPV types—31, 33, 45, 52, and 58 which cause about 20% of cervical cancers and are not covered by previously marketed HPV vaccines.
- Gardasil 9v approved for females ages 9 through 26 and males ages 9 through 15 can prevent cervical, vulvar, vaginal, and anal cancers caused by HPV types 16, 18, 31, 33, 45, 52, and 58, and genital warts caused by HPV types 6 or 11.
- Cervarix (2vHPV) remains equivalent to Gardasil 9 in the prevention of HPV infections and precancers of any HPV type in countries where there has been high coverage.
- 2v Cervarix also has 91% efficacy in women older than 25 years and demonstrated sustained high antibody titers for at least 10 years.
- 2vHPV (Cervarix) has been removed from the schedule because it is no longer available and all available doses expired on January 1, 2018.
- Follow-up studies 8–10 years after HPV4 and HPV2 vaccination have shown no waning of protection. Long-term follow-up studies are being conducted to determine the duration of efficacy for all HPV vaccines.
- HPV vaccines reduce abnormal screening tests, colposcopies, and excisions. However, women who have received an HPV vaccine must continue to have regular Pap tests performed.

Shortly, hopefully, one dose of Cervarix will protect against HPV 16/18 infection with robust antibody titers well above natural infection titers. This may offer the easiest and most cost-effective vaccination program over time, especially in low and lower-middle-income countries. Cervical cancer screening must continue to control cancer incidence over the upcoming decades.

The United States Preventive Services Task Force (USPSTF) recommends cervical cancer screening in women aged 21–65 years with cytology (Pap smear) every 3 years or screening with a combination of cytology and HPV testing every 5 years in women aged 30–65 years.

The two doses of HPV vaccine have efficacy equivalent to the three-dose schedule for 9- to 14-year-olds. The revised two-dose schedule is as immunogenic and effective as the three-dose schedule with no evidence of waning immunity seen 10 years after immunization. A two-dose immunization is a win-win situation, providing an equal immune response from one less trip to the doctor. This saves the cost of a visit and it will increase the proportion of 9- to 14-year-olds who are considered to be fully HPV immunized. Even, a single-dose HPV vaccine would have a big impact on cancer prevention.

The WHO SAGE review concluded that a single-dose HPV vaccine delivers solid protection against HPV compared to two-dose schedules. This could be a game-changer for the prevention of the disease; seeing more doses of the life-saving jab reach more girls.

The SAGE recommends updating dose schedules for HPV are as follows:
- One or two-dose schedule for the primary target of girls aged 9–14
- One or two-dose schedule for young women aged 15–20
- Two doses with a 6-month interval for women older than 21.

The HPV vaccine is now available for adults. In October 2018 the US, FDA announced that the HPV vaccine is expanding for use for adults up to age 45. The vaccine is for men and women between the ages of 27 and 45. Previously, the vaccine was only available for those between the ages of 9 and 26.

The 9vHPV vaccine demonstrated sustained immunogenicity and effectiveness through ~10 years post three doses of 9vHPV vaccination of boys and girls aged 9–15 years. Commencing vaccination between the ages of 9 and 12 holds paramount significance. Before the onset of sexual activity, the immune system can develop robust defenses against the virus, ensuring long-term protection. Delayed initiation may necessitate additional doses and could result in reduced effectiveness. Accumulated safety data from large post-marketing surveillance studies and epidemiologic studies have been consistent with the safety profile in clinical trials.

Dispelling common misconceptions, HPV vaccination is not exclusive to girls. Recent research underscores its significant value in protecting boys as well. The vaccine acts as a safeguard against penile cancer, anal cancer, and head and neck cancers, thereby significantly reducing the risk of these life-threatening diseases.

New evidence shows why the HPV vaccine is as important for boys as girls. A study published in Cell Host & Microbe found that a gender-neutral HPV vaccination strategy is more effective than a girls-only strategy or no strategy. The long-term study involving 60,000 women from 33 Finnish communities found that if both boys and girls are vaccinated, only 50% of children need to be immunized each year to nearly eliminate the occurrence of high-oncogenic HPV types, compared with 90% of girls under a girls-only strategy, and screening protocols might need to be changed where a significant percentage of the population has been vaccinated.

Human Papillomavirus Vaccine Futuristic (Prophylactic → Therapeutic Vaccine)

Current HPV vaccines are extremely effective at preventing infection and neoplastic diseases; however, they are prophylactic and do not clear established infections or lesions. As a result, there is an urgent need for the development of therapeutic HPV vaccines, to treat existing infections, and to prevent the development of HPV-associated cancers.

The WHO also advises the inclusion of routine HPV vaccination in national immunization programs, considering public health priorities, program feasibility, sustainable financing, and cost-effectiveness.

Therapeutic vaccines which trigger cell-mediated immune responses for the treatment of established infections and malignancies are therefore required. DNA vaccines have great potential for the treatment of HPV infections and HPV-associated cancers due to their safety, stability, simplicity of manufacturability, and ability to induce antigen-specific immunity.

About 90% of HPV infections have been effectively prevented with the implementation of vaccines worldwide. However, no significant therapeutic effect has been observed on the already existing infections and lesions. A therapeutic vaccine designed for oncoprotein E6/E7 activates cellular immunity rather than focusing on neutralizing antibodies, which is considered an ideal immune method to eliminate infection.

Vaccine Hesitancy a Big Challenge

Despite the proven benefits of HPV vaccination, certain misconceptions have led to hesitancy among individuals and communities. Addressing these concerns and providing accurate information is essential for informed decision-making.

The vaccine stands as a pivotal defense against a spectrum of cancers caused by HPV, including cervical cancer. One common misconception is that HPV vaccination encourages early sexual activity, a claim debunked by extensive research emphasizing the vaccine's preventive nature. Additionally, both genders benefit from the vaccine, providing protection against HPV-related cancers for boys and girls and reducing overall virus transmission. It is crucial to dispel myths such as the vaccine causing severe side effects or exclusively benefiting girls. Research consistently affirms its safety, with mild and temporary side effects.

The vaccine's efficacy extends to long-term protection, contrary to the belief in its limited duration. Studies confirm enduring defense against HPV-related cancers, reinforcing its sustained effectiveness. Misconceptions about age restrictions for vaccination are debunked, emphasizing its benefits for individuals up to age 26 for females and age 21 for males. Moreover, those already infected with HPV can still receive the vaccine, offering protection against other HPV strains.

The vaccine's targeted approach stimulates antibody production, activates immune responses, prevents HPV infection, and provides cross-protection against multiple HPV strains. Crucially, it contributes to reducing overall HPV transmission, creating a herd immunity effect that safeguards both vaccinated and unvaccinated individuals from potential virus exposure.

Influenza Vaccine for 2023–2024 Season

According to the WHO, there are around a billion cases of seasonal influenza annually. This includes 3-5 million cases of severe illness. The flu causes 290,000–650,000 respiratory deaths annually.

The cornerstone of influenza prevention and epidemic control is strain-specific vaccination.

Since influenza viruses are subject to continual antigenic changes ("antigenic drift"), vaccine updates are recommended by the WHO each September for the Northern Hemisphere and each February for the Southern Hemisphere.

An influenza pandemic occurs when a new flu virus emerges ("antigenic shift") for which humans have little or no immunity. This allows the virus to spread easily from person to person worldwide. Four pandemics have occurred in the last 100 years, in 1918, 1957, 1968, and 2009. Scientists predict that another pandemic will happen, although they cannot say exactly when.

Prevention and control of the 2023–2024 flu season should include routine use of vaccines and antiviral medications.

Updated Flu Vaccine for 2023–2024

Flu viruses are constantly changing. The composition of US flu vaccines is reviewed annually by the US FDA Vaccines and Related Biological Products Advisory Committee and updated as needed to best match the flu viruses for the upcoming season. The 2023–2024 season US flu vaccines contain an updated influenza A(H1N1) pdm09 component:

- A/Victoria/4897/2022 (H1N1)pdm09-like virus for egg-based vaccines and
- A/Wisconsin/67/2022 (H1N1)pdm09-like virus for cell-based or recombinant vaccines.

How well the flu vaccine works can depend in part on the match between the vaccine viruses and circulating viruses. Preliminary estimates show that last season, people who were vaccinated against flu were about 40–70% less likely to be hospitalized because of flu illness or related complications.

Flu Vaccination for People with Egg Allergies

The ACIP voted that people with egg allergy may receive any flu vaccine (egg-based or non-egg-based) that is otherwise appropriate for their age and health status. Additional safety measures are no longer recommended for flu vaccination beyond those recommended for receipt of any vaccine.

The best way to prevent flu and its potentially serious complications is by getting a yearly flu vaccine. Even when flu vaccination does not prevent illness entirely, it has been shown in several studies to reduce the severity of illness in people who get vaccinated but still get sick.

Importance of the "Cocooning" Effect

Immunization of close contacts of children at high risk reduces their risk of contagion. Immunizing mothers and all family members is especially important to protect infants younger than 6 months because they are too young to receive an influenza vaccine.

Minimum age: 6 months for inactivated influenza vaccine (IIV) either trivalent or quadrivalent type. There is no preference and both can be used for annual seasonal immunization with anticipated strains. The CDC, ACIP, and WHO recommend the annual use of IIVs in all people 6 months and older. IIVs contain no live virus and now are available in both trivalent (IIV3) and quadrivalent (IIV4) formulations. IIV4 is likely to offer broader protection than IIV3, especially if the circulating B strain is not included in the IIV3. Neither inactivated vaccine formation is preferred over the other.

- Both trivalent and quadrivalent vaccines can be used and both vaccine types are safe to use in pregnancy.
- Children 6 months through 8 years of age need two doses—the interval between the two doses should be at least 4 weeks. Some children in this age group who have been vaccinated previously will also need two doses. 9 years and older need only one dose of IIV either trivalent or quadrivalent vaccine.
- IIV should be administered to all women who will be pregnant during the influenza season, regardless of trimester.
- For most healthy, nonpregnant persons aged 2 through 49 years, either live-attenuated influenza vaccine (LAIV) or IIV may be used.
- Vaccination should not be delayed to obtain a specific product for either dose. Any available, age-appropriate trivalent or quadrivalent vaccine can be used.

An ID formulation of IIV4 is licensed for use in people 18 through 64 years of age. This method of delivery involves a microinjection with a needle 90% shorter than needles used for IM administration. There is no preference for IM or ID immunization with IIV4 in people 18 years or older.

An intranasal quadrivalent LAIV4 is licensed by the FDA for healthy people 2 through 49 years of age. The 4 vaccine strains in LAIV4 are attenuated, cold-adapted, and temperature-sensitive viruses that replicate in the cooler temperature of the upper respiratory tract and stimulate both an IgA and IgG antibody response.

Vaccine for Adults 65 Years and Older (Senior Flu Shot)

The CDC recommends a higher dose flu vaccine or an adjuvanted flu vaccine (one with an additional ingredient called an adjuvant that helps create a stronger immune response. These vaccines are potentially more effective than the standard flu vaccine for people in this age group. (*Fluzone* high-dose quadrivalent inactivated flu vaccine, *FluBlok* quadrivalent recombinant flu vaccine, and *Fluad* quadrivalent adjuvanted inactivated flu vaccine.)

Senior flu shots contain four times as much flu virus antigen as the regular flu shot. This stimulates a boosted immune response. Side effects of the senior flu shot are often mild and may include pain and redness at the injection site, headache muscle aches, and fatigue.

This high-dose inactivated (HD-IIV3 or 4) influenza vaccine is an adjuvanted trivalent inactivated (aIIV3 or 4) influenza vaccine that is now approved and available for use.

Measles, Mumps, and Rubella Vaccine (Minimum Age: 12 Months for Routine Vaccination)

The WHO technical adviser on measles and rubella voiced alarm at the rapid spread of measles, with >306,000 cases reported worldwide last year—a 79% increase from 2022. To get more accurate figures, the UN health agency models the numbers each year, with its latest estimate indicating that there were 9.2 million cases and 136,216 measles deaths in 2022.

Given the ballooning case numbers, "WHO anticipate an increase in deaths in 2023 as well", and pointing out that 92% of all children who die from measles live among less than a quarter of the global population, mainly in very low-income countries. This year 2024 is going to be very challenging; some 142 million children are estimated to be susceptible to falling ill. This emphasizes the need for on-time vaccination throughout childhood is essential because it helps provide immunity before children are exposed to potentially life-threatening diseases. Vaccines are tested to ensure that they are safe and effective for children to receive at the recommended ages.

Routine Vaccination

A two-dose series of MMR vaccine is given at ages 12 through 15 months and 4 through 6 years. The second dose may be administered before age 4 years, provided at least 4 weeks have elapsed since the first dose.

In an area where disease is high, consider, one dose of either monovalent measles vaccine (preferred) or MMR vaccine to infants aged 6 through 11 months. These children should be revaccinated with two doses of MMR vaccine, the first at age 12 through 15 months and the second dose at least 4 weeks later.

Rubella monovalent vaccine is only given to females in grade 9.

A clinical scenario query answered by the authors on missed MMR doses:

Question: Children between 6 and 18 years who had missed their childhood measles vaccination, how will they get vaccinated? How many doses and when?

Answer: Ensure these unvaccinated school-aged children and adolescents get two doses of MMR catch-up vaccines; the second dose of vaccine is administered at least 4 weeks later.

Word of caution: Measles-antigen alone containing measles vaccine no longer is available in many countries including the United States. At present measles vaccine is available in combination formulations; which include MMR, measles–rubella (MR), and/or MMRV antigen-containing vaccines.

Meningococcal (*Neisseria meningitidis*) Conjugate Vaccines

Neisseria meningitidis, the cause of invasive meningococcal disease (iMD), can result in death within 24 hours of symptom onset, even when diagnosed and treated with antibiotics. Although all age groups can be affected, the prevalence of iMD is highest among young children and adolescents. The pathogen rapidly multiplies once it enters the bloodstream, triggering the release of cytokines and prolific recruitment of immune cells. Despite this robust immune response, 4–20% of children who develop the disease will die from circulatory collapse or brain edema and herniation. Therefore, the best approach to prevent disease and death is through immunization.

New Pentavalent Meningococcal Vaccine

The US FDA has approved a meningococcal vaccine against the five most common serogroups causing disease in children and young adults.

The new formulation called Penbraya is manufactured by Pfizer and combines the components from two existing meningococcal vaccines, Trumenba the group B vaccine, and Nimenrix groups A, C, W-135, and Y conjugate vaccine. This is the first pentavalent vaccine for meningococcal disease and is approved for use in people aged 10–25.

There are basically three groups of vaccines available for meningococcal disease prevention namely:
1. Polysaccharide vaccines (Menomune) were discontinued in 2017
2. Conjugated quadrivalent ACWY vaccine, Menactra
3. Serogroup MenB vaccine

These vaccines are not routinely recommended for healthy children <11 years of age.

The meningococcal polysaccharide vaccine is indicated for military recruits, college students, patients with asplenia or persistent complement deficiencies, those with relevant occupational exposures (e.g., microbiologists), and those who travel to or live in countries in which meningococcal disease is hyperendemic or epidemic. The vaccine is not indicated for patients who are immunosuppressed. It is no longer in use in the USA.

Conjugated Vaccines

- Menactra (MenACWY-D quadrivalent conjugated vaccine) is recommended for infants 9 months of age and older who are at increased risk for meningococcal disease due to serogroups A, C, W, and Y and 2 months for MenACWY-CRM (Menveo).
- Hib-MenCY (MenHibrix)—only cover C and Y serotypes—not ideal for Haj attending.

Administer a single dose of Menactra or Menveo vaccine at age 11 through 12 years, with a booster dose at age 16 years. Adolescents aged 11 through 18 years with HIV infection should receive a two-dose primary series of Menactra or Menveo with at least 8 weeks between doses. In patients with sickle cell disease, meningococcal immunization should not occur until after all pneumococcal immunizations have been completed due to interference in pneumococcal antibody production in some of the pneumococcal serotypes when the two vaccines are given at the same time.

MenHibrix is recommended for infants 6 weeks through 18 months of age who are at increased risk for meningococcal disease due to serogroups C and Y. This is an acceptable Hib vaccine alternative in children at increased risk for meningococcal groups C and Y disease. MenHibrix is not appropriate for protection against meningococcal disease for those traveling to the "meningitis belt" in sub-Saharan Africa or the Hajj. Meningococcal serogroup A is commonly the causative agent in these locations.

Serogroup B (MenB) vaccine series should be administered to persons >10 years of age at increased risk of meningococcal disease (category A). This includes persons with:
- Persistent chronic C3, C5-9, properdin, factor D and H, taking eculizumab (Soliris)
- Anatomic and functional asplenia including sickle cell disease
- Microbiologists routinely exposed to *N. meningitidis* isolates persons identified to be at increased risk because of serogroup B outbreak
- College students living in dorms or any activity that could put young adults in close proximity for extended periods of time are at heightened risk for meningitis B infections.

Two serogroup B meningococcal (MenB) vaccines are approved by the CDC for use in persons 10 through 25 years of age. These vaccines are distinct from MenACWY conjugate vaccines because protection is based upon developing immunity to bacterial proteins rather than capsular polysaccharides.
1. MEN B-F HbP (*Trumenba, Pfizer*) vaccine is a bivalent recombinant lipoprotein vaccine given as a three-dose series for everyone between the age 10 and 25 years.
2. Men B-4C (*Bexsero-Novartis, now GSK*) is a multicomponent vaccine given as two doses.

Pneumococcal Vaccines

In contrast to the conjugated Hib vaccine, pneumococcus disease prevention is complex because of its many serotypes, over, and clinical diversity.

Traditionally, 23 serotype-containing vaccine formulas called polysaccharide 23-valent (PPSV23) vaccine have been in use for over three decades for high-risk adults and for children over 2 years of age. The PPSV23 is not protective for children under 2 years of age. Therefore, conjugated pneumococcal vaccines are developed for universal childhood immunization of infants and children as young as 6 weeks of age for routine childhood immunization to protect children against life-threatening invasive pneumococcal diseases (IPDs) such as sepsis, meningitis, and bacteremic pneumonia.

The 7-valent pneumococcal conjugate vaccine (PCV7) was used in the past, but it has been largely replaced by the 13-valent version (PCV13), 15-valent (PCV15), 20-valent (PCV20), and the 23-valent polysaccharide vaccine (PPSV23) for most vaccination programs.

The minimum age for vaccination is 6 weeks. The PCV13 covers almost 80% of serotypes that cause IPDs and covers 100% of the platelet-rich plasma (PRP) strain causing IPD's in children <5 years of age.

The pneumococcal vaccine formulation is composed of the following pneumococcal capsular variants serotypes namely:
- *7v vaccine composed of 4, 6B, 9V, 14, 18C, 19F, 23F:* Not manufactured any longer.
- *13v composed of additional 6 capsular serotypes that are highlighted: 1, 3, 4, 5, 6A, 6B, 7F, 9V, 14, 18C, 19A, 19F,* and 23F.
- PCV13 or PCV15 is recommended for all infants and children 2 through 59 months of age. There is no preference for one of these vaccines over the other, and they can be used interchangeably. PCV20 is preferred among adults.
- *PCV20:* Serotypes covered in the vaccine for adults aged 18 years and older (Pfizer's 20vPnC) include the 13 serotypes contained in Prevnar 13 (1, 3, 4, 5, 6A, 6B, 7F, 9V, 14, 18C, 19A, 19F, and 23F) *plus* seven additional serotypes (8, 10A, 11A, 12F, 15BC, 22F, and 33F).
- Also, PCV 10v [(PHiD-CV); Synflorix, GSK, serotype 1, 4, 5, 6B, 7F, 9V, 14, 18C, 19F, and 23F] vaccine is a pneumococcal nontypeable *Haemophilus influenzae* protein D conjugate vaccine, currently licensed for the prevention of IPD in many European countries. This decision was based on independent, well-designed studies showing its effectiveness and cross-protection against 19A IPD.

Routine Childhood Immunization with PCV13 or 15v

Administer a four-dose series of PCV13 vaccine at ages 2, 4, and 6 months and at age 12 through 15 months. For children ages 14 through 59 months who have received an age-appropriate series of PCV7, administer a single supplemental dose of PCV13.

Adults' Vaccination with PCV20 Vaccine

Together, all of the 20 serotypes included in 20vPnC are responsible for the majority of currently circulating pneumococcal disease in adults in the US and globally. 14,15,16,17,18

All seven of the new serotypes included in 20vPnC are global causes of IPD,1,2,3,4,5, and six of the seven serotypes (8, 10A, 11A, 15BC, 22F, and 33F) 6,7,8,9 are associated with high case-fatality rates. In addition, four of these serotypes (11A, 15B/C, 22F, and 33F) are associated with antibiotic resistance 5,10,11 and/or meningitis (10A, 15B/C, 22F, and 33F). 12,13

Note: All children who may have received PCV7 as part of a primary series have now aged out of the recommendation for pneumococcal vaccine and PCV7 will eventually be removed from marketing.

24-Valent Pneumococcal Conjugate Vaccine (VAX-24)

A new vaccine candidate, VAX-24, using cell-free protein synthesis to produce a variant of cross-reactive material 197 (eCRM) as the carrier protein, increasing serotype coverage while minimizing carrier suppression. The recent clinical trial to assess the safety, tolerability, and immunogenicity of three different doses of VAX-24 compared to the PCV20 has been encouraging. Need further trails before reaching FDA approval.

23-Valent Polysaccharide Pneumococcal Vaccine

This formulation contains the following capsular serotypes: 1, 2, 3, 4, 5, 6B, 7F, 8, 9N, 9V, 10A, 11A, 12F, 14, 15B, 17F, 18C, 19F, 19A, 20, 22F, 23F, and 33F.

Pneumonia and invasive diseases such as bacteremia and meningitis remain an important source of morbidity and mortality in adults, especially among older adults and those with high-risk clinical situations including immunocompromising conditions and asplenia.
- Almost 40% of IPD in this high-risk person was caused by serotypes in PCV13 and another 33% was caused by serotype in PPSV23 that are not in the PCV13.
- Otitis media episodes and pressure equalization tube (PET) insertions have dropped since the introduction of the PCV13.

Summary

- PCV13 now is recommended routinely for all children 2–71 months of age.
- PCV is not recommended for healthy children 6 through 18 years of age due to their low risk of IPD.
- High-risk children 6 through 18 years of age are eligible for a single dose of PCV13 regardless of whether they have received before the PCV7 or the PPSV23 vaccine.
- PCV20 for the prevention of IPD and pneumonia in adults aged 18 years and older.
- PPSV23 is indicated for 19 years of age and older with immunocompromising conditions and administered a single dose of PCV13 1 year later.
- A single revaccination with PPSV23 should be administered 5 years after the first dose to children with sickle cell disease or other hemoglobinopathies; anatomic or functional asplenia; congenital or acquired immunodeficiencies; HIV infection; chronic renal failure; nephrotic syndrome; diseases associated with treatment with immunosuppressive drugs or radiation therapy, including malignant neoplasms, leukemias, lymphomas, and Hodgkin's disease; generalized malignancy; solid organ transplantation; or multiple myeloma.
- For adults aged 50 through 64 years of age and older both PCV20 and PPSV23 should be given. If the patient has already received PPSV23, administer PCV13 at least 1 year later.

Polio (OPV/IPV) Vaccines

The first polio vaccine to be widely used in humans, known as IPV or Salk vaccine, was developed in the early 1950s.

In India, vaccination against polio [oral polio vaccine (OPV)] started in around 1972 with the EPI. In 1985, the Universal Immunization Program (UIP) was launched to cover all the districts of the country. By 1999, it covered around 60% of infants, giving three doses of OPV to each.

Oral Polio Vaccine

Birth dose used in many developing countries plus routine primary four doses <15 months of age. High scientific evidence shows that the OPV schedules starting with a birth dose are at least as immunogenic as otherwise comparable OPV schedules starting at 6–8 weeks of age.

ACIP recommends only IPV (minimum age: 6 weeks): A four-dose series of IPV is given at ages 2, 4, 6 through 18 months, and 4 through 6 years. The final dose in the series should be administered on or after the fourth birthday and at least 6 months after the previous dose.

WHO: The OPV and IPV vaccines given in sequential order may be the key for the global polio eradication effort. Current studies demonstrate that IPV substantially boosts both mucosal and serological immunity in children previously vaccinated with OPV are historic and have major operational implications for the global polio eradication effort.

- If both OPV and IPV were administered as part of a series, a total of four doses should be administered, regardless of the child's current age.
- If only OPV were administered, and all doses were given before 4 years of age, one dose of IPV should be given at 4 years or older, at least 4 weeks after the last OPV dose.

Rotavirus Vaccine

The United States FDA licensed Rota Shield on August 31, 1998. This product is a live-attenuated rhesus rotavirus-based tetravalent vaccine (RRV-TV). India introduced the rotavirus vaccine (RV) on March 26, 2016, becoming the first country in the WHO's Southeast Asia region to do so. These oral drop vaccines were introduced in a phased approach across India.

Currently, available RV oral drop are:
- Rotarix (RV_1) is administered in a two-dose series at 2 and 4 months of age.
- RotaTeq (RV_5) is administered in a three-dose series at ages 2, 4, and 6 months.

The maximum age for the first dose in the series is 14 weeks, 6 days; vaccination should not be initiated for infants aged 15 weeks, 0 days, or older. The maximum age for the final dose in the series is 8 months, 0 days.

The first dose of rotavirus vaccine should be given before a child is 15 weeks of age. Children should receive all doses of rotavirus vaccine before they turn 8 months of age.

The IAP has revised RV1 to 10 and 14 weeks from existing 6 and 10 weeks of age. Only two doses of RV1 (Rotarix) are recommended at present.

Rabies: Active Immunization (Postexposure)

According to the WHO, the actual number of rabies deaths in India may be far higher than we know because of unreported or untreated cases and the paucity of literature at the national level. The Global Alliance for Rabies Control (GARC) states that India bears the world's heaviest rabies burden, accounting for 35% of all deaths due to the disease. While the number of reported dog bite cases in the country has risen, there's very little awareness among the public and even healthcare practitioners about the protocols for rabies vaccination, say experts—a major challenge as India attempts to achieve its target of eliminating the disease by 2030.

Rabies is almost always fatal after symptoms have developed, and no proven treatment exists. This is why prevention is so critical and should consider the need for PEP when evaluating patients who have had animal contact such as a bite, cut, or scratch. One should always consider whether the exposure is a risk for rabies transmission.

Human diploid cell vaccine (HDCV) and purified chicken embryo cell vaccine (PCECV) are available for use. For a previously unvaccinated immunocompetent person, receive on the first day of PEP (day 0), and repeated doses are given on days 3, 7, and 14 after the first dose, for a total of four doses, with one dose of human rabies immunoglobulin (HRIG) given on day 0 **(Table 4)**.

The highly immunogenic and less reactogenic HDCV and HRIG for PEP have always been in shortage even for countries such as the US, and Europe with relatively fewer rabies incidences. To address these issues, MassBiologics and the US CDC developed the anti-rabies monoclonal antibody to be used in place of HRIG or equine RIG (eRIG). MassBiologics then partnered with serum institute to develop and manufacture the antibody in India because of the high rabies clinical burden round the year.

Why the Monoclonal Antibody?

Human rabies immunoglobulin derived from human blood is an expensive product and carries a potential risk of contamination with bloodborne pathogens. The eRIG, derived from horse serum, is used in many parts of the world but its use is associated with significant adverse effects such as anaphylaxis or serum sickness. Both products are often in short supply and costly for people in places around the world where rabies is endemic. In India alone, it is estimated that only 2% of patients who require the rabies immune globulin receive appropriate postexposure treatment.

To address these issues, MassBiologics and the US CDC developed the anti-rabies monoclonal antibody to be used in place of HRIG or eRIG. MassBiologics then partnered with serum institute to develop and manufacture the antibody in India. Rabishield and TwinRab are the two brands available in India.

Serologic testing to document seroconversion after administration of a rabies vaccine series usually is *not necessary* but occasionally has been advised for recipients who may be immunocompromised or for people with deviations from the recommended vaccination schedule. Immune response should be assessed by performing serologic testing 7–14 days after administration of the final dose in the series. Clinical studies evaluating the efficacy or frequency of adverse reactions when the series is completed with a second product have not been conducted.

Intradermal Use of Rabies Vaccines

The WHO promotes the use of ID administration of rabies vaccines for PEP and offers an equally safe and efficacious alternative to IM. The ID vaccination reduces the volume of vaccine used by 60–80%, is less costly, and has the potential to mitigate vaccine shortages. It requires only one to two vials of vaccine to complete a full course of PEP.

Short Intradermal Use of Postexposure Prophylaxis

The existing 4-week pre-exposure rabies vaccination schedule is costly and often not practicable. Shorter effective schedules would result in wider acceptance. In healthy adults, the ID administration of a double dose of 0.1 mL of HDCV over two visits (days 0 and 7) was safe and not inferior to the single-dose three-visit schedule.

Respiratory Syncytial Virus

Respiratory syncytial virus can cause substantial morbidity and mortality among younger infants and older adults with diseases ranging from mild upper respiratory symptoms to severe lower respiratory tract disease. Also, older adults are at increased risk for RSV-related complications and death owing to age-related higher prevalence of underlying conditions.

After many decades of challenges, a single dose of the mRNA-1345 vaccine resulted in success in preventing RSV diseases for infants from birth up to 6 months of age by active immunization of pregnant individuals at 32 through 36 weeks gestational age and for adults 60 years of age or older (CDC, AAP October, 2023).

TABLE 4: Licensed rabies vaccines and rabies immunoglobulin (RIG) products.

Immunoprophylaxis category	Vaccine products available at KIMS	Manufacturer	Dose and route
Human rabies vaccine	• Human diploid cell vaccine (HDCV) • Purified chicken embryo cell vaccine (PCECV) • Rabies vaccine adsorbed (RVA) is licensed but no longer distributed in the United States	• Sanofi Pasteur • Novartis	1 mL IM. The dose volume is not decreased for children
Human RIG (HRIG)*	There are two products: 1. Imogam Rabies-HT (Sanofi Pasteur) 2. HyperRab S/D (Talecris Biotherapeutics)	Sanofi Pasteur and Alecris Bio	20 IU/kg*, half the amount infiltrated locally
mAb against rabies (two products available)	Rabishield* and Twinrab brand	Serum Institute of India	Refer insert label
Equine RIG	In case HRIG is not available. 40 IU/kg		<1% chance of serum sickness, may require desensitization

*Infiltrate around the wound, any remaining volume should be administered intramuscularly.

Smallpox or Monkeypox Vaccine (JYNNEOS™)

The last naturally occurring case of smallpox occurred in Somalia in 1977. In 1980, the WHO declared that smallpox (variola virus) had been eradicated successfully worldwide, and no subsequent human cases have been confirmed. Monkeypox is a rare disease with symptoms that are similar to but milder than the symptoms of smallpox. The WHO declared the ongoing monkeypox outbreak to be a public health emergency of international concern on July 23, 2022, in the context of the COVID-19 pandemic. The rapidly increasing number of confirmed cases could pose a threat to the international community. Current epidemiological data indicate that a high frequency of human-to-human transmission could lead to further outbreaks, especially among men who have sex with men. In addition, strategies for prevention, such as vaccination of smallpox vaccine, are also included.

A live, nonreplicating vaccinia vaccine (Jynneos™) was approved by the FDA in 2019 for the prevention of smallpox and monkeypox in people 18 years and older who are at high risk for smallpox or monkeypox. Jynneos™ can help protect against smallpox, monkeypox, and other diseases caused by orthopoxviruses, including the vaccinia virus. The CDC recommends vaccination for people who have been exposed to monkeypox and people who may be more likely to get monkeypox.

Jynneos™ is usually administered as a series of two injections, 4 weeks apart. People who have received smallpox vaccine in the past might only need one dose. Booster doses are recommended every 2 or 10 years if a person remains at continued risk for exposure to smallpox, monkeypox, or other orthopoxviruses.

ACAM2000 is a licensed live virus vaccine to prevent smallpox which is a lyophilized vaccine that does not contain the variola virus but rather the related vaccinia virus, different from the virus initially used for immunization by Benjamin Jesty and Edward Jenner from 1774 to 1796. ACAM2000 is grown in tissue culture, highly effective in preventing smallpox. Jynneos™ is approved by the FDA for the prevention of smallpox and monkeypox disease in adults at high risk for smallpox or monkeypox infection. Vaccine protection wanes with time but substantial protection has been observed up to 15–20 years after immunization.

Typhoid Immunization

Around 120 years after the development of the first generation of vaccines, typhoid fever remains a major health threat globally. Currently, available typhoid vaccines fall short in two major characteristics, namely long-term protection and protection for children below 2 years of age, the population that needs it the most. With the newly recommended tetanus toxoid conjugated vaccine (TYBAR-TCV) there are three kinds of vaccine against typhoid disease available. These are:

1. Ty21a (Vivotif®), an oral, LAV; protection lasts 5 years; minimum age for administration to over 6 years of age.
2. Vi-capsular polysaccharide (VICPS, Typhim Vi®) an IM injection (traveler vaccine); given at age 2 years and above including adult protection lasts 2 years.

3. Thirdly, the first conjugate vaccine (Tybar-TCV) for typhoid for children over 6 months of age in endemic countries.

Typhoid conjugate vaccines (TCVs) are of particular interest to the global health community because they have the potential to overcome many of the challenges that prevent the uptake of earlier vaccines. TCVs are more effective and may provide longer-lasting protection, require one dose, and are suitable for children younger than 2 years of age, allowing for inclusion in routine childhood immunization programs.

Indian Academy of Pediatrics Recommendation

Considering the epidemiology of typhoid in India, there is a definite need for protection against typhoid fever below 2 years of age. Therefore, the IAP recommends and includes TCV for primary immunization at 9–12 months of age. There are currently two TCV (Typbar-TCV and PedaTyph) licensed in the country. Those who received a dose of conjugate vaccine at 9–12 months can be prescribed a booster of either Vi polysaccharide (Vi-PS) or the conjugate vaccine at 2 years of age. Those who have received Vi-PS vaccine will need revaccination every 3 years till the intended duration of protection.

These two conjugate vaccines (Typbar-TCV and PedaTyph) are not licensed in the United States. However, if families with children younger than 2 years of age are traveling to live in areas of South Asia where extensively drug resistant (XDR) *Salmonella typhi* is circulating, parents of infants and toddlers can be advised to contact local pediatricians to have their young children vaccinated with this vaccine. It is widely available in India and available in Pakistan in parts of Sindh Province, the center of the XDR *S. Typhi* outbreak.

Protection Against S. Paratyphi A and S. Paratyphi B

Neither Ty21a nor ViCPS vaccine provides reliable protection against *S. paratyphi* A. Results of two field trials suggest that Ty21a may provide partial cross-protection against *S. paratyphi* B.

A Case Scenario: Typhoid Vaccines Interference with the Interpretations of the Widal Test

November 25, 2023: New query on Pediatric Oncall in your expertise category of "Infectious disease".

Dear Sayenna Uduman,

Question: "Respected doctor, how to interpret a positive Widal test after typhoid vaccination? Whether it is positive due to the disease itself or due to previous typhoid vaccination?

Our response:

- A single Widal test is not very clinically relevant, especially in endemic areas such as Africa, Southeast Asia, and the Indian subcontinent. A false-positive Widal test can be caused by past infection, vaccination, and previous exposure to cross-reactive antigens.
- The Widal test measures antibody to O and H antigens; neither Vi vaccine nor oral vaccine induces these antibodies. Therefore, these two vaccines do not interfere with the interpretation of the results of the Widal test.
- A positive Widal test result indicates that someone has been infected with the *Salmonella enterica* serovar typhi bacteria. The test is positive if the typhi O antigen titer is more than 1:160 in an active infection. In past infections or immunized people, the test is positive if the typhi H antigen titer is >1:160.
- The CDC does not recommend using serologic tests, such as the Widal test, to diagnose acute typhoid because these tests are difficult to interpret in endemic populations and where previous *Salmonella* infection or vaccination may result in a false-positive result. Isolate recovery remains important for guiding antimicrobial therapy for enteric fever. Serologic testing may be helpful in the identification of chronic carriers in outbreak situations.

Varicella Vaccine (Minimum Age: 12 Months)

Both monovalent varicella vaccine and MMRV combos have been licensed for use for healthy children 12 months through 15 months of age and 4 through 6 years. The second dose may be administered before age 4 years, provided at least 3 months have elapsed since the first dose. If the second dose was administered at least 4 weeks after the first dose, it can be accepted as valid.

Thirteen years or older healthy individuals, without evidence of immunity should receive two 0.5 mL doses of monovalent varicella vaccine, separated by at least 28 days.

Vaccine—Breakthrough Varicella Disease

Breakthrough disease is defined as a case of infection with wild-type varicella-zoster virus (VZV) occurring >42 days after immunization. Varicella in vaccine recipients usually is very mild, with rash frequently atypical (predominantly maculopapular with a median of fewer than 50 lesions), a lower rate of fever, and faster recovery than disease in unimmunized children. It may be mistaken for other conditions, such as insect bites or poison ivy. Vaccine recipients with mild breakthrough disease are approximately one-third as contagious as unimmunized children. However, approximately 25–30% of breakthrough cases are not mild, with clinical features similar to those in unvaccinated people.

Yellow Fever Vaccine

Yellow fever is a largely zoonotic disease endemic to South America's tropical regions and Africa's sub-Saharan regions. The yellow fever virus belongs to the *Flavivirus* genus and causes acute febrile hemorrhagic fever and jaundice. It is transmitted to humans through *Haemagogus* and *Aedes* mosquito vectors and has a high fatality rate. Current efforts to control the disease are largely through preventative measures such as vaccinations.

The LAV against yellow fever was developed 80 years ago, and its implementation has been widespread. It is known to elicit long-lasting and robust immune responses, with 94% neutralizing antibodies being detected in the recipients even after 3 months from vaccination. Based on recommendations from expert advisory groups, the WHO stated that no booster doses of the yellow fever vaccine were required except in special cases.

A recent study found that among individuals in non-endemic regions who mostly got vaccinated to travel, one dose of the yellow fever vaccine elicited long-lasting protection against the virus 10–60 years after the first dose. Lower observed seroprotection rates among residents of endemic areas were partly explained by the use of a higher cutoff for seroprotection that was applied in Brazil. Studies from sub-Saharan Africa were scarce and of low quality; thus no conclusions could be drawn for this region.

Zoster Vaccination

The burden of herpes zoster increases as a person ages, with steep increases occurring after age 50 years. Older persons >60 years are much more likely to experience postherpetic neuralgia (PHN), hospitalizations, and activities of daily living (ADL) restriction.

A recent global report conducted by GlaxoSmithKline has shed light on a concerning trend among Indian adults aged 50 years and above a lack of awareness regarding shingles and their potential impact. Surprisingly, the report indicates that over 80% of this demographic in India underestimate the risks associated with the disease despite being most susceptible.

There are two approved zoster vaccines namely (1) LAV (Zostavax) and (2) a recombinant subunit vaccine (Shingrix).

Zostavax

The first, live-attenuated herpes zoster (HZ) vaccine (ZVL) reduces the incidence of herpes zoster (shingles) and the incidence and severity of PHN.

A single dose of the vaccine is recommended only for individuals aged >60 years, including those with a previous episode of herpes zoster or a chronic medical condition. Nonetheless Zostavax has short term efficacy among those aged 50 through 59 years. In adults vaccinated age ≥60 years, vaccine efficacy wanes within the first 5 years after vaccination, and protection beyond 5 years is uncertain.

Although the vaccine is contraindicated in significantly immunocompromised patients, it can be administered to those with milder immunosuppression, such as those receiving low-dose glucocorticoids or methotrexate. The use of hydroxychloroquine is not a contraindication. *Zostavax is no longer available for use in the United States, as of November 18, 2020.*

Herpes Zoster Subunit Vaccine (HZ/su) (Shingrix)

Shingrix won US regulatory approval in 2017 to help prevent shingles in adults 50 years and older. Shingrix subunit vaccine appears to be more effective and less costly than Zostavax.

Shingrix is now the preferred vaccine for the prevention of zoster and contains an additional added immune response boosting "adjuvant" known as AS01B. Adjuvants are a common component of many vaccines and are classified as a "molecule that can boost the potency, quality, or longevity of a specific immune response". Zostavax does not contain an immune-boosting adjuvant.

Shingrix is different from Zostavax and the differences between these two drugs are summarized as follows:
- Shingrix is not a live vaccine, unlike Zostavax, which is live.
- Shingrix contains an "adjuvant", boosting vaccine effectiveness while Zostavax does not.

- Shingrix is more effective (97% effective) than Zostavax in preventing cases of herpes zoster.
- Shingrix is recommended for all individuals aged 50 years old and over. Zostavax is recommended for healthy individuals aged 60 years old and over.
- Shingrix is given via an IM injection while Zostavax is given via a SC injection.
- Shingrix is given as a two-dose series, with doses spaced 2–6 months apart. Zostavax is given as a single dose.
- Shingrix does not need to be stored frozen. Zostavax needs to be stored in the freezer.

A two-dose HZ/su (Shingrix) vaccine, administered 2 months apart, is more effective.

CONCLUSION

Ongoing research is crucial for improving vaccines and ensuring their safety and efficacy. Approved vaccines are subjected to continuous monitoring and evaluation as new data emerges. This could lead to updates in vaccine components, dosing schedules, or even the development of entirely new vaccines to address emerging variants or gaps in coverage. It's part of the dynamic nature of public health efforts to stay ahead of evolving infectious diseases.

Regulatory bodies, such as the US Food and Drug Administration (FDA) and the European Medicines Agency (EMA), have established processes for reviewing and approving changes to vaccine formulations. These processes ensure that any modifications maintain or improve the vaccine's safety, efficacy, and quality.

SUGGESTED READING

1. Abramson A, Kirtane AR, Shi Y, Zhong G, Collins JE, Tamang S, et al. Oral mRNA delivery using capsule-mediated gastrointestinal tissue injections. Matter. 2022;5: 975-87.
2. Castiglia P, Pradelli L, Castagna S, Freguglia V, Palù G, Espositoe S. Overall effectiveness of pneumococcal conjugate vaccines: An economic analysis of PHiD-CV and PCV-13 in the immunization of infants in Italy. Hum Vaccin Immunother. 2017;13(10):2307-15.
3. CDC, Green Book, and Red Book USA 2023.
4. Clark RA, Weerasuriya CK, Portnoy A, Mukandavire C, Quaife M, Bakker R, et al. New tuberculosis vaccines in India: Modelling the potential health and economic impacts of adolescent/adult vaccination with M72/AS01E and BCG-revaccination. medRxiv. 2023.
5. Covián C, Retamal-Díaz A, Bueno SM, Kalergis AM. Could BCG vaccination induce protective trained immunity for SARS-CoV-2? Front Immunol. 2020;11:970.
6. Ghany MG. A glimmer of hope for an orphan disease. N Engl J Med. 2023;389:81-82.
7. Halstead SB. Three Dengue Vaccines—What Now. N Engl J Med. 2024;390:464-5.
8. Hamiel U, Kozer E, Youngster I. SARS-CoV-2 rates in BCG-vaccinated and unvaccinated young adults. JAMA. 2020;323(22):2340-1.
9. Hepatitis B Foundation. Vaccine Non-Responders. Available from: https://www.hepb.org/prevention-and-diagnosis/vaccination/vaccine-non-responders/. [Last accessed April, 2024].
10. Huang Y, Mu L, Wang W. Monkeypox: epidemiology, pathogenesis, treatment and prevention. Signal Transduct Target Ther. 2022;7(1):373.
11. Immunize.org. Ask the Experts: Hepatitis B. Available from: https://www.immunize.org/askexperts/experts_hepb.asp. [Last accessed May, 2024].
12. Kallás EG, Cintra MAT, Moreira JA, Patiño EG, Braga PE, Tenório JCV, et al. Live, attenuated, tetravalent butantan-dengue vaccine in children and adults. 2024. N Engl J Med. 2024;390:397-408,
13. Khurana A, Allawadhi P, Khurana I, Allwadhi S, Weiskirchen R, Banothu AK, et al. Role of nanotechnology behind the success of mRNA vaccines for COVID-19. Nano Today. 2021;38:101142.
14. Kumar D, Peter RM, Joseph A, Kosalram K, Kaur H, et al. Prevalence of viral hepatitis infection in India: a systematic review and meta-analysis. J Educ Health Promot. 2023; 12:103.
15. Lynch JA, Lim JK, Asaga PEP, Wartel TA, Marti M, Yakubu B, et al. PLoS Negl Trop Dis. 2023;17(1):e0010969.
16. McIntyre PB, Edwards KM. Genetically modified pertussis toxin: a quantum leap? Lancet Infect Dis. 2018;18(11): 1169-71.
17. MediNexus. (2024). Report: Majority of Indian Adults Underestimate Shingles. Available from: https://www.emedinexus.com/post/40796/. [Last accessed April, 2024].
18. Meites E, Kempe A, Markowitz LE. Use of a 2-Dose schedule for human papillomavirus vaccination—updated recommendations of the advisory committee on immunization practices. MMWR Morb Mortal Wkly Rep. 2016;65:1405-8.
19. Mitchell R, Cayen J, Thampi N, Frenette C, Bartoszko J, Choi KB, et al. Trends in severe outcomes among adult and pediatric patients hospitalized with COVID-19 in the Canadian Nosocomial Infection Surveillance Program, March 2020 to May 2022. JAMA Netw Open. 2023;6(4):e239050.
20. Mo Y, Ma J, Zhang H, Shen J, Chen J, Hong J, et al. Prophylactic and therapeutic HPV vaccines: current scenario and perspectives. Front Cell Infect Microbiol. 2022;12:909223.
21. Pediatric Oncall. (2024). MCQ Quiz. Available from: https://www.pediatriconcall.com/quiz. [Last accessed April, 2024].

22. Ravi Kumar KL, Ganaie F, Ashok V. Circulating serotypes and trends in antibiotic resistance of invasive streptococcus pneumoniae from children under five in Bangalore. J Clin Diagn Res. 2013;7(12):2716-20.
23. Schillie S, Harris A, Link-Gelles R, Romero J, Ward J, Nelson N. Recommendations of the Advisory Committee on Immunization Practices for Use of a Hepatitis B Vaccine with a Novel Adjuvant. MMWR Morb Mortal Wkly Rep. 2018;67(15):455-458.
24. Schnyder JL, de Jong HK, Bache BE, Schaumburg F, Grobusch MP. Long-term immunity following yellow fever vaccination: a systematic review and meta-analysis. Lancet Glob Health. 2024;12(3), e445-56.
25. Shahzad D, Mudassar T, Yasir M. Review on Recombinant Vaccines. Int J Sci Eng Res. 2019;70(8):1473-87.
26. Singh AK, Netea MG, Bishai WR. BCG turns 100: its nontraditional uses against viruses, cancer, and immunologic diseases. J Clin Invest. 2021;131(11):e148291.
27. Soentjens P, Andries P, Aerssens A, Tsoumanis A, Ravinetto R, Heuninckx W, et al. Preexposure intradermal rabies vaccination: A noninferiority trial in healthy adults on shortening the vaccination schedule from 28 to 7 days. Clin Infect Dis. 2019;68(4):607-14.
28. Sonkar A, Bishwal SC, Sharma RK, Barde PV. Prevalence of Hepatitis D virus antibodies in Hepatitis B patients treated at tertiary care unit at Jabalpur Central India. Indian J Med Microbiology. 2022;40(1):132-4.
29. Sridhar S, Luedtke A, Langevin E, Zhu M, Bonaparte M, Machabert T, et al. Effect of dengue serostatus on dengue vaccine safety and efficacy. N Engl J Med. 2018;379(4): 327-40.
30. Wassil J, Sisti M, Fairman J, Davis M, Fierro C, Bennett S, et al. Evaluating the safety, tolerability, and immunogenicity of a 24-valent pneumococcal conjugate vaccine (VAX-24) in healthy adults aged 18 to 64 years: a phase 1/2, double-masked, dose-finding, active-controlled, randomised clinical trial. Lancet. 2024;24(3):308-18.
31. Wiese AD, Huang X, Yu C, Mitchel EF, Kyaw MH, Griffin MR, et al. Changes in otitis media episodes and pressure equalization tube insertions among young children following introduction of the 13-valent pneumococcal conjugate vaccine: a birth cohort-based study. Clin Infect Dis. 2019;69(12):2162-9.

CHAPTER 5

Pediatric Immunizations

■ INTRODUCTION

Immunization strategic principles are on-time routine immunization of all children and adolescents according to the currently updated recommended "Child and Adolescent Immunization Schedule".

Since children are susceptible to specific diseases at certain stages of their development, vaccinations are most effective when administered at the appropriate age and dosage. Children who are not vaccinated or are undervaccinated are left unprotected and face an increased risk of contracting life-threatening illnesses.

A general overview of the childhood vaccination schedule beyond birth doses is as follows:
Birth dose Bacillus Calmette–Guérin (BCG)/coronavirus disease-2019 (COVID-19)/dengue/diphtheria, tetanus, and pertussis (DTP)/*Haemophilus Influenzae* type b (Hib)/hepatitis A virus (HAV)/hepatitis B virus (HBV)/human papillomavirus (HPV)/influenza/Japanese encephalitis/measles, mumps, and rubella (MMR)/meningococcus/polio/rotavirus/respiratory syncytial virus (RSV)/*Streptococcus pneumoniae*/typhoid vaccines/varicella (chickenpox).

These vaccines can be given as monovalent vaccines or in a combination (combo) preparations, i.e., as pentavalent-shot to protect against [diphtheria, tetanus, and pertussis (DTaP)-Hib-hepatitis B] or as the hexavalent vaccine protection against [DTaP-Hib- inactivated polio vaccine (IPV)-hepatitis B] into one injection.

Vaccination schedules and specific vaccines recommended may vary depending on the country and regional health guidelines. It is important to consult with your pediatrician to ensure that your child or adolescent receives the appropriate vaccinations according to your local Health Ministry recommendations.

Additionally, new vaccines may have been developed or existing recommendations may have changed since my last update, so staying current with the latest information is essential for protecting your child's health.

Childhood immunizations are important because they provide immunity to potentially life-threatening diseases. They can prevent common childhood diseases that used to seriously harm or even kill infants, children, and adults. Children who are not vaccinated can spread diseases to others, particularly to those who are too young to be vaccinated, or people with weakened immune systems.

Timing and spacing of vaccines are two of the most important considerations for the appropriate use of vaccines. Specific circumstances commonly encountered in immunization practice are the intervals between doses of the same vaccine. For routine vaccination, vaccine doses should not be administered earlier than the minimum age or at less than the minimum intervals (starting at 6 weeks of age and administered at 4–8 weeks intervals) for primary vaccination series.

■ RATIONALE BEHIND VACCINE ADJUVANT ACTION

A new era of vaccine development is presently emerging through novel combined therapy comprising adjuvants, which specifically activate and drive immune responses. Traditionally, incorporating an adjuvant into a vaccine presents certain benefits, such as a reduced quantity of doses administered, leading to altered immune responses of greater quality, with minimal side effects. A prime example of frequently used adjuvants includes alum adjuvants, which are readily available in the market today, as this compound assists in promoting humoral immunity in an individual.

It is essential to consult with your pediatrician to ensure that your child receives the appropriate vaccinations based on their specific needs and age. In this chapter, the authors have provided a general overview of some common vaccines and principles of routine childhood vaccinations that children and adolescents should receive.

Reference Resources

The Advisory Committee on Immunization Practices (ACIP) is a group of medical and public health experts who develop recommendations on how to use vaccines. The ACIP's recommendations are public health guidance for the safe use of vaccines and related biological products.

The ACIP workgroup endorsements were forwarded to the US Centers for Disease Control and Prevention (CDC) for vaccine recommendations using an explicit evidence-based method. These recommendations are referenced and appropriated in our discussions in this "Pediatric Vaccination Chapter".

The Indian Academy of Pediatrics (IAP) is committed to the improvement of the health and well-being of all children. In collaboration with WHO and as a part of the Universal Immunization Program (UIP), the IAP Committee on Immunization (IAPCOI) 2023–2024, is one of the vital interventions for the protection of children from life-threatening conditions by providing vaccination. The major changes include recommendation of HPV vaccine for boys; a 2-dose schedule of 9vHPV for boys and girls aged 9–14 year; a dose of Td vaccine at 16–18 year; guidance for injectable polio vaccine (IPV) for those patients who are changing from National Immunization Program to IAP schedule **(Table 1)**.

Childhood vaccines that are incorporated in recommended immunization schedules are given as follows.

Bacillus Calmette–Guérin and Hepatitis B Vaccine

These are given shortly after birth, before discharge from the newborn nursery. BCG is one of the most widely used vaccines in the world; a single intradermal dose, usually on the upper left arm, is recommended in healthy babies as soon after birth as possible. BCG vaccine rarely is administered to children in areas where tuberculosis (TB) is not common, only children at high risk are typically immunized. BCG vaccine has a documented protective effect against meningitis and disseminated TB in children.

BCG Vaccination in Preterm and Low Birth Weight Infants

- Currently, evidence from clinically stable infants who were born after >30 weeks of gestational age and/or weighing >1.5 kg seems to support BCG vaccination within 7 days of birth.

TABLE 1: WHO/Indian Academy of Pediatrics Committee on Immunization (IAPCOI) 2023–2024 recommendations: part of the Universal Immunization Program (UIP).

Age	Vaccine
Birth	BCG, hepatitis B1, OPV
6 weeks	DTwP/DTaP1, Hib-1, IPV-1, hepatitis B2, PCV1, Rota-1
10 weeks	DTwP/DTaP2, Hib-2, IPV-2, hepatitis B3, PCV2, Rota-2
14 weeks	DTwP/DTaP3, Hib-3, IPV-3, hepatitis B4, PCV3, Rota-3
6 months	Influenza-1
7 months	Influenza-2
6–9 months	Typhoid conjugate vaccine
9 months	MMR-1 (mumps, measles, and rubella)
12 months	Hepatitis A-1
12–15 months	PCV booster
15 months	MMR-2 and varicella
16–18 months	DTwP/DTaP, Hib, IPV
18–19 months	Hepatitis A2, Varicella 2
4–6 years	DTwP/DTaP, IPV, MMR-3
9–15 years (girls)	HPV (two doses)
10–12 years	Tdap/Td
2nd, 3rd, 4th, and 5th year	Annual influenza vaccine

(BCG: bacillus calmette guérin; DTwP: diphtheria, tetanus, and whole-cell pertussis; DTaP: diphtheria, tetanus, and acellular pertussis; HepB: hepatitis B; Hib B: hemophilus influenzae B; IPV: injectable polio vaccine; MMR: measles mumps rubella; OPV: oral poliovirus vaccines; PCV: pneumococcal conjugate vaccine)

- In countries with a significant number of TB patients in the community, children are vulnerable to getting TB infection early in life (WHO, IAP, and CDC 2022). Therefore, the practice of birth dose that is given should be continued and is highly beneficial for developing nations.

Birth dose hepatitis B: All medically stable infants with a birth weight of at least 2,000 g are recommended to receive the first dose of the vaccine within 24 hours of birth.

This is followed by two more monovalent hepatitis B doses or a series of three combo-containing doses given before the child reaches 18 months of age.

Birth dose polio vaccine: Since 1985, the WHO has recommended oral polio vaccine (OPV) or IPV at the time of birth, particularly in countries where early induction of polio immunity is imperative. There is great variability in the immunogenicity of a birth dose of OPV for reasons largely unknown.

The utility of a birth dose of IPV has higher seroconversion rates in newborns and may be a superior choice in countries that can afford IPV, but there have been few studies of an IPV dose for newborns. The birth dose is to be followed by three more doses given at the recommended gap of 4–8 weeks each interval to complete the primary vaccination series before 18 months of age. Doses may be administered at 4-week intervals when accelerated protection is indicated.

COVID-19 Vaccination [Minimum Age: 6 Months (Moderna and Pfizer-BioNTech mRNA COVID-19 vaccines), 12 Years (Novavax COVID-19 Vaccine)]

- The best hope to move forward from the COVID-19 pandemic is the introduction of COVID-19 vaccines.
- The American Academy of Pediatrics (AAP) and the CDC recommend updated COVID-19 vaccines for everyone age 6 months and older. Nearly all kids are eligible for the 2023–2024 COVID-19 vaccine.

Recommended Dose and Type of Vaccines

The messenger ribonucleic acid (mRNA) vaccines from Pfizer-BioNTech and Moderna are available for children age 6 months and older. For children at least 12 years old who cannot receive the mRNA vaccines, they may be eligible for the updated protein subunit COVID vaccine from Novavax.

Primary Series

Age 6 months to 4 years:
- Two-dose series at 0, 4–8 weeks (Moderna) or three-dose series at 0, 3–8, 11–16 weeks (Pfizer-BioNTech)
- They are up to date when they get three doses of the Pfizer-BioNTech vaccine or two doses of the Moderna vaccine. At least one dose should be an updated Pfizer-BioNTech or Moderna COVID vaccine.

Age 5–11 years:
- Two-dose series at 0, 4–8 weeks (Moderna) or two-dose series at 0, 3–8 weeks (Pfizer-BioNTech)
- They are up to date when they get one dose of the updated Pfizer-BioNTech vaccine or when they get one dose of the updated Moderna COVID vaccine.

Age 12–18 years:
- Two-dose series at 0, 4–8 weeks (Moderna) or two-dose series at 0, 3–8 weeks (Novavax, Pfizer-BioNTech)
- They are up to date when they get 1 dose of updated Pfizer-BioNTech or Moderna COVID vaccine or two doses of updated Novavax vaccine or one dose of any updated COVID vaccine after any original or bivalent COVID vaccine.

For booster dose recommendations, see www.cdc.gov/vaccines/covid-19/clinical-considerations/interim-considerations-us.html.

Persons Who Are Moderately or Severely Immunocompromised

- *Primary series:*
  - *Age 6 months to 4 years:* Three-dose series at 0, 4, 8 weeks (Moderna) or three-dose series at 0, 3, 11 weeks (Pfizer-BioNTech)
  - *Age 5–11 years:* Three-dose series at 0, 4, 8 weeks (Moderna) or three-dose series at 0, 3, 7 weeks (Pfizer-BioNTech)
  - *Age 12–18 years:* Three-dose series at 0, 4, 8 weeks (Moderna) or two-dose series at 0, 3 weeks (Novavax) or three-dose series at 0, 3, 7 weeks (Pfizer-BioNTech)
- *Booster dose:* See www.cdc.gov/vaccines/covid-19/clinical-considerations/interim-considerations-us.html.
- Pre-exposure prophylaxis [monoclonal antibodies (mAbs)] may be considered to complement COVID-19 vaccination. See www.cdc.gov/vaccines/covid-19/clinical-considerations/interim-considerations-us.html#immunocompromised.

Contraindications

Anaphylactic or allergic reaction to a previous dose of COVID-19 vaccine.

Recommended Action

Do not vaccinate with the same COVID-19 vaccine type. May administer the alternate COVID-19 vaccine type.

Precautions

- In persons with a history of any bleeding or coagulation disorder (e.g., clotting factor deficiency and coagulopathy of platelet disorder)

- History of multisystem inflammatory syndrome in children or in adults (MIS-C or MIS-A)
- History of myocarditis or pericarditis within 3 weeks after a dose of any COVID-19 vaccine.

Recommended Action

A subsequent dose of any COVID-19 vaccine should generally be avoided.

Dengue Virus Vaccination (Minimum Age: 9 Years)

As of our current knowledge in October 2023, there were no widely approved vaccines specifically designed for pediatric age groups to prevent dengue fever. The development of dengue vaccines has been a complex and challenging process due to the nature of the dengue virus (DENV), which has four distinct serotypes (STs). Developing a vaccine that provides long-lasting protection against all four STs has been a significant scientific hurdle.

In the face of the ongoing severe acute respiratory syndrome (SARS) COVID-19 pandemic, coinfection with DENV and severe acute respiratory syndrome coronavirus 2 (SARS-CoV-2) poses a significant health concern and speculation over a possibly more severe course. Indeed, patients coinfected with the two viruses have been shown to have severe disease, a higher rate of intensive care unit (ICU) admission, and greater mortality. This has been attributed to similar pathophysiology of the two viruses for causing cytokine storms, capillary leakage, thrombocytopenia, and coagulopathy; during a coinfection, both the viruses either synergistically or individually cause multiorgan damage.

The development of a vaccine is an urgent priority owing to the lack of a specific antiviral treatment against DENV. Currently, five types of DENV vaccines are under development—live-attenuated vaccines (LAVs), inactivated virus vaccines, recombinant subunit vaccines, viral-vector vaccines, and deoxyribonucleic acid (DNA) vaccines.

The most notable candidate Dengvaxia (CYD-TDV), developed by Sanofi Pasteur, is currently the only marketed dengue vaccine. The WHO has approved Dengvaxia for the age group 9–45 years, living in a dengue-endemic region, and having laboratory-confirmed DENV infection in the past as it could pose safety concerns for individuals who had not been previously exposed to the virus.

Routine Vaccination

Aged 9–16 years living in areas with endemic dengue and have laboratory confirmation of previous dengue infection. Three-dose series administered at 0, 6, and 12 months. Dengvaxia is currently not licensed in India.

(Endemic areas include Puerto Rico, American Samoa, US Virgin Islands, Federated States of Micronesia, Republic of Marshall Islands, and the Republic of Palau).

For updated guidance on dengue-endemic areas and prevaccination laboratory testing, see https://www.cdc.gov/dengue/vaccine/hcp/index.html.

Contraindications and Not Recommended

- Lack of laboratory confirmation of a previous dengue infection
- Severe allergic reaction (e.g., anaphylaxis) after a previous dose or to a vaccine component
- Severe immunodeficiency [e.g., hematologic and solid tumors, receipt of chemotherapy, congenital immunodeficiency, long-term immunosuppressive therapy, or patients with human immunodeficiency virus (HIV) infection who are severely immunocompromised].

Precautions

Pregnancy, HIV infection without evidence of severe immunosuppression, and moderate or severe acute illness with or without fever. The dengue vaccine is not approved for use in US travelers who are visiting but not living in endemic areas. The vaccine is associated with an increased risk for severe dengue in those who experience their first natural infection after vaccination.

Diphtheria, Tetanus, and Pertussis (DTwP, DTaP, and Tdap) Vaccinations

Routine vaccination [minimum age: 6 weeks (4 years for Kinrix® or Quadracel®)]

It is important to adhere to the recommended vaccination schedule to ensure that children are adequately protected against these serious diseases. DTwP, DTaP, and Tdap vaccines are not only important for the individual child but also contribute to community immunity, helping to prevent outbreaks of pertussis, diphtheria, and tetanus.

Primary DTwP and DTaP Vaccination Series

Children should receive a series of these vaccines to protect against diphtheria, tetanus, and pertussis.

This series typically consists of five doses series given at the following ages:

CDC/ACIP/AAP	vs.	WHO/IAP recommendation
2 months		6 weeks
4 months		10 weeks
6 months		14 weeks
15–18 months		Yes 15–18 months
4–6 years		10–12 years

Ideal primary doses are five-dose series at age 2, 4, 6, 15-18 months, and 4-6 years.

The routine schedule for administering DTwP/DTaP to children is a three-dose series at age 2, 4, and 6 months, followed by boosters at age 15–18 months and 4–6 years. The first booster may be given at age 12–15 months as long as there is an interval of at least 6 months from the preceding dose.

Prospectively: Fourth dose may be administered as early as age 12 months of age if at least 6 months have elapsed since third dose.

Retrospectively: A fourth dose that was inadvertently administered as early as age 12 months may be counted if at least 4 months have elapsed since third dose.

Booster vaccinations as per the CDC: After the initial DTwP series, a booster Tdap is recommended every 10 years to maintain protection against tetanus and diphtheria and provides continued protection against these diseases.
- A Tdap booster is recommended at age 11–12 years. If a Tdap vaccine was not administered at age 11–12 years, it should be given at the next healthcare visit.
- Tdap can also be administered to pregnant women during each pregnancy (preferably between 27 and 36 weeks of gestation) to protect both the mother and newborn from pertussis.

Contraindications and Not Indicated

- Severe allergic reaction (e.g., anaphylaxis) after a previous dose or to a vaccine component
- *For DTwP and DTaP only:* Encephalopathy (e.g., coma, decreased level of consciousness, and prolonged seizures) not attributable to another identifiable cause within 7 days of administration of a previous dose of DTwP or DTaP.

Precautions

Guillain-Barré syndrome (GBS) within 6 weeks after a previous dose of tetanus-toxoid-containing vaccine, history of Arthus-type hypersensitivity reactions after a previous dose of diphtheria-toxoid-containing or tetanus-toxoid-containing vaccine, and defer vaccination until at least 10 years have elapsed since the last tetanus-toxoid-containing vaccine.

For DTwP and DTaP only: Moderate or severe acute illness with or without fever, progressive neurologic disorder, including infantile spasms, uncontrolled epilepsy, progressive encephalopathy; defer DTaP until neurologic status is clarified and stabilized.

Special Situation

Wound management in children less than age of 7 years with history of three or more doses of tetanus-toxoid-containing vaccine. For all wounds except clean and minor wounds, administer DTaP if >5 years since last dose of tetanus-toxoid-containing vaccine. *For detailed information,* see www.cdc.gov/mmwr/volumes/67/rr/rr6702a1.htm.

Haemophilus Influenzae Type B Vaccination (Minimum Age: 6 Weeks)

Vaccines are only available for Hib. Hib vaccines do not protect against disease caused by any other *H. influenzae* strains. The first Hib conjugate vaccine, licensed in the United States in 1987, contained polysaccharide conjugated to diphtheria toxoid (PRP-D).

Haemophilus influenzae type b affects 337,000 Indian children every year. A vaccine against Hib was introduced in 2011 as part of the pentavalent vaccine and scaled up nationwide. Importantly, the IAP had already recommended in 2006 the use of Hib vaccine for all children. The use of Hib vaccines in the private sector is widespread in India for almost a decade.

The primary series of Hib vaccination typically consists of three or four doses, depending on the specific vaccine brand used. These doses are usually given at 2, 4, 6, and a booster dose is usually recommended at around 12–15 months of age, with a range of 12–18 months.

Routine Vaccination

ActHIB®, Hiberix®, or Vaxelis®: Four-dose series (three-dose primary series at age 2, 4, and 6 months, followed by a booster dose at age 12–15 months)

Vaxelis® is not recommended for use as a booster dose. A different Hib-containing vaccine should be used for the booster dose.

PedvaxHIB®: Three-dose series (two-dose primary series at age 2 and 4 months, followed by a booster dose at age 12–15 months).

Hib combos: Vaccines, such as DTaP-Hib-IPV (Pentacel®) and Hib-MenCY (MenHibrix), are available, which offer protection against multiple diseases in a single shot.

All immunocompetent children irrespective of their Hib vaccination status develop Hib ST-specific antibodies and lifelong immune and protection against invasive Hib diseases. However, children aged 6 years and over including all adults at high risk from any of the following may need one or more doses if not already vaccinated, such as:

- Immunoglobulin deficiency, early component complement deficiency
- A stem cell or bone marrow transplant
- Sickle cell disease or a damaged spleen
- Surgery to remove the spleen
- Chemo or radiation treatment
- Human immunodeficiency virus.

Contraindications and Precautions

Moderate or severe acute illness with or without fever.

Catch-up Immunization

- *One dose administered at the age of 15 months or older:* No further doses needed
- *Unvaccinated at age 15–59 months:* Administer one dose
- *Previously unvaccinated children age 60 months or older who are not considered high risk:* Do not require catch-up vaccination.

Hepatitis A Vaccination (Minimum Age: 12 Months for Routine Vaccination)

Two-dose series (minimum interval: 6 months) at age 12–23 months.

Contraindications and Precautions

Moderate or severe acute illness with or without fever.

Catch-up Immunization

- Unvaccinated persons through the age 18 years should complete a two-dose series (minimum interval: 6 months).
- Persons who previously received one dose at age 12 months or older should receive dose 2 at least 6 months after dose 1.
- Children and adolescents who have not been vaccinated against hepatitis A and are older than the recommended age for routine vaccination can receive "catchup" doses. Typically, these individuals receive two doses of the hepatitis A vax, spaced at least 6 months apart.
- Adolescents age 18 years or older may receive the hepatitis A and hepatitis B combo vax, Twinrix®, as a three-dose series (0, 1, and 6 months) or four-dose series (three doses at 0, 7, and 21–30 days, followed by a booster dose at 12 months).

For persons traveling to or working in countries with high or intermediate endemic HAV, see http://www.cdc.gov/travel/.

- *Infants age 6–11 months:* One dose before departure; revaccinate with two doses (separated by at least 6 months) between age 12 and 23 months.
- *Unvaccinated age 12 months or older:* Administer dose 1 as soon as travel is considered.

Hepatitis B Vaccination (Minimum Age: Birth)

The hepatitis B vaccine is highly effective in preventing HBV infection, which can lead to serious liver disease. Adhering to the recommended vaccination schedule helps protect pediatric populations from HBV infection and its long-term consequences.

Pediatric Dose Vaccine

10 µg dose (in 0.5 mL suspension) is recommended for neonates, infants, children, and adolescents up to 19 years of age. Three-dose hepatitis B monovalent series at age 0, 1–2, and the minimum age for the final dose is 24 weeks (6 months to 18 months).

Booster doses are not typically needed for individuals who receive the complete series of hepatitis B vaccinations during childhood. However, it is crucial to maintain records of children's immunizations and consult with pediatricians for any additional guidance.

- *Birth weight ≥2,000 grams:* One dose within 24 hours of birth if medically stable
- *Birth weight <2,000 grams:* One dose at chronological age 1 month or hospital discharge (whichever is earlier and even if weight is still <2,000 grams)
- Infants who did not receive a birth dose should begin the series as soon as possible.
- Administration of four doses is permitted when a combo containing hepatitis B is used after the birth dose.

- *Minimum intervals:* When four doses are administered, substitute "dose 4" for "dose 3" in these calculations.
- *Final (third or fourth) dose:* Age 6–18 months (minimum age 24 weeks).

Mother is hepatitis B surface antigen (HBsAg)-positive:
- *Birth dose (monovalent hepatitis B vaccine only):* Administer hepatitis B vaccine and hepatitis B immune globulin (HBIG) (in separate limbs) within 12 hours of birth, regardless of birth weight.
- *Birth weight <2,000 grams:* Administer three additional doses of hepatitis B vaccine beginning at age 1 month (total of four doses).
- *Final (third or fourth) dose:* Administer at age 6 months (minimum age 24 weeks)
- *Test for HBsAg and anti-HBs antibody at age 9–12 months.* If hepatitis B series is delayed, test 1–2 months after final dose. Do not test before age 9 months.

Mother is HBsAg-unknown: If other evidence suggestive of maternal hepatitis B infection exists (e.g., presence of HBV DNA, hepatitis B e antigen (HBeAg)-positive, or mother known to have chronic hepatitis B infection), manage infant as if mother is HBsAg-positive.

Birth dose (monovalent hepatitis B vaccine only):
- *Birth weight ≥2,000 grams:* Administer *hepatitis B vaccine* within 12 hours of birth. Determine mother's HBsAg status as soon as possible. If mother is determined to be HBsAg-positive, administer *HBIG* as soon as possible (in separate limb), but no later than 7 days of age.
- *Birth weight <2,000 grams:* Administer *hepatitis B vaccine* and *HBIG* (in separate limbs) within 12 hours of birth. Administer three additional doses of *hepatitis B vaccine* beginning at age 1 month (total of four doses)
- *Final (third or fourth) dose:* Administered at age 6 months *(minimum age 24 weeks)*
- If the mother is determined to be HBsAg-positive or if status remains unknown, test for HBsAg and anti-HBs at age 9–12 months. If the hepatitis B series is delayed, test 1–2 months after the final dose. Do not test before age 9 months.

Contraindications and Precautions

Moderate or severe acute illness with or without fever.

Catch-up Immunizations

- Unvaccinated persons should complete a three-dose series at 0, 1–2, and 6 months for minimum intervals
- Adolescents aged 11–15 years may use an alternative two-dose schedule with at least 4 months between doses (adult formulation Recombivax HB® only).
- *Adolescents age 18 years or older may receive:*
  - *Heplisav-B®:* Two-dose series at least 4 weeks apart
  - *PreHevbrio®:* Three-dose series at 0, 1, and 6 months
  - *Combined hepatitis A and hepatitis B vaccine, Twinrix®:* Three-dose series (0, 1, and 6 months) or four-dose series (three doses at 0, 7, and 21–30 days, followed by a booster dose at 12 months).

Special Situations

- Revaccination is not generally recommended for persons with a normal immune status who were vaccinated as infants, children, adolescents, or adults.
- *Postvaccination serology testing and revaccination* (if anti-HBs < 10 mIU/mL) is recommended for certain populations, including:
  - Infants born to HBsAg-positive mothers
  - Persons who are predialysis or on maintenance dialysis
  - Other immunocompromised persons.

For detailed revaccination recommendations, see http://www.cdc.gov/vaccines/hcp/acip-recs/vacc-specific/hepb.html.

Note: Heplisav-B and PreHevbrio are not recommended in pregnancy due to a lack of safety data in pregnant persons.

Human Papillomavirus Vaccination (Minimum Age: 9 Years)

Human papillomavirus vaccination is essential for preventing HPV-related cancers and is most effective when administered before individuals become sexually active. HPV vaccination recommendations for pediatric age groups vary by country and medical guidelines.

The WHO now recommends a one- or two-dose schedule for girls aged 9–14 years, a one- or two-dose schedule for girls and women aged 15–20 years, and two doses with a 6-month interval for women older than 21 years.

The CDC recommends routine HPV vaccination for both boys and girls starting at age 11 or 12. The vaccine series can be started as early as age 9 years and catch-up for all persons through age 18 years if not adequately vaccinated.

- *Two- or three-dose series depending on age at initial vaccination:*
  - *Age 9–14 years at initial vaccination:* Two-dose series at 0, 6–12 months (minimum interval: 5 months; repeat dose if administered too soon)

- *Age 15 years or older at initial vaccination:* Three-dose series at 0, 1–2 months, 6 months (minimum intervals: dose 1 to dose 2: 4 weeks/dose 2 to dose 3: 12 weeks/dose 1 to dose 3: 5 months; repeat dose if administered too soon)
- *Interrupted schedules:* If the vaccination schedule is interrupted, the series does not need to be restarted.
- No additional dose is recommended when any HPV vaccine series has been completed using the recommended dosing intervals.
- It is essential to follow your country's specific recommendations and consult with pediatricians for advice on HPV vaccination for pediatric patients.

Special Situations

- *Immunocompromising conditions, including HIV infection:* Three-dose series, even for those who initiate vaccination at age 9 through 14 years.
- *History of sexual abuse or assault:* Start at age 9 years. *Pregnancy:* Pregnancy testing not needed before vaccination; HPV vaccination not recommended until after pregnancy; no intervention is needed if vaccinated while pregnant.

Contraindications and Precautions

- Moderate or severe acute illness with or without fever
- HPV vaccination is not recommended during pregnancy.

Safety and Immunogenicity Among Vaccinated Boys and Girls

The 9vHPV vaccine demonstrated sustained immunogenicity and effectiveness through ~10 years post three doses of 9vHPV vaccination of boys and girls aged 9–15 years. In a recently published study showed that immunogenicity, effectiveness, and safety were demonstrated through 10 years postvaccination. Rates of persistent infection and disease related to vaccine-targeted HPV types were within expected ranges, compared with vaccinated cohorts of similar age in previous HPV vaccine efficacy studies.

Influenza Vaccination [Minimum Age: 6 Months (IIV), 2 Years (LAIV4), 18 Years (Recombinant Influenza Vaccine, RIV4)]

Routine Immunization

- Use any influenza vaccine appropriate for age and health status annually.
- Two doses, separated by at least 4 weeks, for *children age 6 months to 8 years* who have received fewer than two influenza vaccine doses before July 1, 2022, or whose influenza vaccination history is unknown (administer dose 2 even if the child turns 9 years between receipt of dose 1 and dose 2)
- One dose for *children aged 6 months to 8 years* who have received at least two influenza vaccine doses before July 1, 2022.
- One dose for all persons age 9 years or older.
(For the 2022–2023 season, see www.cdc.gov/mmwr/volumes/71/rr/rr7101a1.htm. For the 2023–2024 season, see the 2023–24 ACIP influenza vaccine recommendations.)

Special Situations

- *Egg allergy, hives only:* Any influenza vaccine appropriate for age and health status annually.
- *Egg allergy with symptoms other than hives (e.g., angioedema and respiratory distress) or required epinephrine or another emergency medical intervention:* Any influenza vaccine appropriate for age and health status may be administered. If using egg-based IIV4 or LAIV4, administer in a medical setting under the supervision of a healthcare provider who can recognize and manage severe allergic reactions.
- Severe allergic reaction (e.g., anaphylaxis) to a vaccine component or a previous dose of any influenza vaccine.
- *Close contacts (e.g., caregivers and healthcare personnel) of severely immunosuppressed persons who require a protected environment:* These persons should not receive LAIV4. If LAIV4 is given, they should avoid contact with/caring for such immunosuppressed persons for 7 days after vaccination.

Influenza, Cell Culture-based Inactivated Injectable (ccIIV4, Flucelvax® Quadrivalent)

- Severe allergic reaction (e.g., anaphylaxis) to any ccIIV of any valency, or to any component of ccIIV4
- GBS within 6 weeks after a previous dose of any type of influenza vaccine
- Persons with a history of severe allergic reaction (e.g., anaphylaxis) after a previous dose of any egg-based IIV, RIV, or LAIV of any valency. If using ccIV4, administer in medical setting under supervision of healthcare provider who can recognize and manage severe allergic reactions. May consult an allergist.
- Moderate or severe acute illness with or without fever.

Influenza, Recombinant Injectable (RIV4, Flublok® Quadrivalent)

- Severe allergic reaction (e.g., anaphylaxis) to any RIV of any valency, or to any component of RIV4
- GBS within 6 weeks after a previous dose of any type of influenza vaccine
- Persons with a history of severe allergic reaction (e.g., anaphylaxis) after a previous dose of any egg-based IIV, ccIIV, or LAIV of any valency. If using RIV4, administer in medical setting under the supervision of a healthcare provider who can recognize and manage severe allergic reactions. May consult an allergist.
- Moderate or severe acute illness with or without fever.

Influenza, Live Attenuated (LAIV4, Flumist® Quadrivalent)

- Severe allergic reaction (e.g., anaphylaxis) after previous dose of any influenza vaccine (i.e., any egg-based IIV, ccIIV, RIV, or LAIV of any valency)
- Severe allergic reaction (e.g., anaphylaxis) to any vaccine component (excluding egg)
- Children age 2–4 years with a history of asthma or wheezing
- Anatomic or functional asplenia
- Immunocompromised due to any cause including medications and HIV infection
- Close contacts or caregivers of severely immunosuppressed persons who require a protected environment
- Pregnancy
- Cochlear implant
- Active communication between the cerebrospinal fluid (CSF) and the oropharynx, nasopharynx, nose, ear or any other cranial CSF leak
- Children and adolescents receiving aspirin or salicylate-containing medications
- Received influenza antiviral medications oseltamivir or zanamivir within the previous 48 hours, peramivir within the previous 5 days, or baloxavir within the previous 17 days
- GBS within 6 weeks after a previous dose of any type of influenza vaccine
- Asthma in persons aged 5 years old or older
- Persons with underlying medical conditions (other than those listed under contraindications) that might predispose to complications after wild-type influenza virus infection [e.g., chronic pulmonary, cardiovascular (except isolated hypertension), renal, hepatic, neurologic, hematologic, or metabolic disorders (including diabetes mellitus)]
- Moderate or severe acute.

All persons ages ≥6 months with egg allergy should receive the influenza vaccine. Any influenza vaccine (egg-based or non-egg-based) that is otherwise appropriate for the recipient's age and health status can be used.

Japanese Encephalitis Virus Vaccine

The vaccination against JE *is not recommended for routine use*, but only for individuals living in endemic areas. Though occasional cases have been reported from urban areas in few districts. JE virus transmission is seasonal. Human disease usually peaks in the summer and fall. In the subtropics and tropics, transmission can occur year-round, often with a peak during the rainy season.

Japanese encephalitis virus is a *Flavivirus* related to dengue, yellow fever and West Nile viruses, and is spread by mosquitoes. JE is the main cause of viral encephalitis in many countries of Asia with an estimated 68,000 clinical cases every year. Safe and effective vaccines are available and are approved for people 2 months of age and older. It is recommended for people who plan to live in a country where JE occurs or planning to visit a country where JE occurs for long periods (e.g., 1 month or more).

The WHO recommends that JE vaccination be integrated into national immunization schedules in all areas where JE disease is recognized as a public health issue. In India, JE vaccine is provided subnational in select JE endemic districts. As per Government of India guidelines, two doses of JE vaccines have been approved in routine immunization for endemic districts—one along with measles at the age of 9 months and the second with diphtheria, pertussis, and tetanus (DPT) booster at the age of 16–24 months.

JENVAC is a single-dose inactivated JE vaccine. This Vero cell-derived vaccine is prepared from an Indian strain (Kolar-821564XY) of the JE virus. JENVAC has been developed in collaboration with the National Institute of Virology, India.

The vaccine should be administered by intramuscular route. The preferred sites are anterolateral aspect of the thigh for children or the deltoid muscle of upper arm for adults. Anyone who has a severe (life-threatening) allergy to any component of JE vaccine should not get the vaccine.

The JE vaccines are contraindicated in people who have had anaphylaxis after a previous dose of any JE vaccine anaphylaxis after any component of a JE vaccine.

Measles, Mumps, and Rubella Vaccination (CDC, ACIP, and AAP Recommend a Minimum Age of 12 Months for Routine Vaccination)

- Two-dose series at age 12–15 months, age 4–6 years, MMR or measles, mumps, rubella, and varicella (MMRV) may be administered.

Note: For dose 1 in children age 12–47 months, it is recommended to administer MMR and varicella vaccines separately. MMRV may be used if parents express a preference.

In India, the minimum age for the MMR vaccine is 9 months. The recommended schedule is: First dose: 9–12 months, second dose: 15–18 months, and third dose: 4–6 years. The second dose can be given as early as 4 weeks after the first dose. Both doses must be given after the child's first birthday. The IAP recommends the MMR vaccine for all parents who can afford it.

Catch-up Immunization

- *Unvaccinated children and adolescents:* Two-dose series at least 4 weeks apart
- The maximum age for use of MMRV is 12 years
- *Minimum interval between MMRV doses:* 3 months

Special Situations

- *International travel:*
  - *Infants age 6–11 months:* One dose before departure; revaccinate with two-dose series at age 12–15 months (12 months for children in high-risk areas) and dose 2 as early as 4 weeks later.
  - *Unvaccinated children age 12 months or older:* Two-dose series at least 4 weeks apart before departure.
- In mumps outbreak settings, for information about additional doses of MMR (including third dose of MMR), see www.cdc.gov/mmwr/volumes/67/wr/mm6701a7.htm.

Contraindicated or Not Recommended

- Severe allergic reaction (e.g., anaphylaxis) after a previous dose or to a vaccine component
- Severe immunodeficiency (e.g., hematologic and solid tumors, receipt of chemotherapy, congenital immunodeficiency, long-term immunosuppressive therapy or patients with HIV infection who are severely immunocompromised)
- Pregnancy
- Family history of altered immunocompetence, unless verified clinically or by laboratory testing as immunocompetent.

Precautions

- Recent (≤11 months) receipt of antibody-containing blood product (specific interval depends on product)
- History of thrombocytopenia or thrombocytopenic purpura
- Need for tuberculin skin testing or interferon-gamma release assay (IGRA) testing
- Moderate or severe acute illness with or without fever
- *For MMRV only:* Personal or family (i.e., sibling or parent) history of seizures of any etiology.

Meningococcal Vaccine

Meningococcal serogroup A, C, W, Y vaccination [minimum age: 2 months (MenACWY-CRM, Menveo), 9 months (MenACWY-D, Menactra), 2 years (MenACWY-TT, MenQuadfi)]

Note: Meningococcal serogroup B vaccination [minimum age: 10 years (MenB-4C, Bexsero®; MenB-FHbp, Trumenba®)].

The meningococcal vaccine (MCV) is not mandatory in India. However, it is recommended for children at risk, such as those with immune deficiencies.

The meningococcal conjugate vaccine (MenACWY) protects against four types of meningococcal bacteria (types A, C, W, and Y). The CDC recommends routine MenACWY vaccination for all preteens and teens at 11–12-year-old with a booster dose at 16-year-old.

Children and adults at increased risk for meningococcal disease and parents should consult their pediatrician to decide its appropriateness for their child.

Catch-up Vaccinations

- *Age 13–15 years:* One dose now and booster at age 16–18 years (minimum interval: 8 weeks)
- *Age 16–18 years:* One dose

Special Situations

Anatomic or functional asplenia (including sickle cell disease), HIV infection, persistent complement

component deficiency, and complement inhibitor (e.g., eculizumab and ravulizumab) use:
- Menveo®*:
  - *Dose 1 at age 2 months:* Four-dose series (additional three doses at age 4, 6, and 12 months)
  - *Dose 1 at age 3–6 months:* Three- or four-dose series [dose 2 (and dose 3 if applicable) at least 8 weeks after previous dose until a dose is received at age 7 months or older, followed by an additional dose at least 12 weeks later and after age 12 months]
  - *Dose 1 at age 7–23 months:* Two-dose series (dose 2 at least 12 weeks after dose 1 and after age 12 months)
  - *Dose 1 at age 24 months or older:* Two-dose series at least 8 weeks apart
- Menactra®:
  - Persistent complement component deficiency or complement inhibitor use:
    - *Age 9–23 months:* Two-dose series at least 12 weeks apart
    - *Age 24 months or older:* Two-dose series at least 8 weeks apart
  - Anatomic or functional asplenia, sickle cell disease, or HIV infection:
    - *Age 9–23 months:* Not recommended
    - *Age 24 months or older:* Two-dose series at least 8 weeks apart
    - Menactra® must be administered at least 4 weeks after completion of pneumococcal conjugate vaccine (PCV) series.
- MenQuadfi®:
  - *Dose 1 at age 24 months or older:* Two-dose series at least 8 weeks apart.

Travel to countries with hyperendemic or epidemic meningococcal disease, including countries in the African meningitis belt or during the Hajj (see www.cdc.gov/travel/):
- Children less than age 24 months:
  - Menveo®* (age 2–23 months):
    - *Dose 1 at age 2 months:* Four-dose series (additional three doses at age 4, 6, and 12 months)
    - *Dose 1 at age 3–6 months:* Three- or four-dose series [dose 2 (and dose 3 if applicable) at least 8 weeks after previous dose until a dose is received at age 7 months or older, followed by an additional dose at least 12 weeks later and after age 12 months]
    - *Dose 1 at age 7–23 months:* Two-dose series (dose 2 at least 12 weeks after dose 1 and after age 12 months)
  - Menactra® (age 9–23 months):
    - Two-dose series (dose 2 at least 12 weeks after dose 1; dose 2 may be administered as early as 8 weeks after dose 1 in travelers)
- *Children age 2 years or older:* 1 dose Menveo®*, Menactra®, or MenQuadfi®

First-year college students who live in residential housing (if not previously vaccinated at age 16 years or older) or military recruits: One dose Menveo®*, Menactra®, or MenQuadfi®

Adolescent vaccination of children who received MenACWY prior to age 10 years:
- Children for whom boosters are recommended because of an ongoing increased risk of meningococcal disease (e.g., those with complement component deficiency, HIV, or asplenia): Follow the booster schedule for persons at increased risk.
- *Children for whom boosters are not recommended (e.g., a healthy child who received a single dose for travel to a country where meningococcal disease is endemic):* Administer MenACWY according to the recommended adolescent schedule with dose 1 at age 11–12 years and dose 2 at age 16 years.

Note: Menactra® should be administered either before or at the same time as DTaP. MenACWY may be administered simultaneously with MenB vaccines if indicated, but at a different anatomic site, if feasible.

For MenACWY booster dose recommendations, see www.cdc.gov/mmwr/volumes/69/rr/rr6909a1.htm.

Contraindicated or Not Recommended

Severe allergic reaction (e.g., anaphylaxis) after a previous dose or to a vaccine component

Precautions

- Pregnancy
- For MenB-4C only: Latex sensitivity
- Moderate or severe acute illness with or without fever. The new formulation called *PENBRAYA* is manufactured by Pfizer and combines the components from

---

Menveo has two formulations: Lyophilized and liquid. The liquid formulation should not be used before age 10 years.

two existing MCVs, Trumenba the group B vaccine and Nimenrix groups A, C, W-135, and Y conjugate vaccine.

Now, with the newly approved vaccine, children can easily be protected against the five leading meningococcal serogroups (A, B, C, W, and Y) with PENBRAYA, the first and only pentavalent (5-in-1) vaccine to provide the broadest protection with the fewest injections.

The first and only pentavalent PENBRAYA (5-in-1) MenABCWY vaccine is approved for use and indicated for active immunization to prevent invasive disease caused by *Neisseria meningitidis* serogroups A, B, C, W, and Y.
- PENBRAYA is approved for use in individuals 10 through 25 years of age.

The safety and effectiveness of PENBRAYA have not been established in pregnant individuals. Children with certain complement deficiencies and individuals receiving treatment that inhibits terminal complement activation are at increased risk for invasive disease caused by *N. meningitidis* groups A, B, C, W, and Y, even if they develop antibodies following vaccination with PENBRAYA.

Poliovirus Vaccination (Minimum Age for Routine: 6 Weeks)

Routine Vaccination

Four-dose series at ages 2, 4, 6–18 months, 4–6 years; administer the final dose on or after age 4 years and at least 6 months after the previous dose.

Four or more doses of IPV can be administered before age 4 years when a combination vaccine containing IPV is used. However, a dose is still recommended on or after age 4 years and at least 6 months after the previous dose.
- In the first 6 months of life, use minimum ages and intervals only for travel to a polio-endemic region or during an outbreak.
- IPV is not routinely recommended for US residents age 18 years or older.

Series containing OPV, either mixed OPV-IPV or OPV-only series:
- Total number of doses needed to complete the series is the same as that recommended for the US IPV schedule. See www.cdc.gov/mmwr/volumes/66/wr/mm6601a6.htm.
- Only trivalent OPV (tOPV) counts toward the US vaccination requirements:
  - Doses of OPV administered before April 1, 2016, should be counted (unless specifically noted as administered during a campaign).
  - Doses of OPV administered on or after April 1, 2016, should not be counted.
  - For guidance to assess doses documented as "OPV", see www.cdc.gov/mmwr/volumes/66/wr/mm6606a7.htm.

Special Situations
- *Adolescents aged 18 years at increased risk of exposure to poliovirus with:*
  - No evidence of a complete polio vaccination series (i.e., at least three doses): Administer remaining doses (one, two, or three doses) to complete a three-dose series
  - Evidence of completed polio vaccination series (i.e., at least three doses): May administer one lifetime IPV booster

For detailed information, see www.cdc.gov/vaccines/vpd/polio/hcp/recommendations.html.

Contraindication

Severe allergic reaction (e.g., anaphylaxis) after a previous dose or to a vaccine component.

Precautions
- Pregnancy
- Moderate or severe acute illness with or without fever

Rotavirus Vaccination (Minimum Age: 6 Weeks)

Two rotavirus vaccines are licensed for use among infants; a live, oral human-bovine reassortant pentavalent rotavirus [RV5 (RotaTeq®, Merck & Co. Inc.)] vaccine, given as a three-dose series and a live, oral human-attenuated monovalent rotavirus [RV1 (Rotarix®, GlaxoSmithKline)] vaccine, given as a two-dose series. The products differ in composition and schedule of administration. The AAP and the CDC do not express a preference for either vaccine.
- *Rotarix®:* Two-dose series at age 2 and 4 months
- *RotaTeq®:* Three-dose series at age 2, 4, and 6 months
- If any dose in the series is either RotaTeq® or unknown, default to three-dose series.

Catch-up Vaccination
- Do not start the series on or after age 15 weeks, 0 days.
- The maximum age for the final dose is 8 months, 0 days.

Contraindications

- Severe allergic reaction (e.g., anaphylaxis) after a previous dose or to a vaccine component
- Severe combined immunodeficiency (SCID)
- History of intussusception.

Precautions

- Altered immunocompetence other than SCID
- Chronic gastrointestinal disease
- *RV1 only:* Spina bifida or bladder exstrophy
- Moderate or severe acute illness with or without fever.

Respiratory Syncytial Virus Vaccination

Respiratory syncytial virus is a common seasonal causing bronchiolitis; more common in the cool winter and or in monsoon rains seasons, especially in India. The virus is common in children under 2 years, though people of all ages can get it. Illness caused by RSV is often more severe for young and premature infants, as well as older adults with poor health development. Attempts to develop an RSV vaccine for children began in the 1960s with an unsuccessful formalin inactivated RSV. As of this time (December 2023), there are no immunizing tools to protect infants and older adults from illness and death due to RSV.

In 2023, two RSV vaccines for older adults, one of which is also approved for use in pregnant persons, and a long-acting mAb to protect infants and some toddlers up to 19 months of age were approved by the FDA and recommended by the ACIPs of the CDC, USA.

One RSV vaccine (Abrysvo by Pfizer) has been licensed and recommended during weeks 32 through 36 of pregnancy to protect infants.

However, for most infants, either the maternal RSV vaccine or the preventive antibody is recommended to prevent RSV disease, but not both.

Two RSV mAbs products can help prevent severe RSV disease in infants and young children: Nirsevimab (Beyfortus) and Palivizumab (Synagis).

Palivizumab is given monthly injection during RSV seasons; in contrast, Nirsevimab is a single dose for a season *(AstraZeneca's Nirsevimab—not a vaccine but a long-acting mAb that protects infants from RSV)*

The CDC recommends prioritizing available Nirsevimab 100 mg doses for infants at the highest risk for severe RSV disease, i.e., young infants (age <6 months) and infants with underlying conditions that place them at the highest risk for severe RSV disease.

Recommendations for using 50 mg doses are for infants weighing ≥5 kg (≥11 pounds) at this time.

Nirsevimab comes with new challenges alongside its benefits. As high-income countries begin to implement the administration of Nirsevimab, equally importance is its affordability, availability, and accessibility of healthcare access, especially in low- and middle-income countries, where RSV-associated morbidity and mortality are highest.

Streptococcus Pneumococcal Vaccinations [Minimum Age: 6 Weeks (PCV13), (PCV15), and (PCV20), and Over 2 Years (PPSV23)]

Routine Vaccination with PCV

Four-dose series at 2, 4, 6, 12–15 months.

Catch-up Vaccination with PCV

- Healthy children age 24–59 months with any incomplete* PCV series: One dose PCV

Note: PCV13 and PCV15 or PCV20 can be used interchangeably for children who are healthy or have underlying conditions. PCV15 is not indicated for children who have received four doses of PCV13 or another age appropriate complete PCV13 series.

Expert Opinion

In recent reports, PCV15 demonstrated a safety profile that is comparable to PCV13 in infants and children. Immunogenicity of PCV15 is comparable to PCV13 for all shared STs except ST 3, where PCV15 demonstrated superior immunogenicity. Higher immune responses were demonstrated for PCV15 STs 22F and 33F.

Results of the ongoing study to evaluate PCV15 efficacy against vaccine-type pneumococcal acute otitis media (AOM) and anticipated real-world evidence studies will support assessment of vaccine effectiveness and impact, with an additional question of whether higher ST 3 immunogenicity translates to better protection against ST 3 pneumococcal disease.

Special Situations

Underlying conditions below: When both PCV and PPSV23 are indicated, administer PCV first. PCV and PPSV23 should not be administered during the same visit.

- Chronic heart disease (particularly cyanotic congenital heart disease and cardiac failure); chronic lung

disease (including asthma treated with high-dose, oral corticosteroids); diabetes mellitus:
- *Age 2-5 years:*
  - *Any incomplete* series with:*
    - Three PCV doses: One dose PCV (at least 8 weeks after any prior PCV dose)
    - Less than three PCV doses: Two doses PCV (8 weeks after the most recent dose and administered 8 weeks apart)
  - *No history of PPSV23:* One dose PPSV23 (at least 8 weeks after completing all recommended PCV doses)
- *Age 6-18 years:*
  - *Any incomplete* series with PCV:* No further PCV doses needed
  - *No history of PPSV23:* One dose PPSV23 (at least 8 weeks after completing all recommended PCV doses)

■ *Cerebrospinal fluid leak, cochlear implant:*
- *Age 2-5 years:*
  - *Any incomplete* series with:*
    - Three PCV doses: One dose PCV (at least 8 weeks after any prior PCV dose)
    - Less than three PCV doses: Two doses PCV (8 weeks after the most recent dose and administered 8 weeks apart)
  - *No history of PPSV23:* One dose PPSV23 (at least 8 weeks after completing all recommended PCV doses)
- *Age 6-18 years:*
  - No history of either PCV or PPSV23: One dose PCV, one dose PPSV23 at least 8 weeks later
  - Any PCV but no PPSV23: One dose PPSV23 at least 8 weeks after the most recent dose of PCV
  - PPSV23 but no PCV: One dose PCV at least 8 weeks after the most recent dose of PPSV23

■ *Sickle cell disease and other hemoglobinopathies; anatomic or functional asplenia; congenital or acquired immunodeficiency; HIV infection; chronic renal failure; nephrotic syndrome; malignant neoplasms, leukemias, lymphomas, Hodgkin disease, and other diseases associated with treatment with immunosuppressive drugs or radiation therapy; solid organ transplantation; multiple myeloma:*
- *Age 2-5 years:*
  - *Any incomplete* series with:*
    - Three PCV doses: One dose PCV (at least 8 weeks after any prior PCV dose)
    - Less than three PCV doses: Two doses PCV (8 weeks after the most recent dose and administered 8 weeks apart)
  - *No history of PPSV23:* One dose PPSV23 (at least 8 weeks after completing all recommended PCV doses) and a dose 2 of PPSV23 5 years later
- *Age 6-18 years:*
  - *No history of either PCV or PPSV23:* One dose PCV, two doses PPSV23 (dose 1 of PPSV23 administered 8 weeks after PCV and dose 2 of PPSV23 administered at least 5 years after dose 1 of PPSV23)
  - *Any PCV but no PPSV23:* Two doses PPSV23 (dose 1 of PPSV23 administered 8 weeks after the most recent dose of PCV and dose 2 of PPSV23 administered at least 5 years after dose 1 of PPSV23)
  - *PPSV23 but no PCV:* One dose PCV at least 8 weeks after the most recent PPSV23 dose and a dose 2 of PPSV23 administered 5 years after dose 1 of PPSV23 and at least 8 weeks after a dose of PCV

For guidance on determining which pneumococcal vaccines a patient needs and when, please refer to the mobile app, which can be downloaded from here: www.cdc.gov/vaccines/vpd/pneumo/hcp/pneumoapp.html.

PCV Contraindications
■ Severe allergic reaction (e.g., anaphylaxis) after a previous dose or to a vaccine component
■ Severe allergic reaction (e.g., anaphylaxis) to any diphtheria-toxoid-containing vaccine or its component.

PPSV23 Contraindications
■ Severe allergic reaction (e.g., anaphylaxis) after a previous dose or to a vaccine component
■ General precautions are like any other vaccines
■ Moderate or severe acute illness with or without fever.

---

*Incomplete series: Not having received all doses in either the recommended series or an age-appropriate catch-up series, see ACIP pneumococcal recommendations at www.cdc.gov/mmwr/volumes/71/wr/mm7137a3.htm.

TABLE 2: Commercially available typhoid vaccines in the United States.

Typhoid vaccine	Type	Route	Minimum age of receipt, years	No of doses*	Doses frequency, years
Ty21a	Live attenuated	Oral	6	4	5
ViCPS	Polysaccharide	Intramuscular	2	1	2

*Primary immunization. For further information on dosage, schedules, and adverse events, see text.

Typhoid Vaccine

Protection against *Salmonella typhi* is enhanced by typhoid immunization, but currently licensed vaccines do not provide complete protection to children and adults. Two typhoid vaccines are licensed for use in the United States **(Table 2)**, one for use in people 6 years and older and the other in people 2 years and older.

The demonstrated efficacy of the two vaccines licensed by the FDA ranges from 50 to 80%, but the duration of protection differs notably between the vaccines. Vaccine is selected on the basis of age of the child, need for booster doses, and possible contraindications.

Adverse Events

The oral Ty21a vaccine is very well tolerated, but mild adverse reactions may occur; these include abdominal pain, nausea, diarrhea, vomiting, fever, headache, and rash or urticaria. Reported adverse reactions to ViCPS vaccine also are minimal and include fever, headache, malaise, myalgia, and local reaction of tenderness and pain, erythema, or induration of 1 cm or greater.

Precautions and Contraindications

A contraindication to the administration of intramuscular ViCPS vaccine is a history of hypersensitivity to any component of the vaccine. No safety data have been reported for typhoid vaccines in pregnant women. The oral Ty21a vaccine is a LAV and should not be administered to immunocompromised people, including people known to be infected with HIV; to have a phagocytic cell defect; or to have chronic granulomatous disease.

As per the IAP Advisory Committee on Vaccines and Immunization Practices (ACVIP): Recommendations (2021-2022):

- *6-9 months of age typhoid conjugate vaccine:* As of available data, there is no recommendation for a booster dose.

A recent study conducted by researchers at the University of Maryland School of Medicine's (UMSOM) Center for Vaccine Development and Global Health and Malawi-Liverpool Wellcome Trust (MLW) has demonstrated the enduring effectiveness of a single dose of the typhoid conjugate vaccine, Typbar TCV, in a single dose of the typhoid conjugate vaccine, Typbar TCV, in preventing typhoid fever in children aged 9 months to 12 years.

Varicella (Chickenpox) Vaccination (Minimum Age: 12 Months)

Routine Vaccination

- Two-dose series at age 12-15 months and 4-6 years
- Varicella or MMRV may be administered*
- Dose 2 may be administered as early as 3 months after dose 1 (a dose inadvertently administered after at least 4 weeks may be counted as valid).

Catch-up Vaccination

- Ensure persons age 7-18 years without evidence of immunity (see MMWR at www.cdc.gov/mmwr/pdf/rr/rr5604.pdf) have a two-dose series:
  - *Age 7-12 years:* Routine interval: 3 months (a dose inadvertently administered after at least 4 weeks may be counted as valid)
  - *Age 13 years and older:* Routine interval: 4-8 weeks (minimum interval: 4 weeks)
  - The maximum age for use of MMRV is 12 years.

Contraindications

- Severe allergic reaction (e.g., anaphylaxis) after a previous dose or to a vaccine component
- Severe immunodeficiency (e.g., hematologic and solid tumors, receipt of chemotherapy, congenital immunodeficiency, long-term immunosuppressive therapy or patients with HIV infection who are severely immunocompromised).

Note: For dose 1 in children age 12-47 months, it is recommended to administer MMR and varicella vaccines separately. MMRV may be used if parents or caregivers express a preference.

- Pregnancy
- Family history of altered immunocompetence, unless verified clinically or by laboratory testing as immunocompetent.

Precautions
- Recent (≤11 months) receipt of antibody-containing blood product (specific interval depends on product)
- Receipt of specific antiviral drugs (acyclovir, famciclovir, or valacyclovir) 24 hours before vaccination (avoid use of these antiviral drugs for 14 days after vaccination)
- Use of aspirin or aspirin-containing products
- Moderate or severe acute illness with or without fever
- If using MMRV, *see MMR/MMRV* for additional precautions.

CONCLUSION

In this chapter, the pediatric vaccines and vaccination aspects are detailed for children from birth through adolescence. Adherence to the national recommended schedule is essential for children health and the community's well-being. The schedules may vary by country and may change over time based on scientific research and public health recommendations. Vaccination is a critical part of public health efforts to prevent the spread of infectious diseases (IDs) and protect the well-being of all children and adults. Childhood immunizations offer a wide range of benefits for both individual children and the community as a whole. Therefore, it is essential to consult with pediatricians and pediatric ID specialists for the most up-to-date information on vaccinology. Please keep in mind that new vaccines or changes to the schedule may occur at periodic interval. Your child's healthcare provider will help you determine the specific schedule and vaccines your child needs.

SUGGESTED READING

1. American Academy of Pediatrics. (2023). Pediatric COVID-19 Vaccine Dosing Quick Reference Guide. Available from: https://aap.org/covidvaccineguide. [Last accessed April, 2024].
2. Centers for Disease Control and Prevention. (2023). Prevention and Control of Seasonal Influenza with Vaccines: Recommendations of the Advisory Committee on Immunization Practices—United States, 2023–24 Influenza Season. Available from: https://www.cdc.gov/mmwr/volumes/72/rr/rr7202a1.htm. [Last accessed April, 2024].
3. Centers for Disease Control and Prevention. Immunization Schedules. Available from: https://www.cdc.gov/vaccines/schedules/hcp/imz/child-adolescent.html. [Last accessed April, 2024].
4. Chapman TJ, Olarte L, Dbaibo G, Houston AM, Tamms G, Lupinacci R, et al. PCV15, a pneumococcal conjugate vaccine, for the prevention of invasive pneumococcal disease in infants and children. Expert Rev Vaccines. 2024;23(1):137-47.
5. Human vaccines and immunotherapeutics news: January 2022. Hum Vaccin Immunother. 2022;18(1):2039552.
6. Restrepo J, Herrera T, Samakoses R, Reina JC, Pitisuttithum P, Ulied A, et al. Ten-Year Follow-up of 9-Valent Human Papillomavirus Vaccine: Immunogenicity, Effectiveness, and Safety. Pediatrics. 2023;152(4):e2022060993.

CHAPTER 6

Adult Immunizations for Ages 19 Years or Older

CLINICAL SCENARIO ON ANSWERED ADULT-VACCINE QUERY

Q. I am a paramedical staff in a busy hospital, What vaccines do adults need? Do adults need vaccines, can you tell me, sir?

Author's Answer

Yes, you deserve to have all your "adult vaccinations" kept updated as per your institute's policy of "Immunization of Health-Care Workers (HICC)".

To my knowledge, there have been no national adult immunization guidelines in India. Adults are particularly vulnerable during outbreaks, due to a lack of immunization, waning immunity, age-related factors (e.g., chronic conditions and immunosenescence), and epidemiological swings.

The USA Centers for Disease Control and Prevention (CDC) does recommend vaccines for adults based on age, prior vaccinations, health, lifestyle, occupation, travel destinations, etc. Adults without compromised immunity who received all their childhood vaccinations are eligible for:

- *Tetanus and diphtheria Td or Tdap (pertussis added)* booster every 10 years. One dose of the Tdap vaccine is advised during each pregnancy, ideally between weeks 27 and 36.
- *Annual flu (influenza) shot* for everyone ages 6 months or older. Adults aged 50 and older should not get the nasal spray flu vaccine *along with pneumococcal vaccines* at age 65.
- *COVID-19 vaccines and booster shots* are a safe and effective way to extend protection against variants of concern. Mixing vaccines may enhance the immune response.
- *Human papillomavirus (HPV) vaccine:* HPV vaccine—Gardasil 9 for males and females ages 9–45. A recent study provided additional evidence that one shot of the vaccine is highly effective over 3 years, if not longer.
- With recently rising rates of acute hepatitis B (HepB), the CDC recommends *universal HepB vaccination for all adults aged 19–59 years* without a record of previous HepB infection or vaccination.
- *Shingrix* a recombinant herpes zoster vaccine at age 50 for healthy adults at age 50 and older given in two doses.
- *Respiratory syncytial virus (RSV) vaccine* recently approved Arexvy, a vaccine against RSV for adults aged 60 years or older.
- *Also, on its horizon, maternal group B Streptococcus (GBS) and RSV* vaccines given during third trimester of pregnancy are effective at preventing severe infections in newborns (Refer to Chapter 7: Maternal Immunization during Pregnancy and Lactation).

Adults are particularly vulnerable during outbreaks, due to a lack of immunization, waning immunity, age-related factors (e.g., chronic conditions and immuno-senescence), and epidemiological swings. Immunization is an essential part of care for adults, including pregnant women. Vaccination is as important for adults as it is for children, an additional routine vaccine for adults is now on the horizon.

Q. Why do adults too need vaccines?

Author's Answer

Young and healthy adults can get sick, as diseases know no age. Vaccines are recommended for adults starting at 19 years old.

- Many adults were not fully immunized as a child and/or may no longer be protected by vaccines received in childhood.
- Booster doses for some vaccines (e.g., DPT) are recommended to remain life-long protected.
- Adults getting immunized protects not just themselves, but other vulnerable people in their community, such as babies too young to get vaccinated. Also, in other households' older grandparents, and family members are protected.

- Some "newer" vaccines are just for adults and teens. Herpes-Zoster (Shingle) is a good example of a painful disease (postherpetic neuralgia) with possible life-long misery and one can avoid it by getting vaccinated.
- Human papillomavirus vaccine (depending on type) can prevent cervical cancer in young women and genital warts/anal cancer in both sexes.
- Adults are, in general, too busy with work activities, responsibilities, traveling, etc.
- Maternal vaccinations during or prior to getting pregnant are not just to protect pregnant mothers during pregnancy but also protect unborn fetuses and babies' protection during their early infancy period.
- Those with asthma, heart/lung disease, or diabetes and those with HIV/weakened immune system or chronic kidney/liver diseases can get more likely very sick if they are not vaccine protected.
- Older adults are at higher risk for contracting and developing serious complications due to their weakened immune systems, illnesses such as influenza, invasive pneumococcal disease, and shingles will become vulnerable to infections.
- Vaccines are safe, but vaccine-preventable diseases (VPDs) kill tens of thousands of US adults each year.
- Just like eating wholesome foods and exercising regularly, vaccines play a vital role in helping the immune system and keeping adults healthy.

COMMON ADULT VACCINES AND IMMUNIZATIONS

In recent years, there has been a growing recognition of the importance of adult vaccinations concerning public health. Compared with the complicated and ever-changing recommended vaccine schedule for infants and children, vaccines for adults have been straightforward. All adults should make sure they are up to date on these routine vaccines:

- *Influenza (flu) vaccine:* It is typically recommended for all adults, pregnant women, and including individuals with certain medical conditions.
- Diphtheria, tetanus, and pertussis (*DTP*) is prevented by a childhood vaccine, called DTaP/DTP and a vaccine for adolescents *and adults, called Tdap or Td booster* should be taken every 10 years (Tdp/Td are reduced diphtheria and pertussis adult dose). It should give Tdap in every pregnancy at 27–36 weeks.
- *SARS-CoV-2 vaccine:* COVID-19 vaccines have become a critical part of adult immunization. Booster shots and updates to vaccine recommendations may change over time. Everyone aged 6 months or older needs a dose of the updated COVID-19 vaccine. Specifics of who needs what (and when) depend on what they have already received, as well as their immune status.
- *Pneumococcal vaccine:* Adults over 65, and younger adults with specific health conditions, may need pneumococcal vaccinations.
- *Shingles (herpes zoster) vaccine:* Adults over 50, particularly those aged 60 and older, should consider the shingles vaccine.
- *Hepatitis B vaccine:* Recommended for adults at risk of HepB virus (HBV) infection, such as healthcare workers, people with multiple sexual partners, and those with certain medical conditions. The CDC has updated its guidance for HepB testing for the first time since 2008 and now recommends that all adults in the US be tested for HBV at least once in their lifetime.
- *Measles, mumps, rubella (MMR) vaccine:* Adults born after 1957 who have not had two doses of MMR or do not have evidence of immunity should consider vaccination.
- *Varicella (chickenpox) vaccine:* Adults who have never had chickenpox or the vaccine may need this immunization.
- *Meningococcal vaccine:* Recommended for adults with certain risk factors, such as college students living in dorms and people with compromised immune systems.
- *Hepatitis A vaccine (HAV):* Recommended for travelers to certain countries and people at risk of hepatitis A.
- *Typhoid vaccine:* The typhoid conjugate vaccine is recommended for use in children from 6 months of age and in adults up to 45 years or 65 years (depending on the vaccine).
- *Human papillomavirus vaccine:* Protection works best when the vaccine is given during adolescence. Recommended for adults up to age 45 for certain individuals who have not previously received it.
- *Haemophilus influenzae type b (Hib) vaccine:* Not a routine vaccine; in some cases, adults with certain medical conditions may need this vaccine.
- *RSV and GBS vaccine*—recommended for pregnant mothers to prevent early childhood RSV bronchiolitis. RSV vaccine recommended for adults over 60 years of

age and also give vital details about RSV vaccines and GBS vaccines for pregnant people.
- *Mpox vaccines:* All adults in any age group at increased risk of getting Mpox should get a two-dose series of the vaccine. The mpox vaccine notes include a list of mpox risk factors.

Adults may also need other vaccines, based on:
- Based on their age **(Table 1)**
- Life events, jobs, or travel. These include healthcare workers, pregnancy, international travelers, etc.
- Individual health conditions—type 1 and 2 diabetes, heart or cardiovascular diseases, asplenia without a

TABLE 1: Recommended adult immunization schedule by age groups (CDC, USA 2023) (19–26 years of age, 27–49 years of age, 50–64 years of age, and over 65 years of age).

Vaccines	19–26 years	27–49 years	50–64 years	>65 years
Influenza inactivated—IIV4 or recombinant-RIV4	1 dose, annually	1 dose, annually	1 dose, annually	1 dose, annually
Influenza: Live attenuated influenza (LAIV4)	1 dose, annually →	1 dose, annually	Not applicable	→
Tdap or Td: Tetanus toxoid, adult diphtheria, acellular pertussis	1 dose Tdap each → pregnancy 1 dose Td or Tdp wound management	→	→	→
MMR	1 or 2 doses as needed (if not received in childhood or born in 1957 or later) →	→	→	→
Varicella	1 or 2 doses as needed (if not received in childhood →	→	2 doses for all	2 doses for all
Zoster recombinant RZV®	2 doses for immunocompromised	2 doses for immunocompromised	2 doses for all	2 doses for all
HPV, human papillomavirus	2 or 3 doses	27 through 45 years only		
Pneumococcal PCV15, PCV20, PPSV23	1 dose PCV15 followed by → PPSV23 or 1dose PCV20	→ ←	→ ←	→ ← lack evidence
HepA	2 or 3 doses depending on Vax and risk factors	→ ←	→ ←	→ ← lack evidence
HepB	2, 3, or 4 doses depending on Vax or condition. Lack evidence	→ ←	→ ←	Consider if there is a risk factor
MenACWY	1 or 2 doses depending on risk, travel indications	→ ←	→ ←	→ ←
MenB	19–23 years clinical indication rest	Rest depends on indications, risk and Vax, 2 or 3 doses	Rest depends on indications, risk and Vax, 2 or 3 doses	Rest depends on indications, risk and Vax, 2 or 3 doses
Hib®	2 or 3 doses with additional risk	2 or 3 doses with additional risk	2 or 3 doses with additional risk	2 or 3 doses with additional risk

Note:
- Hib® = Special situations:
  – Anatomical or functional asplenia (including sickle cell disease): 1 dose if previously did not receive Hib; if elective splenectomy, 1 dose, preferably at least 14 days before splenectomy
  – Hematopoietic stem cell transplant (HSCT): 3-dose series 4 weeks apart starting 6–12 months after a successful transplant, regardless of Hib vaccination history
- Zoster recombinant RZV®:
  – *Pregnancy:* There is currently no ACIP recommendation for RZV use in pregnancy. Consider delaying RZV until after pregnancy
  – *Immunocompromising conditions (including HIV):* RZV is recommended for use in persons age at 19 years or older who are or will be immunodeficient or immunosuppressed because of disease or therapy.

(HepA: hepatitis A; HepB: hepatitis B; Hib: haemophilus influenzae type B; MenACWY: meningococcus serogroup A, C, W, Y; MenB: serogroup B meningococcal; MMR: measles, mumps, rubella; PCV: pneumococcal conjugate vaccine; RZV: recombinant zoster vaccine) functioning spleen, lung [chronic obstructive pulmonary disease (COPD)], liver—end-stage renal disease (ESRD) and human immunodeficiency virus (HIV) infections, etc.

RECOMMENDED ADULT VACCINE AND IMMUNIZATION SCHEDULE BY AGE GROUPS

One should always rely on the latest guidance and updates from healthcare authorities and professionals for the most current adult immunization recommendations. To be familiar with this chapter, commonly used vaccine "Trade name" and abbreviated vaccine names are tabulated **(Table 2)**. The use of trade names is for identification purposes only and does not imply endorsement by the Advisory Committee on Immunization Practices (ACIP) or CDC.

METAPHORS OF ADULTS USED VACCINES

Influenza Vaccine (Flu) Vaccine

For the best protection, everyone 6 months and older including pregnant mothers should get vaccinated annually for two reasons. Because:
- Immune protection from vaccination declines over time, so an annual vaccine is needed for optimal protection.
- Flu virus strains are constantly changing, and so flu vaccines need to be updated from one season to the next to protect against the viruses that research suggests and anticipate to be most common during the upcoming flu season.

The best time to get the annual flu vaccine: Just before flu viruses begin spreading in your community; it takes about 2 weeks after vaccination for antibodies to develop in the

TABLE 2: Recommended adult—vaccines; nature, abbreviated, and commonly encountered trade names.

Vaccines	Abbreviation(s)	Trade Name
SARS-CoV-2	COVID 19	mRNA Pfizer, Moderna, AstraZeneca Covishield, Covaxin, etc.
Haemophilus influenzae type b	Hib	ActHIB®; Hiberix®; and PedvaxHIB®
Hepatitis A vaccine	HepA	Havrix®; Vaqta®
Hepatitis A and hepatitis B vaccine	HepA-HepB	Twinrix®
Hepatitis B vaccine	HepB	Engerix-B® Recombivax HB® Heplisav-B®
Human papillomavirus vaccine	HPV	Gardasil 9®
Influenza vaccine (inactivated)	IIV4	Many brands
Influenza vaccine (live, attenuated)	LAIV4	FluMist® Quadrivalent
Quadrivalent Influenza vaccine (recombinant)	RIV4	Flublok® Quadrivalent
Measles, mumps, and rubella vaccine	MMR	M-M-R II®
Meningococcal serogroups A, C, W, Y vaccine	• MenACWY-D • MenACWY-CRM • MenACWY-TT	Menactra® Menveo® MenQuadfi®
Meningococcal serogroup B vaccine	MenB-4C MenB-FHbp	Bexsero® Trumenba®
Pneumococcal 15-valent conjugate vaccine	PCV15	Vaxneuvance™
Pneumococcal 20-valent conjugate vaccine	PCV20	Prevnar20
Pneumococcal 23-valent polysaccharide vaccine	PPSV23	Pneumovax23
Tetanus and diphtheria toxoids	Td	Tenivac® Tdvax™
Tetanus and diphtheria toxoids and acellular pertussis vaccine	Tdap	Adacel® Boostrix®
Varicella vaccine	VAR	Varivax
Zoster vaccine, recombinant	RZV	Shingrix

body and provide protection against flu. CDC recommends that people get a flu vaccine by the end of October. However, vaccinations should continue to be offered throughout the flu season, even into January or later.

The World health organization (WHO) has just announced the recommendations* for the viral composition of influenza vaccines for the 2023–2024 season in the northern hemisphere and major parts of mainland Asia including Indian subcontinents (*egg-based or cell culture and recombinant-based quadrivalent vaccines).

Vax effectiveness (VE) can vary. Studies show that flu vaccination reduces the risk of flu illness by between 40 and 60% when most circulating flu viruses are well-matched to those used to make flu vaccines. Effectiveness depends on the similarity of vaccine strain(s) to the circulating strain(s), the age and health status of the recipient, and the type of vaccine administered.

Duration of vaccine immunity lost <1 year due to antibody waning (poor efficacy) and antigenic drift (minor mutations) that result in a novel strain, annually. In contrast abrupt, major changes (antigenic shift) in surface antigen(s), may lead to a pandemic (rare) the last pandemic was in 2009.

There are three kinds of influenza vaccines (vaccine composition is reviewed and updated each year):
- Inactivated influenza vaccine (IIV)
- Live, attenuated influenza vaccine (LAIV)
- Recombinant influenza vaccine (RIV).

Inactivated influenza vaccine (Afluria, Fluad, Flublok, Flucelvax, FluLaval, Fluarix, Fluvirin, Fluzone, Fluzone high-dose, Fluzone Intradermal): There are various acronyms for inactivated flu vaccines—IIV3, IIV4, RIV3, RIV4, and ccIIV4.

Live attenuated influenza vaccine called FluMist, an egg-based live attenuated flu nasal spray vaccine (FluMist Quadrivalent) made with attenuated (weakened) live flu viruses, which is approved for use in people 2 years through 49 years. This vaccine is not recommended for use in pregnant people, immunocompromised people, or people with certain medical conditions.

A recombinant vaccine is used to prevent infection caused by influenza viruses in adults 18 years of age and older. These are the Fluzone High-Dose Quadrivalent vaccine, Flublok Quadrivalent recombinant flu vaccine, and Fluad Quadrivalent adjuvanted flu vaccine.

All flu vaccines for the 2023–2024 season will be quadrivalent (four-component). Most will be thimerosal-free or thimerosal-reduced vaccines (91%).

The composition of flu vaccines has been updated. Flu vaccines for the US 2023–2024 season will contain the following:

- *Egg-based vaccines:*
  - An A/Victoria/4897/2022 (H1N1) pdm09-like virus
  - An A/Darwin/9/2021 (H3N2)-like virus
  - A B/Austria/1359417/2021 (B/Victoria lineage)-like virus
  - A B/Phuket/3073/2013 (B/Yamagata lineage)-like virus
- *Cell- or recombinant-based vaccines:*
  - An A/Wisconsin/67/2022 (H1N1)pdm09-like virus
  - An A/Darwin/6/2021 (H3N2)-like virus
  - A B/Austria/1359417/2021 (B/Victoria lineage)-like virus
  - A B/Phuket/3073/2013 (B/Yamagata lineage)-like virus.

These recommendations include *one update* compared to the 2022–2023 US flu vaccine composition. The influenza A (H1N1) pdm09 vaccine virus component was updated for egg-based and cell- or recombinant-based flu vaccines.

People with egg allergy may get any vaccine (egg-based or non-egg-based) that is otherwise appropriate for their age and health status. Previously, it was recommended that people with severe allergies to eggs (those who have had any symptom other than hives with egg exposure) be vaccinated in an inpatient or outpatient medical setting.

Beginning with the 2023–2024 season, additional safety measures are no longer recommended for flu vaccination of people with an egg allergy beyond those recommended for receipt of any vaccine, regardless of the severity of previous reaction to egg. All vaccines should be given in settings where allergic reactions can be recognized and treated quickly.

The onset of the winter 2023–2024 influenza season has brought with it a novel threat of the influenza virus, known as the H9N2 subtype of the influenza A virus. It primarily affects birds, particularly poultry, and has been identified in various avian species globally. While human cases are relatively uncommon, instances have been reported, typically resulting from close contact with infected poultry. Indian health authorities are on alert to handle an emergency related to H9N2, and public health preparedness is a dynamic and ongoing process.

According to the Indian Council of Medical Research (ICMR), the H3N2 virus is the predominant flu strain circulating in India during the 2023 flu season. India has two seasonal influenza peaks each year, one from January to March and the other after the monsoon season during winter peak months.

Multiple experts believe that this winter's respiratory season should more closely resemble prepandemic years than last year's, though it may take several years for typical seasonal viral patterns to re-establish.

Universal Flu Vaccine

Thanks to the mRNA vaccine technology boom of the SARSCoV-2 COVID-19 pandemic. Now, scientists hope to use this technology to pioneer yet another first— "a universal flu vaccine" that can protect us against all flu types, not just a select few.

"The mRNA platform is attractive here given its scalability and modularity, where you can mix and match different mRNAs". "It is all about covering the different flavors of flu in a way the current vaccines cannot do".

Annual shots protect against flu subtypes known to spread in humans. But many subtypes circulate in animals, like birds and pigs, and occasionally jump on humans, causing pandemics. The current vaccines provide very little protection against these other subtypes. Experts say that "to make a vaccine that would provide some level of immunity against essentially every influenza subtype we know about", e.g., that's 20 subtypes altogether. The unique properties of mRNA vaccines make immune responses against all those antigens possible (Scott Hensley Ph.D., a professor of microbiology at UPenn).

The National Institutes of Health has launched the phase I clinical trial of a novel universal influenza vaccine candidate BPL-1357 to study its safety and efficacy in healthy adult volunteers, aged 18–55 years. The single-site trial will be carried out at the NIH Clinical Center in Bethesda, Maryland.

BPL-1357 is an inactivated, whole-virus vaccine and contains four strains of avian influenza viruses:
1. A/Environment /Maryland/261/2006 H7N3
2. A/Mallard /Maryland/802/2007 H5N1
3. A/Pintail/Ohio /339/1987 H3N8
4. A/Mallard/Ohio /265/1987 H1N9).

In preclinical studies, the vaccine was protective against the six different influenza virus strains, including subtypes that were not included in the vaccine.

SARS-CoV-2 Vaccine

2 plus 1 booster for all adult vaccinees; underscores the substantial enhancement of viral immunity achievable by any kind of COVID vaccine including Indian home breed CoviShield through a third booster injection, which is particularly advantageous for healthcare professionals who face heightened exposure risks. In Oct 2023, the US CDC launched a campaign urging people to get their annual "flu shots and the new "bivalent" updated mRNA boosters" shots at the same time, including for pregnant women and children.

January 2024 Updated: The COVID-19 vaccine note embraces the updated 2023–2024 formula. Everyone aged 6 months or older needs a dose of the updated COVID-19 vaccine. Specifics of who needs what (and when) depend on what they have already received, as well as their immune status. Detailed recommendations for both mRNA and protein-based adjuvanted versions are included in the notes.

We need to be up to date on vaccines and boosters because those seem to reduce the risk for long COVID.

Tdap (Tetanus Toxoid, Reduced Dose Diphtheria Toxoid, and Acellular Pertussis)

One dose (Tdap) to be taken every 10 years till the age of 65. This can be administered in place of the Td vaccine. Recommended for everyone, especially individuals with weakened immune systems.

There are many acellular pertussis component-combo vaccines, e.g.:
- DTaP (Daptacel, Infanrix)
- Tdap (Adacel, Boostrix) containing tetanus toxoid, reduced diphtheria toxoid, and acellular pertussis vaccine
- DTaP-IPV (Kinrix, Quadracel)
- DTaP-HepB-IPV (Pediarix)
- DTaP-IPV/Hib (Pentacel)
- DTaP-IPV-Hib-HepB (Vaxelis).

■ TYPHOID VACCINE

Typhoid conjugate vaccine, consisting of the purified Vi antigen linked to a carrier protein, is given as a single injectable dose in children from 6 months of age and in adults up to 45 years or 65 years (depending on the vaccine).

Two typhoid conjugate vaccines have been pre-qualified by WHO since December 2017 and are being introduced into childhood immunization programs in typhoid-endemic countries.

Two additional vaccines have been used for many years in older children and adults at risk of typhoid, including travelers. These vaccines do not provide long-lasting immunity (requiring repeat or booster doses) and are not approved for children younger than 2 years old:

There is a live attenuated oral vaccine in capsule formulation for people aged over 6 years.

Pneumococcal Vaccines

There are two types: a conjugate vaccine consisting of 7 variant strains, 13 variant strains, 15 variant strains, 20 variant strains, etc., and a polysaccharide vaccine containing 23 variant strains of the pneumococcus bacteria (PPSV23). Recommended, once an individual turns 50 years and those living with chronic illness, sickle cell disease, cochlear implants, transplanted organs, and immunosuppressed people should consider taking this vaccine.

The old recommendation was complicated and confusing. The new one is much more straightforward, *"Fryhofer, an internist in Atlanta, told ID Medical News—now there are only two options"*—(1) a two-vaccine series of PCV15 (vaxneuvance), in combination with the already familiar PPSV23 polysaccharide vaccine (pneumovax 23), and (2) a single dose of the new PCV20, Prevnar 20".

Meningococcal Vaccines (MenACWY and Serogroup B Vaccine)

These are of either polysaccharide versus conjugated types. In adults with anatomic or functional asplenia or complement component/deficiency, microbiologists routinely exposed to isolates of *Neisseria meningitides*.

The first and only pentavalent PENBRAYA (5-in-1) MenABCWY vaccine is approved for use and indicated for active immunization to prevent invasive disease caused by *Neisseria meningitidis* serogroups A, B, C, W, and Y.

PENBRAYA is approved for use in individuals 10 through 25 years of age.

The safety and effectiveness of PENBRAYA have not been established in pregnant individuals. Individuals with certain complement deficiencies and individuals receiving treatment that inhibits terminal complement activation are at increased risk for invasive disease caused by *N. meningitidis* groups A, B, C, W, and Y, even if they develop antibodies following vaccination with PENBRAYA.

Guillain-Barré syndrome (GBS) has been reported in temporal relationships following the administration of another US-licensed meningococcal quadrivalent polysaccharide conjugate vaccine. The decision by the healthcare professional to administer PENBRAYA to individuals with a history of GBS should take into account the expected benefits and potential risks.

Measles, Mumps, and Rubella Vaccine Components

People who have not gotten their MMR vaccine and have never had measles should receive two doses of MMR vaccine or one dose of measles followed by one dose of MMR vaccine. It is a live vaccine and hence pregnant women are not given this vaccine. Also, people with HIV or AIDS, Onco-Hemo blood disorders, and those immunosuppressed are to avoid it.

Mpox Vaccine

Mpox, formerly known as monkeypox, had spread rapidly in the third year of the COVID-19 pandemic when awareness of public health was at a maximum. After a year in which nearly 90,000 people got infected with mpox, and 140 people died, the WHO downgraded the disease in May 2023 from its status as a global health emergency. By mid-December 2023, the WHO was sounding the mpox alarm again that an epidemic of mpox in the Democratic Republic of Congo (DRC) could spread internationally as it had detected a rise in sexual transmissions.

During the global outbreak that began in 2022, the virus mostly spread through sexual contact while mpox can be transmitted sexually, experts do not describe the disease as a sexually transmitted infection (STI). But sex is one of the main transmission routes. The WHO's official states that mpox is spread by close contact with an infected person. That includes talking and breathing near an infected person—via "droplets" as we learned during the COVID pandemic, but also via sexual activity.

There is an antiviral medication called tecovirimat SIGA, which is used to treat monkeypox, cowpox, and smallpox—the latter is an eradicated disease. Tecovirimat interferes with a protein (called VP37) found on the surface of the virus and slows down its ability to spread.

There are three vaccines against mpox—derived through research into smallpox.

Currently, the WHO does not advise mass vaccination against mpox. It is only people who are at risk, i.e., those who have close contact with an infected person—including but not limited to sexual partners and healthcare workers.

The CDC recommends two doses of the JYNNEOS vaccine to prevent monkeypox.

The second dose should be given 28 days after the first dose but can be given up to 35 days later (subcutaneous or intradermal doses).

The vaccine should be administered within four days of exposure to prevent the disease. If administered up to 14 days after exposure, the vaccine may not prevent the disease but could reduce symptoms.

The CDC/WHO also recommends:
- Primary preventive (preexposure) vaccination for individuals at high risk of exposure, i.e., gay, bisexual, and other men who have sex with men (MSM) with multiple sexual partners are at the highest risk of exposure.
- People with immune system-related illnesses, such as HIV, and infants younger than 12 months should not receive ACAM2000.

Varicella (Chickenpox) Vaccine

It is also a live-attenuated vaccine (LAV) hence all the precautions and contraindications like the MMR vaccines. All adults without evidence of immunity to varicella or previous infection should receive two doses of single-antigen vaccine or the second dose of single-antigen vaccine if they have received only one dose.

Herpes Zoster or Shingles Vaccine

There are two kinds of herpes zoster or shingles vaccine include (1) single dose Zostavax vaccine for >60 years and (2) a two dose Shingrix vaccine is a significantly better vaccine, and you can now get that even if.

The single dose of Zostavax is a lyophilized preparation of the OKA strain of live attenuated varicella-zoster virus (VZV). The vaccine could potentially cause necrotizing retinitis. No longer available for use in the United States, as of November 18, 2020 and is now discontinued.

The two doses of recombinant and adjuvanted Shingrix are recommended for adults aged 50 and over.

The Shingrix (recombinant and adjuvanted vaccines)—this vaccine also protects from postherpetic neuralgia, which is a complication that brings about burning pain after the symptoms of shingles subside. CDC recommends two doses of Shingrix separated by 2–6 months for immunocompetent adults aged 50 years and older.

The zoster vaccine now is recommended for use in everyone aged 19 years and older who is or will be immunodeficient or immunosuppressed through disease or therapy. The new purple color bar reflects ACIP's new two-dose series regimen for immunocompromised adults aged 19–49

Should consider Shingrix:
- Whether or not they report a prior episode of herpes zoster.
- Whether or not they report a prior dose of Zostavax, a shingles vaccine that is no longer available for use in the United States.
- It is not necessary to screen, either verbally or by laboratory serology, for evidence of prior varicella.
- Shingrix, can be administered concomitantly, at different anatomic sites, with other adult vaccines, including COVID-19 vaccines. Coadministration of RSV with adjuvanted influenza vaccine (Fluad) and COVID-19 vaccines is being studied.
- Another difference is that Shingrix is injected into the muscle while Zostavax is injected underneath the skin.

Who should get it—all adults above 50 years of age should get this vaccine. People who have had chicken pox should also get this vaccine, even people who have already had shingles should get the Herpes Zoster Vaccine.

Human Papillomavirus Vaccination

There is a lack of knowledge on the HPV, which is the main cause of cervical cancer, in several regions of India. Cervical cancer has witnessed a concerning rise in India, raising alarm bells within the public health sector. The number of cancer cases in the country is projected to go up from 14.6 lakh in 2022 to 15.7 lakh in 2025, according to the ICMR-National Cancer Registry Program (NCRP).

One primary reason is the lack of awareness and education regarding cervical cancer and its preventive measures and a general ignorance of the significance of routine screenings and vaccines.

The HPV vaccination is recommended for all persons through age 26 years: two- or three-dose series depending on age at initial vaccination or condition.

The HPV vaccine safeguards from a series of infections that can lead to cervical, vulvar, and vaginal cancer in women and penile cancer in men. HPV can also lead to anal cancer, genital warts, and throat cancer.

- *Age 15 years or older at initial vaccination:* Three-dose series at 0, 1–2 months, 6 months (*minimum intervals: dose 1 to dose 2: 4 weeks/dose 2 to dose 3: 12 weeks/dose 1 to dose 3: 5 months; repeat dose if administered too soon*).
  - *Age 9–14 years* at initial vaccination and received 1 dose or 2 doses <5 months apart: 1 additional dose
  - *Age 9–14 years* at initial vaccination and received two doses at least 5 months apart: HPV vaccination series complete, no additional dose needed.

Interrupted schedules: If the vaccination schedule is interrupted, the series does not need to be restarted:
- No additional dose is recommended when any HPV vaccine series has been completed using the recommended dosing intervals.
- *Some adults aged 27–45 years:* Based on shared clinical decision-making, two- or three-dose series as above.

Special Situations

- Age ranges recommended above for routine and catchup vaccination, or shared clinical decision-making also apply in special situations.
- *Immunocompromising conditions, including HIV infection:* Three-dose series, even for those who initiate vaccination at age 9 through 14 years.
- *Pregnancy testing is not needed* before vaccination; HPV vaccination is not recommended until after pregnancy; no intervention is needed if inadvertently vaccinated while pregnant.

Maternal Respiratory Syncytial Virus

Two RSV vaccines are available for adults including pregnant women. Arexvy is made by GSK (formerly GlaxoSmithKline) and Abrysvo™ is made by Pfizer. Both vaccines are made of a single surface protein from the virus, called protein F.

The RSV vaccines do not contain a whole virus or a live virus and are safe for pregnant mothers including people with cancer who are eligible to get the shot. Nonlive vaccines contain a part of the RSV virus (called a protein F). The RSV vaccine cannot cause an infection in people with a weakened immune system.

- Pregnant people can receive this vaccine to help protect their infant after birth. 1 dose of maternal RSV vaccine during weeks 32 through 36 of pregnancy, administered immediately before or during RSV season. Abrysvo is the only RSV vaccine recommended during pregnancy.
- This protection is especially important during the baby's first 6 months when they are at high risk for severe RSV.
- Contact your care team if you have questions about whether you should get the vaccine.
- Older adults are at high risk for severe disease. This includes those with heart and lung disease or weakened immune systems. Adults and elderly 60 years or older, should talk to your ID staff in vaccinology for RSV vaccine eligibility.

In addition to Pfizer's maternal RSV vaccine, the FDA in July 2023 approved AstraZeneca's monoclonal antibody nirsevimab (Beyfortus) for the prevention of RSV in neonates and infants entering their first RSV season, and in children up to 24 months who remain vulnerable to severe RSV disease through their second RSV season.

NO Polio Booster Needs for Adults

If people have already gotten their childhood four polio doses of OPV and/or IPV childhood immunization, CDC/WHO does not recommend a booster polio doses for adults. *"The childhood polio vaccine generates strong and durable T-cell immunity against polio and durable memory B-cells".* This helps protect most people against severe disease for a lifetime.

ADENO, ANTHRAX, DENGUE, GROUP B STREPTOCOCCUS, AND ALSO VACCINES AGAINST MALARIAL PARASITES

Adults may need other vaccines such as adeno, anthrax, dengue, GBS, and also vaccines against malarial parasites based on:

Human Adenovirus Vaccine

Currently, there is no human adenovirus (AdHu) vaccine available for the general public.

A live, oral vaccine against AdHu types 4 and 7 is approved by the U.S. FDA military personnel ages 17 through 50 who may be at higher risk for infection from these two adenovirus types. One dose of Two tablets (1 of adenovirus type 4 and 1 of adenovirus type 7), orally.

Comments:
- Tablets should be swallowed whole, without chewing, to avoid releasing the virus in the upper respiratory tract.
- Postpone for vomiting and/or diarrhea; vaccine effectiveness depends upon viral multiplication within the intestinal tract.

The vaccine is recommended by the US Department of Defense for military recruits entering basic training to prevent acute respiratory disease. It may also be recommended for other military personnel at high risk for adenovirus infection.

Anthrax Vaccine

Anthrax bacillus anthracis is a disease of animals, both domestic and wild. Transmission of anthrax is animal-soil-animal transmission through direct inoculation of spores in skin breach, inhalation of spores, and ingestion of contaminated food. Usually, the prevalence among Asian countries is much higher. Anthrax has gained its importance because of biological warfare.

There is a vaccine to prevent anthrax, but it is not typically available to the general public. Anyone who is at increased risk of being exposed to anthrax, including certain military personnel, laboratory workers, and some people who handle animals or animal products (such as veterinarians who handle infected animals), may get the vaccine.

In 1881, Louis Pasteur successfully developed an anthrax vaccine. Later in 1935, Max Stern developed attenuated live vaccine, which is used in livestock; but it is not safe for human use because of virulence. At present, the ACIP recommends five doses of AVA (anthrax vaccine adsorbed). Primary dose of 0.5 mL intramuscular (IM) at 0, 4 weeks, and later 6, 12, and 18 months (preexposure prophylaxis) followed by annual booster dose. This vaccine is recommended for unvaccinated people, but those exposed to anthrax should be given three subcutaneous doses. First one as soon as possible, second and third doses at 2nd and 4th week after the first dose. In pregnant women, the timeline will be the same with subcutaneous administration.

Chikungunya Virus Vaccine

The chikungunya virus (CHIKV) is an "emerging global health threat" due to its growing prevalence and geographic range. The CHIKV disease has been associated with an increased risk of death in adults after symptom onset, including deaths from cerebrovascular diseases, ischemic heart diseases, and diabetes. This highlights the need for equitable access to approved vaccines and effective anti-CHIKV therapeutics and reinforces the importance of robust vector-control efforts to reduce viral transmission.

The US Food and Drug Administration (FDA) recently (Nov 2023) greenlit the first CHIKV vaccine "Ixchiq" (Valneva Austria), for adults at risk of exposure to the virus. The company (Valneva's) will focus on selling the first-in-class vaccine to US travelers heading to countries in the tropics and subtropics where the disease is endemic.

Ixchiq is a single-dose vaccine that contains a live, weakened version of the CHIKV. It may cause symptoms in vaccine recipients similar to those experienced by people who have CHIKV illness.

In its approval, the FDA noted that transmission of CHIKV to newborn babies from pregnant individuals with viremia at delivery has been reported and can cause severe, potentially fatal CHIKV in newborns. The prescribing information includes a warning to inform that it is not known if the vaccine virus can be transmitted from pregnant individuals to newborns, nor is it known if the vaccine virus can cause any adverse effects in the newborn.

Dengue Virus

An important mosquito-borne (*Aedes aegypti* and *Aedes albopictus*) viral disease, caused by four viral serotypes—dengue virus (DENV) V1–V4. It is endemic in tropic and subtropic (at least in 100 countries), often when the rainfall is optimum for mosquito breeding. The WHO estimates 50–100 million infections, including 5 lakh dengue hemorrhagic fever and 22,000 deaths happen among children. The majority of dengue dengue-infected patients may not be symptomatic but can infect mosquitoes after entry into the blood meal. It requires 8–10 days for transmission to another host. In rare cases, it can be transmitted by organ transplant or blood transfusion and vertical transmission.

Indian Dengue Scenarios: Even though the DENV was isolated in 1945 in Calcutta, no vaccine is available yet on the market. A LAV known as Dengvaxia, developed by Sanofi, was licensed in 2015. Following this, long-term follow-up of the Sanofi phase III efficacy trial participants has revealed potential safety concerns. However, this vaccine appears to predispose dengue-naïve recipients to an increased risk of hospitalization. It is recommended by the WHO that DENV vaccination is recommended only for adults with a history of prior DENV infection.

Also, following DENV infection with one type, there is short-lived immunity and cross-protection against disease caused by the other three DENV types. Ideally, any candidate vaccine should produce protective immunity against all four DENV types (tetravalent immunity).

The DENV vaccine must be administered as a three-shot series over a period of 6 months (at 0, 6, and 12 months) to children and adults between the ages of 9 and 45 years old, with a history of prior dengue infection or serological testing for past dengue infection. At least seven DENV vaccines have undergone different phases of clinical trials; however, only three of them (Dengvaxia®, TV003, and TAK-003) have shown promising results.

India is poised now to test out two different dengue vaccine candidates in clinical trials—an LAV, TetraVax-DV, and a recombinant protein-based vaccine, DSV4 can India afford to rule out prior infection in every case before recommending the routine administration of the DENV vaccine is the only major concern!? Since waning immunity might also increase the risk for severe disease in vaccine recipients, the aim should be only to have long-lived vaccine-induced protective.

Japanese Encephalitis Virus (JEV) Vaccine

Japanese encephalitis virus (JEV) belonging to the RNA family Flaviviridae is transmitted to humans through the bite of infected *Culex* species mosquitoes, particularly *Culex* tritaeniorhynchus. The virus is maintained in a cycle between mosquitoes and vertebrate hosts, primarily pigs, and wading birds (also referred to as amplifying hosts or natural reservoirs).

When a mosquito bites an animal (such as pigs or waterbirds) that has the JEV virus and then this mosquito bites a human. Humans are not able to give the JEV to other humans.

The JEV is a public health problem, not only for Asia but for the entire world. However, JE incidence may be rising throughout India because the disease may go largely unobserved, and clinical awareness is typically noticed only after outbreaks. Whether these vaccines will translate into a reduced disease burden remains to be seen.

The JEV risk areas and transmission season in India are Andhra Pradesh, Arunachal Pradesh, Assam, Bihar, Goa, Haryana, Jharkhand, Karnataka, Kerala, Maharashtra, Manipur, Meghalaya, Nagaland, Odisha, Punjab, Tamil Nadu, Telangana, Tripura, Uttar Pradesh, Uttarakhand, and West Bengal. Peak season May–November, especially in northern India; the season may be extended or year-round in some areas, especially in southern India.

India launched a vaccine to prevent JE on October 4, 2013. The Vero cell-derived purified inactivated JE vaccine—JENVAC, which received manufacturing and marketing approvals from the Drug Controller General of India, is the first vaccine to be manufactured in the public-private partnership mode between the ICMR and Bharat Biotech. It is administered in a two-dose schedule to children 1 year of age onwards. The second dose is given at least 4 weeks after the first dose. In the clinical trials, JENVAC showed superior safety and immunogenicity, in comparison to live vaccine. It met all its primary and secondary endpoints in the age group of 1–50 years, after 1 or 2 doses of vaccination.

The inactivated Vero cell culture-derived JEV (manufactured as IXIARO) is the only JEV licensed and available in the United States. Given as a two-dose series, with the doses spaced 28 days apart. Adults aged 18–65 years can get the second dose as early as 7 days after the first dose. The last dose should be given at least 1 week before travel. A booster dose (third dose) should be given if a person has received the two-dose primary vaccination series 1 year or more previously and there is a continued risk for JEV infection or potential for reexposure. For adults and children aged 3 years or older, each dose of IXIARO is 0.5 mL. For children aged 2 months through 2 years, each dose is 0.25 mL.

Reactions to IXIARO are generally mild and include pain and tenderness, mild headaches, myalgia (muscle aches), and low-grade fevers.

Yellow Fever Vaccine

Yellow fever (YF) does not occur in India. Yet, the conditions for transmission of YF are very conducive in India, e.g., presence of mosquito vectors in abundance and susceptible population. The government of India has been following a strict YF vaccination program to prevent the entry of YF in India.

900 million people in 44 endemic countries are at risk for YF (Africa, 31 countries; Latin America, 13 countries).

YF is difficult to diagnose, especially during the early stages; it can be confused with severe malaria, dengue or other hemorrhagic fevers, leptospirosis, viral hepatitis, and other conditions, as well as poisoning.

Yellow fever vaccine is an LAV vaccine that has been available since the 1930s. No vaccine efficacy studies have been performed with YF vaccine. However, the number of YF disease cases was substantially reduced following the introduction of the vaccine supporting it being protective in humans. A single dose provides lifelong immunity. it should be taken 10–14 days before travel to endemic areas (Refer to immunization section).

Yellow fever vaccine is recommended for persons aged ≥9 months who are traveling to or living in areas at risk for YF virus transmission in South America and Africa. YF vaccine may be required for entry into certain countries.

Individuals traveling to and from YF endemic countries (countries where YF disease persists) are required to have a "Valid Yellow Fever Vaccination Certificate" issued by authorized and designated vaccination centers in India.

India has no risk for YF and the CDC has no recommendations for travelers to receive the YF vaccine before going to India.

Zika Virus Vaccine

The challenges in developing a safe and effective vaccine include limiting side effects such as GBS, a potential consequence of Zika virus infection. The Zika virus is a mosquito-borne virus that can cause various health issues, including birth defects in infants born to mothers who were infected during pregnancy.

Efforts to develop a Zika virus vaccine were underway, but progress can change rapidly in the field of medical research.

Malarial Vaccines

In a significant stride toward combating malaria, the WHO has approved the R21/Matrix-M malaria vaccine, jointly developed by the University of Oxford in the United Kingdom and the Serum Institute of India. The R21/Matrix-M vaccine, aimed at curbing the transmission of this life-threatening disease carried by certain mosquito species, is expected to be accessible to the public by mid-2024.

The first approved vaccine for malaria is RTS, S known by the brand name Mosquirix. As of April 2023, the vaccine has been given to 1.5 million children living in areas with moderate-to-high malaria transmission. It requires at least three doses in infants by age 2, and a fourth dose extends the protection for another 1–2 years. The vaccine reduces hospital admissions from severe malaria by around 30%.

Research continues with other malaria vaccines. The most effective malaria vaccine is the R21/Matrix-M, with a 77% efficacy rate shown in initial trials and significantly higher antibody levels than with the RTS, S vaccine which is the first vaccine that meets the WHO goal of a malaria vaccine with at least 75% efficacy.

In a significant stride toward combating malaria, the WHO has approved the R21/Matrix-M malaria vaccine, jointly developed by the University of Oxford in the United Kingdom and the Serum Institute of India. The R21/Matrix-M vaccine, aimed at curbing the transmission of this life-threatening disease carried by certain mosquito species, is expected to be accessible to the public by mid-2024.

■ CONCLUSION

Active participation in adult vaccination programs is crucial for public health and community well-being. Despite the heavier burden of IDs among adults across, most pronouncedly in developing countries including India, vaccines recommended for adults are not widely used. Adult immunization is selective, not universal, different vaccines have different target groups. There are social and cultural deterrents; adults are harder to reach through the public health system and hence vaccination of this age group becomes difficult. You should always consult an infectious diseases physician before vaccination to ensure you receive the appropriate vaccines based on age, health conditions, and lifestyle.

Certainly, adults too need to boost the efficacy of childhood vaccines and aid immunity for newer concurrent medical conditions and morbidities. Adult immunization and boosting afford protection when immunity is suppressed due to acquired illnesses. There is a limited perception on the part of the healthcare providers and beneficiaries that adult vaccine-preventable diseases are significant health problems. By getting vaccinated, adults contribute to the overall community herd immunity which helps protect those who may be more vulnerable, such as individuals with compromised immune systems or allergies to vaccines.

Vaccinations are now for noncommunicable diseases (NCD) on the horizon! Like traditional vaccines, NCD vaccines work by modulating the human immune system, but they target the cells, proteins, or other molecules that are associated with the NCD in question rather than pathogens or pathogen-infected cells. These aspects are discussed in details in our book Chapter 12 NCD.

■ SUGGESTED READING

1. CDC. (2022). Use of Recombinant Zoster Vaccine in Immunocompromised Adults Aged ≥19 Years: Recommendations of the Advisory Committee on Immunization Practices — United States, 2022. Available from: http://www.cdc.gov/mmwr/volumes/71/wr/mm7103a2.htm [Last accessed April, 2024].
2. CDC. (2023). What Vaccines are Recommended for You. Available from: https://www.cdc.gov/vaccines/adults/rec-vac/index.html#other [Last accessed April, 2024].
3. CDC. (2024). Updates to the ACIP Flu Vaccine Recommendations for the 2023-2024 season. Available from: https://www.cdc.gov/flu/season/faq-flu-season-2023-2024.htm [Last accessed April, 2024].
4. Cerqueira-Silva T, Pescarini JM, Cardim LL, Leyrat C, Whitaker H, Antunes de Brito CA, et al. Risk of death following chikungunya virus disease in the 100 million Brazilian Cohort, 2015-18: a matched cohort study and self-controlled case series. Lancet Infect Dis. 2024: S1473-3099(23)00739-9.
5. Kulkarni R, Sapkal GN, Kaushal H, Mourya DT. Japanese Encephalitis: a Brief Review on Indian Perspectives. Open Virol J. 2018;12:121-30.
6. Medscape. (2024). One Step Closer to Universal Flu Protection. Available from: https://www.medscape.com/viewarticle/985832 [Last accessed April, 2024].

CHAPTER 7

Pregnancy and Lactation Periods' Vaccinations

■ INTRODUCTION

Immunizing pregnant women to protect the mother, fetus, and infant from infection has increasingly been used over the last decade. Protection against newborn infections are protected mainly by maternal antibodies transferred transcendently both during pregnancy or after delivery via breastfeeding. Both the transplacental- and breast milk-(BM)-derived maternal antibodies function as the primary source of protection against IDs in neonates during the first vulnerable weeks of life.

During recent ID outbreaks [influenza, severe acute respiratory syndrome coronavirus 2 (SARS-CoV-2), pertussis, and Zika] and for other IDs [cytomegalovirus (CMV) and Guillain–Barré syndrome (GBS)], and pregnant women are increasingly identified as an important target for vaccination. For some of these diseases, vaccines are already on the market and recommended during pregnancy. For others, vaccines are currently under development; furthermore, some are even specifically designed to be administered during pregnancy.

This chapter's guidance for vaccine recommendations in pregnant and breastfeeding women dealt with the following aspects, for example, the practice of vaccinating pregnant individuals to protect both the mother and the developing fetus from certain IDs. Vaccines recommended for pregnant individuals have undergone rigorous testing to ensure their safety during pregnancy and breastfeeding periods. Yes, it is safe to get the vaccines recommended during pregnancy except for live attenuated vaccines (LAV).

■ HIGHLIGHTS

- Women of reproductive age should be screened for their immunization status and any indicated immunizations should be administered according to published adult immunization schedules.
- All LAV should be avoided during pregnancy unless the risk of disease exposure exceeds the potential risk of immunization.
- In general, inactivated vaccine immunizations present a low risk for adverse outcomes in pregnant women and their offspring.
- Except for yellow fever and smallpox, LAV vaccines are relatively contraindicated in pregnancy.
- Maternal immunization has been demonstrated to be a safe and effective strategy for protecting both pregnant women and their infants from severe vaccine-preventable diseases, including SARS-CoV-2, influenza, and pertussis.
- Tetanus toxoid, diphtheria toxoid, and acellular pertussis (Tdap) is recommended in every pregnancy, between 27 and 36 weeks of gestation.
- Influenza vaccine is recommended in each pregnancy and can be administered in any trimester.
- RSV vaccine is recommended for during pregnancy at 32–36 weeks' gestation.
- GBS vaccine is now added for during pregnancy.
- Other vaccines may be indicated in special circumstances due to medical comorbidities, travel, or workplace exposures.
- Smallpox and yellow fever vaccines should be avoided in pregnant women unless the risk of disease exceeds the risk of immunization. All other vaccines are safe to administer to breastfeeding women.
- To increase the uptake of vaccines, prenatal care providers should strongly recommend, stock, and administer vaccines in their offices.
- Many vaccines are recommended for breastfeeding individuals and are generally considered safe.

September 27th, 2023: A query on Pediatric Oncall Journal was answered in the expertise category of "Vaccine".

"Hello Sir, I need your advice for my obstetric patient 19-year-old primigravid woman GA 20 weeks plus. What vaccinations are safe and needed for her as her childhood immunization records are not available"?

Author's response:

The World Health Organization (WHO), Advisory Committee on Immunization Practices (ACIP), and

American College of Obstetricians and Gynecologists (ACOG) recommend that pregnant women get two vaccines during every pregnancy—the inactivated flu shot (not the live nasal flu vaccine) and also the Tdap vaccines.

Flu shots can be given during any trimester of pregnancy because the influenza virus poses a danger to pregnant people. Flu shot prevents serious maternal flu illnesses and protects newborns during the first few months of life when they are most vulnerable to influenza infections.

Also, pregnant individuals receive Tdap during the 27th through 36th week of each pregnancy, preferably during the earlier part of this period. This time frame is recommended because it provides the most protection for the pregnant woman and the fetus. It also maximizes the antibodies present in the newborn at birth to protect from pertussis.

Experts now recommend that coronavirus disease 2019 (COVID-19) vaccination shots should be given during any trimester to maintain maternal and fetal health. Scientific studies to date have shown no safety concerns for babies born to people who were vaccinated against COVID-19 during pregnancy.

To conclude, it is strongly advised to screen this mother for rubella antibody [immunoglobulin G (IgG)] serology soon after her delivery. Seronegative mothers are not immune to rubella and should receive the postpartum measles, mumps, and rubella (MMR) vaccination to prevent congenital rubella syndrome (CRS) occurrence in future pregnancy.

MATERNAL VACCINATION

Maternal vaccination is generally considered safe for both the pregnant individual and the developing fetus. The benefits of vaccination in preventing serious infections usually outweigh the potential risks.

Pregnant individuals with well-documented, age-appropriate vaccination against MMR should not be revaccinated, even if serology test results show a negative or equivocal titer. Rubella testing is routinely ordered as part of a prenatal panel, which is a group of tests used to find infections and other problems early in pregnancy. As part of this panel, rubella testing is used to check the pregnant person for immunity to rubella.

Serology testing can be performed to determine immunization status and help determine whether vaccination is required. Rubella IgG serology testing should be used for assessing rubella immunity, including before and/or after pregnancy.

Generally, if patients do not know whether they have been vaccinated against MMR, the Centers for Disease Control and Prevention (CDC) recommends revaccination without serology testing.

Maternal immunization is an important approach to prevent serious infections in newborns in the first few weeks of life until they can start receiving their vaccinations. Appropriate vaccination can prevent serious complications from IDs for pregnant women, the fetus, and newborns.

This stratagem can provide passive immunity to newborns, as antibodies produced by the mother's immune system in response to the vaccine can be transferred transplacentally to the developing fetus. In this way, maternal immunizations protect newborns during the first few months of life when they are most vulnerable to infections. This is especially important for diseases such as pertussis, which can be life-threatening for infants.

Common vaccines given to pregnant individuals include the influenza (flu) vaccine and the Tdap vaccine. The flu vaccine is typically administered during flu season, while the Tdap vaccine is recommended during each pregnancy, ideally between weeks 27 and 36, to protect against pertussis. Both the flu and Tdap vaccines are safe and effective for pregnant individuals and their babies.

The US CDC and professional medical organizations, including the ACOG and the Society for Maternal–Fetal Medicine, strongly recommend COVID-19 vaccination at any point in pregnancy, as well as booster doses when it is time to get one.

- The vaccines recommended for maternal immunization can vary by region and may change over time.
- It is essential for individuals who are pregnant or planning to become pregnant to stay informed about the latest guidance from healthcare professionals and public health authorities.
- The decision to receive vaccines during pregnancy should be based on individual circumstances and health considerations.
- The timing of maternal immunization is crucial. Healthcare providers typically recommend specific windows during pregnancy when these vaccines should be administered to maximize the transfer of protective antibodies to the fetus.

TABLE 1: Immunization recommendations for pregnant mom and during lactation.

Vaccines	Indicated during every pregnancy	In certain people may be given during pregnancy	Contraindicated during pregnancy	Can be given postpartum or when breastfeeding or both
COVID-19	Explained as further			
Flu inactivated	Yes			Yes
Tdap	Yes			Yes
Pneumococcal		Yes		Yes
GBS				
MenACYW and serogroup B		Yes		Yes
HAV		Yes		Yes
HBV		Yes		Yes
HPV				Yes
MMR			Yes	Yes
Varicella			Yes	Yes
RSV	Yes			

(COVID-19: coronavirus disease 2019; GBS: Guillain–Barré syndrome; HAV: hepatitis A virus; HBV: hepatitis B virus; HPV: human papillomavirus; MenACYW: meningococcal conjugate; MMR: measles–mumps–rubella; RSV: respiratory syncytial virus; Tdap: tetanus toxoid, adult dose diphtheria toxoid, and acellular pertussis)

Public health agencies and medical organizations also regularly update their guidelines on the following table may be used to find a "general" recommendation for vaccinating a pregnant woman with a particular vaccine. It is essential to stay informed about the latest updated recommendations **(Table 1)**.

COVID-19 Vaccine Recommended for Pregnant Women

- Pregnant individuals are at a higher risk of experiencing severe illness if they contract COVID-19 and studies have shown a significant risk of transplacental and/or vertical transmission to the fetus and the newborn during the delivery process.

Unvaccinated women who contract COVID-19 during pregnancy are at increased risk for pregnancy loss and neonatal death. Unlike numerous pathogens that kill the fetus by infecting it directly, SARS-CoV-2 causes "widespread and severe" destruction of the placenta that deprives the fetus of oxygen. A team of 44 researchers in 12 countries concluded after examining 64 stillbirths and four neonatal deaths in which the placentas were infected with the virus. Therefore, vaccination during pregnancy can protect moms from getting very sick from COVID-19. Overall, maternal immunization against COVID-19 has been an important tool in protecting pregnant individuals and their infants from the potential risks of COVID-19.

Antibodies generated by the vaccinated mother can be transferred to the fetus through the placenta and to the infant through BM, providing a degree of passive immunity during the critical early months of life. Maternal messenger ribonucleic acid (mRNA) COVID-19 vaccination was associated with a lower risk of Omicron infection among infants aged ≤6 months only if the vaccine was given during the antenatal period.

Further, "if corroborated by other studies that the lower risk was only maintained in infants when their mothers were vaccinated during pregnancy may suggest a need for maternal SARS-CoV-2 vaccination at each pregnancy similar to current recommendations for maternal influenza and pertussis vaccination", the authors concluded.

Pregnant individuals who received a booster dose had substantially more antibodies against SARS-CoV-2, both in their blood and in their cord blood, suggesting that boosting also increased their newborns' immune defenses against COVID-19.

Multiple studies and real-world data have shown that COVID-19 vaccines, such as those developed by Pfizer-BioNTech, Moderna, Johnson & Johnson, and others, are generally safe for pregnant individuals. The vaccines have undergone rigorous testing to ensure their safety and efficacy. For those who have not been vaccinated, they may receive any COVID-19 vaccine products available to them.

- mRNA or Novavax vaccines are preferred over the J&J/Janssen COVID-19 vaccine for primary series, additional doses (for immunocompromised persons), and for booster vaccination.
- Professional medical organizations, including the ACOG and the Society for Maternal–Fetal Medicine, recommend COVID-19 vaccination at any point in pregnancy. Vaccination can be given during any trimester to maintain maternal and fetal health.
- Pregnant women exposed to the mRNA COVID-19 vaccine before 12 weeks of gestation did not have an increased risk of congenital malformation compared to women exposed outside the teratogenic window. As vaccination is safe and effective, emphasis must be placed on promoting vaccination during pregnancy.
- Pregnant and recently pregnant people up to 6 weeks postpartum should receive a bivalent mRNA COVID-19 vaccine booster dose following completion of their last primary vaccine dose or monovalent booster. COVID-19 vaccine is recommended for postpartum and/or lactating individuals who were not vaccinated before.

Rare Adverse Effects

Vaccination against COVID-19 *with vector vaccines* seems to increase slightly the risk of GBS. GBS is a rare but serious immune-mediated neurological condition characterized by damage to the peripheral nervous system. Two thirds of cases of GBS are diagnosed following infection; however, vaccination has also been linked to GBS pathogenesis. GBS occurring following vaccination does differ in characteristics from GBS during the pre-COVID-19 era.

Nonmenstruating women were more likely to experience unexpected vaginal bleeding after receiving COVID-19 vaccinations, according to a new study. Researchers suggested it could have been connected to the SARS-CoV-2 spike protein in the vaccines. The study was published in Science Advances.

After vaccinations became widely available, many women reported heavier menstrual bleeding than normal. Researchers at the Norwegian Institute of Public Health in Oslo examined the data, particularly among women who do not have periods, such as those who have been through menopause or are taking contraceptives.

Addendum

Hybrid SARS-CoV-2 immunity in pregnancy: Immunity from a prior infection plus vaccination—is associated with a greater likelihood of protection at delivery for mothers and infants compared with a prior infection alone. According to results published data "showed that at delivery, fewer unvaccinated participants (87% antispike IgG+, 86% neutralizing antibodies) and their infants (86%, 75%) had antispoke IgG+ or neutralizing antibodies compared with vaccinated participants and their infants (100% for all)".

Flu (Influenza) Vaccines

Flu vaccines have been given to millions of pregnant women over the years and scientific evidence shows that it is safe. The flu shot, which is an inactivated vaccine, is the recommended choice for pregnant women as a safe and effective way to protect both the mother and her unborn baby from the flu and its complications. Inactivated vaccines do not contain live viruses and cannot cause flu illness.

Pregnant women can receive the flu vaccine at any stage of pregnancy. It is safe and recommended during all trimesters. Influenza viruses change from year to year, so pregnant women need to get vaccinated annually to ensure they are protected against the most current strains.

- An inactivated flu vaccine can be given during any trimester of pregnancy and should be given each flu season as soon as the vaccine is available.
- Although flu seasons vary in their timing, the CDC recommends getting vaccinated by the end of October, if possible. Getting vaccinated later during flu season, though, can still be beneficial.
- Side effects of the flu vaccine are generally mild and may include soreness at the injection site, low-grade fever, or mild body aches. Serious allergic reactions are rare.
- The nasal spray version of the flu vaccine, known as FluMist® (quadrivalent influenza vaccine live, intranasal) *is not recommended* for pregnant women. Pregnant women should receive the injectable flu vaccine.

It is important to consult with a healthcare provider to address any specific questions or concerns about receiving the influenza vaccine during pregnancy.

Tetanus–Diphtheria–Acellular Pertussis/Tetanus–Diphtheria Vaccine

The Tdap vaccine is a combination vaccine that provides immunity against three bacterial infections namely tetanus toxoid, reduced diphtheria toxoid, and acellular pertussis.

The Tdap vaccines are generally considered safe and effective. Maternal immunization with the Tdap vaccine is an important aspect of prenatal care to protect both the pregnant woman and her newborn baby.

Especially, the amount of whooping cough antibodies in the body decreases over time. That is why the CDC recommends women get Tdap during each pregnancy, even if their pregnancies are only a year or two apart. Doing so allows each of their babies to get the greatest number of protective antibodies and the best protection possible against these infections.

The antibodies produced by the mother in response to the Tdap vaccine are transferred to the baby, protecting during the first few months of life when the baby is too young to receive the pertussis vaccine themselves.

Pertussis vaccination in pregnancy is beneficial for infants: A study published in pediatrics found that a maternal pertussis vaccination near 28 weeks' gestation was associated with a 66% lower risk of infection among infants ages 6–8 months. Researchers also observed that vaccine effectiveness from maternal vaccination in infants younger than 2 months was 70.4%, but for infants ages 7–8 months, vaccine effectiveness from maternal pertussis declined to 43.3%, and after 8 months, it was no longer effective.

Recommended during every pregnancy, regardless of how long it has been since you previously received the Tdap vaccine, only one dose is recommended during each pregnancy.

Timing of Tdap Vaccination During Pregnancy

- Pregnant women who never received a primary tetanus and diphtheria (Td) series should receive three doses. Give Td/Tdap at intervals of 0, 1, and 6 months. One of the three doses should be Tdap, preferably given between 27 and 36 weeks.
- Pregnant women are encouraged to get the Tdap vaccine at any time during pregnancy, but optimally during the third trimester (preferably between 27 and 36 weeks) of each pregnancy, preferably as early as in the 27 to the 36-week window as possible.

This way, the maternal immune response is boosted and maximizes the passive transfer of antibodies to protect the newborn at the time of delivery.

- If a mom did not get a Tdap vaccine during pregnancy and has never gotten it, the CDC recommends that she gets the vaccine immediately after giving birth.

Tdap can be safely administered earlier in pregnancy if needed.

- Pregnant women should receive Tdap instead of Td, anytime during pregnancy if it is indicated for wound care or during a community pertussis outbreak.
- If Tdap is administered earlier in pregnancy, it should not be repeated between 27 and 36 weeks' gestation; only one dose is recommended during each pregnancy.

It is safe for women to receive most vaccines right after giving birth, even are safe during breastfeeding.

Pneumococcal Vaccines

Pneumococcal vaccines are important for protecting against infections caused by *Streptococcus pneumoniae* bacteria, which can lead to serious illnesses such as pneumonia, meningitis, and bloodstream infections. Maternal immunization with pneumococcal vaccines is a strategy aimed at protecting both pregnant individuals and their newborns from these potentially life-threatening infections.

The two main types of pneumococcal vaccines are the pneumococcal polysaccharide vaccine (PPSV23) and the pneumococcal conjugate vaccine (PCV), for example, PCV13, PCV15, and PCV20. ACIP currently has no recommendation for PCV vaccination, but ACOG recommends vaccination in pregnant patients at high risk for severe pneumococcal disease. The PCV13 is usually preferred for maternal immunization because it provides broader protection and is better at preventing invasive pneumococcal disease. However, no adverse consequences have been reported among newborns whose mothers were inadvertently PPSV23 vaccinated during pregnancy.

- ACIP recommends that pregnant women with medical risk factors for invasive pneumococcal disease be immunized with PPSV23 in pregnancy.
- The safety of pneumococcal immunization in the first trimester has not been established, though no adverse events have been reported.
- No guideline has been published regarding the use of PCV13 in pregnancy.

The timing of maternal pneumococcal vaccination is typically during the third trimester of pregnancy. This allows for the development of protective antibodies in the mother, which can be passed to the baby through the placenta.

Specific recommendations for maternal pneumococcal vaccination may vary by country and region. Healthcare providers typically follow guidelines provided by public health authorities.

Safety: Maternal pneumococcal vaccination is generally considered safe for both the pregnant individual and the developing fetus. The benefits of vaccination in preventing serious infections usually outweigh the potential risks.

Contraindications: Some individuals may have contraindications to certain vaccines. Pregnant individuals should consult their healthcare provider to determine if pneumococcal vaccination is appropriate.

Meningococcal Conjugate and Serogroup B Vaccines

Meningococcal diseases can lead to serious conditions such as meningitis and septicemia, which can have severe consequences, including death. Adolescents and young adults are among the groups most susceptible to meningococcal disease. Vaccination efforts have targeted this. The WHO has supported vaccination campaigns in regions with high disease prevalence.

There are different types of meningococcal vaccines available, such as the conjugate vaccines [e.g., meningococcal conjugate (MenACWY) and meningococcal B (MenB)] and the polysaccharide vaccines. The choice of vaccine may depend on the specific strains of Neisseria meningitidis prevalent in the region and the mother's vaccination history.

Maternal vaccination against meningococcal diseases is an approach to protect newborns and infants from this potentially life-threatening bacterial infection. Vaccination should be deferred in pregnant and lactating women unless the woman is at increased risk. If indicated, quadrivalent vaccination during pregnancy should not be barred because the benefits of vaccination are considered to outweigh the potential risks.

Timing of Vaccination

Maternal vaccination is typically recommended during the third trimester of pregnancy. This timing allows for the transfer of protective antibodies to the fetus before birth.

Maternal health: It is important to consider the mother's health and vaccination history when determining whether maternal vaccination is appropriate. Certain vaccines may not be recommended for all pregnant women and the decision should be made in consultation with a healthcare provider.

Maternal vaccination recommendations may vary by country and region, so it is essential to follow local healthcare guidelines to determine the most appropriate vaccination strategy based on individual health and regional guidelines.

Postpartum vaccination: Even if a mother receives a meningococcal vaccine during pregnancy, it is often recommended that the infant receives their meningococcal vaccinations according to the regular childhood vaccination schedule.

Group B Streptococcus (Guillain–Barré Syndrome) Vaccine

Background: GBS can cause invasive disease [invasive GBS (iGBS)] in young infants, typically presenting as sepsis or meningitis and is also associated with stillbirth and preterm birth. GBS vaccines are under development, but their potential health impact and cost-effectiveness have not been assessed globally.

Most GBS disease cases among newborns result from mother-to-infant transmission during labor and delivery. Many women are asymptomatically colonized by GBS in the genital and gastrointestinal tracts. About half the infants born to colonized mothers are themselves colonized on the skin and mucosal surfaces as a result of passage through the birth canal or as a result of GBS ascending into the amniotic fluid. The majority of colonized infants (98%) are asymptomatic. About 2% will develop early-onset disease, presenting with sepsis, pneumonia, or meningitis in the first few days of life **(Fig. 1)**.

As of this time (2023), pregnant women who test positive for colonization of GBS in their third trimester are treated with intrapartum antibiotic prophylaxis, which is more than 80% effective in the prevention of early-onset disease in infants during the first 6 days after birth but is not effective against late-onset disease at 7–89 days.

Studies have shown that a vaccine given during pregnancy produced antibodies against GBS that were

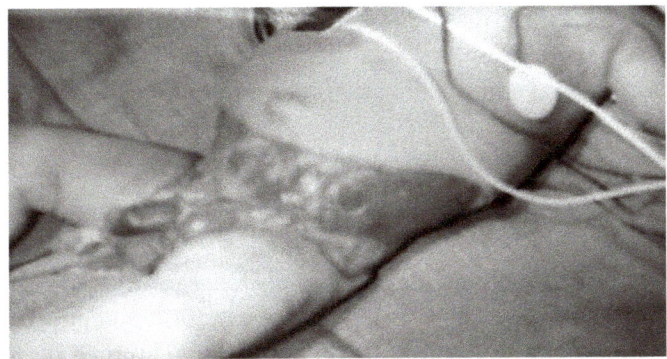

Fig. 1: Guillain–Barré syndrome (GBS) causing necrotizing fasciitis in a 3-month-old infant and invasive GBS (iGBS) and death.

transferred to infants at IgG thresholds associated with a reduced risk of invasive GBS diseases. Maternal GBS vaccine given during pregnancy could potentially prevent both early- and late-onset disease and mitigate the need for intrapartum antibiotic prophylaxis in otherwise healthy women.

In studies, among pregnant women who received a conjugated hexavalent (GBS6) capsular polysaccharide (CPS) vaccine-induced antibody concentrations were associated with a reduced risk of invasive newborn diseases.

Such a vaccine could be beneficial because intrapartum antibiotic prophylaxis may contribute to antimicrobial resistance (AMR) and disrupt the development of the infant microbiome.

It is important to note that the maternal GBS vaccine would provide a much-needed measure in the prevention of GBS infection worldwide and to a substantial percentage of pregnant women living in resource-limited community settings where microbiologic screening and intrapartum antibiotic prophylaxis are unavailable.

In an editorial comment, Carol Baker, MD, of the McGovern Medical School at the University of Texas Health Science Center in Houston, noted that commercial apathy toward vaccinating pregnant women has slowed the development of maternal vaccines, but that may be reaching a turning point.

To conclude, hexavalent maternal vaccination (GBS6) has been associated with anti-CPS IgG levels in newborns associated with reduced risk of invasive GBS diseases. Maternal GBS vaccination could have a large impact on infant morbidity and mortality. Globally, a GBS maternal vaccine at a reasonable price is likely to be a cost-effective intervention.

Respiratory Syncytial Virus Vaccines and Maternal Respiratory Syncytial Virus

Respiratory syncytial virus is a common cause of illness in children and infants are among those at highest risk for severe disease, which can lead to hospitalization. On August 21st, 2023, the Food and Drug Administration (FDA) approved first vaccine for pregnant individuals to prevent RSV in infants. This approval provides an option for healthcare providers and pregnant individuals to protect infants from this potentially life-threatening disease.

Respiratory syncytial virus is a highly contagious virus that causes respiratory infections in individuals of all age groups. It is the most frequent cause of lower respiratory tract disease (LRTD) in infants worldwide. In most parts of the United States (US), RSV circulation is seasonal, typically starting during the fall and peaking in the winter.

The virus is especially common in children and most individuals can be expected to be infected with RSV by the time they reach 2 years of age. While RSV most often causes cold-like symptoms in infants and young children, it can also lead to serious LRTDs such as pneumonia and bronchiolitis. In infants and children, the risk of RSV-associated LRTDs is highest during the first year of life. According to the CDC, RSV is the leading cause of infant hospitalization in the US.

In May 2023, there were two RSV vaccines approved for adults ages 60 years and older—RSVpreF3 (Arexvy, GSK) and RSVpreF (Abrysvo, Pfizer).

Additionally, on May 18, 2023, an FDA panel of advisers voted that data supported the efficacy and safety of a candidate maternal RSV vaccine, given to pregnant women to protect infants aged up to 6 months.

Clinical trials have shown that this vaccine can generate an immune response in pregnant women and transfer protective antibodies to their infants. This passive immunity can help protect newborns from severe RSV infection during the first few months of life when they are most vulnerable.

- RSV vaccine recently approved Pfizer's Abrysvo, a vaccine against the RSV for adults aged 60 years or older. Also, on its horizon, maternal RSV and GBS (group B Strep) vaccines are effective at preventing severe infections in newborns.

The American Academy of Family Physicians (AAFP) RSV recommendations for pregnant people and adults 60 years and older—the bivalent RSVpreF maternal RSV vaccine for pregnant people during 32 through 36 weeks gestation, using seasonal administration, to prevent RSV lower respiratory tract infection in infants.

Pfizer's Abrysvo, the company's bivalent RSV prefusion F (RSVpreF) vaccine, is administered as a single-dose injection into the muscle, approved for use at 32 through 36 weeks gestational age of pregnancy. Also, the FDA approved Abrysvo in May for the prevention of LRTD caused by RSV in individuals 60 years of age and older.

Maternal RSV vaccination has been shown to reduce the risk of severe RSV infections in infants, especially those born prematurely or with other risk factors for severe RSV disease.

The most commonly reported side effects by pregnant individuals who received Abrysvo were pain at the injection site, headache, muscle pain, and nausea.

Safety: The safety of maternal RSV vaccination has been demonstrated in clinical trials and it is generally considered safe for both the pregnant individual and the developing fetus. Like any medical intervention, there can be rare side effects, so it is essential to discuss the risks and benefits with a healthcare provider.

In addition to Pfizer's maternal RSV vaccine, the FDA in July 2023 approved AstraZeneca's monoclonal antibody (mAb) nirsevimab (Beyfortus) for the prevention of RSV in neonates and infants entering their first RSV season and in children up to 24 months who remain vulnerable to severe RSV disease through their second RSV season.

Maternal RSV Vaccine could Significantly Reduce Clinical Visits and Costs

Data derived from Hanau et al. shows that maternal RSV vaccination could reduce medical costs by $691.8 million and nonmedical costs by $110 million. The study also projects infant hospitalizations due to RSV would fall by 51%.

Maternal Immunization Task Force joint statement: Obstetric care professionals recommend RSV vaccine for pregnant individuals.

AstraZeneca's nirsevimab—not a vaccine but a long-acting mAb that protects infants from RSV.

Hepatitis Vaccines

The most common cause of jaundice in pregnancy is acute viral hepatitis. Viral hepatitis may present the same in pregnant and nonpregnant patients, but the overall impact on maternal and fetal health is important as perinatal transmission may occur in all types of hepatitis. Therefore, prevention, treatment, and control of infection during pregnancy is of paramount importance to prevent perinatal transmission.

Hepatitis A Virus Vaccines

Hepatitis A virus (HAV) vaccine is the most common cause of acute hepatitis but is *rarely reported during pregnancy*. Most people who get hepatitis A during pregnancy do not experience serious complications. Studies have shown an increased chance of preterm labor (labor that begins before 37 weeks of pregnancy) following HAV infection during pregnancy.

Hepatitis A virus infection brings no known risks to a developing fetus but can cause pregnancy complications, such as premature contractions or problems with the placenta. This risk of exposure might be higher if one travels to areas with a high prevalence of hepatitis A or work in healthcare or other professions where one might be exposed to the virus.

The HAV vaccine is recommended for pregnant people who are at risk of contracting hepatitis A and is generally considered safe during pregnancy. It is an inactivated vaccine, generally considered safer during pregnancy. There are different brands of hepatitis A vaccines, so your healthcare provider will determine which one is most appropriate for your situation.

- Any person who wants to be protected from HAV or indicates to use may receive the vaccine during pregnancy or the postpartum period.
- *Timing:* During pregnancy, it is usually given in the second or third trimester. This is to minimize any potential risks to the developing fetus.

Hepatitis B Virus Vaccine

Pregnant women are screened for HepB surface antigen (HBsAg). If a woman is found to be HBsAg positive (carriers), she is considered infectious and can potentially transmit the virus to her baby.

If a pregnant person develops acute type B hepatitis infection, that may cause serious liver disease and the virus can pass from them to the baby during or after birth. If a baby gets HepB, there is a 90% chance that they will develop a lifelong infection. HBV vaccines can reduce the risk of a person developing HBV and complications from the virus in both the pregnant person and the fetus.

The HBV vaccine is a safe and effective way to prevent infection. It is an inactivated virus, so there is no evidence of any risks from vaccination during pregnancy to the fetus or nursing. There is also no evidence of any risks from vaccinating against HBV during pregnancy or nursing.

Maternal HepB vaccination, also known as maternal HepB immunoprophylaxis, is a medical practice designed to prevent the transmission of the HepB virus (HBV) from mother to newborn during childbirth.

Based on the CDC's 2022 adult immunization schedule and its supporting evidence of benefit, the ACOG recommends HepB vaccination for all unvaccinated pregnant adults.

Vaccination: If the pregnant woman is HBsAg positive or her HepB status is unknown, she is typically given the HepB vaccine during her pregnancy. This helps protect both the mother and the newborn from HBV infection.

Remember that even if a mother receives the HepB vaccine during pregnancy, her baby will have to be vaccinated after birth. The protective antibodies are not transmitted from the mother to her baby. Therefore, all infants born to HBsAg carrier mothers are also started on the HepB vaccination series, usually within 24 hours of birth. The vaccine is administered in multiple doses, typically at birth, at 1–2 months, and at 6 months of age.

Hepatitis B Immune Globulin

In addition to the vaccine, infants born to HBsAg-positive mothers are usually given HepB immune globulin (HBIG) within 12 hours of birth. HBIG is a concentrated form of antibodies against HBV, providing immediate protection to the baby.

By administering the HBIG to newborns, the risk of HBV transmission is significantly reduced. This strategy has been highly effective in preventing perinatal (mother-to-child) transmission of HepB and it is considered a crucial step in reducing the burden of HepB infection worldwide.

The specific vaccination and testing protocols may vary by region and healthcare guidelines, so it is important to consult with a healthcare professional for the most up-to-date information and guidance.

Importantly, PreHevbrio and Heplisav-B are not recommended during pregnancy due to a lack of safety data. Due to the more powerful adjuvant, Heplisav-B requires only two doses separated by 1 month. PreHevbrio is recommended for those 18 years and older. It is administered in three doses using a schedule similar to most other hepatitis vaccines. The second dose is given 1 month after the first and the third dose is administered 6 months after the first dose.

Hepatitis B virus vaccine side effects during pregnancy: Hepatitis B virus vaccine causes common side effects in around 1 in 10 people who have it. The most common side effects, according to a 2014 study, include discomfort around the injection site and mild-to-moderate fever.

Uncommon side effects include: Swelling at the injection site, fatigue, headache, and erythema, an immune reaction of the skin that can cause a rash.

Most side effects are mild and will go away on their own. However, an individual should consult a doctor as soon as possible if uncommon or rare side effects occur.

Hepatitis E virus vaccine: In rare cases, acute hepatitis E virus (HEV) can be severe and result in fulminant hepatitis (acute liver failure) and these patients are at risk of death. Pregnant women with HEV, particularly those in the second or third trimester, are at increased risk (up to 20–25%) of acute liver failure, fetal loss, and mortality.

A vaccine to prevent HEV infection has been developed and is licensed in China but is not yet available elsewhere. The efficacy of 93.3% [95% confidence interval (CI) 78.6-97.9] in the perprotocol set was confirmed within 4.5 years of follow-up. The highly efficacious hepatitis E vaccine may hold great promise for reducing the high mortality and multiple adverse outcomes associated with HEV infection in pregnant women.

Human Papillomavirus Vaccines

- Not recommended to be given during pregnancy, but if you inadvertently receive it, this is not a cause for concern.

The human papillomavirus (HPV) vaccines are typically recommended for individuals before they become sexually active, as they are most effective when given before exposure to the virus.

However, if someone becomes pregnant and has not completed the recommended HPV vaccine series, it is generally recommended to postpone any remaining doses until after pregnancy. The vaccine can be resumed after childbirth or once they are no longer pregnant.

Postpartum vaccination: After giving birth and if not breastfeeding, individuals can receive any remaining doses of the HPV vaccine. It is safe to start or complete the vaccine series during the postpartum period.

Breastfeeding: The HPV vaccines are not known to pose a risk to breastfeeding mothers or their infants. Therefore, it is generally safe to receive or continue the vaccine series while breastfeeding.

Human papillomavirus vaccine is recommended for all people aged 26 years or younger, so if you are in this age group, make sure you are vaccinated before or after your pregnancy.

People aged 27 through 45 years may also be vaccinated against HPV after a discussion with their healthcare professional. The vaccine is given in two or three doses (depending on the age at which the first dose is given) over 6-month period.

Safety during pregnancy: The HPV vaccines, which include Gardasil 9 and Cervarix, have not been specifically tested for safety during pregnancy. Therefore, healthcare providers generally advise against administering these vaccines to pregnant individuals, especially during the first trimester when the fetus is developing rapidly. The concern is mainly about potential risks to the developing fetus, although no significant safety concerns have been reported when the vaccine was inadvertently given during pregnancy.

Measles, Mumps, Rubella and Varicella Vaccinations During Pregnancy

Live attenuated vaccines including the MMR and varicella (MMRV) vaccines including live attenuated influenza vaccine are contraindicated for pregnant individuals. Theoretically, the live attenuated virus (LAV) in a vaccine could cross the placenta and result in viral infection of the fetus. Owing to this concern, most LAV vaccines are contraindicated during pregnancy.
- If indicated (i.e., for seronegative individuals), the MMRV should be given during the postpartum period.
- Inadvertent administration during pregnancy has not been associated with CRS or congenital varicella syndrome (CVS).

Measles: A measles infection during pregnancy can cause miscarriage, premature birth, and low birth weight. Pregnant individuals should not be vaccinated for measles until after childbirth.
- The measles vaccine is typically not administered during pregnancy. If a pregnant person is not immune to measles and needs the vaccine, it is usually recommended to wait until after giving birth to receive the MMRV vaccine.

Mumps: Like measles, the mumps component of the MMR should not be given to pregnant people and is generally not given during pregnancy. It is usually recommended to wait until after pregnancy to receive MMR vaccine but should be given to them before or after pregnancy if indicated.

Rubella: Infection in pregnancy can be serious for the baby, especially during the first 3 months of gestation. Rubella can cause a miscarriage or serious birth defects in a developing baby if a woman is infected while she is pregnant. Having rubella during pregnancy increases the risk of CRS—this is a condition that happens when a pregnant person passes rubella to their baby during pregnancy **(Fig. 2)**. The most common birth defects from CRS can include: Cataracts, deafness, heart defects, microcephaly, intellectual disabilities, etc.

A woman's rubella immunity (IgG antibody presence) must be tested before pregnancy to make sure they are immune to rubella. If you are not immune, the MMR vaccine is not recommended during pregnancy.

Getting vaccinated against rubella during pregnancy is not recommended. This is why it is best to get vaccinated before starting to get pregnant. Women who are not immune require two doses of vaccine a minimum of 28 days apart and should avoid pregnancy for at least 28 days after immunization.

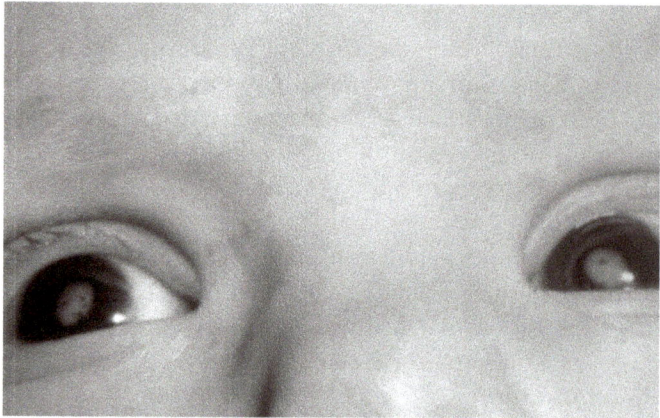

Fig. 2: Infant with congenital rubella has clouding of the eyes (cataracts) due to congenital rubella syndrome.
Courtesy: Immunization Action Coalition.

Rubella IgG serology testing should be used for assessing rubella immunity, including before, during, and after pregnancy. Testing for rubella IgG avidity can be used to distinguish between recent exposure to rubella and a more distant exposure.

Routine IgM screening of pregnant people is not recommended and should be limited to suspected rubella cases. It is not recommended for screening asymptomatic people.

Varicella (Chickenpox)

Congenital varicella with short-limb syndrome and scarring of the skin—the mother had varicella during the first trimester of pregnancy **(Fig. 3)**.
- Getting chickenpox during pregnancy, especially early pregnancy, increases the risk of birth defects.
- The varicella vaccine is a live vaccine and is generally not recommended during pregnancy. The vaccine can sometimes cause congenital varicella infection, a rare group of birth defects that can cause scars and problems with the arms, legs, brain, and eyes.

Pregnant women should avoid the varicella vaccine in the 30 days before trying to get pregnant unless they have been exposed to chickenpox.

It is recommended that one should wait until 3 months after the second dose of the vaccine before trying to conceive, if one is not sure of pregnancy.

If a pregnant person is not immune to chickenpox and is at risk of exposure, they should consult their healthcare provider for guidance. In certain situations, postexposure prophylaxis with varicella–zoster immune globulin (VZIG) may be recommended.

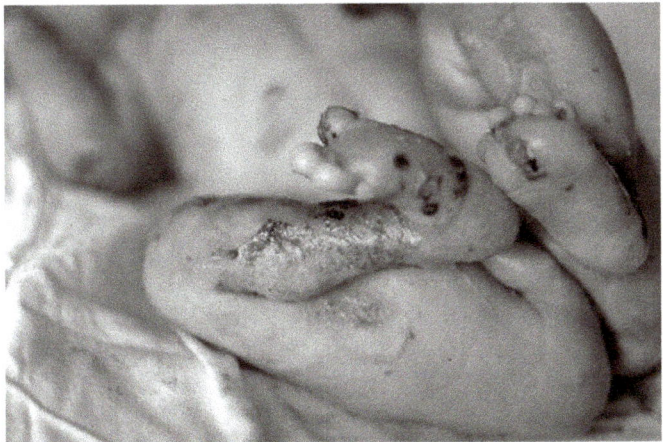

Fig. 3: Newborn with congenital varicella syndrome.

It is essential for pregnant individuals to discuss vaccination with their healthcare provider. They can assess the individual's specific circumstances, immunity status, and potential risks of exposure to IDs to make appropriate recommendations.

Zoster (Shingles) Vaccination During Pregnancy

Zoster vaccine is not recommended for pregnant women. The zoster vaccine is primarily designed to prevent shingles in adults aged 50 years and older, as well as those with weakened immune systems. While the vaccine is generally safe for most people, it is not recommended during pregnancy due to potential risks to the developing fetus.
- There is currently no ACIP recommendation for recombinant zoster vaccine (RZV) use in pregnancy. Consider delaying RZV until after pregnancy.

Parvovirus B19 (Erythema Infectiosum, Fifth Disease)

No specific antiviral therapy or vaccine is presently available for parvovirus B19 (PB19V) infection, but efforts in the search for compounds inhibiting PB19V replication are now being pursued.

New virus-like particle-based PB19Vs vaccine candidates, produced by coexpressing VP2 and either wild-type VP1 or phospholipase-negative VP1 in a regulated ratio from a single plasmid in *Saccharomyces cerevisiae* have been developed and show sufficient promise to test in humans.

Parvovirus B19 infection occurring during pregnancy can cause fetal hydrops, intrauterine growth restriction, isolated pleural and pericardial effusions, and death, but the virus is not a proven cause of congenital anomalies. The risk of fetal death is between 2% and 6% when infection occurs during pregnancy. The greatest risk appears to occur during the first half of pregnancy.

Pregnant women who discover that they have been in contact with children who were in the incubation period of erythema infectiosum (EI) or with children who were in aplastic crisis should have the relatively low potential risk of infection explained to them.

The ACOG recommends that pregnant women exposed to PB19V should have serologic testing performed to determine susceptibility and possible evidence of acute PB19V infection. Pregnant women with evidence of acute infection should be monitored closely (e.g., serial ultrasonographic examinations) by their obstetric provider. In pregnant women with suspected or proven intrauterine infection, amniotic fluid and fetal tissues should be considered infectious and contact precautions should be used in addition to standard precautions if exposure is likely.

Children with EI may attend childcare or school because they no longer are contagious once the rash appears (**Fig. 4**).

Zika Virus Vaccine Needs

Zika virus (ZIKV) is primarily transmitted to humans through the bite of infected Aedes mosquitoes, but it can also be sexually transmitted. Unlike the mosquitoes that spread malaria, this type of mosquito mainly bites during the day from sunrise to sunset.

Infection during pregnancy resulting in transplacental virus transmission can lead to birth defects such as microcephaly and other neurological complications in infants. This is called "congenital zika syndrome." ZIKV infection can also cause pregnancy complications, including stillbirth or premature delivery.

- Currently, there are no FDA-approved vaccines for ZIKV despite its impact on the health of millions of people worldwide.
- Assessment of heterologous flavivirus vaccination is important given the cocirculation of Japanese encephalitis virus (JEV) and yellow fever virus with ZIKV.

Zika virus is a single-stranded, RNA virus in the genus *Flavivirus* that is related antigenically to dengue, yellow fever, West Nile, St Louis encephalitis, and JEV. Two major lineages, African and Asian, have been identified through phylogenetic analyses.

As evidenced by recent epidemics, both Ebola and ZIKV infections are potentially catastrophic when occurring in pregnant women. Ebola virus causes extremely high rates of mortality in both mothers and infants; the ZIKV is a TORCH (toxoplasmosis, rubella, cytomegalovirus, herpes simplex, and other organisms) infection that produces a congenital malformation syndrome and pediatric neurodevelopmental abnormalities.

Zika virus can be passed from a pregnant person to a fetus. It primarily spreads through bites from infected mosquitoes. One can also get Zika through sex without a condom with someone infected by ZIKV. Protection against mosquito bites during the day and early evening is a key measure to prevent ZIKV virus infection, especially among pregnant.

There are many clinical similarities between maternal rubella and ZIKV infections. Both are febrile rash illnesses and both have arthropathy, or arthritis, as manifestations, especially among women of pregnant age groups. Also, like rubella, there is an asymptomatic component to Zika, so not everyone knows when they are infected with rubella or with ZIKV. The most devastating effects have been neurotropic, with microcephaly in the newborns of ZIKV-infected mothers (**Figs. 5 to 7**). The mode of infections, transmission route, and clinical resemblances

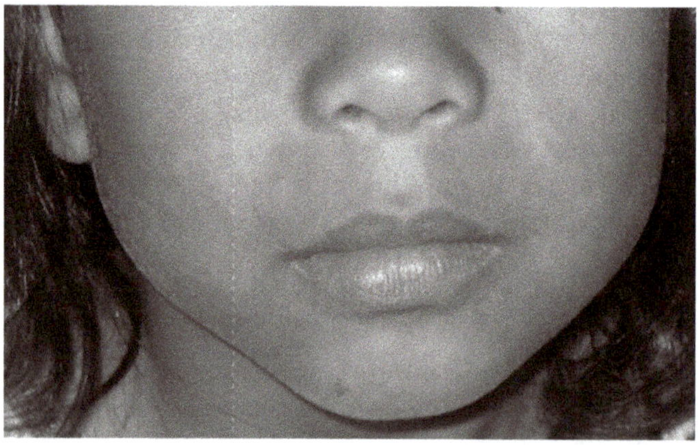

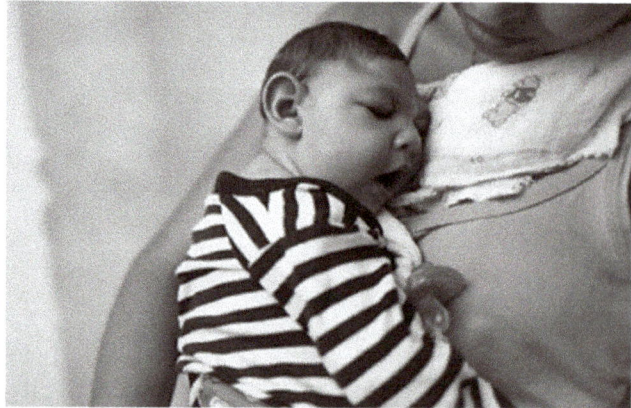

Fig. 4: A healthy 6-year-old school-attending girl developed an asymptomatic symmetrical red papular eruption on the face, extremities, and trunk, which became confluent on the face 1 week earlier.
Courtesy: H Cody Meissner, MD, FAAP.

Fig. 5: The World Health Organization/Pan American Health Organization (WHO/PAHO)—a mother holding her baby outside the reference center in the care and monitoring of children with microcephaly.
Courtesy: SA Uduman. ZIKA, KIMS Health Booklet, 2017.

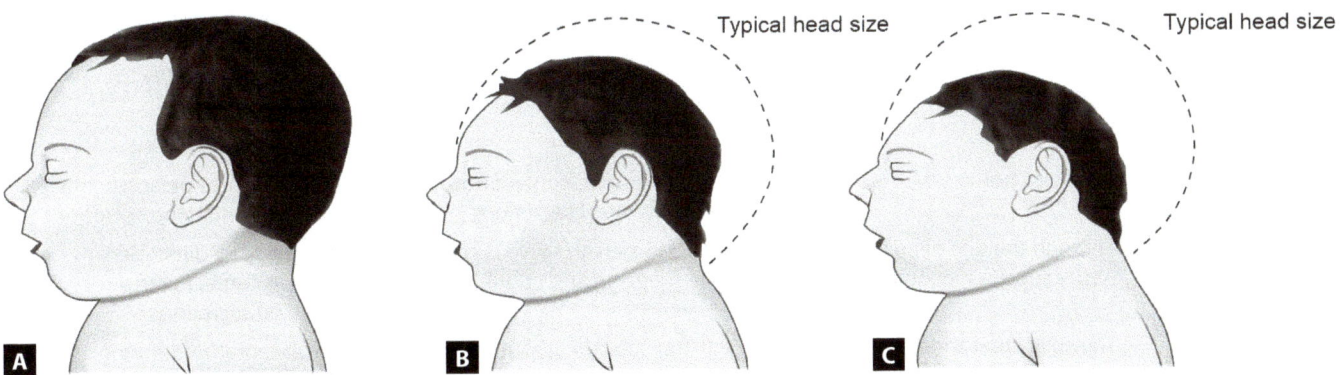

Figs. 6A to C: Range of zika virus (ZIKV) microcephaly: (A) Baby with typical head size; (B) baby with microcephaly; and (C) baby with severe microcephaly (CDC responds to Zika).
Courtesy: SA Uduman. ZIKA, KIMS Health Booklet, 2017.

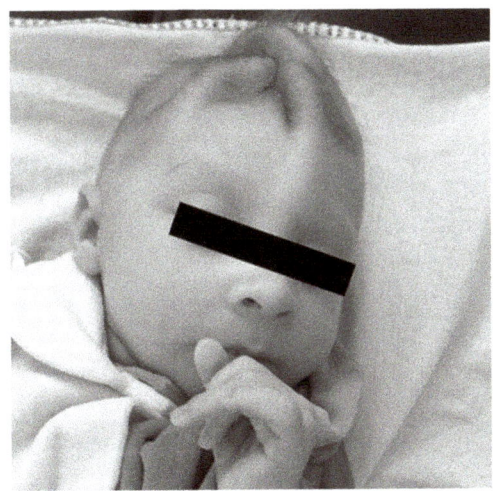

Fig. 7: Zika virus (ZIKV) wreaks havoc on the baby's brain, causing the skull to collapse in on itself. Ventriculomegaly is found to infect most Brazilian babies suffering from ZIKV. Almost complete agyria and internal hydrocephalus of lateral ventricles are seen.
Courtesy: SA Uduman. ZIKA, KIMS Health Booklet, 2017.

including congenital infection aspects are tabulated in **Table 2**.

Zika virus infection is a threat to at-risk populations, causing major birth defects and serious neurological complications. The development of a safe and efficacious ZIKV vaccine is, therefore, a global health priority.

There is little doubt that the development of an effective Zika vaccine will have its greatest benefit in preventing pregnant women from congenital infections. Zika purified inactivated virus (ZPIV) was previously shown to be protective in nonpregnant mice and rhesus macaques. Although recent Aripo virus (ARPV)/ZIKV vaccine demonstrates exceptional safety and efficacy, very little is known about (1) the minimal and/or optimal dose for achieving complete protection from ZIKV-induced disease; (2) the impact of boosters on vaccine-induced immunity; or (3) the influence of vertebrate-infectious flaviviruses (VIFs) during coinfection with ARPV/ZIKV in vertebrate cells.

Zika vaccine candidates (2023)—VLA1601 is a highly purified, inactivated, adjuvanted zika vaccine candidate adsorbed on aluminum hydroxide that has completed a phase 1 clinical trial, on the original manufacturing platform of the Japanese encephalitis vaccine IXIARO. Assessment of heterologous flavivirus vaccination is important given the cocirculation of JEV and yellow fever virus with ZIKV.

Several ZIKV vaccine candidates are in clinical development, one of which is a ZPIV that has shown useful safety and immunogenicity in clinical trials. However, neutralizing antibody titers produced after vaccination have been low compared with those from ZIKV convalescent patients. As the ZIKV shares a sizeable proportion of its antigens with other flaviviruses, it is possible that priming with other flavivirus vaccines could potentiate the immunogenicity of ZPIV.

Cytomegalovirus Vaccine Needs

Cytomegalovirus, a member of the herpes family [human herpesvirus 5 (HHV5)], is an often harmless viral infection that can cause mild flu symptoms, if any, in healthy people. But in pregnancy, a CMV can be passed onto a woman's unborn baby through the placenta and cause developmental delays, miscarriage, stillbirth, hearing loss, and mental disability. The prevalence of congenital CMV (cCMV) infection at birth ranges from 0.2 to 2.2% and is

TABLE 2: Comparisons between zika, rubella, and CMV infections (maternal and newborn infection aspects).

	Zika—seasonal	Rubella—endemic in those unvaccinated	CMV—no seasonality Ubiquitous
Virus	RNA	RNA	DNA
Primarily	Mosquito borne	Direct or droplet contact from nasopharyngeal secretions	Direct person-to-person contact with virus-containing secretions
Maternal infection	Through the bite of an infected Aedes species mosquito	Person-to-person saliva contact while sneezing and coughing	Horizontally by direct person-to-person contact with virus-containing secretions
Maternofetal transmission	Transplacental and during intrapartum and postnatally	Only transplacental route up to 16 weeks GA	Transplacental and during intrapartum and postnatally
Other transmission mode	Sexual, blood transfusion	?	Blood, platelet, WBC transfusion, organ and HSCT
Infected persons remain contagious	1 week before onset symptoms and the virus is found in high titer in urine, tears, and semen longer than blood in asymptomatic men	Up to 1 week before and 1 week after rash onset	Seropositive individuals are lifelong infectious
Diagnosis	PCR blood, urine, cervical and vaginal smear, IgM	IgG and IgM; IgG avidity assay	IgG, M, shell vial culture, IgG avidity assay, PCR
Seropositive IgG individuals	Probably protective. Sero-negative are at risk of infection	Are immune and protective (natural or vaccine-induced)	Are infectious
Newborn aspects			
System affected	Brain—neurotrophic	CVS, eye, ear, hematopoietic, CNS	Hematopoietic, ear, CNS
Viral excretion period	? Indefinite—waiting data	Infectious up to 1 year	Indefinite
NB diagnosis	PCR: Cervical, vaginal seminal secretion, blood, urine, CSF	Blood, urine, and CSF	Blood, cervical secretion saliva, urine, and CSF
Vaccine prevention	*No* licensed vaccine yet. (on phase I and II clinical trial)	*Yes*, since 1969. Yet, globally about 300 infants a day are born with CRS	No, many candidate vaccines are under clinical trials

(CMV: cytomegalovirus; CNS: central nervous system; CSF: cerebrospinal fluid; CRS: congenital rubella syndrome; CVS: congenital varicella syndrome; DNA: deoxyribonucleic acid; GA: gestational age; HSCT: hematopoietic stem cell transplantation; IgG: immunoglobulin G; PCR: polymerase chain reaction; RNA: ribonucleic acid; WBC: white blood cell)

higher in low-income communities. Approximately, 10% of affected infants are symptomatic at birth and disability develops in up to 25% by the age of 2 years. There are no in utero treatments recommended in the US to improve outcomes of pregnancies in persons with primary CMV infection.

Cytomegalovirus infection may be acquired prenatally or perinatally and is the most common congenital viral infection. Signs at birth, if present, are intrauterine growth restriction, prematurity, microcephaly, jaundice, petechiae, hepatosplenomegaly, periventricular calcifications, chorioretinitis, pneumonitis, hepatitis, and sensorineural hearing loss. If acquired later in infancy, signs may include pneumonia, hepatosplenomegaly, hepatitis, thrombocytopenia, sepsis-like syndrome, and atypical lymphocytosis. Diagnosis of neonatal infection is best made by viral detection via culture or polymerase chain reaction (PCR) testing. Treatment is mainly supportive. Parenteral ganciclovir or oral valganciclovir may prevent hearing deterioration and improve developmental outcomes and is given to infants with symptomatic disease identified in the neonatal period.

The highest risk to an unborn baby occurs when a woman who has never had CMV before is infected with the virus for the first-time during pregnancy. This is especially risky if the infection occurs during the first half of the pregnancy. Recent pieces of literature do not support the use of maternal CMV hyperimmune globulin to improve outcomes in the children of women with primary CMV infection in early pregnancy. A vaccine that prevents CMV infection in seronegative women could reduce the incidence of cCMV infection, a major cause of neurodevelopmental disability.

There is no vaccine available to prevent cCMV. A vaccine that was based on CMV envelope glycoprotein B (gB) with a new adjuvant, MF59 (a squalene-in-water emulsion), entered clinical trials, which demonstrated that the vaccine was immunogenic and had acceptable profiles of adverse events and side effects. The gB/MF59 vaccine can boost antibody and $CD4^+$ responses to CMV for at least 1 year.

In recent periods, the mRNA-1647 vaccine has shown promise in clinical evaluations. Safety and efficacy of a replication-defective investigational CMV vaccine, V160, in clinical trials in seronegative women were generally well tolerated and immunogenic; however, three doses of the vaccine did not reduce the incidence of primary CMV infection in CMV-seronegative women compared with placebo. This study provides insights into the design of future CMV vaccine efficacy trials, particularly for the identification of CMV infection using molecular assays.

SEXUALLY TRANSMITTED INFECTIONS DURING PREGNANCY

Sexually transmitted infection (STI) is a bacterial or viral illness acquired from having vaginal, oral, or anal sex with someone who is infected. Untreated STIs can cause serious health problems for a mom and her baby. The most common STIs that can affect pregnancy include chlamydia, genital herpes, gonorrhea, HepB, hepatitis C (HepC), human immunodeficiency virus (HIV)/acquired immunodeficiency syndrome (AIDS), HPV, syphilis, and trichomoniasis (Trich).

Maternal infections can pass to the fetus transplacentally or at the time of delivery during labor and/or during the breastfeeding period. Some maternal STIs can be transmitted to fetuses during pregnancy or transvaginal delivery. Syphilis can cross the placenta, whereas gonorrhea, chlamydia, HepB, HIV, and herpes can be acquired by the newborn during labor.

One important prevention tool against STIs is the vaccination given to mothers. Currently, vaccines are available for three of the most common STIs including HPV, hepatitis A, and HBV. Other vaccines are under development, including those for HIV and herpes simplex viruses (HSVs) and syphilis during pregnancy can cause problems for both to mom and the fetus.

- As of now, there are no approved vaccines available for gonorrhea, chlamydia, or syphilis.

Syphilis

- Congenital syphilis is arguably the worst manifestation of syphilis and can be prevented with appropriate maternal screening and treatment.

Syphilis is a sexually or vertically (mother to fetus) transmitted disease caused by the infection of *Treponema pallidum* (TPA). The incidence of syphilis has increased over the past years even though this bacterium is an obligate human pathogen; the infection route is well known and the disease can be successfully treated with penicillin.

Over the course of almost a decade, there has been a continued increase in the three nationally reportable STIs in the US—chlamydia, gonorrhea, and syphilis—including a large spike in cases of congenital syphilis that has alarmed experts in the USA.

The number of reported rates of congenital syphilis cases has continued to rise in the past and is now up by 937%. In 2022 alone, there were 3,755 cases of babies born with congenital syphilis in the US.

Escalating rates of congenital syphilis predated the coronavirus disease 2019 (COVID-19) pandemic but increased further as public health programs shifted to respond to COVID-19. The effect of untreated syphilis on maternal and neonatal health outcomes is profound and the rate of congenital syphilis in the US was the highest it has been in nearly 30 years.

Intrauterine infection with *TPA* can result in stillbirth, hydrops fetalis, or preterm birth or may be asymptomatic at birth. Infected infants can have hepatosplenomegaly, snuffles (copious nasal secretions), lymphadenopathy, hemolytic anemia, or thrombocytopenia at birth or within the first 4–8 weeks of age. Untreated infants, including those asymptomatic at birth, may develop late manifestations, which usually appear after 2 years of age and involve the central nervous system (CNS), bones and joints, teeth, eyes, and skin. Late manifestations can be prevented by treatment of early infection.

An effective vaccine for syphilis remains elusive. A variety of strategies have been tested, including inactivated bacteria and subunit recombinant proteins, even though with limited success.

In the last century, several vaccine prototypes have been tested in preclinical studies, mainly in rabbits. While none of them protected against infection, some prototypes prevented bacteria from disseminating to distal organs, attenuated lesion development, and accelerated their healing. Despite these promising results, there is still some controversy regarding the identification of vaccine candidates and the characteristics of a syphilis-protective immune response.

The ideal syphilis vaccine should protect against TPA infection. However, even if the vaccine is unable to completely prevent infection, it could still be worth considering as a means of limiting bacteria dissemination and tissue invasiveness, blocking the establishment of latency, or preventing the disease from progressing to secondary and tertiary stages.

Most importantly, a vaccine that prevents TPA transplacental invasion might also reduce the number of congenital syphilis in endemic areas, where the number of nondiagnosed infected individuals might be high and access to healthcare may be limited.

Recently, there has been evidence that TPA can be cultured *in vitro* and that genetic manipulation of this pathogen can be accomplished. These scientific advances are likely to open the gateway to new research lines that can shed light on the current controversies.

Syphilis Prevention During Pregnancy

The risk for antepartum fetal infection or congenital syphilis at delivery is related to the syphilis stage during pregnancy. All women should be screened serologically for syphilis at the first prenatal care visit or should be performed at the time of pregnancy testing. Antepartum screening can be performed by manual nontreponemal antibody testing [e.g., rapid plasma reagin (RPR)].

Pregnant women with positive treponemal screening tests should have additional quantitative nontreponemal testing because titers are essential for monitoring treatment response. Serologic testing should also be performed twice during the third trimester—at 28 weeks' gestation and at delivery for pregnant women who live in communities with high rates of syphilis and for women who have been at risk for syphilis acquisition during pregnancy.

Penicillin G is the only known effective antimicrobial for treating fetal infection and preventing congenital syphilis. Pregnant women should be treated with the recommended penicillin regimen for their stage of infection.

Gonorrhea

Gonorrhea among pregnant women has been associated with risk for spontaneous abortion, intrauterine growth restriction, premature rupture of membranes, preterm birth, low infant birthweight, chorioamnionitis, and postpartum endometrial infection. However, precise risks for each outcome have not been well-defined. Perinatal transmission of *Neisseria gonorrhoeae* (*N. gonorrhoeae*) can result in neonatal conjunctivitis, a frequent cause of blindness before the institution of topical ocular antibiotic prophylaxis for neonates globally.

Renewed interest in developing vaccines against N. gonorrhoeae has been sparked by the increasing threat of gonococcal AMR and growing optimism that gonococcal vaccines are biologically feasible. *Evidence suggests* serogroup B *Neisseria meningitidis* vaccines might provide some cross-protection against *N. gonorrhoeae* and new gonococcal vaccine candidates based on several approaches are currently in preclinical development.

Chlamydia

Chlamydia vaccine development has been hindered by its intracellular lifestyle and the need to elicit both humoral and cell-mediated immunity. Chlamydia is easily treated with a course of antibiotics, but there is currently no vaccine to prevent the disease.

All pregnant women aged <25 years as well as older women at increased risk for chlamydia should be routinely screened for *Chlamydia trachomatis* at the first prenatal visit. Pregnant women who remain at increased risk for chlamydial infection also should be retested during the third trimester to prevent maternal postnatal complications and chlamydial infection in the neonate. Pregnant women identified as having chlamydia should be treated immediately and have a test of cure to document chlamydial eradication by a nucleic acid amplification test (NAAT) 4 weeks after treatment. All persons diagnosed with a chlamydial infection should be rescreened 3 months after treatment.

GENERAL MATERNAL CARE AGAINST SEXUALLY TRANSMITTED INFECTION PREVENTION

The CDC recommends that every pregnant woman should get screened for syphilis, HIV, HepB, and HepC during the first prenatal visit. The CDC also suggests screening for chlamydia and gonorrhea at your first visit if you are under 25 years and/or you have risk factors.

Get vaccinated against HPV and HepB—the HPV vaccine is not safe to get when you are pregnant, so get it before pregnancy if possible. The HepB vaccine may be safe during pregnancy, depending on your situation.

Depending on the type of STI, these can be treated by antibiotics that treat infections caused by bacteria, such as chlamydia, gonorrhea, and syphilis. Many antibiotics are safe in pregnancy, including beta-lactams, such as penicillin and amoxicillin, clindamycin, metronidazole, nitrofurantoin, vancomycin, and cephalosporin.

- Antibiotics such as fluoroquinolones and tetracyclines are generally not recommended during pregnancy.
- Maternal antiviral medicine and other treatments can relieve symptoms and may reduce the risk of passing the virus to the baby.

HIV-INFECTED MOTHERS—MATERNAL AND NEWBORN IMMUNOPROPHYLAXIS

In the absence of breastfeeding, the risk of HIV infection for infants born to untreated women living with HIV (WLHIV) in the US is approximately 25%, with most transmission occurring near the time of delivery. Maternal viral load is the critical determinant affecting the likelihood of mother-to-child transmission (MTCT) of HIV, although transmission has been observed across the entire range of maternal viral loads.

Pregnant WLHIV should receive antiretroviral therapy (ART) regimens, both for treatment of HIV infection and for prevention of MTCT of HIV. Sustained virologic suppression is the goal both during pregnancy and following delivery. Detailed recommendations for use of antiretrovirals (ARVs) in pregnant WLHIV can be found online.

Because children born to HIV-infected mothers passively acquire maternal antibodies, antibody assays are not informative for the diagnosis of infection in children younger than 18 months unless assay results are negative. Therefore, laboratory diagnosis of HIV infection during the first 18 months of life is based on HIV NAATs [Refer to Chapter 3: Innovative Infectious Diseases Vaccines (The Future of Vaccines).

TRAVEL VACCINES DURING PREGNANCY (YELLOW FEVER, TYPHOID FEVER, AND JAPANESE ENCEPHALITIS VACCINES)

- Certain travel vaccines are generally not recommended during pregnancy.

The safety of vaccines during pregnancy is a critical consideration because some vaccines may pose risks to the developing fetus.

Yellow Fever Vaccine

The yellow fever vaccine is a LAV. While yellow fever can be a serious disease, the vaccine is generally not recommended during pregnancy unless the risk of contracting yellow fever is very high. In such cases, the decision to vaccinate should be made after carefully weighing the potential risks and benefits with a healthcare provider.

Having the yellow fever vaccine might be considered necessary if travel to an area where yellow fever is common cannot be avoided during pregnancy. Your doctor is the best person to help you decide what is right for you and your baby.

In rare cases, the yellow fever vaccine can have serious and sometimes fatal side effects. There are concerns for the babies of pregnant and nursing women who receive yellow fever vaccines.

Yellow fever vaccine has been given to many pregnant women without any apparent adverse effects on the fetus. However, since the vaccine is a live virus vaccine, it poses a theoretical risk. Pregnant women should avoid or postpone travel to an area where there is a risk of yellow fever.

Typhoid Fever Vaccine

There are two types of typhoid vaccines—(1) the injectable (Vi CPS) and (2) the oral (live attenuated) vaccine. Neither of these vaccines is typically recommended during pregnancy unless the risk of typhoid infection is high and cannot be mitigated by other means.

The CDC recommends a typhoid vaccine for travelers to parts of the world where typhoid is common. However, the vaccine is not 100% effective and should not be used as a substitute for being careful about what you eat or drink.

Pregnant women are usually offered an injectable nonlive typhoid vaccine instead of the live vaccine, which is taken as a tablet. The inactivated Vi polysaccharide vaccine may be preferable in pregnancy due to the theoretical risk of fetal infection from live vaccines.

The typhoid vaccine should be given at least 1 month before traveling, but it can be given closer to your travel date if necessary. Booster vaccinations are recommended every 3 years.

Even if you are fully vaccinated, taking additional hygiene and food and water precautions is important as neither of these vaccines offers 100% protection.

Japanese Encephalitis Virus Vaccine

The JEV vaccine is also a LAV. Like other live vaccines, it is generally avoided during pregnancy due to the theoretical risk of transmitting the weakened virus to the fetus. In areas where JEV is prevalent, healthcare providers will assess the risk of exposure and consider vaccination, taking into account the individual circumstances of pregnant women.

In general, if a pregnant woman is planning international travel to areas where these diseases are endemic, it is crucial to consult with a healthcare provider who can evaluate the specific risks and benefits and provide personalized recommendations. In many cases, pregnant women may be advised to postpone travel to high-risk areas until after giving birth or to take other precautions to reduce the risk of infection.

It is important to note that vaccine recommendations can change over time, so it is essential to consult with a healthcare provider or travel medicine specialist for the most up-to-date information and guidance regarding travel vaccines during pregnancy.

■ VACCINATION DURING LACTATION

Background query that was answered by authors on December 28, 2022—was posted by professor Mohamud Sheikh, Community medicine from Al Ain, College of Medine and Health Sciences, UAE University.

"China inactivated COVID vaccine, should a pregnant and breastfeeding be vaccinated with the Chinese inactivated vaccine that UAE Health Ministry has just approved"?

Author's response:
The available data on the Sinovac-CoronaVac vaccine for COVID-19 in pregnant women are insufficient to assess either vaccine efficacy or possible vaccine-associated risks in pregnancy. However, this vaccine is an inactivated vaccine with an adjuvant that is commonly used in many other vaccines with a well-documented safety profile, such as HepB and tetanus vaccines, including in pregnant women.

The effectiveness of the Sinovac-CoronaVac vaccine for COVID-19 in pregnant women is therefore expected to be comparable to that observed in nonpregnant women of similar age. Further studies are expected to evaluate safety and immunogenicity in pregnant women.

In the interim, the WHO recommends the use of the Sinovac-CoronaVac vaccine for COVID-19 in pregnant women when the benefits of vaccination to the pregnant woman outweigh the potential risks. To help pregnant women make this assessment, they should be provided with information about the risks of COVID-19 in pregnancy, the likely benefits of vaccination in the local epidemiological context, and the current limitations of safety data in pregnant women. The WHO does not recommend pregnancy testing prior to vaccination nor delaying pregnancy or considering terminating pregnancy because of vaccination.

Vaccine effectiveness is expected to be similar in lactating women as in other adults. The WHO recommends the use of the COVID-19 vaccine Sinovac-CoronaVac in lactating women as in other adults. The WHO does not recommend discontinuing breastfeeding after vaccination.

Lactating Women's Severe Acute Respiratory Syndrome Coronavirus 2 Vaccination Effects

Many vaccines are recommended for breastfeeding individuals and is generally considered safe. The benefits of vaccination often outweigh the potential risks as vaccines can protect both the breastfeeding mother and infant from vaccine-preventable diseases.

Here are some commonly recommended vaccines for breastfeeding individuals:

- *Influenza (flu) vaccine:* The flu vaccine is safe during lactation and is usually recommended. It can help prevent influenza in both the breastfeeding parent and the infant.
- *Tdap vaccine:* Tdap vaccination is recommended for postpartum individuals, even while breastfeeding, to protect against whooping cough and to boost immunity to Td.
- *SARS-CoV-2 vaccination is recommended for breastfeeding parents* as it can protect against severe illness and transmission of the virus to the infant through BM (BM) A recent study has shown trace mRNA amounts were detected in the whole BM and BM extracellular vehicles (EVs) up to 45 hours postvaccination. However, these EVs neither expressed SARS-CoV-2 spike protein nor induced its expression in the

HT-29 cell line. Linkage analysis suggests vaccine mRNA integrity was reduced to 12–25% in BM EVs. Nevertheless, since the minimum mRNA vaccine dose to elicit an immune reaction in infants <6 months is unknown, a dialogue between a breastfeeding mother and her healthcare provider should address the benefit/risk considerations of breastfeeding in the first 2 days after maternal vaccination.

- *HPV vaccine:* The HPV vaccine is typically safe during lactation.
- *Pneumococcal vaccine:* Depending on individual risk factors, some people may be advised to receive the pneumococcal vaccine during lactation.
- *Meningococcal vaccine:* If you have specific risk factors, a healthcare provider may recommend the meningococcal vaccine during lactation.
- *Hepatitis A and HepB vaccines:* If not already vaccinated, these vaccines can be administered during lactation to protect against hepatitis.

Always consult your ID expert in vaccinology before getting any vaccine during lactation as individual circumstances and health history may affect the recommendations. Additionally, some vaccines may have specific contraindications or precautions, so it is crucial to discuss to ensure the safety and health of both mom and her baby. Physicians can provide guidance on which vaccines are appropriate based on individual basic and specific situations.

COVID-19 VACCINES DURING PREGNANCY AND BREASTFEEDING

- COVID-19 vaccines do not cause infection with the COVID-19 virus, including in pregnant women or their babies. None of the USA FDA-approved COVID-19 vaccines contain the live virus that causes COVID-19. Also, keep in mind that mRNA COVID-19 vaccines do not alter your DNA or cause genetic changes.
- The ACOG, the CDC, and other national organizations are recommending vaccination in women of reproductive age group nor is a pregnancy test needed before administering the vaccines.
- Pregnant women after receiving the first dose of a COVID-19 vaccine that requires two doses, it is recommended that they get their second shot. Pregnant women may also receive a COVID-19 booster shot. If anyone has concerns, they should talk to their healthcare provider about the risks and benefits.
- Getting a COVID-19 vaccine can protect you from severe illness due to COVID-19. Vaccination can also help pregnant women build antibodies that might protect their exclusively breastfed babies.

IMMUNOTHERAPY AND CANCER TREATMENT DURING PREGNANCY

The cases of cancer diagnosed during pregnancy are an ever-increasing trend nowadays.

Oncological drugs used for various types of gestational cancer during the first 3 months of a pregnancy should be avoided as far as possible because they can cause fetal death and fetal teratogenic (and other) serious complications. Various studies have shown that the administration of oncological drugs should be postponed until at least after the first trimester of pregnancy.

Further research is needed to reveal its efficacy during pregnancy. Data must be extracted and analyzed dutifully by physicians and, more specifically, by oncologists to be sure of the application of immunotherapy to pregnant women.

BREASTFEEDING AND MATERNAL HUMAN IMMUNODEFICIENCY VIRUS

Transmission of HIV by breastfeeding accounts for one third to one half of MTCT of HIV worldwide. Because of social and cultural reasons, the WHO recommends breastfeeding their infants exclusively for the first 6 months of life because infant morbidity associated with formula feeding is unacceptably high and safe alternatives to human milk may not be readily available.

- Whenever possible, an HIV-infected mother and her infant should be referred to a facility providing HIV-related services for women and children.

In 2021, 2.4 million Indians were living with HIV. Of all HIV infections, 39% (930,000) are among women. The NB delivered to HIV-positive untreated mothers has an extremely high risk for MTCT of HIV. It is more likely among mothers who acquire HIV infection late in pregnancy or during the postpartum period. In these clinical situations, the WHO recommends that all infants receive postnatal prophylaxis for HIV as soon as possible and preferably within 6–12 hours of birth.

The recommended empiric regimen for prevention of MTCT in infants who are not breastfed in a resource-rich setting is zidovudine plus lamivudine plus either nevirapine or raltegravir for 6 weeks. In resource-limited settings, zidovudine plus nevirapine for 6 weeks is the recommended regimen *(CDC, 2023)*. Three-drug regimens are safe in neonates; however, there is no evidence that they are more effective than two-drug regimens in high-risk infants.

MONOCLONAL ANTIBODY USED IN PREGNANCY AND LACTATION

Immunotherapy is becoming an increasingly common component of cancer therapy and the incidence of cancer in pregnancy is on the rise. Therefore, it is of great importance to understand the effect of immunotherapy exposure on maternal and fetal outcomes.

Increasingly, pregnant patients with inflammatory or autoimmune diseases use mAb biologics before conception, during pregnancy, and while breastfeeding. However, a minority of biologicals may lead to immunological and hematological abnormalities in the exposed infant.

- mAb infusion therapy can be used to help lessen the severity of COVID-19 for both pregnant women and their unborn babies if the woman tests positive for COVID-19 and is experiencing mild-to-moderate symptoms within the first 10 days of symptom onset.
- The administration of immune checkpoint inhibitors (ICIs) during pregnancy is associated with an increased incidence of pregnancy complications, prematurity, and low birth weight. The administration of these regimens is not recommended during gestation.

Since the approval of ipilimumab in 2011, ICIs have become the backbone of treatment for a growing number of malignancies. There have been few case reports on ICI exposure during pregnancy. A cancer diagnosis in pregnancy is uncommon, complicating 0.02–0.1% of all pregnancies. Breast cancer, hematological malignancies, cervical cancer, and melanoma are among the most diagnosed cancers in pregnancy. Despite the relatively low number of cases, the occurrence of several age-dependent malignancies in pregnancy is expected to rise as decisions to delay childbearing are becoming increasingly common.

Given the lack of data, all patients undergoing immunotherapy treatment be counseled about dual contraceptive methods, which should be used both during treatment and for an established period after the cessation of treatment. Whenever applied, close monitoring of the mother and the fetus is required.

DOS AND DON'TS TO REMEMBER

When it comes to vaccinations during pregnancy and lactation, here are some general dos and don'ts to keep in mind: Discuss the benefits and potential risks of each vaccine with your obstetricians and neonatologist to ensure moms are up-to-date on the recommended vaccinations during pregnancy and lactation. They can provide personalized advice based on maternal-specific health conditions and any potential risks associated with the vaccine.

Dos

- Do follow the recommended vaccination schedule—consult with your obstetrician and this may include vaccines such as the annual influenza vaccine and the Tdap vaccine during each pregnancy. Influenza can be particularly severe during pregnancy, so it is recommended to receive the influenza vaccine during flu season to protect both you and your baby.
- Getting vaccinated against COVID-19 is beneficial and is recommended during pregnancy or during the postpartum period. None of the COVID-19 vaccines contain live virus.
- Yes, mothers who are vaccinated against COVID-19 should be encouraged to continue breastfeeding. This can help protect both the mom and her newborn after birth to protect their infants. Unlike COVID-19 disease, vaccine-induced mother's immunity can pass through BM to her baby.
- There has been no evidence to suggest that COVID-19 vaccines are harmful to have received a vaccine and are breastfeeding or to their babies. COVID-19 vaccines cannot cause COVID-19 in anyone, including breastfeeding people and their babies.

The ACOG now recommends COVID-19 vaccines for everyone pregnant or breastfeeding. However, the WHO Strategic Advisory Group of Experts on Immunization (SAGE) acknowledged the lack of data for recommending the vaccine to lactating women. Given the importance of breastfeeding, researchers are encouraged to prioritize this topic and provide data on the safety of these vaccines for breastfeeding mothers and their infants.

Don'ts

- *Do not receive live vaccines during pregnancy:* Live vaccines, such as the MMR vaccine and the varicella vaccine, are generally not recommended during pregnancy due to theoretical risks to the developing fetus. It is advisable to receive these vaccines before pregnancy if needed.

- *Do not assume all vaccines are safe during pregnancy:* While many vaccines are considered safe during pregnancy, it is important to consult with your obstetricians to determine which vaccines are recommended and safe for you.
- *Do not delay necessary vaccinations:* Should receive necessary vaccinations during pregnancy and lactation to protect yourself and your baby from vaccine-preventable diseases. Delaying vaccinations may leave you and your baby vulnerable to infections.

CONCLUSION

Vaccination during pregnancy and lactation is an important aspect of maternal and infant health. Certain vaccines are recommended during pregnancy to protect both the mother and the unborn child, while others should be avoided due to potential risks.

Pregnant individuals and those breastfeeding should communicate openly with their obstetricians about their vaccination status and any concerns they may have. It is crucial to note that recommendations may evolve and new vaccines may be introduced over time. Every individual's health situation is unique and decisions regarding vaccines should be made based on a thorough discussion with the hospital's ID specialists.

SUGGESTED READING

1. Ávila-Nieto C, Pedreño-López N, Mitjà O, Clotet B, Blanco J, Carrillo J. Syphilis vaccine: challenges, controversies and opportunities. Front Immunol. 2023;14: 1126170.
2. Baker CJ. Group B streptococcal vaccine—sisyphus reconciled. N Eng J Med. 2023;389:275-7.
3. Centers for Disease Control and Prevention. Guidelines for Vaccinating Pregnant Women. Available from: https://www.cdc.gov/vaccines/pregnancy/hcp-toolkit/guidelines.html#pcv [Last accessed April, 2024].
4. Clinicalinfo.hiv.gov. (2024). Recommendations for the Use of Antiretroviral Drugs During Pregnancy and Interventions to Reduce Perinatal HIV Transmission in the United States. Available from: https://clinicalinfo.hiv.gov/en/guidelines/perinatal/whats-new-guidelines [Last accessed April, 2024].
5. Cooper L; Lessons from the USA, 1964-2013. The Hidden Burden: Rubella and Congenital Rubella Syndrome, WHO Region of Europe Immunization Managers Meeting, Antalya, Turkey, 15 March 2014.
6. Crispino P, Marocco R, Di Trento D, Guarisco G, Kertusha B, Carraro A, et al. Use of monoclonal antibodies in pregnant women infected by COVID-19: a case series. Microorganisms. 2023;11(8):1953.
7. Das R, Blázquez-Gamero D, Bernstein DI, Gantt S, Bautista O, Beck K, et al. Safety, efficacy, and immunogenicity of a replication-defective human cytomegalovirus vaccine, V160, in cytomegalovirus-seronegative women: a double-blind, randomised, placebo-controlled, phase 2b trial. Lancet Infect Dis. 2023;23(12):1383-94.
8. Edwards KM. Impact of vaccination during pregnancy on infant pertussis disease. Pediatrics. 2023;152(5): e2023063067.
9. Goh O, Pang D, Tan J, Lye D, Chong CY, Ong B, et al. mRNA SARS-CoV-2 vaccination before vs during pregnancy and omicron infection among infants. JAMA Netw Open. 2023;6(11):e2342475.
10. Gottlieb SL, Ndowa F, Hook EW 3rd, Deal C, Bachmann L, Abu-Raddad L, et al.; Gonococcal Vaccine PPC Expert Advisory Group. Gonococcal vaccines: Public health value and preferred product characteristics; report of a WHO global stakeholder consultation. Vaccine. 2020;38(28): 4362-73.
11. Hanna N, De Mejia CM, Heffes-Doon A, Lin X, Botros B, Gurzenda E, et al. Biodistribution of mRNA COVID-19 vaccines in human breast milk. EBioMedicine. 2023;96: 104800.
12. Hughes BL, Clifton RG, Rouse DJ, Saade GR, Dinsmoor MJ, Reddy UM, et al.; Eunice Kennedy Shriver National Institute of Child Health and human development maternal–fetal medicine units network. a trial of hyperimmune globulin to prevent congenital cytomegalovirus infection. N Engl J Med. 2021;385:436-44.
13. Hughes BL, Clifton RG, Rouse DJ, Saade GR, Dinsmoor MJ, Reddy UM, et al. Randomized trial of hyperimmune globulin for congenital CMV infection—2-year outcomes. N Engl J Med. 2023;389:1822-4.
14. IDWeek. Abstract 1942. Boston: IDWeek; 2023. pp. 11-5.
15. The J of Infectious Diseases. 2024; 229(1):1-297.
16. Koutras A, Ntounis T, Fasoulakis Z, Papalios T, Pittokopitou S, Prokopakis I, et al. Cancer treatment and immunotherapy during pregnancy. Pharmaceutics. 2022;14(10):2080.
17. Maertens K, Orije MRP, Van Damme P, Leuridan E. Vaccination during pregnancy: current and possible future recommendations. Eur J Pediatr. 2020;179(2):235-42.
18. McDonald R, O'Callaghan K, Torrone E, Barbee L, Grey J, Jackson D, et al. Vital Signs: Missed opportunities for preventing congenital syphilis—United States, 2022. MMWR Morb Mortal Wkly Rep. 2023;72(46):1269-74.
19. Medical News Today. (2023). Should you get an HBV vaccine during pregnancy? Available from: https://www.medicalnewstoday.com/articles/hep-b-vaccination-during-pregnancy#overview [Last accessed April, 2024].

20. Medscape. Vaccination/immunization during pregnancy. Available from: https://emedicine.medscape.com/article/2500098-overview#a5 [Last accessed April, 2024].
21. Ogunjimi OB, Tsalamandris G, Paladini A, Varrassi G, Zis P. Guillain-Barré Syndrome Induced by Vaccination Against COVID-19: A Systematic Review and Meta-Analysis. Cureus. 2023;15(4):e37578.
22. Pfizer. (2022). Annaliesa Anderson, Ph.D., Will Lead Pfizer's Vaccine Research & Development. Available from: https://www.pfizer.com/news/press-release/press-release-detail/annaliesa-anderson-phd-will-lead-pfizers-vaccine-research [Last accessed April, 2024].
23. Salehi I, Porto L, Elser C, Singh J, Saibil S, Maxwell C. Immune checkpoint inhibitor exposure in pregnancy: a scoping review. J Immunother. 2022;45(5):231-8.
24. Shanes ED et al. Am J Clin Pathol. 2020 May 22
25. Stafford IA, Workowski KA, Bachmann LH. Syphilis complicating pregnancy and congenital syphilis. N Engl J Med. 2024;390:242-53.
26. Venkatesan P. (2023). First RSV vaccine approvals. Available from: https://www.thelancet.com/journals/lanmic/article/PIIS2666-5247(23)00195-7/fulltext [Last accessed April, 2024].
27. Weldon R. (2023). 'Crisis': Congenital syphilis increasing at 'heartbreaking rate.' Available from: https://www.healio.com/news/pediatrics/20231107/crisis-congenital-syphilis-increasing-at-heartbreaking-rate?utm_source=selligent&utm_medium=email&utm_campaign=news [Last accessed April, 2024].

CHAPTER 8: Vaccines for the Elderly (Older Adults) (Senior Care Vaccinations)

▪ INTRODUCTION

Elderlies over 60 years of age should make sure to protect themselves as much as possible by keeping their vaccinations up-to-date. As people age, their immune systems change, making them more vulnerable to severe complications from preventable diseases, a condition known as immunosenescence. Thus, vaccination programs for seniors aged 60 years and above are imperative for promoting overall health and longevity.

Vaccinations for seniors against influenza, pneumonia, shingles, and hepatitis B (HepB) are specifically designed for older people and are known to be more effective than the standard vaccines. While vaccines do not guarantee complete immunity, they significantly reduce the risk of severe complications, thereby building a resilient and healthy elderly community.

Likewise, disseminated (Zoster) shingles is rare but can be more serious than localized shingles. **(Fig. 1)** Older adults and people with a weakened immune system may be at higher risk of developing disseminated shi. ngles.

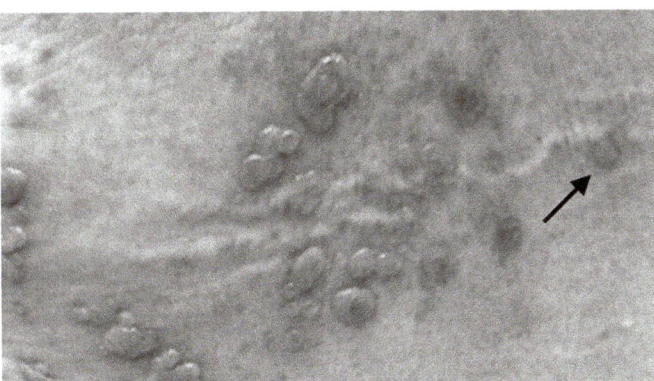

Fig. 1: Disseminated Zoster in an elderly individuals, a 67-year-old woman, with a medical history of controlled hypertension and diabetes mellitus presented to the emergency room (ER) with a painful rash for approximately 1 week. There were lesions on the left flank and backcrossing midline. [Also, erythematous patches and vesicles on her face and trunk, back and buttocks, and lower extremities (not shown in this figure)].
(Courtesy: Immunization Action Coalition)

Prompt treatment with antiviral medication can help treat disseminated shingles and prevent complications.

Elderly who have ongoing health conditions such as diabetes or heart disease, getting vaccinated is especially important. Vaccines can protect you from serious diseases (and related complications), so aged individuals can stay healthy as they age.

▪ SENIOR CARE VACCINATIONS

Seven vaccines that older adults need include:
1. The annual seasonal flu vaccine
2. Booster dose of the tetanus toxoid, adult dose diphtheria toxoid, and acellular pertussis (Tdap) or tetanus and adult diphtheria toxoids (Td)
3. Coronavirus disease 2019 (COVID-19) vaccines
4. HepB vaccine
5. Pneumococcal vaccines
6. Two-dosed Shingrix shingles vaccine (zoster)
7. Respiratory syncytial virus (RSV) vaccine.

The most important vaccinations seniors should discuss with their physicians include the flu vaccine, pneumococcal vaccine to prevent pneumonia, shingles vaccine, and Tdap vaccine.

Annual Seasonal Flu Shot

Older adults are at a higher risk for developing serious complications from the flu, such as pneumonia. A flu vaccine is especially important if one has a chronic health condition such as heart disease or diabetes. The flu is highly contagious and can easily be transmitted from person to person. The virus also changes over time, which means flu illness can occur again and again. To ensure flu vaccines remain effective, the vaccine is updated every year.

Everyone aged 6 months and older should get an annual flu vaccine, but the protection from a flu vaccine can lessen with time, especially in older adults. Vaccinated individuals are less likely to become seriously ill or hospitalized with the flu if they get the shot annually.

Ideally, one should get a flu vaccine by the end of October each year for optimal protection when the flu season starts. It takes at least 2 weeks for the vaccine to be effective. However, if the vaccine is not received by the end of October, it is not too late as flu season typically peaks in December or January. As long as the flu virus is spreading, getting vaccinated will help protect those who got vaccinated.

There are flu vaccines designed specifically for older adults: The Centers for Disease Control and Prevention (CDC) recommends that people aged 65 years and older receive a higher-dose flu vaccine or an adjuvanted flu vaccine (one with an additional ingredient called an adjuvant that helps create a stronger immune response. These vaccines are potentially more effective than the standard flu vaccine for people in this age group. (*Fluzone*—high-dose quadrivalent inactivated flu vaccine, *FluBlok*—quadrivalent recombinant flu vaccine, and *Fluad*—quadrivalent adjuvanted inactivated flu vaccine).

The high-dose recombinant vaccine conferred more protection against polymerase chain reaction-(PCR)-confirmed influenza than an egg-based standard-dose vaccine among adults between the ages of 50 and 64 years.
- If none of the recommended high-dose flu vaccines are available, any other age-appropriate influenza vaccine should be used.

The senior flu shot contains four times as much flu virus antigen as the regular flu shot. This stimulates a boosted immune response. Side effects of the senior flu shot are often mild and may include pain and redness at the injection site, headache, muscle aches, and fatigue.

Side effects of the senior flu shot are often mild:

Flu vaccine side effects are generally mild and go away on their own within a few days. Some side effects that may occur from a flu shot include soreness, redness, and/or swelling where the shot was given, headache (low grade), fever, nausea, muscle aches, and fatigue.

Tdap or Td Booster Shot Every 10 Years

Vaccines are recommended for adults, including the elderly, to provide protection against these diseases. Most people get vaccinated as children, but the elderly also need booster shots as they get older to stay protected against these diseases. The CDC recommends that adults get a Tdap or Td booster shot every 10 years.

The Tdap vaccine contains a lower dose of diphtheria and pertussis antigens along with tetanus toxoid. It helps boost immunity and provides protection against these diseases, which can have serious complications for individuals of all ages, including the elderly.

COVID-19 Vaccines for Elderlies—the First Priority Groups

The COVID-19 vaccines have been a crucial tool in combating the COVID-19 pandemic, especially for vulnerable populations such as the elderly. The older they are, the more immune dysfunction they have. Older adults are more likely than younger people to get very sick for longer durations, which causes them to have a higher risk of complications and death from COVID-19.

In many countries, elderly individuals were among the priority groups to receive the COVID-19 vaccine due to their increased vulnerability to the virus. Protecting the elderly has been a primary focus of vaccination efforts. Vaccines are highly effective in preventing severe illness, hospitalization, and death from COVID-19, including in the elderly population. Vaccination significantly reduces the risk of severe disease and its associated complications. The authorized vaccines have demonstrated a strong safety profile in the elderly population.

The United States (US) CDC recommends that older adults stay up-to-date with COVID-19 vaccines, including booster shots. Different COVID-19 vaccines may have varying levels of effectiveness and safety profiles. Both of the messenger ribonucleic acid (mRNA) COVID-19 vaccines authorized for use in the US Pfizer/BioNTech and Moderna have been shown in studies to be about 94–95% effective in preventing COVID-19 infection in all patients. But are they just as safe and effective for those 80 years and older?

Booster shots or additional doses of COVID-19 vaccines were being recommended for elderly individuals and those with weakened immune systems to enhance and prolong their protection. The need for booster shots may vary based on the evolving situation and updated recommendations from health authorities.

The 2023/2034 updated COVID-19 vaccines—made by Pfizer-BioNTech, Moderna, and Novavax—provide a high level of protection against the virus. Older adults should receive one dose of the updated vaccine at least 2 months after the last dose of any COVID-19 vaccine.

Recently (2023), the CDC recommended everyone 6 months and older get an updated COVID-19 Pfizer-BioNTech and Moderna booster shot. This updated bivalent mRNA booster vaccine prevents the spike protein of the original SARS-CoV-2 and the Omicron BA.4/BA.5 SARS-CoV-2. These additional doses aim to enhance and prolong the immune response, especially in individuals with weakened immune systems.

In a paper published this week in the Journal of the American Medical Association (JAMA), scientists also found that older adults (average age 76 years) who received Moderna had a 14% lower risk of being diagnosed with COVID-19 compared with those who received Pfizer. These results were not surprising given that Moderna contains 100 µg of mRNA, while Pfizer contains 30 µg.

Getting the vaccine into the arms of as many older adults as possible is important. Also, everybody needs to continue taking precautions after being vaccinated against COVID-19, including wearing a mask, practicing social distancing, and washing hands frequently.

People aged 75 years or older who have not had a COVID-19 vaccination in 6 months should have a booster dose. It is crucial for healthcare providers to educate and encourage the elderly population to receive COVID-19 vaccination. Vaccination plays a vital role in protecting the elderly from severe illness and reducing the impact of COVID-19 on this vulnerable population.

Hepatitis B Vaccine

Hepatitis B special situations: Age 60 years or older and at risk for HepB virus infection: Two-dose (heplisav-B) or three-dose (Engerix-B, Recombivax HB) series or three-dose series hepatitis A (HepA)—HepB (Twinrix) as mentioned above.

Chronic liver disease [e.g., persons with hepatitis C, cirrhosis, fatty liver disease, alcoholic liver disease, autoimmune hepatitis, alanine aminotransferase (ALT), or aspartate aminotransferase (AST) level greater than twice upper limit of normal].

Human immunodeficiency virus (HIV) infection—sexual exposure risk [e.g., sex partners of HepB surface antigen- (HBsAg)-positive persons, sexually active persons not in mutually monogamous relationships, persons seeking evaluation or treatment for a sexually transmitted infection, and men who have sex with men].

Current or recent injection drug use—percutaneous or mucosal risk for exposure to blood (e.g., household contacts of HBsAg-positive persons; residents and staff of facilities for developmentally disabled persons; healthcare and public safety personnel with reasonably anticipated risk for exposure to blood or blood-contaminated body fluids; hemodialysis, peritoneal dialysis, home dialysis, and predialysis patients; and patients with diabetes).

Incarcerated persons—travel in countries with high or intermediate endemic HepB.

Also, note that anyone aged 60 years or older who does not meet risk-based recommendations may still receive HepB vaccination.

Pneumococcal Vaccines for the Elderly

Pneumococcal conjugate vaccine (PCV) is now approved in India for those >50 years for the prevention of pneumonia and invasive pneumococcal disease (IPD) caused by 13 pneumococcal serotypes (STs). Pneumococcal vaccines are important for protecting elderly individuals against infections caused by the bacterium *Streptococcus pneumoniae*, also known as *pneumococcus*. This bacterium can cause a range of illnesses, including pneumonia, meningitis, and bloodstream infections, which can be particularly severe in older adults. There are two main types of pneumococcal vaccines recommended for the elderly, namely capsular polysaccharide [pneumococcal polysaccharide vaccine 23 (PPSV23)] and conjugated pneumo (PCV many types).

- Although progress has been made to decrease the incidence of IPD, it remains a serious risk to adults aged 65 years and older. In 2019, ~1 in 7 cases in the US resulted in death.

There are ~100 known *Streptococcus pneumoniae* STs, but they do not all contribute equally to the burden of IPD.

Pneumococcal conjugate vaccines are highly effective at protecting against disease from STs included in the vaccine. PCVs contain selected pneumococcal polysaccharides that are individually conjugated to carrier proteins. The first PCV, licensed in 2000, contained seven STs (PCV7), while the most recently approved contains 20 (PCV20), with several other higher valency PCVs in development. Increasing valency has obvious benefits in terms of broader disease coverage but comes at the cost of decreasing immunogenicity due to carrier suppression. Sooner or later, conjugated 24 valent (VAX 24) vaccine is expected to be introduced, although it will be important to understand any cost implications of this new cell-free protein synthesis technology.

Centers for Disease Control and Prevention says there are four pneumococcal vaccines licensed for use in the US by the Food and Drug Administration (FDA):

1. PCV13 (Prevnar 13®)

2. PCV15 (Vaxneuvance®)
3. PCV20 (Prevnar 20®)
4. PPSV23 (Pneumovax23®).

20 valent PCVs contain STs: 1, 3, 4, 5, 6A, 6B, 7F, 8, 9V, 10A, 11A, 12F, 14, 15B, 18C, 19A, 19F, 22F, 23F, and 33F.

Please note that PCV24 vax is on clinical trials and is *not* FDA approved.

For those who have never received any PCV, the CDC recommends PCV15 and PCV20 for adults aged 65 years or older and adults aged 19 through 64 years old, with certain medical conditions or other risk factors.

Adults who received an earlier PCV (PCV13 or PCV7) should talk with a vaccine provider to learn about available options to complete their pneumococcal vaccine series.

Adults aged 65 years or older have the option to get PCV20 if they have already received (but not PCV15 or PCV20) at any age and PPSV23 at or after the age of 65 years old. These adults can talk with their doctor and decide, together, whether to get PCV20.

For older adults who do not have an immunocompromising condition, cochlear implant, or cerebrospinal fluid leak—give one dose of PCV20 or PPSV23. Regardless of the vaccine used, their series is complete. The PCV20 dose should be given at least 5 years after the last pneumococcal vaccine.

Studies show that getting at least one shot of PCV13 protects:
- At least 8 in 10 babies from serious infections called IPD
- 3 in 4 adults aged 65 years or older against IPD
- 9 in 20 adults aged 65 years or older against pneumococcal pneumonia

June 1, 2022, Harvard School Public Health published:
- PCV13 and PPSV23—a person who has not received one of these earlier vaccines (PCV13 and PPSV23) should have a single dose of the new PCV20 or PCV15, followed by a year or more later with a "chaser" of PPSV23. (This period can be shortened to 8 weeks for people at high risk.)

People who have had one of the earlier vaccines should follow these guidelines:
- PPSV23 recipients should have one of the new PCVs (PCV15 or PCV20), at least a year after their PPSV23 vaccination.
- PCV13 recipients do not need one of the new PCVs at this time, but if not already received, they should get a PPSV23 vaccination 6–12 months later.

TABLE 1: Serotypes (STs) contributing to the burden of IPD in adults aged 65+ years changed over time.

Year	PCV STs	Non-PCV STs
1998	10%	90%
2010	41%	59%
2019	47%	53%

(IPD: invasive pneumococcal disease; PCV: pneumococcal conjugate vaccine)

Nearly one in two cases of IPD in adults aged 65+ years were due to STs not included in current PCV vaccines (US 2019). STs contributing to the burden of IPD in adults aged 65+ years changed over time **(Table 1)**.

2020 Active Bacterial Core surveillance epidemiology data ("ABC data") reflect:
- 56% of cases due to PCV STs and 44% of cases due to non-PCV serotypes, about one in two cases of IPD in adults aged 65+ years, though CDC noted historic decreases in the burden of IPD monitored by ABC data were likely due to the associated mitigation measures implemented during the COVID-19 pandemic.

Zoster (Shingles) Shingrix Vaccine for Older Adults

Zoster is caused by the varicella-zoster virus (VZV), the same virus causing chickenpox (varicella). For individuals who have had chickenpox, the virus is still in a dormant stage throughout life in the human system. As people get older, the dormant virus could become reactivated again and cause shingles.

Routine Vaccination of People Aged 50 Years and Older

The CDC recommends Shingrix [a recombinant zoster vaccine (RZV)] given in two doses for the prevention of herpes zoster (HZ) (shingles) and related complications such as postherpetic neuralgia.

Also, healthy adults aged 50 years and older should get vaccinated with the Shingrix vaccine (RZV), which is given in two doses separated by 2–6 months for immunocompetent adults aged 50 years and older.

The long-term efficacy of the vaccine is especially important because older adults are now living much longer than in previous years. People live these days into their 80s and even 90s. Therefore, it is really important to have a long-lasting vaccine. According to a new study published in the Annals of Internal Medicine, two doses of the RZV are effective against HZ for 4 years after vaccination.

Zostavax, a single-dose live attenuated zoster vaccine, *is no longer available for use.*

Shingrix can be administered concomitantly, at different anatomic sites, with other adult vaccines, including COVID-19 vaccines. Coadministration of RZV with adjuvanted influenza vaccine (Fluad) and COVID-19 vaccines is being studied.

Zoster vaccine should not be given to people who are immunocompromised, pregnant women, or those who have previously had anaphylaxis to the vaccine (either Zostavax or varicella vaccine) or its components (including gelatin or neomycin).

Note of Cautions

- One should get a shingles vaccine (Shingrix) even if you have already had chickenpox or the chickenpox vaccine or if you do not remember whether one had chickenpox.
- One should also get the shingles vaccine (Shingrix) if you have already had shingles, i.e., zoster illness or received Zostavax.
- There is no specific amount of time *one* needs to wait before administering Shingrix to patients who have had HZ. However, you should not give Shingrix to patients who are experiencing an acute episode of HZ and/or are sick and have a fever, weakened immune system, or have had an allergic reaction to Shingrix.

Just like with any other vaccine, patients sometimes have concerns about the potential side effects of RZV, said Tien. But those effects, such as muscle pain, nausea, and fever, are mild compared to shingles.

Two doses of RZV are recommended for the prevention of shingles and related complications in adults aged ≥19 years who are or will be immunodeficient or immunosuppressed because of disease or therapy. The second dose of RZV should typically be given 2–6 months after the first. However, for persons who are or will be immunodeficient or immunosuppressed and who would benefit from completing the series in a shorter period, the second dose can be administered 1–2 months after the first.

The CDC currently (January 2024) recommends two doses of RZV separated by 2–6 months for patients aged 50 years and older. Adults older than 19 years who are immunocompromised should receive two doses of RZV separated by 1–2 months

For more detailed clinical guidance, see www.cdc.gov/shingles/vaccination/immunocompromised-adults.html

Respiratory Syncytial Virus Vaccine for Older Adults

The RSV infection is a common virus that usually causes mild, cold-like symptoms. However, the clinical spectrum of RSV disease ranges from mild upper respiratory symptoms to severe lower respiratory tract disease. It has a higher risk of developing severe symptoms and can cause life-threatening pneumonia and bronchiolitis. Older adults are at increased risk for RSV-related complications and death owing to age-related immunosenescence and a higher prevalence of underlying conditions.

Especially high risk for RSV-associated hospitalization are those with comorbidities such as congestive heart failure, chronic obstructive pulmonary disease, asthma, coronary artery disease, cerebrovascular disease, diabetes mellitus, and chronic kidney disease, as well as immunocompromised patients, including those who have undergone solid organ or bone marrow transplant. In addition, for those who are frail and have an advanced age (especially ≥75 years), the illness can be particularly dangerous. Older adults who get very sick from an RSV infection may need to be hospitalized and the illness can even be life-threatening.

According to the US CDC, up to 120,000 adults aged 65 years or older are hospitalized with RSV annually and as many as 10,000 die. The annual incidence of RSV infection is estimated to range from 3% to 10% among older adults, depending on underlying risk factors, with frail older persons also at risk for severe RSV infection. Consequently, the societal burden and healthcare utilization that are associated with RSV infection in older adults are substantial.

In India, RSV disease epidemiology among adults and elderly is lacking. The rates of RSV detection in various hospital- and community-based studies mostly done in children vary from 5% to 54% and from 8% to 15%, respectively. As the worldwide population ages, the burden of RSV infection is expected to increase a situation that highlights the need for an RSV vaccine in this population. Thus far, the RSV circulation is seasonal, typically starting during the fall and peaking in the winter.

RSV vaccines are available now for 2023–2024 to protect older adults from the serious health problems that can occur with RSV infection.

On May 03, 2023, the FDA approved the first RSV vaccine GSK's *"Arexvy"*—an adjuvanted RSV PreF3 vaccine, for individuals 60 years of age and older. The CDC recommends adults aged 60 years and older may receive a single dose of the RSV vaccine; RSV vaccine may be given at the same time as other vaccines.

The American Academy of Family Physicians' (AAFP) recommendation is consistent with recommendations from the Advisory Committee on Immunization Practices (ACIP) and the CDC, which have both endorsed the use of new RSV vaccines for people aged 60 years and older. Patients over 60 years should talk to their family physician or other clinician about whether or not RSV vaccination is right for them.

Respiratory syncytial virus vaccine is composed of a part of the virus component (called a protein F) that does not contain a whole virus or a live virus and is safe for pregnant mothers including people with cancer who are eligible to get the shot. The RSV vaccine cannot cause an infection in people with a weakened immune system.

Like the flu, RSV infections are most common in the fall and winter months, so consider getting vaccinated before RSV season starts. However, you can benefit from the RSV vaccine at any time of year.

A single dose of the mRNA-1345 vaccine resulted in no evident safety concerns and led to a lower incidence of RSV-associated lower respiratory tract disease and of RSV-associated acute respiratory disease than placebo among adults 60 years of age or older. ACIP recommends a dose of either vaccine for adults aged 60 years or older.

Quick take: In older adults, the mRNA-1345 vaccine is a lipid nanoparticle-encapsulated mRNA-based vaccine encoding the membrane-anchored RSV-F glycoprotein, derived from an RSV A strain and stabilized in the preF conformation.

■ VACCINE SAFETY AND SIDE EFFECTS

- Vaccines are very safe, and they can help keep you from getting serious or life-threatening diseases. The most common side effects for all these vaccines are mild and may include pain, swelling, or redness where the vaccine was given.
- Should keep individual vaccination records, listing the types and dates of shots, taken along with any side effects or problems.

■ CONCLUSION

The population in India over the age of 60 years has tripled in the past 50 years and will relentlessly increase shortly. The elderly population in the world is increasing

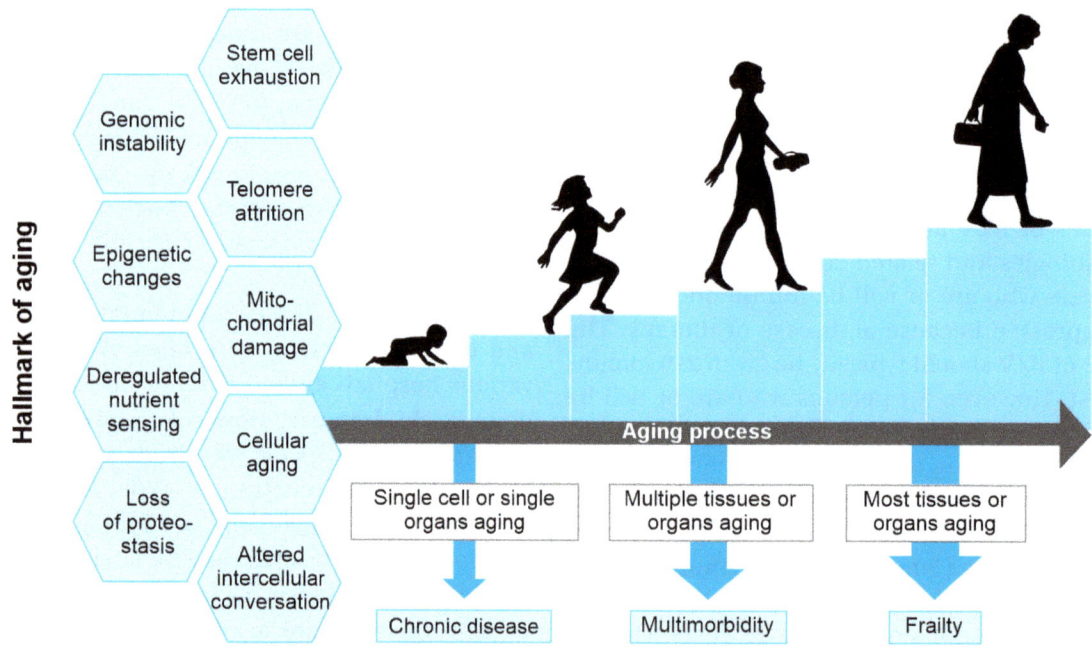

Fig. 2: Largely age-related clinical syndrome characterized by the physiological decline in several body systems, resulting in an increased vulnerability to poor health outcomes and death.

rapidly due to an extended life expectancy. Currently, around 8.5% of the world's population (or about 617 million people) are 65 years or older.

Among the many infections to which the elderly are prone, some can be prevented by administration of appropriate vaccines. Vaccination of the elderly is one of the most effective means of preventing disease, disability, and death from infectious diseases.

- *Frailty is highly prevalent in the elderly* and is associated with an impaired immune response, a higher propensity to infection, and a lower response to vaccines **(Fig. 2)**.

Additionally, the presence of uncontrolled comorbid diseases in the elderly also contributes to sarcopenia and frailty. Literature studies have shown that conventional vaccines only yield suboptimal protection for the elderly, which wanes rapidly in a shorter time.

To solve these problems: More immunogenic vaccine formulations using larger doses of antigen, stronger vaccine adjuvants, recombinant subunit, or protein-conjugated vaccines are needed. Further, newly developed mRNA vaccines, giving booster shots, and exploring alternative routes of administration are our future.

SUGGESTED READING

1. CDC. (2023). 2016-2020 Serotype Data for Invasive Pneumococcal Disease Cases by Age Group from Active Bacterial Core Surveillance. Available from: https://data.cdc.gov/d/qvzb-qs6p [Last accessed April, 2024].
2. CDC. (2023). Pneumococcal Vaccination: What Everyone Should Know. Available from: https://www.cdc.gov/vaccines/vpd/pneumo/public/index.html [Last accessed April, 2024].
3. The Lancet Infectious Disease J. 2023;23(12)1323-1428, e506-e567.
4. Harris DA, Hayes KN, Zullo AR, Mor V, Chachlani P, Deng Y, et al. Comparative Risks of Potential Adverse Events Following COVID-19 mRNA Vaccination Among Older US Adults. JAMA Netw Open. 2023;6(8):e2326852.
5. Hsiao A, Yee A, Fireman B, Hansen J, Lewis N, Klein NP. Recombinant or Standard-Dose Influenza Vaccine in Adults under 65 Years of Age. N Engl J Med. 2023;389:2245-55.
6. Wilson E, Goswami J, Baqui AH, Doreski PA, Perez-Marc G, Zaman K, et al. Efficacy and Safety of an mRNA-Based RSV PreF Vaccine in Older Adults. N Engl J Med. 2023;389:2233-44.
7. Zerbo O, Bartlett J, Fireman B, Lewis N, Goddard K, Dooling K, et al. Effectiveness of Recombinant Zoster Vaccine Against Herpes Zoster in a Real-World Setting. Ann Intern Med. 2024;177(2):189-95.

Immunotherapies: Preventive and Therapeutic Advancements

SECTION 2

Mohd Uduman, Jr Uduman, AK Uduman

9. **Immunotherapy and Gene Therapy Approaches in Disease Prevention and Treatments**
   Mohd Uduman

10. **Immunization in Special Clinical Circumstances Including Solid Organ Transplant (Immunocompromised and Immunosuppressed SOT and HSCT Recipients)**
    Jr Uduman, AK Uduman

11. **Cancer Vaccines: Preventive and Therapeutics**
    Mohd Uduman, Jr Uduman, AK Uduman

12. **Vaccines and Immunotherapies against Noncommunicable Diseases**
    Jr Uduman, AK Uduman

13. **Innovative Infectious Diseases Vaccines (The Future of Vaccines)**
    Mohd Uduman

Immunotherapy and Gene Therapy Approaches in Disease Prevention and Treatments

Mohd Uduman

■ INTRODUCTION

Immunotherapy marks a transformative breakthrough in medicine, revolutionizing how we combat diseases by fine-tuning the immune system to either stimulate aspects of its activity or suppress it. This innovative strategy employs antibodies, T-cells, and cytokines to precisely target a wide array of conditions, from cancers to autoimmune disorders.

The evolution of immunotherapy underscores its critical role as a major advancement beyond conventional treatment methods. In oncology, it has made significant strides, utilizing the body's immune defenses to pinpoint and eliminate cancer cells. This approach is noted for its precision and comparatively favorable side-effect profile, contrasting with the more traditional chemotherapy and radiation therapy. Immunotherapy has shown remarkable potential in improving survival rates across a variety of cancers and in generating long-lasting responses, thereby reducing the need for ongoing treatment.

In addition to cancer treatment, immunotherapy offers promising prospects in managing autoimmune conditions such as rheumatoid arthritis and type 1 diabetes by regulating the immune system to prevent it from attacking the body's own cells. The development of vaccines through immunotherapeutic techniques, aimed at pathogens such as the human papillomavirus (HPV), demonstrates the versatility of this method in combating infectious diseases (IDs) as well.

Despite these advancements, the field of immunotherapy is not without its challenges. The effectiveness of these treatments can vary widely among individuals, a phenomenon that underscores the importance of ongoing research and clinical trials aimed at enhancing the precision and efficacy of immunotherapy. The high costs associated with these treatments and the potential for immune-related adverse effects, such as inflammation in healthy tissues, are significant hurdles. These challenges emphasize the critical need for continued innovation in this area. This includes the exploration of biomarkers to better predict treatment responses and the development of strategies to minimize side effects, leveraging the advancements in precision medicine to create more targeted, effective, and patient-specific therapeutic options.

Cutting-edge research in immunotherapy is exploring avenues such as chimeric antigen receptor (CAR)-T-cell therapy for blood cancers and the potential of combination therapies, which pair immunotherapy with other treatment modalities to enhance efficacy and overcome resistance. These efforts promise to further expand the therapeutic landscape, offering hope for treatments that are more effective, personalized, and accessible.

Recent developments and advancements in immune and gene therapies for both infectious and non-communicable diseases have shown promising potential in enhancing treatment strategies and improving patient outcomes. These progressions represent a significant shift towards more personalized and targeted treatment approaches, utilizing the body's own immune system and genetic interventions to fight diseases more effectively **(Fig. 1)**.

■ ADVANTAGES OF IMMUNOTHERAPY

- *Enhanced effectiveness:* Immunotherapy has demonstrated remarkable effectiveness in treating advanced gastrointestinal (GI) cancers, frequently resulting in prolonged survival and higher response rates compared to conventional therapies.
- *Durable responses:* Immunotherapy can trigger sustained immune responses against cancer, sometimes leading to remission or even a cure in certain instances.
- *Fewer side effects:* Immunotherapy generally produces fewer and less severe side effects than chemotherapy and radiation, significantly improving the quality of life for patients undergoing treatment.
- *A critical addition to cancer treatment:* Immunotherapy is increasingly recognized as a vital fourth pillar of

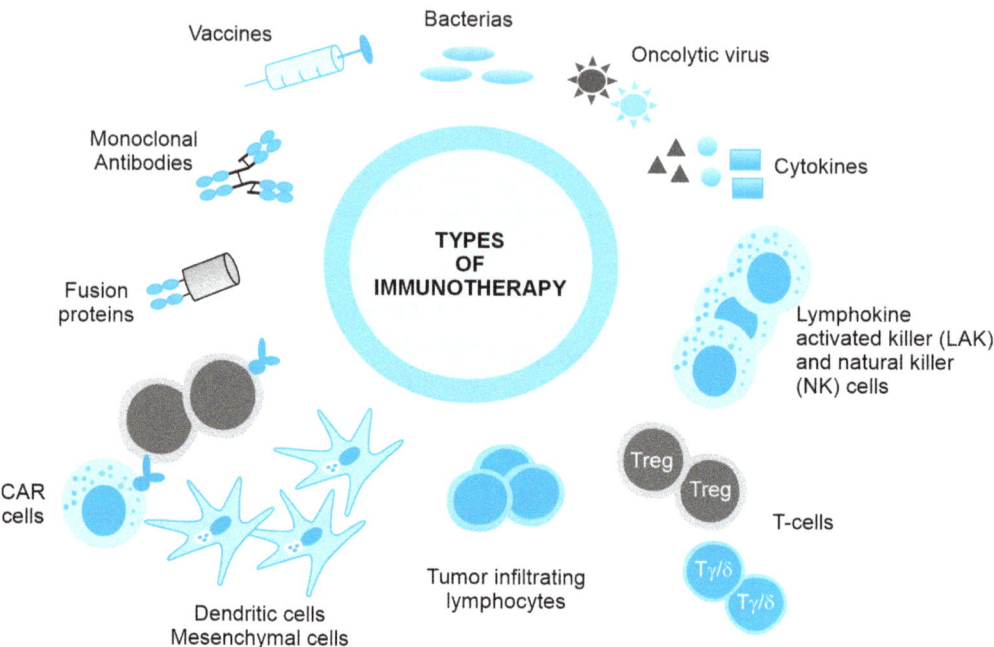

Fig. 1: Diverse modalities of immunotherapy. This diagram categorizes the key types of immunotherapies used in clinical settings, illustrating the breadth of strategies that harness the immune system to fight disease. It includes targeted antibodies, cell-based therapies, cytokines, oncolytic viruses, and vaccines, among others, each playing a distinct role in immune system modulation for therapeutic purposes.

cancer treatment, complementing surgery, radiation, and chemotherapy, and offering a new avenue to combat cancer.

■ BENEFITS OF IMMUNOTHERAPY:

- *Improved efficacy:* Immunotherapy has shown significant efficacy in treating advanced GI cancers, often leading to longer-term survival and improved response rates compared to traditional therapies.
- *Robust responses:* Immunotherapy can induce long-lasting immune responses against cancer cells, potentially leading to remission and even cure in some cases.
- *Reduced side effects:* Compared to chemotherapy and radiation, immunotherapy typically has fewer and milder side effects, improving patients' quality of life during treatment. Immunotherapy has come to be recognized as a major fourth arm that can be used to attack cancers, adding to surgery, radiation, and chemotherapy.

■ VACCINES

Vaccine therapy, a cornerstone in the battle against IDs for centuries, has achieved monumental successes, including the eradication of smallpox and the control of polio worldwide. Today, this field extends beyond traditional microorganism-based vaccines to embrace a wider spectrum of immunotherapeutic strategies, encompassing cytokines, and poly- and monoclonal antibodies (mAbs). These innovations mark a significant shift toward leveraging both innate and adaptive immune responses, heralding a new era in medical treatment.

Cytokines, small proteins crucial for cell signaling in immune responses, and mAbs, engineered to target specific antigens, are at the forefront of this evolution. They contrast with polyclonal antibodies, which are derived from different immune cells and target multiple antigens. This precision in targeting disease mechanisms underpins the latest advances in cellular immunotherapy.

Particularly notable are cancer vaccines such as sipuleucel-T (Provenge) for prostate cancer, which activates the immune system against cancer cells, and vaccines against the HPV, which prevent the onset of HPV-related cancers. These successes demonstrate the efficacy of targeted immune activation, offering new hope to patients and showcasing the potential of immunotherapy to not only treat but also prevent disease.

Immunotherapy seeks to harness the host's adaptive and innate immune responses to achieve the long-lived elimination of diseased cells. It can be broadly categorized into active approaches, including vaccine therapy and allergen-specific immunotherapy, and passive approaches, which encompass adoptive cell transfers and antibody-based therapies. This division highlights the field's multifaceted nature and its potential to address a wide range of diseases.

The advent of mRNA vaccine technology represents a pivotal breakthrough, offering rapid development and deployment capabilities, as evidenced by its critical role in addressing the COVID-19 pandemic. Looking forward, research into personalized cancer vaccines, which tailor treatment to the individual's unique tumor antigens, promises to revolutionize oncology by making therapy more effective and reducing side effects.

These advancements underscore a broader implication for global health—the potential to significantly reduce the burden of both infectious and non-IDs, thereby improving the quality of life for millions worldwide. As the field of vaccine therapy and immunotherapy continues to evolve, it stands as a testament to human ingenuity and the relentless pursuit of better health outcomes for all.

■ PASSIVE-MEDIATED IMMUNOTHERAPY

Passive immunotherapy involves the direct administration of prepared immune elements, such as antibodies or immune cells, that have been generated outside the body (ex vivo) to patients. These elements are ready to target and neutralize pathogens or diseased cells immediately upon administration, without the need to stimulate the patient's own immune system to mount a response. This approach offers the advantage of providing immediate protection or therapeutic effects, making it especially valuable in urgent situations where the body does not have the time to develop its own defensive response.

Antibodies used in passive immunotherapy, for example, can be monoclonal, targeting a specific pathogen or cancer cell antigen with high precision, or polyclonal, offering a broader range of target engagement. The use of immune cells, such as T-cells engineered to express CAR T-cells, represents another cutting-edge application of passive immunotherapy, harnessing the power of the immune system to directly attack cancer cells.

In contrast, active immunotherapy seeks to engage and boost the patient's own immune system, encouraging it to develop a long-lasting defense mechanism against diseases. This is achieved through the stimulation of the patient's immune response, leading to the development of specific immune effectors, such as immunoglobulins (Igs) (antibodies produced by B-cells) and T-cells, which are tailored by the immune system to recognize and combat specific pathogens or abnormal cells. Active immunotherapy not only aims to fight current infections or diseases but also to establish an immunological memory, providing long-term protection against future threats.

This distinction between passive and active immunotherapy underscores the versatility and adaptability of immunotherapeutic strategies in modern medicine. Each approach offers unique benefits and challenges, with passive immunotherapy providing immediate, albeit temporary, protection, or treatment, and active immunotherapy focusing on generating a durable, adaptive immune response. The integration of these strategies, tailored to individual patient needs and disease specifics, highlights the complexity and dynamism of contemporary immunotherapeutic practices, paving the way for more personalized and effective treatments.

■ MONOCLONAL ANTIBODIES

Monoclonal antibodies represent a groundbreaking class of therapeutic agents, designed with unparalleled specificity to target unique epitopes on cells or molecules. These engineered proteins closely mimic the function of natural human antibodies but with enhanced selectivity and efficacy. Produced by clones of a single parent immune cell, mAbs are homogeneous entities, which justifies their designation as "monoclonal". The journey of mAbs in the realm of medical therapy began with the US Food and Drug Administration's (FDA) approval of Orthoclone OKT3 in 1986, a milestone that marked the advent of mAbs for clinical use, primarily to prevent the rejection of transplanted organs. Since this pioneering approval, the landscape has broadened significantly, with over 150 mAbs receiving FDA approval, addressing a wide spectrum of noncommunicable diseases including various cancers, autoimmune diseases, and a range of inflammatory conditions.

The utilization of mAbs in combating IDs is a relatively recent but rapidly expanding application. Traditionally, vaccines have played a pivotal role in offering long-term protection against infectious agents, yet they typically require weeks to elicit a full protective immune response. In contrast, mAbs can confer immediate immunity, a critical advantage in acute infection scenarios or outbreak interventions. Initially, out of the first 100 antibody-based therapeutics approved in the United States, only a handful were designated for IDs. This scenario is changing dramatically, underscored by the approval of mAbs for combating Ebola, the development of refined antibodies against the respiratory syncytial virus (RSV), and the strategic deployment of mAbs during the COVID-19 pandemic. The horizon looks promising, with ongoing research aiming to extend mAb therapies to a broader array of infectious threats, including malaria, Dengue fever (DENV), human immunodeficiency virus (HIV), and other pathogens with pandemic potential (see below in details).

Immune Checkpoints and their Inhibitors

Immune checkpoints are critical regulatory pathways in the immune system that maintain self-tolerance and modulate the duration and amplitude of physiological immune responses. However, cancer cells can exploit these pathways, effectively "turning off" the immune response against the tumor.

Immune checkpoint inhibitors (ICPIs) are a class of drugs that block checkpoint proteins from binding with their receptors, allowing T-cells to attack cancer cells. This approach has transformed the treatment landscape for several types of cancer, marking a significant advancement in oncology. Proteins such as programmed death-ligand 1 (PD-L1) on tumor cells and programmed death 1 (PD-1) on T-cells are pivotal in modulating immune responses, often resulting in the inhibition of T-cell activity against tumor cells. ICPIs, by targeting checkpoints such as PD-L1 or PD-1, disrupt this inhibitory signal, thereby reactivating T-cells to recognize and destroy tumor cells **(Figs. 2A and B)**.

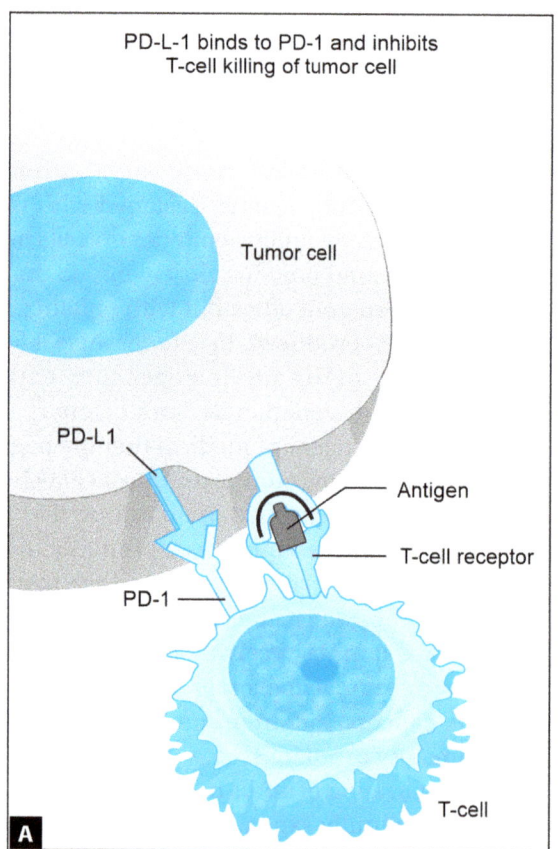
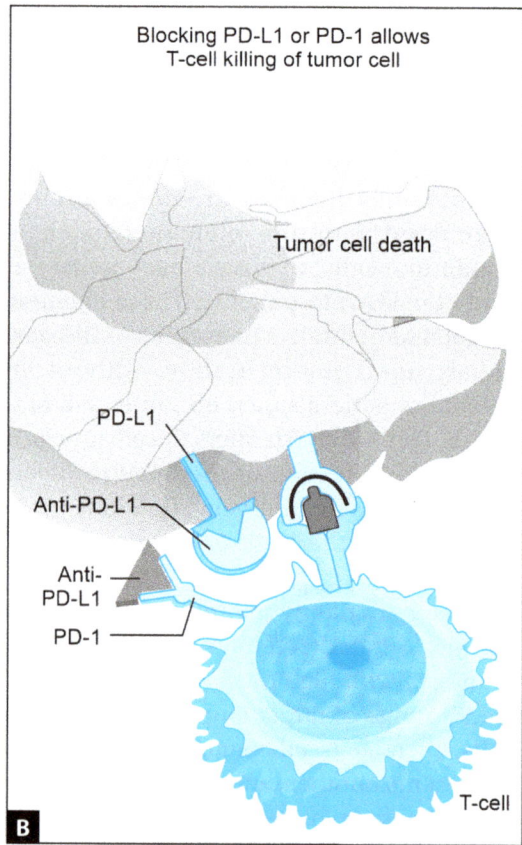

Figs. 2A and B: Immune checkpoint inhibitor mechanism. (A) Illustrates how the interaction between PD-L1 on the surface of tumor cells and PD-1 receptors on T-cells inhibits T-cell activity, preventing the immune-mediated destruction of tumor cells; (B) Demonstrates the action of immune checkpoint inhibitors, specifically anti-PD-1 and anti-PD-L1 antibodies, which block the PD-1/PD-L1 interaction. This blockade reinstates the T-cells' ability to recognize and eliminate tumor cells, thereby enhancing the immune response against the cancer. (PD-L1: programmed death-ligand 1; PD-1: programmed death 1)

This innovative therapeutic class, encompassing drugs such as pembrolizumab (Keytruda), nivolumab (Opdivo), and ipilimumab (Yervoy), has demonstrated efficacy against a variety of cancers, including melanoma, lung cancer, and bladder cancer, by enhancing the immune system's ability to target cancer cells. The integration of ICPIs with other modalities of cancer treatment—such as chemotherapy, radiation therapy, and targeted therapy—has further amplified their effectiveness, offering synergistic benefits that lead to improved immune responses against tumors and enhanced clinical outcomes for patients.

The advent of mAbs and ICPIs exemplifies the remarkable strides in medical science toward harnessing the immune system's innate capabilities, offering hope for more effective treatments against a wide array of diseases, including those once deemed intractable. As research continues to unravel the complexities of the immune system, these therapies are poised to redefine the paradigms of disease management, heralding a new era of precision medicine.

Bispecific Antibodies

Bispecific antibodies (BsAbs) represent a pioneering advancement in the realm of mAbs, distinguished by their innovative engineering to bind simultaneously to two distinct epitopes or antigens. This dual-targeting capability enables BsAbs to offer enhanced specificity and efficacy in therapeutic applications. By engaging two separate antigens—potentially on the same or different cells—BsAbs facilitate a novel approach to immunotherapy, particularly in the field of oncology.

The principle behind BsAbs is not just to improve target specificity by binding two antigens on a single cell but also to bridge immune cells to cancer cells. This bridging function orchestrates a more directed and potent immune attack against cancer cells, enhancing the efficacy of immune-mediated eradication of tumors. Among the several BsAbs in development or clinical use, blinatumomab stands out as a notable example. Approved for the treatment of acute lymphoblastic leukemia (ALL), blinatumomab has also shown promise in certain types of lymphoma. Its mechanism—binding to both CD19 on B-cells (a common antigen in B-cell malignancies) and CD3 on T-cells—exemplifies the potential of BsAbs to redirect and activate the immune system against cancer cells.

The advent of BsAbs marks a significant leap beyond traditional mAbs, offering a strategic advantage in tumor immunotherapy. The clinical outcomes associated with BsAbs have demonstrated superior efficacy compared to conventional mAbs, underlining their potential in treating various cancers. Their ability to engage multiple targets simultaneously opens up new avenues for therapeutic intervention, not only in oncology but also in the treatment of a wide range of diseases where multitarget engagement could prove beneficial.

Furthermore, the development of BsAbs complements the broader revolution in immunotherapy, which includes the use of cytokines and recombinant fusion proteins. As the scientific community continues to explore and refine this technology, the potential applications of BsAbs are expanding, promising a new era of precision medicine where therapies are tailored to harness and direct the body's immune system with unprecedented specificity and effectiveness.

■ FUSION PROTEINS

Fusion proteins represent a cutting-edge class of biopharmaceuticals, crafted by combining two or more distinct protein entities to form novel molecules with enhanced therapeutic potential. This innovative approach to drug design has paved the way for the development of antibody-cytokine fusion proteins, among others, which have significantly advanced the field of targeted cancer immunotherapy. These fusion proteins are engineered to deliver a one-two punch against cancer by not only directly enhancing tumoricidal (tumor-killing) activity but also by activating secondary antitumor immune responses, offering a multifaceted attack on cancer cells.

The design of fusion proteins often involves linking a targeting component, such as an antibody or a fragment thereof, with a potent effector molecule, such as a cytokine, toxin, or enzyme. The antibody component directs the fusion protein to specific antigens expressed on the surface of cancer cells, ensuring high specificity and minimizing off-target effects. Once bound to the cancer cell, the effector domain of the fusion protein is activated, which can directly induce cell death or modulate the tumor microenvironment in a way that promotes an immune-mediated attack on the tumor.

Antibody-cytokine fusion proteins, for instance, harness the targeting capability of antibodies to deliver cytokines directly to the tumor site. Cytokines are critical communicators in the immune system, capable of enhancing immune cell infiltration into tumors and stimulating a more robust immune response against cancer cells. By concentrating cytokine activity precisely where it is needed, these fusion proteins can significantly boost the immune system's ability to fight cancer, while reducing the systemic toxicity often associated with cytokine therapy.

The strategic advantage of fusion proteins lies in their modular design, which allows for the combination of various functional elements to target different aspects of tumor biology. This versatility enables the development of highly specialized therapies tailored to the unique characteristics of different cancers. For example, some fusion proteins are designed to disrupt the tumor's ability to evade the immune system, while others may target the tumor's blood supply or directly trigger cancer cell apoptosis.

As research progresses, the potential of fusion proteins extends beyond oncology, with applications in autoimmune diseases, IDs, and regenerative medicine. The development of these innovative molecules is a testament to the power of biotechnology to create highly effective, targeted therapies that can improve patient outcomes and quality of life. The ongoing exploration and refinement of fusion protein technologies hold promise for the next generation of precision medicine, offering new hope for treatments that are more effective, less toxic, and broadly applicable across a range of diseases.

■ BACTERIA-BASED IMMUNOTHERAPIES

The innovative use of bacteria in cancer therapy marks a radical departure from traditional treatment methodologies, introducing a novel approach within the field of immunotherapy. This strategy capitalizes on the unique capabilities of specific bacterial strains to either directly attack tumor cells or modulate the immune system, thereby enhancing its ability to recognize and destroy cancer. Bacteria's innate propensity to selectively colonize tumors and incite a vigorous immune response against the tumor microenvironment provides a dual-action mechanism in combating cancer.

Bacteria-based immunotherapies deploy live, attenuated bacteria or bacterial components, stimulating the body's immune defense mechanisms against cancer. These therapies stand as potent treatments on their own or when combined with other immunotherapies, chemotherapy, or radiation therapy, potentially augmenting their efficacy and surmounting tumor resistance.

Remarkable strides have been made with strains such as *Listeria monocytogenes* and *Salmonella typhimurium*, genetically modified to serve as vectors for cancer therapy. These bacteria are meticulously engineered to target and proliferate within tumor sites safely. Their presence within tumors serves a dual purpose—directly attacking cancer cells or disrupting the tumor microenvironment to hinder cancer growth, and acting as powerful adjuvants that draw a robust immune response. This immune engagement, initially against the bacteria, broadens to include a targeted attack on tumor cells.

These engineered bacteria are also designed to deliver therapeutic molecules—such as cytokines that bolster the immune response or genetic material coding for tumor antigens—directly to tumors. This strategic delivery turns the cancer itself into an immune target, facilitating not just tumor mass reduction but also immunological education about the cancer's specific characteristics. This could lead to durable immunity and potentially prevent recurrence.

The promise of bacteria-based immunotherapies lies in their unique mechanism of action, which differs fundamentally from traditional treatments. By employing living organisms that can actively target and penetrate tumors, these therapies offer a dynamic and adaptable approach to cancer treatment. As research progresses, further advancements in genetic engineering and synthetic biology are expected to enhance the specificity, safety, and efficacy of bacteria-based immunotherapies, making them a potent tool in the arsenal against cancer.

One of the most recognized bacteria-based cancer therapies is *Bacillus Calmette-Guérin (BCG)*, which has been used for decades as an effective treatment for nonmuscle invasive bladder cancer. BCG is a live, attenuated strain of *Mycobacterium bovis* that, when instilled directly into the bladder, induces a local immune response capable of attacking bladder cancer cells. Its success in treating bladder cancer and preventing recurrence has made BCG one of the earliest and most enduring examples of bacteria-based immunotherapy in clinical use.

Another innovative application involves the use of *L. monocytogenes*. A modified form of this *Bacterium, Lm-based immunotherapies*, has been engineered to stimulate a potent immune response against cancer cells. For instance, *axalimogene filolisbac (AXAL)* is an investigational therapy using attenuated *Listeria* that has been genetically modified to express HPV-associated antigens. AXAL has shown promise in clinical trials for treating HPV-related cancers, such as cervical cancer, by targeting and stimulating an immune response specifically against HPV-transformed cells.

Similarly, *Salmonella typhimurium* has been genetically modified to create *VNP20009*, a highly attenuated strain designed to target and accumulate within tumors. While VNP20009 has been explored in clinical trials for its ability to directly shrink tumors and stimulate an immune response, ongoing research is aimed at enhancing its efficacy and safety profile for cancer therapy.

The *CVRx-014*, based on a modified *Salmonella* strain, is another example being explored for its potential to deliver anticancer agents directly to tumor sites. This approach aims to leverage the bacteria's natural tumor-targeting properties to improve the delivery and therapeutic index of cancer drugs.

This innovative cancer treatment strategy exemplifies oncology's broader shift toward more personalized, precise therapies. By maximizing therapeutic efficacy and minimizing side effects, bacteria-based immunotherapies promise to redefine cancer treatment paradigms. Ongoing exploration and technological advancements in genetic engineering and synthetic biology are poised to augment the specificity, safety, and efficacy of these therapies, offering new hope in the fight against cancer.

As the scientific community delves deeper into the potential of bacteria-based immunotherapies, their integration into cancer treatment regimens stands as a testament to the field's dynamic evolution, promising transformative impacts on patient care and treatment outcomes.

CYTOKINES

Cytokines are small proteins secreted by cells in response to inflammation, categorized into groups such as chemokines, interleukins (ILs), interferons (IFs), and others. They serve as biomarkers of inflammation and aid in the early diagnosis of diseases.
- *Interleukins* are produced by leukocytes and act on other leukocytes, facilitating cellular communication.
- *Interferons* are pivotal in initiating immune responses to pathogens.
- *Lymphokines*, produced by lymphocytes, and monokines, produced by monocytes, attract immune cells like macrophages and neutrophils, respectively.
- *Chemokines* are specifically involved in directing the migration of immune cells.

The understanding of cytokine roles in immune responses has led to the development of biological therapeutics aimed at modulating these reactions, especially in conditions characterized by excessive cytokine production, such as rheumatoid arthritis and severe IDs.

Biologics such as *Enbrel* (etanercept) and *Kineret* (anakinra) are designed to inhibit cytokine signaling by binding directly to cytokine receptors, preventing cytokine-induced activation of immune responses. Similarly, *Actemra* (tocilizumab) and *Kevzara* (sarilumab) target and bind specifically to IL-6 receptors, effectively dampening the immune system's overreaction.

Another strategy involves the neutralization of cytokines themselves. Tumor necrosis factor-alpha (TNF-α) inhibitors, including drugs like *Remicade* (infliximab), *Humira* (adalimumab), and *Cimzia* (certolizumab pegol), bind directly to the TNF molecule, preventing it from engaging with cell surface receptors. This approach helps in mitigating the adverse effects of excessive cytokine production and is crucial in managing diseases where cytokine storms are a significant pathological factor.

Abnormal cytokine expression or regulation is implicated in various autoimmune diseases, highlighting the potential of targeting cytokines as a therapeutic strategy. Advances in recombinant cytokine and receptor technologies are paving the way for more effective, targeted therapies, offering new hope for patients with immune-mediated disorders.

It is important to highlight a phenomenon known as a "cytokine storm", an overzealous immune reaction marked by the excessive release of cytokines. This can lead to severe inflammation, a hallmark of advanced disease stages in infections such as COVID-19, where it significantly contributes to disease severity and progression. Elevated levels of cytokines like IL-6 are key indicators of a cytokine storm, leading to intense, systemic inflammation, and potential organ damage.

The ongoing exploration and refinement of cytokine-targeted treatments hold the promise of more precise intervention strategies, potentially transforming the management of inflammatory and autoimmune diseases, and providing a foundation for the development of novel therapeutic agents.

Key players in autoimmune therapeutics: When there is an abnormal expression or regulation of cytokines, it can promote autoimmune diseases. Targeting cytokines is an innovative treatment approach against immune disorders. Comprehensive recombinant cytokines and receptors enable scientists to design more effective and targeted therapies.

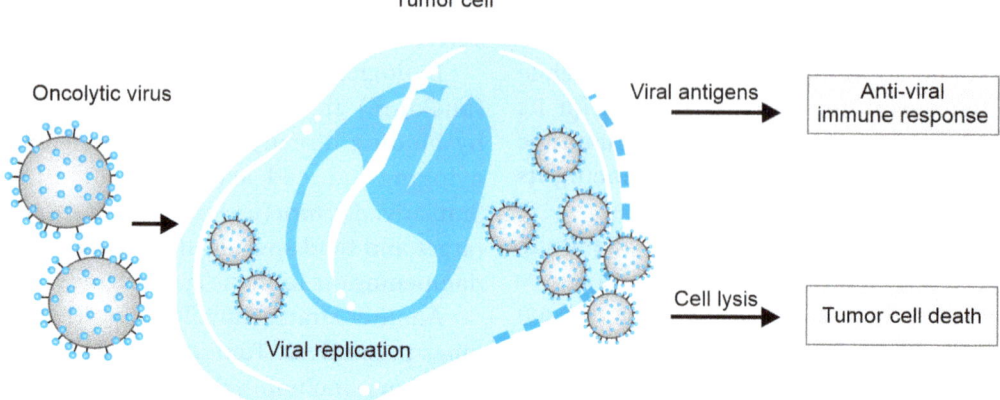

Fig. 3: An illustration of an oncolytic virus replicating within a tumor cell, causing cell lysis and leading to the cell's destruction. This process also initiates an antitumor immune response.

■ ONCOLYTIC VIRUSES

Oncolytic viruses (OVs) are a class of therapeutic agents that use the natural properties of viruses to selectively infect and destroy cancer cells. As they replicate inside tumor cells, they cause cell lysis, leading to the destruction of the cancer cell. This process not only directly impacts tumor cells but also stimulates the host's immune response. The expression of viral antigens upon viral replication within the tumor cells acts as a beacon, triggering an antiviral immune response that can secondarily target and eradicate tumor cells **(Fig. 3)**.

The potential of bacteria in antitumor therapy has been restricted application due to various challenges. In contrast, the therapeutic use of viruses has gained traction. Virus-based therapy was pioneered in the 1990s with the advent of genetically modified adenoviruses. It is only in recent years, however, that these OVs have moved from experimental stages to practical, clinical applications.

Oncolytic viruses are engineered to preferentially target and infect malignant cells, exploiting specific vulnerabilities in cancer cells, such as defective antiviral responses or the presence of oncogenic pathways. Once inside, they replicate until they induce immunogenic cell death (ICD), which not only kills the cell but also releases tumor antigens in an inflammatory context that can potentiate the host's antitumor immunity.

The unique mechanism of OVs—inducing direct oncolysis and eliciting systemic antitumor immunity—has opened new avenues in cancer therapy. By acting both as direct cytotoxic agents and as facilitators of tumor-specific immune responses, OVs represent a dual-modality for treating cancer.

Current research and clinical trials are investigating a range of OVs, each with distinct advantages and specificities. For example, the FDA-approved talimogene laherparepvec (T-VEC), a modified herpes simplex virus (HSV), is used for the treatment of melanoma. The success of T-VEC paves the way for further approvals and the development of a new generation of OVs targeting a variety of cancers.

Challenges remain in optimizing the delivery of OVs, avoiding immune clearance, and ensuring that the viral lytic cycle is completed before the host's immune system can neutralize the therapeutic viruses. Moreover, combining OVs with other treatments such as checkpoint inhibitors, chemotherapy, or radiation therapy, may enhance efficacy and overcome resistance mechanisms deployed by tumors.

As the science of OVs evolves, the future of cancer therapy looks increasingly promising. This innovative approach has the potential to offer less invasive, more targeted treatment options, and to complement or even replace traditional therapies for a variety of malignancies. The next frontier in OV therapy will likely involve personalizing virus selection and engineering to the genetic profile of individual tumors, maximizing therapeutic efficacy, and ushering in a new era of precision oncology.

■ CHIMERIC ANTIGEN RECEPTOR T-CELL THERAPY

Chimeric antigen receptor-T-cell therapy is a transformative approach to cancer treatment, leveraging the body's own immune cells to recognize and combat malignancies. This sophisticated form of immunotherapy involves modifying a patient's T-lymphocytes—key players in the immune response—to target B-cell malignancies such as lymphoma and leukemia with remarkable precision and potency.

The historic breakthrough in CAR T-cell therapy was exemplified by the first patient treated in 2009, who experienced a complete regression of disease and has remained disease-free for over a decade, according to Rosenberg et al. from the NIH Cancer Research in Bethesda, USA. This success story underlines the potential of CAR-T therapy as a durable and potentially curative treatment for certain cancers.

Originally devised for blood cancers, CAR T-cells are now making a groundbreaking transition into the treatment of autoimmune disorders, including multiple sclerosis (MS). With clinical trials underway, the adaptability of CAR T-cells showcases the potential breadth of adoptive cell therapy (ACT), extending its utility beyond oncology.

Cytokines, crucial in immune signaling, play a pivotal role in the culture and success of immune cell-based therapies. They are integral to the activation and expansion of both CAR-T and CAR-Natural Killer (CAR-NK) cells. The interplay of cytokines within the cellular milieu is fundamental to cultivating robust, therapeutic immune cells capable of vigorous expansion and targeted action.

Transitioning from mAbs to CAR T-cells, this form of ACT endows T-cells with the enhanced ability to seek out and eliminate cancer cells. Cell therapy introduces functional cells into the body to combat disease. When these cells are genetically engineered, as in cell-based gene therapy, they are endowed with specialized functions that are not naturally present.

In CAR T-cell therapy, a gene that codes for a specific CAR is introduced into the patient's T-cells, reprogramming them to identify and attack cancer cells. The CAR is a synthetic construct that combines both antigen-binding and T-cell activating functions, enabling T-cells to lock onto specific proteins presented by tumor cells.

Therapies such as tisagenlecleucel (Kymriah) and axicabtagene ciloleucel (Yescarta) have garnered significant attention for their efficacy in treating certain types of leukemia and lymphoma. These treatments exemplify the success of CAR-T therapy in inducing remissions in cancers that were previously resistant to conventional therapies.

As research progresses, the potential of CAR T-cell therapy continues to expand, with efforts focusing on refining the technology to minimize side effects, enhance efficacy, and extend the reach to solid tumors. The integration of precision medicine principles into the development of CAR T-cells may soon allow for personalized immunotherapies tailored to the unique immunological landscape of each patient's cancer, offering the hope of targeted, effective, and long-lasting treatments.

The evolution of CAR T-cell therapy reflects the broader trend of advancing human health through innovation, continuing to redefine the boundaries of what is possible in the treatment of cancer and other diseases.

DENDRITIC CELLS AND MESENCHYMAL STEM CELLS

Dendritic cells (DCs) and mesenchymal stem cells (MSCs) are pivotal to the advancement of cell-based immunotherapies due to their distinct and complementary roles within the immune system.

Dendritic cells are the sentinels of the immune system, with a primary function of processing antigen material and presenting it on their surface to other cells of the immune system, hence initiating a tailored immune response. They act as messengers between the innate and the adaptive immune systems. Therapeutic strategies involving DCs often focus on enhancing their antigen-presenting capabilities to better stimulate T-cells against cancer cells. This approach includes the development of DC vaccines, where cells are loaded with tumor antigens and then reintroduced into the patient to elicit a strong and specific antitumor response.

Dendritic cells (DCs) are the most potent antigen-presenting cells known in the human body that activate T-cells. Their unique physiological advantages have led to the development of DC vaccines, which are popular in cancer treatment. Currently, several DC vaccines have been approved globally for indications such as renal cancer, liver cancer, and prostate cancer

Mesenchymal stem cells are multipotent stromal cells that can differentiate into a variety of cell types. Beyond their regenerative potential, MSCs possess anti-inflammatory and immunomodulatory properties, making them an invaluable tool for cellular-based immunotherapy. Their ability to home to sites of inflammation and tumor environments, coupled with their capacity to evade the immune system, positions them as ideal vehicles for gene and drug delivery.

The MSCs are being explored for their therapeutic potential across a wide spectrum of diseases and disorders. Their role in modulating immune responses is particularly valuable in the treatment of autoimmune diseases, graft-versus-host disease (GvHD), and in enhancing the efficacy of cancer immunotherapies. In addition, their use in tissue engineering and regenerative medicine offers hope for repairing and regenerating damaged tissues and organs.

Combining the unique properties of MSCs and DCs could lead to innovative therapies that leverage the strengths of both cell types. For instance, MSCs could be used to modulate the immune environment to be more receptive to a vaccine based on DCs loaded with cancer antigens, potentially increasing the efficacy of the vaccine.

Furthermore, the intrinsic qualities of MSCs as facilitators of tissue repair and their immunosuppressive capabilities suggest they could play a significant role in mitigating the side effects of conventional treatments such as chemotherapy and radiation therapy. In gene therapy, MSCs can be engineered to express therapeutic genes, providing a targeted approach to delivering treatments directly to affected areas within the body.

As research progresses, the therapeutic applications of DCs and MSCs continue to expand. Clinical trials are underway to further understand the full potential of these cells in treating complex diseases, including various forms of cancer, immune-related disorders, and tissue degeneration. By tapping into the natural abilities of these cells, scientists and clinicians are working toward developing novel treatments that could significantly improve patient outcomes and quality of life.

The potential for DCs and MSCs in medical science reflects a transformative period in treatment modalities, highlighting the power of cellular therapies to address some of the most challenging medical conditions. With continued research and clinical innovation, dendritic and MSCs may provide the foundation for the next generation of therapeutic approaches.

TUMOR-INFILTRATING LYMPHOCYTES THERAPY

Tumor-infiltrating lymphocyte (TIL) therapy represents a personalized form of immunotherapy that harnesses the patient's own immune cells to mount an attack against cancer. TILs are immune cells that have migrated into tumor tissue, indicating a natural immune response against the tumor. These cells, due to their presence in the tumor microenvironment, are believed to be primed to recognize and attack cancer cells.

The process of TIL therapy involves several critical steps. It begins with the surgical removal of a patient's tumor, from which TILs are isolated. These cells are then expanded to large numbers in the laboratory using a variety of cytokines, including IL-2, to enhance their proliferation and activation. Once a sufficient number of TILs are generated, they are infused back into the patient, where they are more capable of targeting and destroying cancer cells due to their prior exposure to the tumor's specific antigens.

TIL therapy has shown significant promise in the treatment of melanoma, where it has resulted in robust and sometimes complete responses in patients with advanced disease. Its effectiveness against melanoma has prompted research into its applicability for other solid tumors, with the aim of providing a targeted and effective treatment option where conventional therapies may fall short.

One of the key advantages of TIL therapy is its specificity. Since the TILs are derived from the patient's own tumor, they are already tailored to recognize and fight the patient's specific cancer cells. This minimizes the risk of the immune system attacking healthy cells, a common side effect in less-targeted immunotherapies.

Moreover, the expansion of TILs outside the body and their subsequent reintroduction into the patient circumvent the immunosuppressive tumor environment that can inhibit immune cell function. This gives TILs a better chance of overcoming the cancer's defenses and leading to tumor regression.

Despite its promise, TIL therapy faces challenges such as the technical complexity of cell expansion, the need for individualized production, and managing the side effects associated with high-dose IL-2 therapy. Additionally, identifying patients who are most likely to benefit from TIL therapy and understanding why some tumors are more infiltrated by lymphocytes than others are critical areas of ongoing research.

Emerging strategies to improve TIL therapy include the use of checkpoint inhibitors to enhance TIL activity, genetic modifications to improve their tumor-targeting capacity, and optimizing protocols for cell expansion to generate more potent TILs. As these techniques evolve, TIL therapy could become a mainstay of treatment for a variety of cancers, offering hope to patients with hard-to-treat solid tumors.

In conclusion, TIL therapy exemplifies the incredible potential of leveraging the immune system in the fight against cancer. With continued advancements in cell culture techniques and immunomodulation, TIL therapy may transform the therapeutic landscape, offering personalized and effective treatment options for cancer patients.

REGULATORY T-CELLS AND GAMMA DELTA T-CELLS

Regulatory T-cells (Tregs) and gamma delta ($\gamma\delta$) T-cells are specialized subsets of T-cells that develop in the thymus and play crucial roles in maintaining immune homeostasis. They are central to the fine balance between effective immune responses and the prevention of autoimmune diseases.

Tregs, a subset of CD4+ T-cells, are essential for maintaining immune tolerance. They suppress immune responses, preventing the immune system from attacking the body's own tissues and reducing inflammation that can cause damage. Tregs function through various mechanisms, including direct cell-to-cell contact and the release of inhibitory cytokines such as IL-10 and TGF-β. Their ability to modulate the activity of DCs, macrophages, neutrophils, and other immune cells is critical for preventing excessive immune reactions and maintaining tolerance.

Gamma delta T-cells represent a less common subset of T-cells characterized by their unique T-cell receptors. Unlike the more common alpha beta ($\alpha\beta$) T-cells, $\gamma\delta$ T-cells can recognize a wide variety of antigens without the need for presentation by major histocompatibility complex (MHC) molecules, allowing them to respond to many different types of pathogens and stressed cells quickly. They are thought to serve as a bridge between the innate and adaptive immune systems, providing rapid responses to infection and potentially contributing to tumor surveillance.

Recent evidence has revealed significant crosstalk between Tregs and other immune cells, including $\gamma\delta$ T-cells, indicating a collaborative network crucial for immune regulation. Treg interactions with DCs, macrophages, neutrophils, and $\gamma\delta$ T-cells facilitate a wide range of immunological outcomes, from the dampening of inflammatory responses to the activation of antimicrobial defenses. These interactions are delicate and finely tuned, and dysregulation can lead to the development of autoimmune disorders or ineffective immune responses.

Understanding the interplay between Tregs and $\gamma\delta$ T-cells is increasingly recognized as important for the development of new therapeutic strategies. By harnessing or modulating the functions of these cells, researchers hope to develop treatments for autoimmune diseases, enhance vaccine efficacy, and improve cancer immunotherapies.

The complexity of the immune system, with its highly integrated network of cells, defies simplistic classification. While it can be useful to consider the functions of individual cell types in isolation, a more comprehensive understanding of immunity emerges when considering the cooperative functionality of cells. The dynamic crosstalk and synergy among various immune cells orchestrate a balanced immune response that can protect against pathogens, cancer, and also maintain self-tolerance to prevent autoimmunity.

As immunology research advances, therapeutic approaches that target Tregs and $\gamma\delta$ T-cells are becoming more sophisticated, with the potential to treat a variety of conditions that stem from immune system dysfunction. The prospect of specifically modulating these cells offers exciting possibilities for precision medicine, where treatments can be tailored to the needs of each patient based on a detailed understanding of their immune system's unique characteristics and requirements.

Lymphocyte-Activated Killer Cells

Lymphocyte-activated killer (LAK) cells are a specialized class of cytolytic lymphocytes that possess the unique ability to target and destroy tumor cells that are resistant to NK-cells. These powerful effector cells can be generated by culturing lymphocytes with activating cytokines, such as IL-2, which endow them with the capacity to recognize and kill a wide range of human tumor cells in vitro.

The activity of LAK cells is notable for its lack of restriction to a specific tumor antigen. They exhibit the remarkable capability to lyse autologous (self-derived) tumor cells as well as modified self and allogeneic (from a genetically non-identical member of the same species) tumors. This broad reactivity makes LAK cells a versatile tool in the field of cancer immunotherapy. The effectiveness of LAK cells is consistent across both populations of cells and at the individual clonal level, where clones of cells are derived from a single common ancestor, suggesting a robust and reproducible antitumor response.

The LAK cells are considered to be part of a broader spectrum of adoptive cellular therapy. When reintroduced into a patient, these cells can home in on and attack tumor cells throughout the body, making them a potential treatment option for metastatic cancers. Their use in immunotherapy is particularly intriguing due to their ability to kill tumor cells that have developed resistance to other forms of immune attack, such as those unresponsive to NK-cells, which are a part of the body's innate immune defense.

The implementation of LAK cell therapy in clinical settings often involves the ex vivo expansion of a patient's lymphocytes, followed by their activation with cytokines, and subsequent reintroduction into the patient's bloodstream. This approach aims to boost the immune system's natural anticancer activities and has been explored in various clinical trials for the treatment of cancers such as melanoma, renal cell carcinoma, and other solid tumors.

However, challenges remain in the therapeutic use of LAK cells. The need for large-scale ex vivo cell expansion, the management of associated toxicities from high-dose cytokine administration, and the variability in patient responses are all areas that require further research and refinement.

Advances in the understanding of LAK cell biology could lead to improved methods of cell activation and expansion, better patient selection criteria, and the development of combination therapies that enhance the efficacy of LAK cells. Combining LAK cell therapy with other immunotherapeutic strategies, such as checkpoint inhibitors or cancer vaccines, may provide synergistic effects, leading to better clinical outcomes.

As the field of cancer immunotherapy continues to evolve, LAK cells offer a promising avenue for treatment, particularly for patients with tumors that have proven refractory to conventional therapies. Future research focused on optimizing LAK cell therapy could significantly enhance its potential as a potent weapon in the fight against cancer.

Natural Killer Cells

Natural killer cells, also known as large granular lymphocytes (LGL), are an essential component of the innate immune system, distinguished by their ability to respond rapidly to a variety of pathological challenges. As a critical part of the diverse family of innate lymphoid cells (ILC), NK-cells comprise approximately 5–20% of all circulating lymphocytes in the human body.

The function of NK-cells is often compared to that of cytotoxic T-cells, which are part of the vertebrate adaptive immune response. While both cell types are capable of destroying target cells, NK-cells do not require prior sensitization to specific antigens. They are equipped with an array of activating and inhibitory receptors, which enable them to discern healthy cells from abnormal cells, such as those that are virus-infected, stressed, or transformed into tumor cells.

The NK-cells are thus instrumental in controlling early signs of infection and are particularly noted for their roles in combating viral infections and tumor growth. They are capable of inducing apoptosis, or programmed cell death, in cells that lack the appropriate markers of self, which are usually expressed by healthy cells and recognized by inhibitory NK-cell receptors. Conversely, cells that exhibit abnormal or stress-induced proteins can be targeted for destruction through activating receptors.

In the context of cancer, NK-cells can recognize and kill certain types of tumor cells without the need for tumor antigen presentation, which is required by cytotoxic T-cells. This allows NK-cells to contribute to tumor surveillance and control. The antitumor activity of NK-cells can be enhanced by various cytokines, such as IL-2 and IL-15, which can increase their proliferation, survival, and cytotoxic potential.

Recent advances in immunotherapy have sought to harness and augment the natural tumor-fighting capabilities of NK-cells. This includes strategies such as adoptive NK-cell transfer, where NK-cells are isolated from either the patient or a donor, activated and expanded ex vivo, and then infused back into the patient. Some approaches involve mAbs that can engage NK-cells and direct their cytotoxic activity toward tumor cells, a method known as antibody-dependent cell-mediated cytotoxicity (ADCC).

Additionally, genetic engineering of NK-cells to express CAR-NK-cells is an emerging area of research. This combines the specificity of CAR T-cell therapy with the innate cancer recognition abilities of NK-cells, potentially creating a powerful form of cancer immunotherapy with broader target recognition and fewer side effects related to off-tumor toxicity.

Ongoing research continues to delve into the complexities of NK-cell biology, seeking to overcome challenges such as tumor-induced immunosuppression, which can dampen the efficacy of NK-cells, and to tailor NK-cell based therapies for a wider range of cancers.

In the vast and dynamic landscape of immunotherapy, NK-cells stand out as promising agents for the development of novel treatments. With their intrinsic ability to target and destroy abnormal cells, NK-cells offer hope for more effective and natural forms of cancer therapy, embodying the innate power of the immune system to combat disease.

■ GENE THERAPY

Gene therapy is a revolutionary medical technique that manipulates genetic material within a patient's cells to treat or prevent disease. By introducing healthy genes into cells, either to replace missing or defective ones or to enhance the body's ability to fight disease, gene therapy offers potential cures for a range of genetic disorders. Since the first successful gene therapy trial in 1989, the field has advanced significantly, with several therapies now approved for clinical use. As advances continue, gene therapy offers hope for those suffering from previously untreatable conditions, flagging the way for a new era of personalized medicine

The principle behind gene therapy is relatively straightforward—it involves the transfer of genetic material—either DNA or RNA—into patient cells. This transfer can compensate for abnormal genes or make a beneficial protein. If a mutated gene causes a necessary protein to be faulty or missing, gene therapy may be able to introduce a normal copy of the gene to restore the function of the protein.

There are several methods and techniques within gene therapy:

- *Gene editing:* This involves making precise changes to the genome of a cell. Techniques like clustered regularly interspaced short palindromic repeats (CRISPR)/Cas9 allow scientists to cut out, add, or replace specific parts of DNA. This method can potentially correct mutations directly in the DNA sequence.
- *Gene replacement:* This strategy aims to replace a faulty gene with a healthy copy. It is particularly useful for diseases caused by a single defective gene.
- *Gene addition:* Rather than replacing a faulty gene, an additional gene is introduced into the body. This extra gene can produce a functioning protein that the person's body needs.
- *Gene inhibition:* Sometimes, the goal is to turn off a gene that is functioning improperly. RNA interference (RNAi) is one technique used to silence genes.

While gene therapy and immunotherapy are distinct, their paths often intersect, particularly in the treatment of cancer. For example, genetic manipulation can be used to enhance the body's immune response against cancer, as seen in CAR T-cell therapy, which modifies a patient's T-cells to attack cancer cells.

The convergence of gene therapy and virotherapy is seen in the use of OVs, which are genetically modified to selectively infect and kill cancer cells while sparing healthy tissues. These viruses can be engineered to carry therapeutic genes, effectively becoming vectors that deliver genetic material directly into cancer cells.

While gene therapy holds tremendous promise, it also comes with risks. Potential complications could include an immune reaction to the introduced vectors, the possibility of inducing tumorigenesis if the genetic material integrates into the wrong section of the genome, or other unforeseen effects. However, recent advances in delivery methods, vector development, and gene editing technologies have significantly mitigated these risks, making gene therapy safer and more precise.

Currently, gene therapy is approved for a handful of genetic disorders and is under investigation for many more, including a variety of cancers. Some therapies aim to eliminate the need for lifelong medication, offering the hope of a one-time cure. With ongoing research, the range of diseases that can be addressed by gene therapy continues to expand, including conditions that have been challenging to treat with traditional methods.

As gene and genetic therapies evolve, they stand at the forefront of a new era in medicine. Each advance brings us closer to realizing their full potential to change the lives of patients with genetic diseases, cancer, and beyond. Their development reflects the cumulative effort of decades of research, and each success story fuels the journey toward innovative treatments that could transform the therapeutic landscape.

■ IMMUNOTHERAPEUTIC ASPECTS

Active Immunization

It typically involves the administration of a primary series of injections of one or more doses of vaccine to "prime" the immune system and generate effector proteins (antibodies) and cells. Typically, "booster" doses of vaccine are administered periodically to enhance the level of specific antibody and effector T-cells.

The immunologic basis of approaches to active immunization is: (1) live-attenuated vaccines (LAVs) and (2) inactivated or detoxified agents or their purified components.

The antibodies elicited in response to antigen by vaccinations are usually polyclonal Abs, secreted by B-cells, and are long-lasting.

For some diseases, such as poliomyelitis and influenza, both approaches have been used. LAVs have the advantage of producing a complex immunologic response simulating natural infection. Commonly, immunity induced by a single dose of an LAV is possibly lifelong, however, the strength of response, particularly the humoral response, usually is less robust than the response following natural infection, and detectable antibodies can wane with time, resulting in some potential loss of protection.

Induction of immunity by LAVs can be inhibited by passive antibodies, whether from transplacental acquisition from the mother or receipt of Ig-containing blood products. Thus, the optimal response depends on ensuring that transplacentally derived passive antibody levels have declined. The examples of the primary measles vaccination at 12 months of age instead of earlier, and the delay of measles vaccination after administration of blood products. In addition, because the response may be only 90–95% after a single-dose, a two-dose or multiple-dose regimen can be necessary to induce higher levels of protection in the community and prevent the spread of disease if the population is exposed (community protection).

Inactivated or purified antigen vaccines induce response only to components present in the vaccine. Generally, multiple doses, usually three or more, are necessary to induce satisfactory antibody levels that persist for long periods; booster doses at longer intervals (e.g., 10 or more years for tetanus and diphtheria toxoids) sometimes are required to ensure lasting protection.

The nature of vaccine responses depends on antigen type. Protein and glycoprotein antigens usually induce both humoral immunity and memory (response through helper T-lymphocytes) after multiple doses, as evidenced by more rapid, broad, and intense (anamnestic) response to successive doses. Polysaccharide antigens by themselves induce only humoral antibodies without T-lymphocyte stimulation and fail to induce an anamnestic response with repeated antigenic challenge. This limitation can be overcome by the conjugation of polysaccharides to protein carriers to induce both a stronger immune response in younger children and immunologic memory, i.e., conjugated *Haemophilus influenzae* type b (Hib), *Pneumococcus* vaccine, etc.

Passive Immunization

Passive immunization entails the administration of preformed antibodies to a recipient and, unlike active immunization, confers immediate protection but for only a short period. This is especially important when that person has a high risk of complications from the disease or when time does not permit adequate protection by active immunization alone [e.g., rabies immunoglobulin (RIG), varicella zoster immunoglobulin (VZIG), hepatitis B immunoglobulin (HBIG)].

Passive immunization can be accomplished with several types of products, i.e., either *polyclonal IgG antibodies or mAb*.

The choice is dictated by the types of products available, the type of antibody desired, the route of administration, timing, and other considerations. These products include standard IgG kind of products; some of which are for intramuscular use [e.g., HBIG, VZIG, RIG, tetanus IG (TIG)], and others are for intravenous (IV) use [e.g., botulism, cytomegalovirus (CMV), vaccinia] **(Table 1)**.

■ MONOCLONAL ANTIBIOTICS

Monoclonal antibiotics are often made from pathogen-specific immune cells of people who have recovered from an infection. They are highly specific and can be designed to identify and attack a particular disease-causing organism. Many copies of the antibody can be made in larger quantities in a laboratory to mimic and are usually given as an IV infusion or in some cases an injection.

One way the immune system protects the body from microorganisms and other foreign substances is by making large numbers of antibodies. An antibody is a protein that sticks to a specific protein called an antigen. Antibodies circulate throughout the body until they find and attach to the antigen. Once attached, they can help other parts of the immune system to destroy the cells containing the antigen.

The mAbs are a type of passive immunity that can aid the immune system in being more targeted and have the potential to protect against IDs (i.e., RSV, COVID-19, CMV, etc.) or treat an illness. The mAbs works almost immediately and its duration of effect may vary. Potential to last many months or longer.

Biological Basis for Antibody Clonality

A monoclonal antibody is a collection of the antibodies secreted by a single B-cell clone, therefore having

TABLE 1: Licensed US antibody products for passive immunity to IDs or toxins [standard immunoglobulins (human)].

Product	Brand names	Made by	Licensed indications
IVIG	Many, e.g., Gammaplex, Gammagard, etc.		Primary humoral immunodeficiency; multifocal motor neuropathy; chronic idiopathic thrombocytopenic purpura; Kawasaki syndrome; and chronic inflammatory demyelinating polyneuropathy
IGSc		CSL Behring Baxter, Behring	Primary humoral immunodeficiency; multifocal motor neuropathy
IGIM	GamaSTAN	G Biotherap	Hepatitis A; measles; varicella; and rubella
Hyper IG (human)			
VZIG	VariZIG		Varicella postexposure prophylaxis in high-risk groups
HBIG–IM and IV use			Prevention and postexposure prophylaxis for hepatitis B—in NB and others. Postliver transplant cases
CMV-IVIG (human)			Prophylaxis of CMV disease associated with organ transplantation
Rabies IG			Postexposure treatment of rabies, given in conjunction with the rabies vaccine
TIG (human)			Prophylactic or therapeutic treatment of tetanus
Anthrax IVIG (human)			Treatment of inhalation anthrax
Botulism IVIG (human)			Treatment of infant botulism (type A or type B *Clostridium botulinum*)
Vaccinia IVIG (human)			Treatment and/or modification of complications resulting from smallpox vaccination

(CMV: cytomegalovirus; HBIG: hepatitis B immunoglobulin; IGIM: immunoglobulin intramuscular; IGSc: Immune globulin subcutaneous; IVIG: intravenous immunoglobulin; TIG: tetanus IG; VZIG: varicella zoster immunoglobulin)

specificity for only one antigenic epitope. They can then make many copies of that antibody in the laboratory and *are known as monoclonal antibodies.*

In contrast, a large number of B-cells can recognize the same antigen, the resulting response involves antibodies secreted by different B-cells targeted toward different epitopes on the same antigen. Such a response is called polyclonal. In other words, a polyclonal antibody is a collection of all the antibodies directed against a given antigen by many different B-cell clones.

Vaccines-elicited antibodies and mAbs are not the same. Both are used in the context of IDs but serve different purposes and work differently. Vaccines contain antigens that stimulate the body's immune system to recognize these antigens as foreign, destroy them, and "remember" them. When the real pathogen tries to invade the body, the immune system quickly recognizes it and destroys it. Essentially, vaccines are a form of primary prevention, used to prevent the onset of a given disease.

The mAbs, on the other hand, are laboratory-created molecules that can mimic the immune system's attack on pathogens. They are engineered to serve as substitute antibodies that can restore, augment, or modulate the immune system's attack on cells. mAbs are typically used for therapeutic purposes, often in the context of treating a disease that is already present. In the context of COVID-19, for example, vaccines (like Pfizer-BioNTech, Moderna, J&J, etc.) are used to train the immune system to recognize and fight off the severe acute respiratory syndrome coronavirus 2 (SARS-CoV-2) virus while mAb treatments (like Regeneron) are used therapeutically in individuals who have already been infected with the virus. The specific role of the treatment is to bind to the virus and prevent it from entering the body's cells, thereby limiting the difference between the two types of antibodies is in the names. "Mono" refers to one and "poly" refers to many **(Table 2)**.

- mAbs are clones of just one antibody, and they bind to one antigen only.
- Polyclonal Abs come from several different types of immune cells and will bind to more than one antigen.

mAbs have varied therapeutic uses and major clinical applications include:

- It is possible to create a mAb against any infective agents that bind specifically to almost any extracellular target, such as cell surface proteins and cytokines.

TABLE 2: Comparison of monoclonal and polyclonal Ig antibody therapy.	
Monoclonal antibiotics (mAbs)	**Polyclonal IgAbs (Vaccine-induced)**
Advantages	
• Abs is secreted by a single B-cell clone and has *high-specific activity for only one* antigenic epitope. Standardized potency • Can be manufactured in vitro at a large scale, with inherently high specificity and lot consistency. Minimal biohazard potential	• Multiple isotypes with different B-cell epitopes—polyvalent specificity • Much simpler to produce than mAbs, the effect can last for a longer time
Disadvantages	
Monovalent specificity: • Limited to single epitope specificity • Potential to select for escape mutants • Usually only last for a few months, thus requiring people to get multiple infusions or injections on a regular schedule	Low-specific activity: • Broad variation in potency • Limited availability • Biohazard risk of human blood products

Source: https://www.astrazeneca.com/what-science-can-do/topics/covid-19/covid-19-difference-between-antibodies-and-vaccines.html#

- mAbs can be used to render their target ineffective (e.g., by preventing receptor binding), to induce a specific cell signal (by activating receptors), to cause the immune system to attack specific cells, or to bring a drug to a specific cell type (such as with radioimmunotherapy which delivers cytotoxic radiation).
- Major applications include cancer, autoimmune diseases, asthma, organ transplants, blood clot prevention, and certain IDs.
- Over 100 mAbs are in development, and their unique features ensure that these will remain a part of the therapeutic pipeline.
- The first licensed monoclonal antibody was Orthoclone OKT3 (muromonab-CD3) which was approved in 1986 for use in preventing kidney transplant rejection. It is a monoclonal mouse IgG2a antibody whose cognate antigen is CD3. It works by binding to and blocking the effects of CD3 expressed on T-lymphocytes.

Although immunotherapy can be used for many diseases (infections, autoimmune diseases, macular degeneration, allergic diseases, etc.), it is being used most expansively in the cancer field. The main goal is to destroy the tumor, either directly or indirectly (by enhancing the patient's immune system), while offering greater specificity and fewer side effects than conferred by conventional therapies.

Major Types of Monoclonal Antibiotics

Four major mAb types are classified by their manufacturing method: These four types of mAbs differ in their composition, origin, and potential immunogenicity. The naming conventions help to identify and classify them based on their structure and development process, providing important information for clinicians and researchers working with these therapeutic agents.

The mAbs have multiple uses in health care; with clinical implications and can be divided into the following categories—(1) murine mAbs, (2) chimeric mAbs, (3) humanized mAbs, and (4) human mAbs.

1. *Murine antibodies* that are fully derived from mice *have a short half-life in vivo* (due to immune complex formation), *limited penetration into tumor sites*, and inadequately recruited host effector functions.

    Understanding proteomics has proven essential in identifying novel tumor targets (Suffix -mab). Proteomics is the study of the interactions, function, composition, and structures of proteins and their cellular activities. Proteomics provides a better understanding of the structure and function of the organism than genomics. Murine mAbs are named using the *prefix "o-" or "-omab"* at the end of the generic name.

2. *Chimeric mAbs:* Chimeric antibodies are molecules made up of domains from different animal species. For example, the Fc region or all the constant regions of a mouse mAb may be replaced with those of a human antibody. With the development of recombinant DNA technology, it has become possible to combine the heavy (H)- and light (L)-chain variable (V) regions of a desired mouse mAb with human constant (C) regions creating *hybrid (chimeric)* antibody molecules.

    This was initially achieved by the production of chimeric *(suffix by ximab)*, humanized antibodies (suffix by Zumab) and human (suffix by Umab). For example, "rituximab", is a chimeric antibody that contains murine variable regions and is used to treat certain types of lymphoma and autoimmune diseases. Likewise "infliximab" is a chimeric antibody that targets TNF-α and is used to treat inflammatory diseases such as rheumatoid arthritis.

3. *Humanized mAbs* have a majority of human sequences, with only a small portion of mouse sequences in the complementarity-determining regions (CDRs). Humanizing results in a molecule of approximately 95% human origin reducing the immunogenicity associated with murine mAbs. Humanized mAbs are named using the *suffix by "zumab"* at the end of the generic name. For example, "trastuzumab" is a humanized mAb used in the treatment of human epidermal growth factor receptor 2 (HER2)-positive breast cancer.

   Chimeric and humanized antibodies have generally replaced the murine, mice mAb in therapeutic antibody applications.

4. *Fully human mAbs:* Fully human mAbs are entirely derived from human sequences, both in the constant and variable regions. They are designed to minimize immunogenicity and maximize compatibility with the human immune system. Fully human mAbs are named using the suffix by *"umab"* at the end of the generic name. For example, "adalimumab" is a fully human antibody that targets TNF-α and is used to treat various autoimmune diseases such as rheumatoid arthritis and psoriasis.

Monoclonal Antibodies: A Game Changer for Disease Prevention and Treatment

Monoclonal antibodies are clones of human antibodies that are made in a laboratory and are meant to stimulate individual immune systems. mAbs as therapies are more targeted than some other types of treatments and have been more successful at treating many types of diseases and disorders, including some cancers. mAbs have shown efficacy in treating a wide range of diseases and disorders including:

- Infectious diseases
- Cancer
- Hemoglobinopathies
- Autoimmune diseases
- Neurological disorders
- Allergic conditions
- Ophthalmic diseases
- Transplant rejection
- Inherited diseases and disorders

List of mAbs and indications are tabulated in **Annexures 1 and 2.**

The first FDA-approved therapeutic mAb was *a murine IgG2a CD3-specific transplant rejection drug, OKT3 (also called muromonab)*, in 1986. This drug found use in solid organ transplant recipients who became steroid-resistant. Hundreds of therapies are undergoing clinical trials. Most are concerned with immunological and oncological targets.

Palivizumab (Synagis) is the first and only FDA-approved mAb for the prevention of severe RSV disease. Synagis was approved for initial use in the US by the FDA in 1998 and 2004 (BLA 103770/S-5059) and in Canada, Europe, the UK, Israel, and India in 2023.

Over two-thirds of mAb products are for transplant rejection, cancer, autoimmune diseases, IDs, antiviral prophylaxis, and antithrombotic treatment. Just a few examples:

- Palivizumab is used for RSV:
- Abciximab—a platelet aggregation inhibitor is used as an adjunct to percutaneous coronary intervention (PCI) for the prevention of acute ischemic cardiac problems.
- Edrecolomab, Recombinant humanized antivascular endothelial growth factor (rhuMAbVEGF), etc., to treat solid tumors.
- Enlimomab, OKT3, etc., used to treat and ameliorate organ transplant rejection.
- Trastuzumab is used in subjects with metastatic breast cancer.
- Rituximab is used for therapy of leukemias and lymphomas.
- Infliximab is used as therapy for Crohn's disease and rheumatoid arthritis.

The number of US-FDA approvals of mAb therapies has been rising since the first mAb drug for humans was approved in 1986.

Monoclonal Antibodies Uses in Infectious Diseases

In the setting of IDs, mAbs have the potential to provide almost immediate effect, making them potentially suitable for use in disease prevention as well as treatment.

Examples of mAbs that have been used, in pediatric practice since 1998 include, e.g., *palivizumab for the RSV* bronchiolitis in infancy and childhood. Fundamentally mAbs can neutralize viruses, prevent their entry into host cells, or facilitate their clearance by the immune system. Palivizumab (Synagis) is the first and only FDA-approved mAb for the prevention of severe RSV disease. Synagis was approved for initial use in the US by the FDA in 1998 and 2004 (BLA 103770/S-5059) and in Canada, Europe, the UK, Israel, and India in 2023.

Human-neutralizing mAbs against viral infections are classified by whether they have an envelope. Antibodies can recognize viral glycoproteins of the envelope on the surface of the virion as target antigens. Enveloped viruses include SARS-CoV, SARS-CoV-2, influenza virus, hepatitis C virus (HCV), Ebola virus (EBOV), Zika virus (ZIKV), DENV, chikungunya virus (CHIKV), and HIV. Neutralizing mAbs against enveloped viruses are created to block the binding of the glycoprotein to the host cell receptor in most cases.

mAb treatment for long–COVID: mAb cocktail casirivimab/imdevimab (Regeneron) given to treat acute COVID-19 infection has also been found to be effective against long-term COVID-19. The research, which assessed the benefits of mAbs, suggests relief may finally be ahead for millions of Americans with long-term COVID-19 for whom treatment has remained elusive.

In contrast, nonenveloped viruses including adenovirus, norovirus, and rhinovirus enter the host via lysis of the membrane or making pore-like structures in the membrane without interaction between a viral glycoprotein and a host receptor. The development of antibodies against nonenveloped viruses has not progressed much.

mAbs against Bacterial Diseases

Bacteria have more complicated structures than viruses. Therefore, fewer therapeutic neutralizing mAbs against bacterial infection have been developed. Depending on the type of bacteria, the major components include DNA, RNA, cytoplasm, cell membranes, and cell walls. Some bacteria have appendages such as flagella, pili, and capsules. Furthermore, gram-negative bacteria have an outer membrane outside of the cell wall.

Antibacterial mAbs could offer more effective ways of addressing antibiotic resistance and bacterial infections by targeting conserved pathways and activating the body's immune system.

mAbs against Parasites

"Very exciting" mAbs Development against Malarial Parasites

Although no mAbs are currently approved for malaria, recent data published at a medical conference demonstrated that one dose of a mAb called CIS43LS safely protected healthy adults from malaria infection during the 6-month malaria season in Mali.

The NIH said researchers are testing a second, more potent antimalarial mAb that is given subcutaneously in smaller doses and has shown promise in adults in early-stage testing. It is being assessed in two phase 2 trials in infants, children, and adults in Mali and Kenya. It will be some time before knowing whether this approach will make sense, but mAbs are an immunologic approach to controlling malaria and the initial results are very exciting.

mAb against Cancers

In oncology care settings, mAbs have revolutionized cancer treatment. mAbs are often used as a targeted therapy to identify and attack specific cancer cells or proteins associated with cancer, inhibiting their growth, promoting immune responses, or delivering cytotoxic agents directly to the tumor. Over 100 mAbs are in development, and their unique features ensure that these will remain a part of the therapeutic pipeline. For cancer treatment, they can be designed to, block growth signals, stop angiogenesis, or recruit and enhance immune responses against cancer cells.

The first licensed mAb antibody was Orthoclone OKT3 (muromonab-CD3) which was approved in 1986 for use in preventing kidney transplant rejection. It is a monoclonal mouse IgG2a antibody whose cognate antigen is CD3. It works by binding to and blocking the effects of CD3 expressed on T-lymphocytes.

Kohler and Milstein produced *murine mAbs from hybridomas* in 1975; a hybrid cell produced by the fusion of an antibody-producing lymphocyte with a tumor cell and used to culture continuously a specific mAb. Although murine mAbs were developed for clinical application, allergic reactions, the induction of antidrug antibodies (ADAs), and short half-life in humans shifted the technology toward chimeric mouse-human and then humanized Abs.

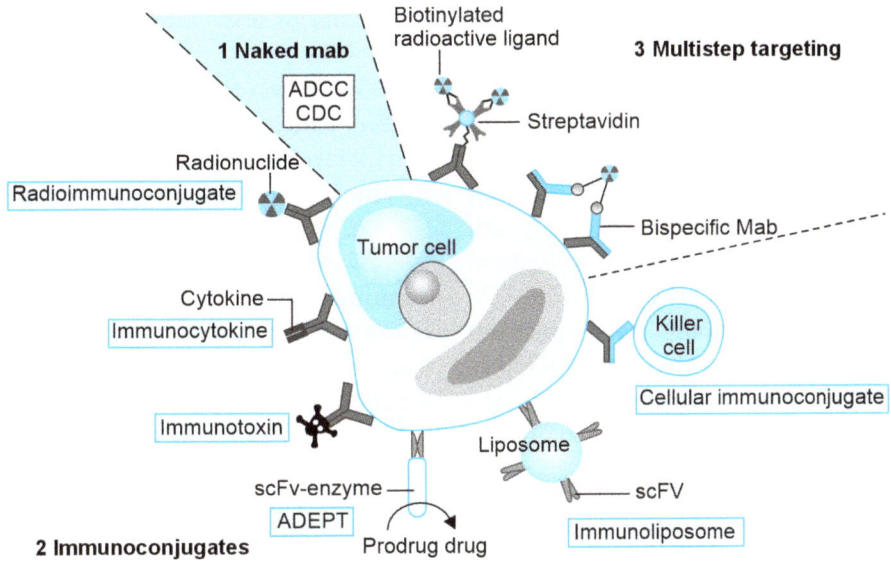

Fig. 4: Cancer mAb uses in clinical practice. (ADEPT: antibody-directed enzyme prodrug therapy; ADCC: antibody-dependent cell-mediated cytotoxicity; CDC: complement-dependent cytotoxicity; scFv: single-chain Fv fragment)

In the chimeric mouse-human Abs, the entire variable regions of a mouse Ab are fused with the constant regions of a human Ab to reduce immunogenicity and extend the half-life, but the tendency of chimeric mAbs to induce ADAs is still substantial.

There are still unmet medical needs in the treatment of many tumors including intracranial aggressive brain tumors including glioblastomas. New effective strategies that can eliminate the residual tumor cells are urgently needed. Immunotherapy offers a precise approach for specifically targeting residual glioblastoma cells with reduced risk of collateral toxicity.

Cancer mAb Uses in Clinical Practice

See **Figure 4**.

For Preventing Transplant Rejection

The mAbs are employed to prevent organ transplant rejection by targeting immune cells or molecules involved in the rejection process. The first FDA-approved therapeutic mAb was a murine IgG2a CD3-specific transplant rejection drug, OKT3 (also called muromonab), in 1986.

Muromonab is a monoclonal anti-CD3 antibody used as immunosuppressive therapy in kidney, heart, and liver transplant patients. This drug found use in solid organ transplant recipients who became steroid-resistant.

mAbs USE IN NONCOMMUNICABLE DISEASES

Autoimmune disorders, neurological disorders and allergic conditions.

There are hundreds of ongoing mAbs therapeutic clinical trials. Most are concerned with immunological and oncological targets. Also, for >30 years, mAbs have been approved and used to treat numerous NCDs such as severe asthma, rheumatoid arthritis, Crohn's disease, MS, and many types of cancer.

- mAbs are used to treat various autoimmune disorders such as rheumatoid arthritis, psoriasis, lupus, and inflammatory bowel diseases. They can modulate the immune response and reduce inflammation associated with these conditions.
- mAbs are being investigated for the treatment of neurological conditions such as Alzheimer's disease (AD), MS, and migraine. They target-specific molecules involved in the pathology of these disorders to potentially slow disease progression or alleviate symptoms.
- mAbs are used to manage allergic diseases, such as asthma and allergic rhinitis. They target molecules involved in the allergic response, reducing inflammation and alleviating symptoms.
- In cardiology, fully human mAbs-directed against proprotein convertase subtilisin/kexin type 9 (PCSK9)

have shown to be effective in reducing low-density lipoprotein cholesterol (LDL-C) in phase II clinical trials among patients with familial hypercholesterolemia (FH).
- mAbs have been developed for the treatment of ophthalmic conditions like age-related macular degeneration and diabetic retinopathy. They can inhibit abnormal blood vessel growth or inflammation in the eye.

These are just a few examples of the broad-spectrum of diseases that can be treated with mAbs. These therapies are successfully used in the clinic and/or in tertiary care hospital settings in repeated high-dose bolus injections imply high costs. The versatility and specificity of mAbs make them valuable therapeutic options across different medical fields.

■ VACCINES AND mAbs

mAbs and vaccines are not considered the same in the context of cancer and or NCD prevention.

mAbs are medicines that directly deliver man-made antibodies against a virus given to help fight off infections. mAbs is an engineered molecule in the laboratory that mimics natural antibodies to imitate the body's normal infection-fighting abilities, i.e., passive short-duration protections.

In contrast, vaccines are made of the parts of a pathogen (capsular material, toxins, and, or a particle) that trigger an immune response against an infection. Lasting protective polyclonal antibodies protection against given vaccination shot.

While both vaccines and mAbs can play roles in cancer prevention and treatment, they are not interchangeable. Vaccines are primarily focused on preventing the development of cancer by targeting specific infectious agents linked to cancer [e.g., HPV and hepatitis B virus (HBV) vaccines], whereas the mAbs are used as part of the treatment strategy after cancer has been diagnosed.

■ CANCER VACCINES

Cancer vaccines are designed to prevent certain types of cancer by stimulating the immune system to recognize and attack cancer cells.

Preventive Cancer Vaccines

- The most well-known cancer vaccine is the HPV vaccine, which can prevent infections with certain strains of HPV known to cause cervical and oral cancers.
- The HBV vaccine is another example that can prevent liver cancer, as chronic infection with HBV is a major risk factor for liver cancer. These vaccines are typically administered before exposure to the causative agents (e.g., HBV and HPV) to provide long-term protection.

However, both vaccines and mAbs are used as part of immunotherapy, which aims to strengthen the immune system's ability to attack cancer. Both are administered therapeutically to help treat existing cancer, but their roles in prevention are different as stated above.

The mAbs are molecules engineered to mimic the immune system's ability to fight off harmful cells such as cancer. For cancer treatment, they can be designed to specifically target cancerous cells and inhibit their growth, deliver cytotoxic agents, block growth signals, stop angiogenesis, or recruit and enhance immune responses against cancer cells. It is important to note that the field of cancer prevention and treatment is vast and evolving, with ongoing research exploring new approaches and therapies.

In the context of COVID-19, for example, vaccines (such as Pfizer-BioNTech, Moderna, and J&J) are used to train the immune system to recognize and fight off the SARS-CoV-2 virus while mAb treatments (like Regeneron) are used therapeutically in individuals who have already been infected with the virus. The specific role of the mAb (Regeneron) treatment is to bind to the virus and prevent it from entering the body's cells, thereby limiting the severity of the disease.

From mAb Therapy to T-cell based Therapy for the Treatment of Human Malignancies (Cancer)

Role of CAR T-cell Treatment as Immunotherapy

The CAR-T treatment generally involves extracting disease-fighting white blood cells known as T-cells from a patient, re-engineering them to attack cancer, and infusing them back into the body.

The CAR T-cells are cells that are genetically engineered (changed) in a laboratory. They have a new receptor so they can bind to cancer cells and kill them. Different types of cancer have different antigens. Each kind of CAR T-cell therapy is made to fight a specific kind of cancer antigen.

As their name implies, T-cells which help orchestrate the immune response and directly kill cells infected by pathogens are the backbone of CAR T-cell therapy. This has transformed the treatment landscape for B-cell malignancies and also is now showing great promise in at least three distinct autoantibody-dependent autoimmune diseases.

CD19-directed CAR T-Cell Therapy in Autoimmune Disease

Although recent data provides new evidence for the short- and long-term safety and efficacy of CD19 CAR T-cell therapy in autoimmune disease, controlled clinical studies are needed. Even though it is premature to judge whether these patients are indeed cured of their autoimmune disease, CD19 CAR T-cells at least appear to be able to achieve sustained disease- and drug-free remission.

CAR T-cell therapy, which is approved for certain cancers, involves removing and modifying a patient's immune cells and is known as a "cell-based gene therapy" (autologous, patient own cells, individualized). Traditional cancer treatments use nonspecific (chemo and radio) drugs and mAbs to target tumor cells. The CAR T-cell therapy, however, leverages the immune system's T-cells to recognize and attack tumor cells. T-cells are isolated from patients and modified to target tumor-associated antigens (TAAs).

Currently, available CAR T-cell therapies are customized for each patient (individualized). They are made by collecting T-cells from the patient and reengineering them in the laboratory to produce proteins on their surface called chimeric antigen receptors or CARs. The CARs recognize and bind to specific proteins, or antigens, on the surface of cancer cells (**Fig. 5**).

This innovative treatment involves modifying a patient's T-cells in the laboratory to enhance their ability to recognize and attack cancer cells. The process includes collecting T-cells from the patient, genetically engineering them to express CARs that specifically target cancer cell antigens, and then infusing these modified cells back into the patient. The engineered CAR T-cells are better

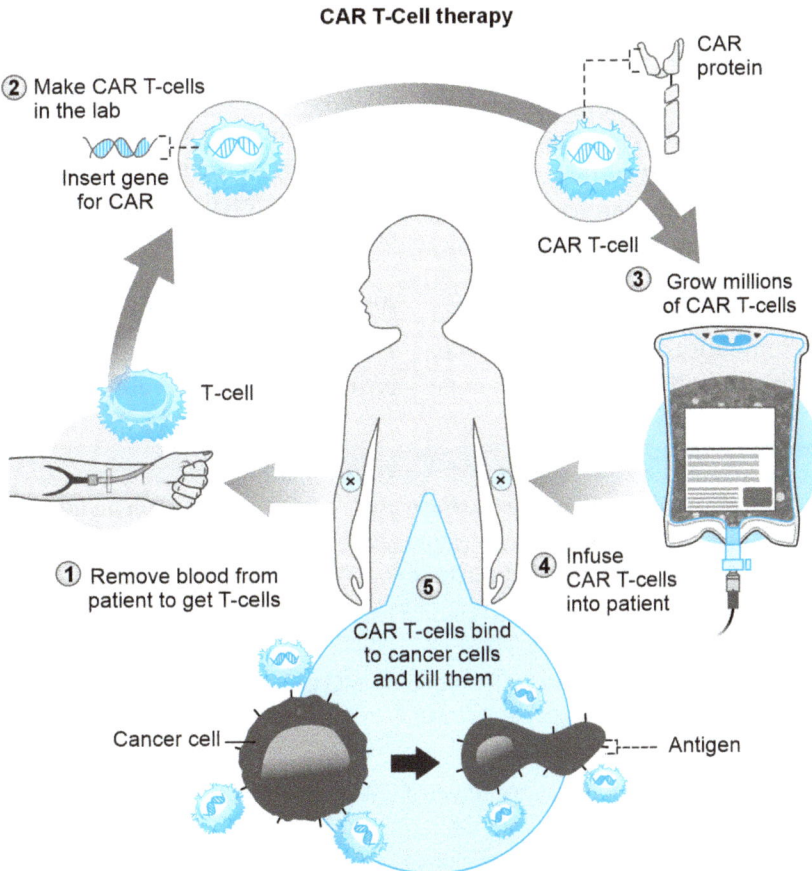

Fig. 5: CAR T-cell therapy, short for chimeric antigen receptor T-cell therapy, is a form of immunotherapy used to treat cancer.

equipped to identify and kill cancer cells, offering a targeted approach to cancer treatment. Currently, CAR T-cell therapies are customized for each patient and have shown promise in treating certain types of cancers, including some blood cancers like leukemia and lymphoma.

A single infusion of autologous CD19-directed CAR T-cell therapy led to persistent, drug-free remission in 15 patients with life-threatening SLE, idiopathic inflammatory myositis, or systemic sclerosis.

Recently reported study data provide evidence for the feasibility, preliminary efficacy, and side-effect profile of CD19 CAR T-cell therapy in patients with severe autoimmune disease. Although these data provide new evidence for the short- and long-term safety and efficacy of CD19 CAR T-cell therapy in autoimmune disease, controlled clinical studies are needed. CD19 CAR T-cell transfer appeared to be feasible, safe, and efficacious in three different autoimmune diseases, providing a rationale for further controlled clinical trials.

The CAR T-cells are now widely available in the United States and other countries and have become a standard treatment for patients with aggressive lymphomas and have become a part of modern medicine. The CAR T-cell therapies approved by the FDA to date target one of two antigens on B-cells, CD19, or B-cell maturation antigen (BCMA). A growing number of CAR T-cell therapies are being developed and tested in clinical studies. Although there are important differences between each specific therapy that can affect how they function in patients, they all share similar components **(Table 3)**.

More than 80% of children diagnosed with ALL that arises in B-cells, the predominant type of pediatric ALL, will be cured by intensive chemotherapy. But effective treatments have been limited for patients whose cancers return, or relapse, after chemotherapy or a stem-cell transplant.

In 2017, however, a new option appeared, with FDA's approval of tisagenlecleucel (Kymriah), the first CAR T-cell therapy to be approved by the agency, based on clinical trials demonstrating it could eradicate cancer in children with relapsed ALL.

CD19-targeted CAR T-cells are also offering hope to adults and children with advanced aggressive lymphomas. Before the development of CAR T-cells, many of these patients "were virtually untreatable. The results in lymphoma to date "have been incredibly successful, and CAR T-cells have become now a frequently used therapy for several types of lymphoma.

Off-the-shelf CAR T-cell therapies: Researchers have also begun to rethink the source of immune cells for CAR T-cell therapies—using T-cells collected not from patients, but from healthy donors (*allogenic, i.e., from other persons*). The goal "off-the-shelf" CAR T-cell therapies that would be immediately available for use rather than having to be manufactured for each patient.

After the overhauled T-cells are "expanded" into the millions in the laboratory, they are then infused back into the patient. If all goes as planned, the CAR T-cells will continue to multiply in the patient's body and, with guidance from their engineered receptor, recognize, and kill any cancer cells that harbor the target antigen on their surfaces.

Autologous versus Allogenic CAR T-Cell Therapy

There are numerous autologous and allogeneic CAR-T products, are in development. Manufacturers of these

TABLE 3: FDA-approved CAR T-cell therapy.

Generics	Brand	Target Ag and disease-targeted	Patient populations
Tisagenlecleucel	Kymriah	CD19 = B-cell acute lymphoblastic leukemia (ALL), B-non-Hodgkin lymphoma (B-NHL)	Children and young adults with refractory or relapsing B-cell ALL
Axicabtagene ciloleucel	Yescarta	CD19 = B-cell NHL Follicular lymphoma (FL)	• Adults with refractory or relapsing B-cell NHL Adults with relapsed or refractory FL
Brexucabtagene autoleucel	Tecartus	CD19 = Mantle cell lymphoma (MCL), B-cell ALL	• Adults with relapsed or refractory MCL • Adults with refractory of relapsed ALL
Lisocabtagene maraleucel	Breyanzi	CD19 = B-cell NHL	Adults with relapsed or refractory MCL
Idecabtagene vicleucel	Abecma	B-cell maturation antigen (BCMA)—multiple myeloma	Adults with relapsed or refractory multiple myeloma
Ciltacabtagene autoleucel	Carvykti	BCMA—multiple myeloma	Adults with relapsed or refractory multiple myeloma

next-generation CAR T-cell products are seeking to improve the efficacy and safety profile of existing therapies for hematologic cancers and to target solid tumors. CAR T-cells are also under investigation for the treatment of nonmalignant conditions, such as autoimmune diseases.

All of the FDA-approved CAR T-cell therapies rely on a disarmed virus to deliver the genetic material into T-cells to produce the CAR. But for the off-the-shelf CAR T-cells now being tested in small clinical trials, gene-editing technologies such as CRISPR are a widely used technology for precise and efficient gene editing in live cells. This genome editing technology is known to function in a variety of host systems, including bacteria, yeast, plants, insects, zebrafish, and mammals.

New treatment options where few existed, the initial development of CAR T-cell therapies focused largely on the most common cancer in children, ALL. >80% of children diagnosed with ALL that arises in B-cells, the predominant type of pediatric ALL, will be cured by intensive chemotherapy. But effective treatments have been limited for patients whose cancers return, or relapse, after chemotherapy or a stem-cell transplant. In 2017, however, a new option appeared, with the FDA's approval of tisagenlecleucel (Kymriah), the first CAR T-cell therapy to be approved by the agency, based on clinical trials demonstrating it could eradicate cancer in children with relapsed ALL.

CD19-targeted CAR T-cells are also offering hope to adults and children with advanced aggressive lymphomas. Before the development of CAR T-cells, many of these patients "were virtually untreatable", said James Kochenderfer, MD, of NCI's Center for Cancer Research, who has led several trials of CAR T-cell therapies in patients with diffuse large B-cell lymphoma. The results in lymphoma to date "have been incredibly successful", and CAR T-cells have become a frequently used therapy for several types of lymphoma.

The mAbs and CAR T-cells are two branches of cancer immunotherapy demonstrate the great ability to completely recognize cancer cell-surface receptors and blockade proliferative or inhibitory pathways. On the other hand, T-cell activation by genetically engineered CAR receptors via the TCR/CD3 and costimulatory domains can induce potent immune responses against specific TAAs. Both of these approaches have beneficial antitumor effects on cancer including colorectal cancer (CRC).

Standard treatments for CRC, including surgery, radiotherapy, and chemotherapy, have many side effects owing to their nonspecificity toward normal cells, leading to toxicity. Immunotherapy using both mAbs and CAR T-cells is effective with minimal side effects and toxicity. Furthermore, clinical trials using CARs could have promising therapeutic outcomes in patients with CRC. Although some challenges and concerns are using both mAbs and CAR T-cells, combinational therapies are expected to improve the antitumor effects and optimize their functions.

Understanding and Managing the Side Effects of CAR-T Cell Therapies

Like all cancer treatments, CAR T-cell therapies can cause severe side effects, including a mass die-off of antibody-producing B-cells and infections. One of the most frequent and serious side effects is cytokine release syndrome (CRS) including dangerously high fevers and precipitous drops in blood pressure.

The other side effect of particular concern with CAR T-cell therapies is neurologic effects, including severe confusion, seizure-like activity, and impaired speech. The precise cause of these neurologic side effects [also called immune effector cell–associated neurotoxicity syndrome, or (ICANS)] is still unclear.

It is important for clinicians caring for people who have received CAR T-cells to report the *occurrence of any new cancer*. At this time, experts recommend that patients and clinical trial participants who receive treatment with these products be monitored for new cancers throughout their lives since owing to the relatively recent widespread introduction of CAR-T products into clinical care we do not yet know how long after treatment people remain at risk for these adverse events.

Different ways of preventing CRS and ICANS are now under intense study. One approach is the prophylactic use of tocilizumab and low-dose steroids. Although further studies are needed, "the data so far are reassuring".

In many patients, both children and adults, mild forms of CRS can be managed with standard supportive therapies, including steroids. And as researchers have gained more experience with CAR T-cell therapy, they have discovered ways to better manage the more serious cases of CRS.

A big part of that management is the drug tocilizumab (Actemra); a drug, initially used to treat inflammatory conditions such as juvenile arthritis, which blocks the activity of IL-6, a cytokine that is often secreted in large amounts by T-cells and macrophages. Although it is

TABLE 4: Common mAb drugs that inhibit the activity of important immune checkpoints.

Immune checkpoint	Immune checkpoint inhibitors (ICPs)	FDA approval
PD-1	• Nivolumab (Opdivo) • Pembrolizumab (Keytruda) • Cemiplimab (Libtayo)	Melanoma, NSCLC, RCC, cHL, HNSCC, urothelial carcinoma, CRC, HCC melanoma, NSCLC, HNSCC, cHL, PMBCL, urothelial carcinoma, CRC, gastric cancer, cervical cancer, HCC, MCC CSCC
PD-L1	• Atezolizumab (Tecentriq) • Durvalumab (Imfinzi) • Avelumab (Bavencio)	Urothelial carcinoma, NSCLC, TNBC NSCLC, urothelial carcinoma MCC, and urothelial carcinoma
CTLA-4	Ipilimumab (Yervoy)	Melanoma

Source: Salehi I, Porto L, Elser C, Singh J, Saibil S, Maxwell C. immune checkpoint inhibitor exposure in pregnancy: A scoping review. J Immunother. 2022;45(5):231-8.

effective for treating CRS, tocilizumab does not seem to help with ICANS. Steroids are currently the best treatment option for severe ICANS, particularly dexamethasone, which is better at penetrating the central nervous system (CNS) than other steroids.

IMMUNE CHECKPOINT INHIBITOR THERAPY

Immune checkpoint inhibitors, a form of cancer immunotherapy, have dramatically contributed to oncologic success. This treatment represents a newer pathway in cancer therapy, effectively enhancing the immune response against tumor cells.

The ICPIs are increasingly utilized for dermatologic diseases such as melanoma, non-small-cell lung cancer (NSCLC) cell lung cancer, and in the GI world for CRC with microsatellite instability.

These inhibitors block the immune checkpoint pathways, which normally regulate the immune responses that our body would intrinsically use to prevent harm from antigens and other immune-related damage. However, in selectively blocking this process, these agents can create tumor lysis.

Currently, Approved ICPIs Target the Molecules CTLA4, PD-1, and PD-L1

- PD-1 is the transmembrane programmed cell death 1 protein (also called PDCD1 and CD279), which interacts with PD-L1 (PD-1 ligand 1, or CD274).
- PD-L1 on the cell surface binds to PD-1 on an immune cell surface, which inhibits immune cell activity.

Among PD-L1 functions is a key regulatory role in T-cell activities. It appears that (cancer-mediated) upregulation of PD-L1 on the cell surface may inhibit T-cells that might otherwise attack. Antibodies that bind to either PD-1 or PD-L1 and therefore block the interaction may allow the T-cells to attack the tumor **(Table 4)**.

The type of immune ICPI therapy may have an association with the risk for immune-related hepatoxicity. There are a couple of different classes of ICPs to consider, including CTLA-4 inhibitors such as ipilimumab, and anti–PD-1/PD-L1 drugs such as pembrolizumab, which is often used in melanoma therapy. However, the relative risk they pose for adverse events does not appear significant.

Role of Microbiome in Immunotherapies

Emerging research suggests that the composition of the gut microbiome can influence responses to cancer immunotherapy. Modulating the microbiome through probiotics, antibiotics, or fecal microbiota transplantation (FMT) may enhance the efficacy of immunotherapy treatments.

GENE (DNA) THERAPY

The term "gene therapy" sometimes appears alongside misinformation about mRNA vaccines, which include the Pfizer and Moderna COVID-19 vaccines. These vaccines contain mRNA, a genetic cousin of DNA that prompts cells to make the coronavirus "spike protein". The vaccines do not alter cells' DNA, and after making the spike, cells break down most of the mRNA.

There are two types of gene therapy:
1. *Somatic gene therapy:* This type usually occurs in the somatic cells of the human body. This is related to a single person and the only person who has the damaged cells will be replaced with healthy cells. In this method, therapeutic genes are transferred

into the somatic cells or the stem cells of the human body. This technique is considered the best and safest method of gene therapy.

2. *Germline gene therapy:* It occurs in the germline cells of the human body. Generally, this method is adopted to treat the genetic, disease-causing variations of genes that are passed from the parents to their children. The process involves introducing healthy DNA into the cells responsible for producing reproductive cells, eggs, or sperm. Germline gene therapy is not legal in many places as the risks outweigh the rewards.

Gene (DNA) therapy works by adding new copies of a gene that is broken, or by replacing a defective or missing gene in a patient's cells with a healthy version of that gene **(Fig. 6)**. Gene therapy in a global context involves the correction of a genetic defect thereby correcting an underlying disease and disorders.

When a gene mutation (a permanent alteration in the DNA sequence) causes a protein to be missing or faulty, gene therapy may be able to restore the normal function of that protein. Thus, gene therapy is understood as the ability of genetic improvement through the correction of altered (mutated) genes or site-specific.

Basically, DNA is located inside the nucleus of each human cell, where it is packaged into chromosomes, and also inside mitochondria, the "power plant" organelles located outside the nucleus.

DNA is a molecule that stores genetic information, and genes are pieces of genetic information that cells use to make a particular product, such as a protein.

Although there are mitochondrial diseases that could someday be cured with gene therapy, currently, the term gene therapy refers to treatments that target nuclear DNA genes on the 23 pairs of chromosomes of chromosomes inside the nucleus **(Fig. 7)**.

Classically, gene therapy has referred to the process of either "knocking out" a dysfunctional gene or adding a copy of a working gene to the nucleus to improve cell function. Gene therapy is currently directed at diseases stemming from a problem with just one gene, or at most

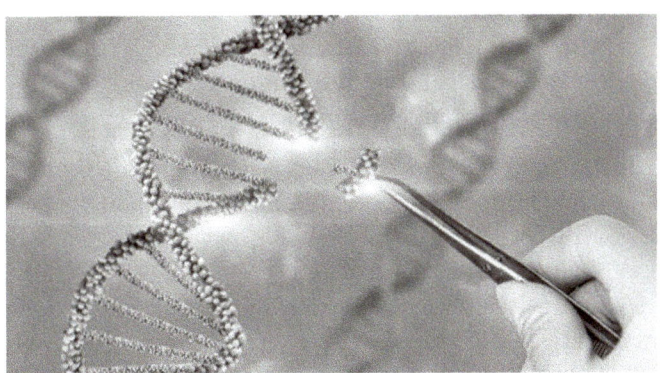

Fig. 6: What exactly is gene therapy and how does it work?
(Courtesy: Natali_Mis via Shutterstock)

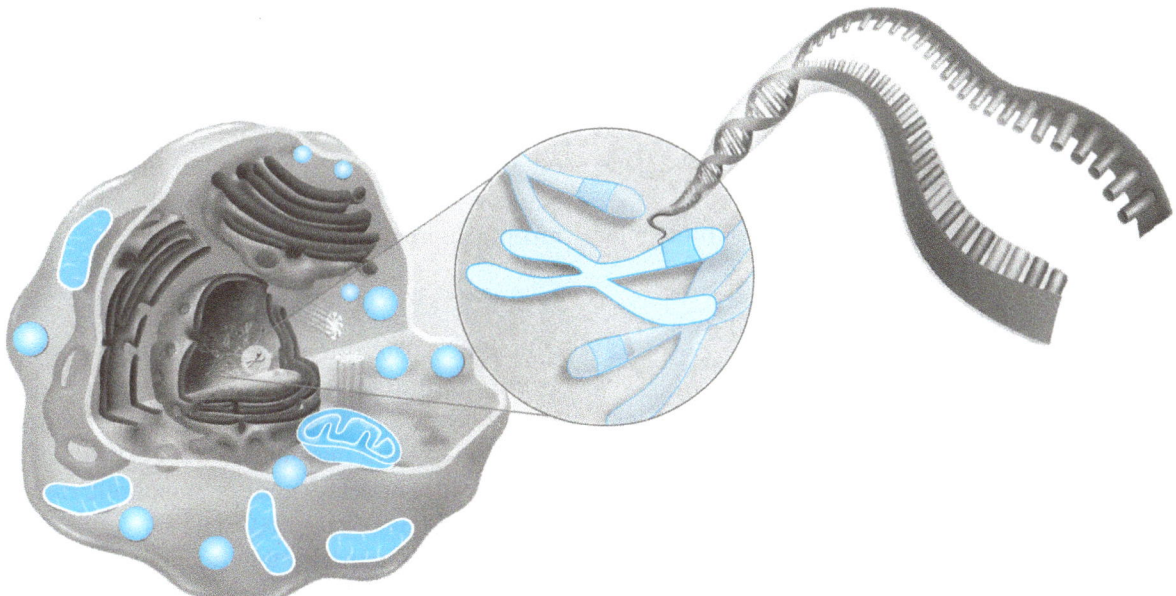

Fig. 7: An illustration of DNA inside chromosomes that are then inside a cell nucleus.
(Courtesy: BSIP/UIG via Getty Images).

a few genes, rather than those that involve many genes. *Ever since mapping the human genome, scientists have envisioned replacing mutated genes with healthy ones to cure genetic diseases.*

However, the field of gene therapy is now expanding to include strategies that do not all fall into the classic categories of knocking out bad genes or adding good genes. For example, researchers are developing genetic techniques for treating Parkinson, Alzheimer, and Huntington's diseases (HDs) that work by ramping up or suppressing the activity of specific genes.

While the treatments may add genes to body cells, knock out genes, or act in some way to change the function of genes, *each gene therapy is directed to the cells of particular body tissues.*

Thus, when scientists and doctors talk about what gene therapy does to DNA, they are not talking about all of the DNA in the body, but only some of it.

The timelines and milestones in developing gene therapy approach: from conception to clinical applications:
1953—discovery of DNA structure
1966—gene therapy approached
1968—viruses are used as carriers of transforming genetic materials
1970—trials of gene replacement therapy in arginase deficiency
1900—first gene therapy trial
1999—Gelsinger, a gene therapy patient, dies after therapy
2002—gene therapy applied for treating X-SKIDS in children
2005—first approved oncolytic virus
2007—Leber's congenital amaurosis, a type of inherited childhood blindness was successfully treated by a gene therapy approach.
2008—first approved gene-based medicines, molecular mechanisms, and clinical indications

Nov 2023—CRISPR Gene Editing Had a Breakthrough Year and it is Only Getting Started

In November 2023, the gene editing tool scored its first clinical approval for treating sickle cell anemia and beta-thalassemia in the United Kingdom. These painful blood disorders are caused by a single genetic typo that distorts blood cells' shape and limits their ability to deliver oxygen.

A few weeks later, the US-FDA greenlighted the therapy for sickle cell and is set to rule on beta-thalassemia by March of 2024. A European Medicines Agency regulatory committee soon followed with an endorsement for the therapy, suggesting it will likely be available across Europe.

Gene therapy can be either ex vivo or in vivo:
- *Ex vivo gene therapy means* that cells are removed from the body, treated, and then returned to the body. This is the approach used to treat genetic diseases of blood cells, because bone marrow can be harvested from the patient, and stem cells from that bone marrow can be treated with gene therapy for instance, to supply a gene that is missing or not working correctly and the transformed cells can be infused back into the patient (**Fig. 8**).
- *In vivo, gene therapy means* that the gene therapy itself is injected or infused into the person. This can be through injection directly to the anatomic site where the gene therapy is needed (a common example being the retina of the eye), or it can mean injection or infusion of a genetic payload that must travel to the body tissues where it is needed.
  - *CRISPR-Cas9 in vivo gene editing of KLKB1 for hereditary angioedema:* Hereditary angioedema is a rare genetic disease that leads to severe and unpredictable swelling attacks. NTLA-2002 is an in vivo gene-editing therapy based on CRISPR-CRISPR-associated protein 9. NTLA-2002 targets the gene encoding kallikrein B1 (KLKB1), with the goal of lifelong control of angioedema attacks after a single dose.

In both *ex-vivo* and *in-vivo* gene therapy, the genetic payload is packaged within a container, called a vector, before being delivered into cells or the body. One such vector is the adeno-associated virus (AAV). This is a group of viruses that exist in nature but have had their regular genes removed and replaced with a genetic payload, turning them into gene therapy vectors.

ONCOLYTIC VIRUSES AND GENE THERAPY

Oncolytic virus therapy, also called virotherapy, is a form of immunotherapy that uses viruses to infect and kill cancer cells. It is a fascinating type of cancer cell and gene therapy and may lead to a breakthrough in treating solid tumors and rare genetic metabolic disorders, e.g., glycogen storage diseases (GSDs).

Viruses are particles that infect or enter our cells and then use the cell's genetic machinery to make copies of themselves and subsequently spread to surrounding uninfected cells. These viruses are programmed not to

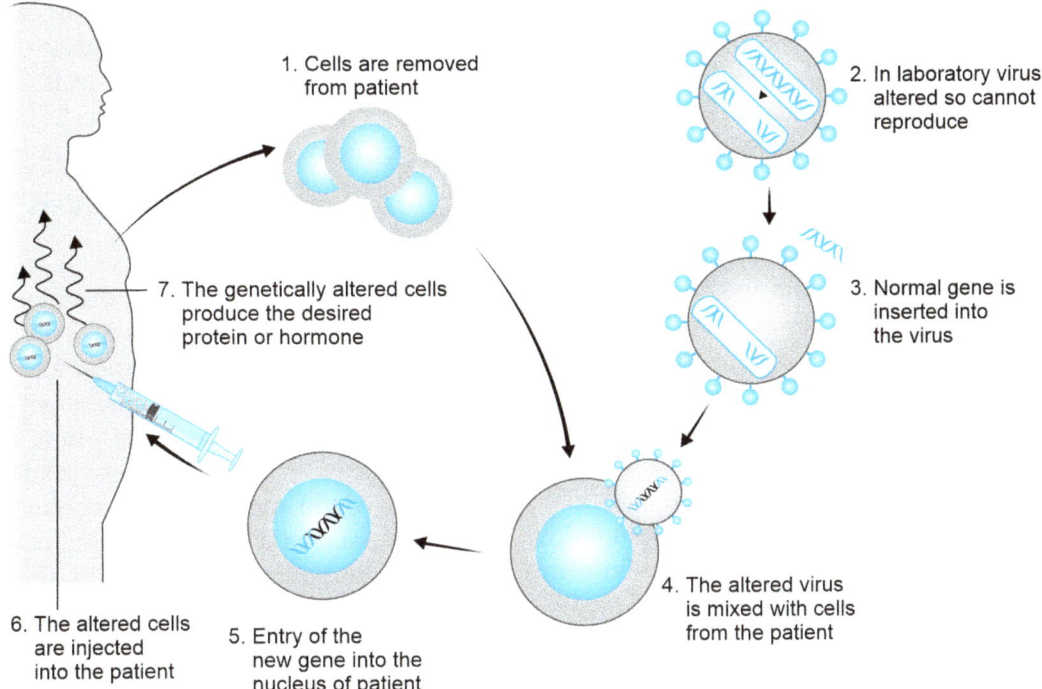

Fig. 8: Gene therapy can involve inserting genes into an individual's cells and tissues to treat a disease. This diagram shows *an example of ex vivo gene therapy*.
Courtesy: Aldona Griskeviciene via Alamy Stock Photo.

attack healthy tissue. Scientists modify them to target specific cells with specific genetics that are linked to the patient's cancer.

With a bit of fine-tuning, viruses can be trained to focus their destructive power on cancer cells (adenoviruses, lentivirus, etc.). OVs offer the attractive therapeutic combination of tumor-specific cell lysis together with immune stimulation, therefore acting as potential in situ tumor vaccines. Moreover, OVs can be engineered for the optimization of tumor selectivity and enhanced immune stimulation and can be readily combined with other agents.

The ability of these agents to control and make use of antitumor immunity appears to be key to their success. The effectiveness of OVs has been demonstrated in many preclinical studies and recently in humans, with US FDA approval in advanced melanoma, a breakthrough for the field.

Several viruses are being considered for potential OV therapy. The most common is the HSV type 1. For example, this virus is currently being used in an OV therapy clinical trial for glioblastoma. Other viruses used for cancer virotherapy include adenovirus, measles, vaccinia virus, etc.

OV therapy has potential for most, if not all, solid tumors. There is one OV therapy approved by the US-FDA for cancer: T-VEC, a modified HSV, for specific types of melanoma cases.

Is gene therapy safe?
Adeno-associated virus has been used to deliver gene therapy for many years because it has a good safety record. It is much less likely to cause a dangerous immune response than other viruses that were used as vectors several decades ago when gene therapy was just getting started. Additionally, packaging genetic payloads within AAV carriers allows for injected or infused gene therapy to travel to particular body tissues where it is needed. This is because there are many types of AAV, and certain types are attracted to certain tissues or organs. So, if a genetic payload needs to reach liver cells, for example, it can be packaged into a type of AAV that likes to go to the liver.

In the early days of gene therapy, which began in 1989, researchers used retroviruses as vectors. These viruses delivered a genetic payload directly into the nuclear chromosomes of the patient. However, there was concern that such integration of new DNA into chromosomes might cause changes leading to cancer, so the strategy was initially abandoned. More recently, scientists have successfully used retroviruses in experimental gene therapies without causing cancer; for example, a retrovirus-based therapy was used to treat infants with "bubble boy disease".

After moving away from retroviruses, researchers turned to adenoviruses, which offered the advantage of delivering the genetic payload as an episome, a piece of DNA that functions as a gene inside the nucleus but remains a separate entity from the chromosomes. The risk of cancer was extremely low with this innovation, but adenovirus vectors turned out to stimulate the immune system in very powerful ways.

In 1999, an immune reaction from adenovirus-carrying gene therapy led to the death of an 18-year-old Jesse Gelsinger, who'd volunteered for a clinical trial. *Gelsinger's death shocked the gene therapy community*, stalling the field for several years, but the current gene therapies that have emerged over the years based on AAV are not dangerous. However, they tend to be expensive and the success rate varies, so they typically are used as a last resort for a growing number of genetic diseases.

What conditions are currently treated with gene therapy?

- *As of January 2024*, gene therapy can treat certain blood diseases, such as hemophilia A, hemophilia B, sickle cell disease (SCD), and beta-thalassemia.
- Gene therapy and genome editing for GSDs. Is close to clinical trials may offer a single administration with permanent, noninheritable, liver cell genome correction, but currently, each pathogenic variant requires a customized validated therapeutic, in a clinical trial.

In the future, genetic therapies may be used to prevent, treat, or cure certain inherited disorders, such as cystic fibrosis (CF), and alpha-1 antitrypsin deficiency, and they also may be used to treat cancers or infections, including HIV.

What these diseases have in common is that the problem comes down to just one gene. This made beta-thalassemia and SCD low-hanging fruits for ex vivo gene therapies that involve removing and modifying bone marrow stem cells, whereas hemophilia A and hemophilia B are treated with in vivo gene therapies that target liver cells. That said, other treatments exist for these blood diseases, so gene therapy is more of a last resort.

Gene therapy has also been useful in treating hereditary retinal diseases, for which other treatments have not been useful.

Numerous enzyme deficiency disorders also come down to one bad gene that needs to be replaced. Cerebral adrenoleukodystrophy, which causes fatty acids to accumulate in the brain, is one such disorder that can be treated with gene therapy, according to Boston Children's Hospital.

Gene Therapy for Patients with Glycogen Storage Diseases

For the rare genetic metabolic disorder, GSD type 1a (GSD1a), liver transplantation is the only potential cure. Patients endure enormous physical and psychological challenges that significantly impact their quality of life. New gene therapies in clinical trials have the potential to replace defective/missing enzymes via adenovirus vector serotype 8 (AAV8) and provide a much-needed treatment option for patients. Clinicians should understand these emerging therapies so they can be prepared to help patients with GSD1a take advantage of these options, when available.

What gene therapies are in development?

Another group of targets for gene therapy are diseases of the nervous system where treatments for genetic forms of neurological disorders are being developed. For example, gene therapies to treat a pair of genetic diseases called Tay–Sachs disease and Sandhoff disease. Both conditions result from organelles called lysosomes filling up with fat-like molecules called gangliosides. The effects of these diseases include delay in reaching developmental milestones, loss of previously acquired skills, stiffness, blindness, weakness, and lack of coordination with eventual paralysis. Children born with Tay–Sachs disease and Sandhoff disease generally do not make it past 2–5 years of age.

Cell-based gene therapy—CAR T-cell therapy, which is approved for certain cancers, involves removing and modifying a patient's immune cells and is known as a "cell-based gene therapy".

■ TO SUM UP

Gene therapy delivery systems are crucial for the successful delivery of therapeutic genes to target cells in the treatment of various diseases, including genetic disorders, certain types of cancer, and viral infections.

Recent advances in gene therapy delivery systems have focused on improving the efficiency, specificity, and safety of gene transfer. These advances can be broadly categorized into developments in viral and nonviral delivery systems:

- *Viral gene delivery systems:* Viral vectors remain a popular choice for gene therapy due to their high efficiency in delivering genetic material into host cells. Recent advancements have focused on engineering safer and more specific viral vectors, such as lentiviruses, adenoviruses, and adeno-associated viruses (AAVs). Efforts have been made to modify these vectors to reduce their immunogenicity and improve their targeting capabilities to specific cell types or tissues.
- *Nonviral gene delivery systems:* Non-viral methods have gained attention due to their lower immunogenicity and potential for repeated administration. Recent innovations include:
  - *Nanoparticle-based systems:* These involve the use of nanoparticles, such as lipid nanoparticles (LNPs), for the delivery of nucleic acids. LNPs have been notably used in mRNA vaccines and are being explored for delivering CRISPR-Cas9 components for gene editing.
  - *Electroporation:* This technique, which uses electrical pulses to transiently permeabilize cell membranes, has been refined for more efficient and less invasive delivery of genetic material.
  - *Hydrogel and scaffold-based delivery:* These systems provide a matrix for the sustained release of genetic material and have applications in tissue engineering and regenerative medicine.
- *Targeted gene silencing and cancer therapy:* Advances in gene silencing technologies, such as RNA interference (RNAi) and CRISPR-Cas systems, have been incorporated into delivery platforms for targeted gene therapy in cancer. Nanoparticle-based delivery systems have been developed to enhance the specificity and efficacy of gene silencing agents.
- *Stimulus-responsive nanocarriers:* These are designed to release their genetic cargo in response to specific stimuli, either internal (e.g., pH, enzyme presence) or external (e.g., light, magnetic field), improving the precision of gene delivery.
- *Bacteria-based delivery systems:* Utilizing genetically modified bacteria to deliver therapeutic genes is an emerging area. These systems exploit the natural ability of certain bacteria to invade human cells, offering a novel approach for targeted gene delivery, particularly in cancer therapy.
- Aerosol and inhalation delivery for for chronic lung diseases

CRISPR AND GENOME EDITING (ERA OF GENE EDITING IN MEDICINE)

CRISPR *(clustered regularly interspaced short palindromic repeats)/Cas9* is a unique genome editing tool, commonly known as '*Genetic Scissors*' that can be easily used in a wide range of applications, including, epigenetics, biotechnology, plant engineering, livestock breeding, gene therapy, diagnostics, and so on, Enhanced CRISPR methods enables stable insertion of better genes into the DNA.

Genome editing machinery has provided the possibility of direct and specific recognition and modification of genomic sequences in practically all eukaryotic cells.

CRISPR gene editing is a powerful technique for modifying DNA that could someday be used in gene therapies. Here is a simplified breakdown of how CRISPR gene editing works (*CRISPR: Clustered Regularly Interspaced Short Palindromic Repeat*).

The future looks hopeful when it comes to gene therapy overall, on account of new technological developments, including CRISPR gene editing. This is an extremely powerful technique for cutting out parts of DNA molecules and even pasting new parts in—analogous to what you do with text in word processing applications.

CRISPR is not the first method that scientists have used to edit DNA, but it is far more versatile than other techniques. It is not yet quite ready for in vivo chromosomal manipulation, but it is advancing exponentially.

Perhaps even closer to the horizon is the prospect of delivering larger genetic payloads into cells. One big drawback of the AAV vector is that each virus particle can carry just a small amount of DNA, but recent research has revealed that a different type of virus, called CMV, can be adapted to carry gene therapies with a much bigger payload than AAV. Not only might this someday expand gene therapy to more diseases requiring larger genes than AAV can carry, but it also could enable more than one gene to be delivered in a single therapy.

CRISPR: A New Tool for Editing Genes

CRISPR—a gene editing technique that enables scientists to make precise cuts in DNA. The first scientific paper about it was published in 2012, and its development by Jennifer Doudna and Emmanuelle Charpentier—won the Nobel Prize in chemistry just 8 years later.

This so-called CRISPR/Cas. Simply, this treatment uses a guide molecule that indicates exactly where the DNA edit needs to be made, along with a Cas enzyme that cuts the DNA to initiate the edit. The US FDA approved a pair of gene editing therapy treatments for SCD and thalassemic recessive hemoglobinopathy diseases:

- Exa-cel—Casgevy is the CRISPR-based treatment.
- Lovo-cel—Lyfgenia uses an older gene therapy approach.

For sickle cell, patients' cells are removed from the body and CRISPR is used to make an edit that turns back on the production of fetal hemoglobin (FHb), a form of the protein that babies make in the womb. Once the edited cells are returned, the FHb can make up for the mutated hemoglobin (Hb) that causes sickle cell.

Fetal hemoglobin has a higher oxygen-carrying capacity than adult Hb or sickle Hb. Making FHb along with sickle Hb renders a patient similar to someone with sickle cell trait, e.g., that's when someone inherits one sickle cell gene and one normal gene, . So they "do not have any of the complications of the disease".

Researchers say that "it is more than good enough". It is known and pointed out that some people naturally have genetic mutations that keep FHb high, "and they do not have symptoms, even if they have the disease". "So it was like a physiologic, demonstrated approach that would work if you could turn on FHb".

Clinical trial results are encouraging and show as that the "longest time without a crisis was 45.5 months, almost 4 years, and researchers will continue to follow these patients. The hope is that the effects could last their entire lives.

The CRISPR-Cas9-mediated genome editing technology brings great promise for inhibiting migration, invasion, and even treatment of tumors. However, the potential off-target effect limits its clinical application, and an effective ethical review is necessary.

Despite the CRISPR-associated nuclease (Cas) system bringing promise for tumor therapy associated with gene mutation; problems such as off-target and ethics need to be resolved. We still have a long way to go until the CRISPR/Cas9 technology is ready to treat cancer-mature.

The second approved SCD therapy, Lyfgenia, uses an older gene therapy approach, and involves an older technology, using a virus to deliver a healthy copy of the gene that produces adult Hb to make up for the one producing the sickled form. It also involves removing the patient's cells and then returning them. It is shown similarly encouraging results. These both bring tremendous benefits to the patients.

December 21, 2023; HuidaGene's gene-editing therapy was named a rare pediatric drug approved by the FDA—CRISPR DNA editing therapy: called HG302, for Duchenne muscular dystrophy (DMD).

Like SCD, DMD is a genetic disorder characterized by progressive muscle degeneration and weakness due to the alterations of a protein called dystrophin that helps keep muscle cells intact. DMD is one of four conditions known as dystrophinopathies. DMD symptom onset is in early childhood, usually between ages 2 and 3. The disease primarily affects boys, but in rare cases, it can affect girls. DMD has an X-linked recessive inheritance pattern and is passed on by the mother, who is referred to as a carrier.

HG302 employs a gene-editing approach to eliminate or skip over, a protein-coding portion of DMD called exon 51 in patients' cells when the transcript is being made. That allows the production of a short but functional dystrophin protein, which is expected to improve muscle function. HG302 uses an enzyme expected to lead to better efficacy and safety.

HG302 is intended to be a one-time therapy, where the gene-editing materials are packaged into a viral carrier that helps it be taken up by muscle cells when delivered as a single IV infusion.

The gene-editing technology employed is called CRISPR/Cas. Simply, this treatment uses a guide molecule that indicates exactly where the DNA edit needs to be made, along with a Cas enzyme that cuts the DNA to initiate the edit. Experts look forward to advancing HG302 into the clinic as soon as possible.

The Difference between mAbs/CAR T-Cell Therapy versus CRISPR

CRISPR is a gene editing technology, while CAR T-cells are cells that have been created using gene editing technology. Until CRISPR was invented, CAR T-cells were generated using other genome engineering technologies.

"Universal" CAR T-cells that have undergone gene editing to allow them to be used off-the-shelf without having to be derived uniquely for each host, an approach that could bring therapy to a much broader range of patients

■ RNA THERAPY

Now and then, medicine changes fundamentally; in 1928 when Fleming discovered penicillin; or in 1953 when Watson, Crick, and Franklin characterized the double-helical structure of DNA. Many diseases and disorders are a problem by proteins (RNA and DNA). In some cases, like hypercholesterolemia, the body produces too much protein; in others, like hemophilia, too little.

Today in medicine, there are essentially two places where we are at a vital turning point.
1. *One is RNA vaccines*; the future of medicines, e.g., mRNA-based vaccines and therapeutics is a bit more incomprehensible and it may be just impactful.
2. The other is RNA therapeutics.

RNA VACCINES: THE RNAISSANCE (REBIRTH)

Until recently most people had never even heard of mRNA vaccines; thanks to decades of mRNA research and innovation. As scientists put it", The whole field of mRNA is just exploding. It is a game changer in medicine. The mRNA vaccines use the synthetic genetic sequence or "code" of the antigen translated into mRNA. It is a ghost of the real thing, fooling the body into creating very real antibodies. The artificial mRNA itself then disappears, degraded by the body's natural defenses including enzymes that break it down, leaving us with only the antibodies.

It is, therefore, safer to produce mRNA vaccines, more quickly and cheaply, compared with traditional vaccines. No longer need huge biosecure laboratories growing deadly viruses inside millions of chicken eggs. Instead, just one laboratory can sequence the proteins of the antigen and email it around the world. With that information, a laboratory could make "a million doses of mRNA in a single 100 mL test tube.

Now scientists believe they may be the key to solving a wealth of health problems and even *gave this new era a name: "the RNAissance" (Rebirth)*.

FUTURE

In addition to making vaccines easier to tolerate, oral capsule-form approach could also be used to deliver other kinds of therapeutic RNA or DNA directly to the digestive tract. There are many immune cells in the GI tract, and stimulating the immune system of the GI tract is a known way of creating an immune response.

Like most vaccines, RNA vaccines have to be injected, which can be an obstacle for people who fear needles. Now, a team of MIT researchers has developed a way to deliver RNA in a capsule that can be swallowed, which they hope could help make people more receptive to them.

Nucleic acids, in particular RNA, can be extremely sensitive to degradation, particularly in the digestive tract. To overcome this challenge, RNA needs to be carried by a new type of protective polymeric nanoparticle (beta-amino esters). These particles, which can deliver RNA with high efficiency, are made from a type of polymer called poly (beta-amino esters). These polymers are more effective than linear polymers at protecting nucleic acids and getting them into cells.

RNA Therapies

Several techniques, called RNA therapies, use pieces of RNA, which is a type of genetic material similar to DNA, to help treat a disorder.

In many of these techniques, the pieces of RNA interact with a molecule called messenger RNA (or mRNA for short). In cells, mRNA uses the information in genes to create a blueprint for making proteins. By interacting with mRNA, these therapies influence how much protein is produced from a gene, which can compensate for the effects of a genetic alteration.

Examples of these RNA therapies include antisense oligonucleotide (ASO), small interfering RNA (siRNA), and microRNA (miRNA) therapies. An RNA therapy called RNA aptamer therapy introduces small pieces of RNA that attach directly to proteins to alter their function.

EPIGENETIC THERAPY

Genetics and epigenetics are both fascinating fields that explore into the details of our genetic material. *Genes are made from DNA* and play a crucial role in determining our traits, characteristics, and susceptibility to various conditions. Genetic information is inherited from parents and passed down through generations.

Epigenetics focuses on physical changes that affect how genes are "expressed". It explores modifications that occur outside the DNA sequence but still influence gene activity. While all cells have the same DNA, epigenetics determines how each cell will function, turning genes on and off to make them appropriate for their specific roles (e.g., liver cells, brain cells, heart cells).

It is another gene-related therapy, called epigenetic therapy, to fix any changes in the DNA that might have caused the medical illnesses. This type of treatment works by using drugs or other epigenome-influencing techniques to treat medical conditions. This helps bring the DNA back to how it was before cancer started, to fix any changes in the DNA that might have caused cancer. Scientists have created drugs that can find changes in cancer cells that are related to how the cells grow.

Epigenetic changes are specific modifications (often called "tags") attached to DNA that control whether genes are turned on or off. Abnormal patterns of epigenetic modifications alter gene activity and, subsequently, protein production. Epigenetic therapies are used to correct epigenetic errors that underlie genetic disorders including cancer, heart disease, diabetes, mental illnesses, etc. Epigenetic therapy offers a potential way to influence those pathways directly.

Epigenetic modifications are reversible and therefore allow excellent opportunities for therapeutic intervention. Nowadays, several epigenetic drugs are used worldwide to treat cancer. Conventional epigenetic drugs can relatively easily reach the tissues of interest, and they are proven to be effective in leukemias.

Interestingly, the CRISPR/dCas9 technology is an extremely promising tool for targeted epigenetic therapy. It can be assumed that, with the development of CRISPR/dCas9-based technologies, the epigenetic editing field will begin to thrive.

Another novel therapeutic strategy for cancer treatment is the application of multitargeting drugs, i.e., drugs that target both an epigenetic enzyme, as well as other cancer-related proteins. Such an approach can simplify the treatment regimens, decrease adverse drug reactions, and reduce the potential mechanisms of drug resistance.

Futuristic New Frontiers

Inhalable lung cancer treatment (nebulizer) is so promising innovative delivery through inhalation.

Lung cancer is one of the most common cancers and has one of the lowest survival rates in the world. Cytokines, which are small signaling proteins, such as interleukin-12 (IL-12), have demonstrated considerable potential as robust tumor suppressors. However, their applications are limited due to a multitude of severe side effects.

The new inhalable treatment uses exosomes (small blue balls), also called extracellular vesicles (EVs) to deliver IL-12 mRNA to lung cancer cells. Researchers are now trying new delivery methods that target tumor cells without affecting healthy tissue. Ke Cheng's team took a new approach, inserting mRNA for IL-12 into exosomes. *(Cheng Lab/Columbia Engineering 11 January 2024, Nature Nanotechnology. DOI: 10.1038/s41565-023-01580-3)*

Exosomes are usually injected systemically into the bloodstream", said Cheng. "In this new study, inhaled exosomes can efficiently reach the lung and deliver an anti-lung cancer cargo, IL-12 mRNA. "This is an interesting study that explores the inhalable delivery of engineered EVs for the treatment of lung cancer and offers insights into focused delivery of EV-based drugs which has one of the lowest five-year survival rates in the world with implications for diseases beyond cancer.

■ A QUICK TAKE

Immunotherapy is one of the most effective therapeutic options for cancer patients. Five specific classes of immunotherapies include: (1) mAb-based targeted therapies; (2) cell-based CAR T-cell, checkpoint inhibitors therapy; (3) cancer vaccines; and (4) OVs.

- mAbs and CAR T-cells are two branches of cancer immunotherapy, approaches to elicit patients' immune responses against tumor cells to eradicate the tumor.
- mAbs can completely recognize cancer cell-surface receptors and blockade proliferative or inhibitory pathways. On the other hand, T-cell activation by genetically engineered CAR-T receptors can induce potent immune responses against specific TAAs, and enhance the therapeutic efficacy against cancers.
- Although some challenges and concerns are by using both mAbs and CAR T-cells, combinational therapies will improve the anti-tumor effects and optimize their functions.

IMMUNOTHERAPY AGAINST INHERITED DISABILITIES

- Authors' communications *dated July 23rd, 2021* focused on the "futuristic gene therapies" for those individuals, plagued with physical and intellectual disabilities.

  This subject has been shared with two top individuals who have dedicated their lives to providing "disability care" Institutes in Ayikudy, Thenkasi, Tamil Nadu (ASSA); they are namely; President Padma Shree Mr Ramakrishnan and Mr Sankar Raman, the Promotor and Cochairman of the ASSA who has also served as President, Indian Muscular Dystrophy Association.
- Yes, there are gene therapy drugs for many variants of inherited neuromuscular disorders including the commonly recognized spinal muscular atrophy (SMA) and DMD: both at a clinical trial under close

supervision with an extremely high price tag of multiple crores in Indian RS equivalents.
- There is one Spinraza (Nusinersen) injection for all kinds of SMA and for other neuromuscular (DMDs) disorders in grown-up people; to stop the disease progression. Said to have very impressive clinical responses. Pleased that; Indian PM Modi has made "rules-relaxation" and opportunities for SMA/DMD folks to receive these USA made gene drug; also some Indian philanthropists are supporting helping to get it for a few, but still, not sure the drug was used for SMA or DMD and their treatment outcome.
  - Spinraza was the first drug approved for children and adults with SMA by the US-FDA in 2016. Spinraza is given an intrathecal route.
- Zolgensma (onasemnogene abeparvovec-xioi) is the second and most effective drug for the disorder given intravenously as a one-time treatment. Zolgensma gene therapy is used to treat children <2-years-old with SMA and was not evaluated in patients with advanced SMA.
- In August 2020, the FDA announced the release of a third drug called Evrysdi (risdiplam) to treat patients as young as 2 months. This is the first oral drug to treat the disease.
- *DMD:* There is a dystrophin gene "microdystrophin", a single IV dose given to DMD adults showed that "good regain motor function" just a web as an example for your views.
- *Nov 23, 2021:* Regenxbio, RGX-202, one-time experimental gene therapy for the treatment of DMD, has been granted orphan drug designation by the US FDA. to support the process of developing new therapeutics, including tax credits for costs associated with clinical trials.

HISTORICAL BACKGROUND OF GENETIC MUSCULAR DISORDERS

Duchenne's muscular dystrophy is caused by mutations in the DMD gene responsible for producing a protein called dystrophin, a protein that normally functions like a shock absorber, helping to cushion the muscles from damage during muscle contractions.

The DMD-causing mutations lead to virtually no functional dystrophin, and as a result, muscles accumulate more wear-and-tear damage over time, leading to symptoms such as muscle loss and weakness.

Children born with this disease suffer progressive muscle degeneration, and existing treatments are limited to a fraction of patients with the condition.

The DMD primarily affects boys, and symptoms usually appear in early childhood. The disorder follows an X-linked recessive inheritance pattern, meaning the faulty gene is located on the X chromosome. Since males have one X chromosome and one Y chromosome, if they inherit the mutated gene on their X chromosome, they will likely develop DMD. Females, with two X chromosomes, are typically carriers and may not show symptoms but can pass the faulty gene to their offspring.

DMD Gene Therapy

Elevidys (delandistrogene moxeparvovec) received FDA approval on June 22, 2023, for DMD children ages 4–5 who can walk and have a confirmed mutation in the *DMD* gene. Hopefully, the Indian Council of Medical Research (ICMR) will allow this gene shot in India and help thousands of Indian DMDs that provide the potential to alter the trajectory of this degenerative disease.

SGT-003, a next-generation gene therapy candidate for DMD being developed by solid biosciences, has been granted orphan drug designation by the US-FDA (Jan 2024). SGT-003 uses a novel viral vector to deliver a genetic payload. The vector has a specifically designed capsid (viral shell) and was created to maximize muscle tropism, basically meaning the vector efficiently delivers genes to muscle cells but not to other cell types.

Limb-Girdle Muscular Dystrophy Type 2E

Children with LGMD2E is a rare form of LGMD with no treatments beyond symptom management. LGMD2E, also known as LGMDR4, is caused by mutations in the *SGCB* gene, which limit the production of beta-sarcoglycan. As a result, the formation of the sarcoglycan protein complex is impaired, leading to muscle weakness and wasting, mainly in the hips and shoulders.

Phase 3 clinical trial of *SRP-9003 gene therapy* in LGMD2E for patients, ages 4 and up, who can or cannot walk, has been promising. Earlier results from the SRP-9003 clinical development program demonstrated, "significant protein expression at both 12 weeks (almost 3 months) and 2 years after treatment as well as functional benefits, including slowing progression of this disease, improving mobility, and enhancing the quality of life for individuals living with LGMD2E".

Current medical practice—many states in the USA have mandatory 30 plus inherited disorders are to be screened, soon after birth in a single drop blood heelprick test including DMD and SMA; if test positive a single dose to the infant will replace the missing *DMD* dystrophin gene and make the child free of these gene-deficient disorders.

Concerns are unaffordable cost to common people and families in the USA to this gene therapy. Even, the Indian medical fraternity and healthcare bureaucrats would need a thorough knowledge of the evolving immunotherapeutic of inherited genetic diseases and disorders. Importantly, each case needs a thorough medical assessment, and application.

Inherited Disabilities

Prevalence of Inherited Genetic Disorders in India

Due to India's large population, high birth rate, and widespread practice of consanguineous marriages within various communities, there is a high prevalence of genetic disorders in the country.

Inherited neuromuscular disorders include amyotrophic lateral sclerosis (ALS), DMD, myasthenia gravis, and SMA.

There can be different causes for these diseases. Many of them are genetic. This means they are inherited, run in families, or are caused by a new mutation in your genes. Some neuromuscular disorders are autoimmune diseases. Sometimes the cause is unknown.

Many neuromuscular diseases have no cure, and their treatment compromises the immune system, thereby increasing the risk of infections and serious illness. Consequently, vaccinations to protect against infections are an important part of the clinical management of these diseases. However, the wide variety of immunotherapies that are currently used to treat neuroimmunology disease particularly MS and neuromyelitis optica spectrum disorders can also impair immunological responses to vaccinations.

The success of vaccination in patients receiving immunotherapy largely depends on the specific mode of action of the immunotherapy. To minimize the risk of infection when using immunotherapy, assessment of immune status and exclusion of underlying chronic infections before initiation of therapy are essential. Selection of the required vaccinations and leaving appropriate time intervals between vaccination and administration of immunotherapy can help to safeguard patients.

Amyotrophic lateral sclerosis (Lou Gehrig disease) is the most common form of motor neuron disease, is a progressive neurodegenerative disorder that affects nerve cells in the brain and spinal cord, gradually leading to muscle weakness, paralysis, and eventually respiratory failure. As the disease progresses, individuals may experience difficulties with speaking, swallowing, and breathing, significantly impacting their quality of life.

While the exact cause of ALS remains unclear, a combination of genetic and environmental factors likely contributes to its development. Currently, there is no cure for ALS, and treatment focuses on managing symptoms, improving quality of life, and providing support for individuals and their families.

Thalassemia and sickle cell anemia is an inherited blood disorder characterized by either reduced production of Hb or abnormal Hb, resulting in sickle-shaped red blood cells. Inheritance follows an autosomal recessive pattern.

Cystic fibrosis is inherited in an autosomal recessive pattern, meaning a child must inherit two abnormal copies of the gene (one from each parent) to develop the condition. Results from a defective gene CF causing the body to produce thick, sticky mucus that obstructs airways and blocks ducts in the pancreas and other organs.

Fragile X syndrome (FXS) is an X-linked condition that affects all over the world and is the most common genetic cause of inherited intellectual disability and autism spectrum disorder (ASD). Males with the mutated gene are more severely affected because they have only one X chromosome, while females, who have two X chromosomes, may have milder symptoms or be carriers of the condition. It results from hypermethylation of the *FMR1* (Fragile X messenger ribonucleoprotein 1) gene leading to function loss of the protein product FMRP.

There is no cure for FXS. However, treatment services can help people learn important skills. Services can include therapy to learn to talk, walk, and interact with others. In addition, medicine can be used to help control some issues, such as behavior problems. While gene therapy for FXS is still in its infancy, recent successes in other single-gene conditions (such as SMA) are setting the ground rules for how such therapies may be employed and what hurdles they need to overcome.

Down syndrome is one of the most common chromosomal disorders observed in India, as it is globally. It is caused by the presence of an extra copy of chromosome 21 (trisomy). This additional genetic material disrupts the normal course of development, leading to physical and intellectual disabilities.

The current treatments for inherited diseases and disorders are mostly symptomatic without affecting the underlying cause of the disease. Emerging evidence supports a potential role for immunotherapy in the management of disease progression. Numerous reports raise the exciting prospect that either the immune system or its derivative components could be harnessed to fight the misfolded and aggregated proteins that accumulate in several neurodegenerative diseases. Passive and active vaccinations using mAbs and specific antigens that induce adaptive immune responses are currently under evaluation for their potential use in the development of immunotherapies, such as vaccination therapy.

Immunotherapy has shown significant promise in the area of cancer treatment. However, applying such principles to inherited or genetic diseases is more complex and currently in the early stages of research. There are some aspects worth considering.

Gene therapy, not to be confused with immunotherapy, is likely the leading area of development when it comes to managing most inherited diseases, and it involves targeting the disease at the genetic level, often by introducing a healthy copy of the affected gene.

Experimental approaches are being explored in the field of gene therapy that could potentially be considered a form of immunotherapy against inherited diseases. Gene therapy involves introducing, removing, or altering genetic material within a person's cells to treat or prevent disease. Experts suggest that gene editing might become a reality in the treatment and prevention of a variety of human diseases in the coming 10 years.

Here are a few ways in which gene therapy might be used to address inherited diseases:

- *Gene editing:* Techniques like CRISPR-Cas9 enable targeted modification of specific genes. In theory, this could be used to correct or replace faulty genes responsible for inherited diseases.
- *Gene silencing:* RNA interference (RNAi) is a process that can selectively silence or downregulate the expression of specific genes. This approach might be used to suppress the effects of mutated genes causing inherited diseases.
- *Gene addition:* In some cases, introducing a functional copy of a gene into the patient's cells might compensate for the defective gene causing the inherited disease.
- *Ex vivo gene therapy:* Cells can be taken from a patient, modified outside the body to correct the genetic defect, and then reintroduced into the patient. This is known as ex vivo gene therapy.

Inherited diseases, such as hemophilia B, which are treated by providing therapeutic proteins, sometimes stimulate an unwanted immune response. Strategies are being developed to modulate and limit this undesired immune response.

Likewise, CAR T-cell immunotherapies that specifically target cells contributing to disease pathology could theoretically be explored. With that being said, immunotherapies for inherited diseases are generally in the early stages of development, and much further research is needed before they are likely to become common treatment options. Currently, as with many diseases, prevention, early detection, and management of symptoms are still key.

It is important to note that these approaches are still largely experimental, and their safety and efficacy are being studied in clinical trials. The specific approach taken would depend on the nature of the inherited disease, the type of genetic mutation involved, and the current state of research and technology. Research in this area is ongoing, and advancements are being made to develop safe and effective treatments for a variety of inherited diseases.

Gene Therapy for Neurodegenerative Disorders

Gene therapy is especially suited for well-validated genetic targets that are not amenable to traditional therapies. It has been well tolerated and shown long-lasting efficacy in clinical trials for various human neurodegenerative diseases, including Parkinson's disease (PD), AD, HD, and aromatic-L-amino-acid (AADC) deficiency.

The sustained, even permanent therapeutic effects of gene therapy are especially appealing for compartmentalized organs such as the eye, cochlea, or CNS, which structures are difficult to treat because most agents cannot breach the physiological barriers such as the blood-cerebrospinal fluid barrier (BCSFB), blood-retina barrier (BRB), and blood-brain barrier (BBB).

Viral and nonviral vectors can successfully direct transgenes that express therapeutic proteins, antibodies, Cas9/gRNA for gene editing, miRNAs, and siRNA to diseased tissues in humans and animals. For neurodegenerative disorders, the most commonly applied

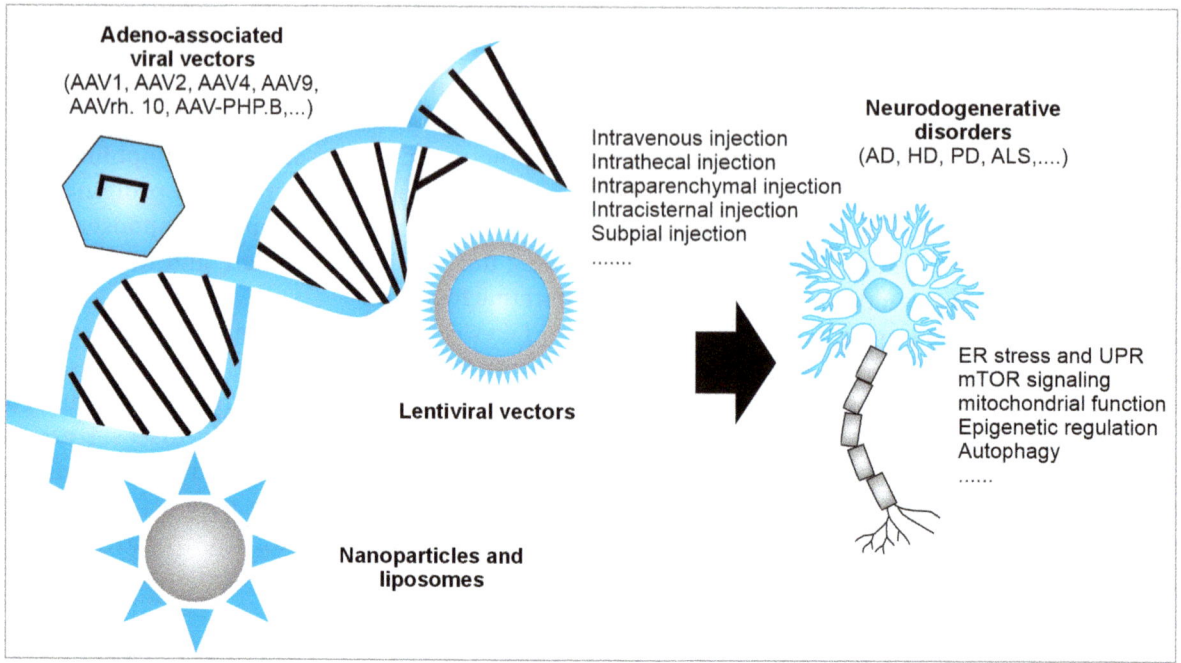

Fig. 9: Gene therapy delivery system can target multiple tissues and cells within the CNS that breach the physiological blood-brainbarriers.

vector is one of the AAVs. Additionally, a large number of capsids can be employed across species to favorably target multiple tissues and cells within the CNS, including oligodendrocytes, astrocytes, and neurons **(Fig. 9)**.

There have been significant advances in developing effective delivery routes, especially for the CNS and eye. Preclinical studies have demonstrated that numerous routes of gene delivery, including subpial, intracerebroventricular, intrathecal, intraparenchymal, intravitreal, and subretinal injection, can attain sufficient gene quantities in diseased tissues. Recently reported vectors have an unequaled capability to transfer genes to the CNS after systemic injection. These vectors are an obvious improvement over AAV9 and potentially enhance our ability to treat additional neurological disorders.

The successful delivery of therapeutic genes must target cells in the treatment of various diseases, including genetic disorders, certain types of cancer, and viral infections. Recent advances in gene therapy delivery systems have focused on improving the efficiency, specificity, and safety of gene transfer.

A better understanding of the onset and progression of neurodegenerative disorders will facilitate prompt diagnosis and target selection, which should allow early treatment for certain of these diseases. As progress continues in optimizing transgene design, delivery, and vectors, the prospects of gene therapy for neurodegenerative disorders will undoubtedly become even brighter.

Hereditary Angioedema

It is an inherited genetic disease that causes severe, painful, and sudden swelling attacks. These disturb normal activities and have the potential to cause airway damage and death. Hereditary angioedema, a rare genetic disorder, was often not correctly diagnosed due to its rarity.

The symptoms of hereditary angioedema result from the dysregulation of the contact activation pathway. *C1 esterase inhibitor (C1-INH)* is a key regulator of the pathway and attenuates the production of bradykinin, a peptide that leads to increased vascular permeability and subsequent tissue swelling, using the inhibition of the proteases factor XIIa and plasma kallikrein. *In the most common types of hereditary angioedema, C1-INH deficiency (in type 1 disease) and C1-INH dysfunction (in type 2 disease) lead to increased bradykinin production and angioedema attacks.*

Inhibitors of plasma kallikrein activity are now approved for long-term prophylaxis. More recently, RNA-silencing therapeutic approaches that reduce the total levels of plasma kallikrein (plasma kallikrein and its zymogen precursor, plasma prekallikrein) have shown promise in early trials.[6,7] Although these and other therapies have substantially improved the management of hereditary angioedema in recent years, lifelong administration of these treatments is necessary.

Gene editing offers hope to patients with inherited disorders. In a recent trial published in the NEJM (February 1, 2024 N Engl J Med. 2024; 390:432-41), a dose-dependent reduction in total plasma kallikrein protein was demonstrated, achieving reductions of up to 95% to treat hereditary angioedema, a genetic disease-causing severe swelling attack.

The investigational therapy, NTLA-2002, used in vivo CRISPR/Cas9 technology to target the *KLKB1* gene, responsible for producing plasma prekallikrein. By editing this gene, the therapy reduced the levels of total plasma kallikrein, effectively preventing angioedema attacks.

Researchers from the University of Auckland, Amsterdam University Medical Center, and Cambridge University Hospitals successfully treated over 10 patients with CRISPR/Cas9 technology. The single-dose treatment appeared to provide a permanent cure for the disabling symptoms of hereditary angioedema patients.

KEY POINTS

- All indicated vaccinations should be administered before initiation of immunotherapy whenever possible; appropriate intervals between vaccination and treatment vary with treatment and vaccination.
- Inactivated vaccines are considered safe in neuroimmunological diseases but live vaccines are generally contraindicated during immunotherapy.
- Vaccination responses during immunotherapy can be diminished or abrogated, depending on the treatment and vaccination; antibody titer testing to monitor responses can be considered where appropriate.
- Vaccinations must be avoided during relapses or exacerbations of neuroimmunological diseases.
- Vaccination against SARS-CoV-2 is recommended for patients with neuroimmunological disease but some immunotherapies limit the immune response; therefore, timing should be considered carefully.

CONCLUSION

Novel and innovative therapeutic strategies are necessary to overcome the challenges typically faced by existing IDs prevention and control methods such as lack of adequate efficacy, drug toxicity, and the emergence of drug resistance. Most recently COVID-19 reinforces the role of immunotherapeutic strategies in the broader field of disease control.

Immunotherapy is also a treatment that uses a person's immune system to fight cancer. cells. While its most general applications are founded in cancer treatment, advances made toward the curative treatment of HIV, tuberculosis, malaria, Zika viruses, etc., are needed

Immunotherapy treatment can reach areas of our body that surgery cannot. As evidenced by recent developments and success through the use of immunotherapies such as vaccines, and mAb-based therapies, and CAR T-cell-based therapies have already shown abundant promise to overcome such limitations while also advancing the frontiers of medicine. Ultimately, the comprehensive specificity, safety, and cost of immunotherapeutics will impact its widespread implementation.

Bottom Line

Immunotherapy is a promising treatment option for people with cancer. The treatment method, administered orally, intravenously, topically, or through your bladder, helps T-cells detect and attack cancer cells, which may help reduce or stop cancer progression.

In some people, immunotherapy may improve overall survival rate and quality of life.

As with any cancer treatment, you may experience unpleasant side effects after receiving immunotherapy. Talking with your doctor about what to expect from the treatment, including possible side effects, is important.

A Query and Answer—Built on Futuristic Genetically Engineered Virus Vaccines

The authors answered a query and concerns on the "Gain of Function Research (GOFR) on Vaccines Uses and Gains in Medicine" on July 23rd, 2021: *This was expressed by a Senior Infectious Diseases Consultant* from a major "Quaternary Health Care Hospital" in India on the "genetically engineered viruses causing pandemics!"

Q. "Gain of Function Research" on Viruses is detrimental to humanity unless strictly regulated. Such genetically engineered viruses have the potential to create epidemics and pandemics.

Ans. Yes. with the strictly stipulated "US-FDA Pharmaceutical Regulations"; the viruses can be genetically engineered for a variety of reasons including gene therapy for the treatment of genetic diseases, cancer-killing viruses, vaccine development, and boosting immune cells.

- Genetically engineering viruses are essentially comprised of a nucleic acid core surrounded by a protein coat. The protein coat contains specific glycoproteins that enable them to bind to receptors in the body, causing them to fuse to the cell membrane and release their nucleic acid sequence to infect the cell.
- The virulent nucleic acid sequence hijacks the cellular machinery to self-replicate, lyse the cell, spread, and infect other cells. Using reverse genetics, the sequence of a viral genome can be identified, including that of its different strains and variants. This enables scientists to identify sequences of the virus that enable it to bind to a receptor, as well as those regions that cause it to be so virulent.

ANNEXURES

1. *List of approved mAbs and Indications are tabulated.*
2. *KIMS health pharmacy stockpiled mAbs utility during Sep-Oct–Nov 2023*

Annexure 1: Therapeutic monoclonal antibodies approved or in regulatory review either in Europe and the USA.

#	mAb	Brand by	Approval date, route	Type and target	Indications
1.	Abciximab KIMS	ReoPro	12/94 IV	Chimeric Fab	Lessen the chance of heart attack in people who need percutaneous coronary intervention (PCI) KIMS 57 use
2.	Adalimumab KIMS	Humira	12/2022 Sc	TNF fully Humanized	TNF, RA
3.	Adalimumab-atto	Amjevita	9/2016, Sc	TNF as above	All arthritis include RA Crohn's diseases
	Aducanumab				Alzheimer's
4.	Ado-trastuzumab emtansine		2/2013 IV	HER2 humanized	Metastatic Ca
	adalimumab-adbm		8/2017 Sc	FH	Arthritis, ulcerative colitis, Crohn's, psoriasis
5	Alemtuzumab (Campath)		5/2001 IV	CD52	B-cell lymphatic leukemia/MS, SOT recipients
6.	Alirocumab	Sanofi	7/2015 Sc	PCSK9 Ful human	Familial cholesterol, Coronary Stenting Trial' use to prevent thrombosis
	Amivantamab,	Rybrevant		Bispecific mAb	Promising efficacy of amivantamab plus chemotherapy in patients with untreated advanced nonsmall-cell lung cancer (NSCLC) with epidermal growth factor receptor (EGFR) exon 20 insertions
7.	Atezolizumab (Tecentriq)		5/2016 IV	human	Urothelial Ca, immune checkpoint inhibitor (ICPs)
8.	Avelumab (Bavencio)		3/2017 IV	Fully human	Metastatic Merkel cell Ca, immune checkpoint inhibitor (ICPs), metastatic blader Ca, chemotherapy or immunotherapy with nivolumab or pembrolizumab are given. Sometimes palliative therapy is offered
9.	Basiliximab (Simulect)	Novartis	12/98 IV	Chimeric	Renal transplant rejects propyl
10.	Belimumab		3/2011 IV	Fully human	SLE
11.	Bevacizumab	Avastin	2/2004 IV	Humanized	Metastatic Colorectal Ca, NSCL, Renal cell Ca, HCC
	Benralizumab not in KIMS		11/2017 Sc	Humanized	For severe asthma, cystic fibrosis benralizumab, an mAb against the interleukin-5α receptor expressed on eosinophils, may be an option for treating EGPA

Contd...

Contd...

#	mAb	Brand by	Approval date, route	Type and target	Indications
12.	Bezlotoxumab		10/2016 IV	Fully human	*Clostridium difficile* toxin prevent
13.	Blinatumomab		12/2014 IV	Mouse bispecific	Inotuzumab ozogamicin followed by blinatumomab achieved excellent outcomes. Adult ALL, lymphoma
14.	Brentuximab vedotin		9/2011 IV	Chimeric, Ab drug conjugate	Hodgkin, lymphoma
15.	Brodalumab		2/17 Sc	Chimeric	Plague psoriasis
	Bezlotoxumab		10/2016 IV	Fully human	*Clostridium difficile* toxin prevent
16.	Bezlotoxumab		10/2016 IV	Fully human	*Clostridium difficile* toxin prevent
17.	Bococizumab Withdrawn in 2016				Evolocumab, alirocumab, and bococizumab hypercholestrlemeia, treatment and prevention of dyslipidemia, hyperlipidemia, hypercholesterolemia, and cardiovascular
18.	Capromab pendetide		10/96 IV	Murine, Radiolab	Diagnostic imaging and post-Ca prostate
	Cemiplimab (Libtayo)				Immune checkpoint inhibitor (ICPs)
	Cocktail casirivimab/ imdevimab (Regeneron)				Long COVID – 19
19.	Certolizumab pegol		4/08 Sc	Fully humanized	Crohn, Rheu arthritis
20.	Cetuximab		2/04 IV	Chimeric	Metastatic, Colorectal Ca
	Cinpanemab				Parkinson disease
	Crizanlizumab				Sickle cell crisis
21.	Daclizumab		12/97 IV	Humanized	Prophy organ rejection, renal transplant
22.	Daclizumab		5/16 Sc	Humanized	MS
23.	Daratumumab		11/15 IV	Humanized	MS, Multiple myeloma
24.	Denosumab		8/2010 Sc	Fully Human	Post-menopausal osteoporosis
	Depemokimab				Cystic fibrosis
25.	Dinutuximab		3/2015 IV	Chimeric	Peds high-risk neuroblastoma
	Dostarlimab				First-line treatment for rectal cancer. 6 months treatment q 3 weeks. 100% of patients showed a complete response. Sept 13, 2022
26.	Dupilumab (not available in KIMS)		3/2017 SC	Fully humanized (FH)	• in alleviating symptoms of prurigo nodularis, atopic dermatitis, asthma. Children with eosinophilic esophagitis (FDA-approved Jan 2024). Cystic fibrosis • Dupilumab, given by injection, is a recombinant human Ig -G4 mAb that inhibits interleukin 4 (IL-4) and IL-13 signaling
27.	Durvalumab (Imfinzi)	KIMS	5/2017 IV	FH	Ovarian Ca, urothelial CA KIMS use NSCL Immune checkpoint inhibitor (ICPs)
28.	Eculizumab (Soliris)		3/2007 IV	Humanized	Management of atypical hemolytic uremic syndrome (aHUS), which may occur in kidney transplant recipients
29.	Elotuzumab		11/2015 IV	Humanized	Multiple myeloma
	Emicizumab	Hemlibra			Hemophilia
	Enfortumab Vedotin				Enfortumab Vedotin and Pembrolizumab in Untreated Advanced Urothelial Cancer
	Epcoritamab				FDA approved Feb 2024, epcoritamab and loncastuximab, diffuse large B-cell lymphoma (DLBCL)
	Erenumab		5/18 Sc	FH	Migraine headache

Contd...

Contd...

#	mAb	Brand by	Approval date, route	Type and target	Indications
30.	Evolocumab		2/2015 Sc	FH	Hypercholesterolemia
	Frexalimab = anti-CD40L mAb				Multiple sclerosis MS . Inhibition of CD40L with Frexalimab in Multiple Sclerosis
	Gemtuzumab	Wyeth	9/2017 IV	Humanized	AML
31.	Golimumab		4/2009 SC	FH	RA, psoriatic arthritis, all arthritis
32.	Ibalizumab		3/2018 IV	Humanized	HIV
33.	Ibritumomab tiuxetan		2/2002 IV	Murine	NHL, B-cell lymphoma
34.	Idarucizumab		10/2015 IV	Humanized	Emergency reversal anticoagulant
	Inclacumab				Sickle cell disease
	Imatinib (Gleevec)				Cancer cell killing
	Ipilimumab				First approved immune checkpoint inhibitor (ICPIs), was combined with nivolumab
35.	Infliximab (Remicade)	KIMS	8/1998 IV	Chimeric	Crohn's and also used in graft versus host disease (GVHD) and autoimmune disorders that may affect transplant recipients
36.	Infliximab-abda		4/2017 IV	Chimeric	All arthritis, ulcerative colitis, Crohn's
	Infliximab-qbtx	Pfizer	12/2017 IV	Chimeric	
	Inotuzumab Ozogamicin	Wyeth	8/2017 IV	Humanized	Inotuzumab ozogamicin followed by blinatumomab achieved excellent outcomes. Adult ALL, lymphoma
37.	Ipilimumab (Yervoy)		3/2011 IV	FH	Metastatic melanoma, immune checkpoint inhibitor (ICPs)
38.	Ixekizumab	Eli lilly	3/2016 SC	Humanized	Plague psoriasis
	Loncastuximab				FDA approved Feb 2024, epcoritamab and loncastuximab, diffuse large B-cell lymphoma (DLBCL)
39.	Ixekizumab	Eli lilly	3/2016 SC	Humanized	Plague psoriasis
	Mepolizumab				Cystic fibrosis, COPD, mepolizumab for eosinophilic granulomatosis with polyangiitis
	Muromonab CD3 (Orthoclone OKT3)		1986	Muraine	The first FDA-approved therapeutic mAb for SOT
40.	Natalizumab		11/2004 IV	humanized	Multiple sclerosis
41.	Necitumumab		22/2015 IV	FH	Lung Ca Squamous cell metastasis
42.	Nivolumab- ICP inhibitors		12/2014 IV	FH	Melanoma, sq cell lung Ca ICP = immune checkpoint inhibitors (ICPs) for renal cell Ca, esophageal CA, metastatic blader Ca, chemotherapy or immunotherapy with nivolumab or pembrolizumab
43.	Obiltoxaximab		3/2016 IV	Chimeric	Inhalation anthrax
44.	Obinutuzumab		11/2013 IV	Humanized	Chronic lymphocytic leukemia
45.	Ocrelizumab		3/2017 IV	Humanized	MS
46.	Ofatumumab		10/2009 IV	FH	Chronic lymphocytic leukemia, MS

Contd...

Contd...

#	mAb	Brand by	Approval date, route	Type and target	Indications
47.	Olaratumab		10/2016 IV	FH	Soft tissue sarcoma
48.	Omalizumab	KIMS	6/2003 Sc	Humanized	Moderate-to-severe persistent asthma shows promise in protecting against severe reactions in children with multiple food allergies, data show Waiting for FDA approval soon, cystic fibrosis
49.	Palivizumab Med Immune		6/1998 IM	Humanized	RSV prophylaxis monthly, nirsevimab 1 shot a season
50.	Panitumumab		9/2006 IV	FH	Metastatic colorectal cancer
51.	Pembrolizumab (Keytruda) = ICP		9/2014 IV	Humanized	Melanoma, uterine Ca ICP, metastatic blader Ca, chemotherapy or immunotherapy with nivolumab or pembrolizumab
52.	Pertuzumab		6/2012	Humanized	Metastatic breast Ca
	Prasinezumab				Prasinezumab and Cinpanemab for Parkinson's diseases
53.	Ramucirumab		4/2014 IV	FH	Gastric Ca
54.	ranibizumab		6/2006 Intra EYE	Humanized	Macular degeneration
55.	Raxibacumab		12/2012 IV	FH	Inhalation anthrax
56.	Reslizumab		3/2016 IV	Humanized	Br asthma, cystic fibrosis
57.	Rituximab (Rituxan)	KIMS	11/97 IC	Chimeric	• Follicular lymphoma, diffuse large B-cell lymphoma • Chronic lymphocytic leukemia. rheumatoid arthritis, MS
	Rituximab and hyaluronidase		6/2017 Sc		CLL, lymphoma, SOT patients
	Rozanolixizumab-noli				A targeted treatment option in *myasthenia gravis*: RYSTIGGO®
	Sarilumab	Sanofi	5/2017 SC	FH	RA
58.	Secukinumab		1/2015 SC	FH	Plague psoriasis
	Sibeprenlimab				Sibeprenlimab is a humanized IgG2 mAb that binds to and neutralizes IgA nephropathy
59.	Siltuximab		4/2014 IV	Chimeric	Castleman disease
	Tildrakizumab-asmn		3/2018 Sc	Humanized	Psoriasis
	Teplizumab			Humanized	Newly diagnosed type 1 diabetes can prevent disease progression is unknown
60.	Tocilizumab	KIMS	1/2010 IV	Humanized	RA and all arthritis
61.	Trastuzumab (Herceptin)		9/1998 IV	Humanized	Metastatic Ca breast, cancer cell killer uterine Ca
	Ublituximab				MS
62.	Ustekinumab		9/2009 SC	FH	Psoriasis
63.	Ustekinumab		9/2016 IV Sc	FH	Plaque psoriasis, psoriatic arthritis, Crohn's disease
64.	Vedolizumab	Entyvio	5/2014 IV	Humanized	Ulcerative colitis, Crohn's disease

Annexture 2: Therapeutic use of monoclonal antibodies at KIMS Health Tertiary Hospital, Thiruvananthapuram, India for a period of 3 months (September, October and November 2023)

SL No	Name of the drug	Brand name	Dosage form	Dose	Manufacture	Uses	Total consumption SEP-NOV
1.	Omalizumab	Omalirel	Injection	150 mg	Reliance	Moderate-to-severe persistent asthma	10
2.	Rituximab	Ristova	Injection	100 mg	Roche	Non-Hodgkin's lymphoma, chronic lymphocytic leukemia, Wegener's granulomatosis, pemphigus vulgaris, and rheumatoid arthritis	69
		Ristova	Injection	500 mg			52
		Reditux RA	Injection	500 mg	DRL		15
		Toritz	Injection	100 mg, 500 mg	Torrent		
		Reditux	Injection	100 mg	DRL		12
		Reditux	Injection	500 mg			21
3.	Infliximab	Remicade	Injection	100 mg	J&J	Crohn's disease and ulcerative colitis	
4.	Adalimumab	Exemptia	Injection PFS	40 mg	Zydus	Inflammation of the joints (rheumatoid arthritis)	3
5.	Tocilizumab	Actemra	Injection	80 mg, 162 mg, 400 mg	Cipla	Treat rheumatoid arthritis and juvenile idiopathic arthritis	
		Actemra	Injection PFS	400 mg 200 mg			1
6.	Durvalumab	IMFINZI	Injection	120 mg, 500 mg	Astra Zeneca	Nonsmall cell lung cancer	
7.	Abciximab	ABCIXIREL	Injection	10 mg	Reliance	Lessen the chance of heart attack in people who need percutaneous coronary intervention (PCI)	57
8.	Cetuximab (anti-EGFR)	ERBITUX	Injection	100 mg, 500 mg	Merck	Treatment for bowel cancer that has spread (advanced bowel cancer) and head and neck cancers	
9.	Trastuzumab (Anti HEV –L therapy)	Herclon	Injection	440 mg	Roche	Treatment of HER2-positive breast cancer	53
		Herclon	Injection	150 mg			1
		Herhope	Injection	150 mg	Torrent		3
		Herhope	Injection	440 mg			53
		Hertraz	Injection	440 mg	Mylan		
		Ujvira	Injection	100 mg	Zydus		57
		Ujvira	Injection	160 mg			11
		Canmab	Injection	150 mg	Biocon		3
		Canmab	Injection	440 mg	Biocon		10
10.	Pertuzumab (anti-Hev-L therapy)	Perjeta	Injection	420 mg	Roche	To treat certain types of breast cancer	

Contd...

CHAPTER 9: Immunotherapy and Gene Therapy Approaches in Disease Prevention and Treatments

Contd...

SL No	Name of the drug	Brand name	Dosage form	Dose	Manufacture	Uses	Total consumption SEP-NOV
11.	Bevacizumab	Bevazza	Injection	100 mg, 400 mg	Lupin	Colon and rectal cancer (cancer that begins in the large intestine)	For glioblastoma 10 mg/kg IV q2 weeks
		Krabeva	Injection	100 mg, 400 mg			
		Bevacirel	Injection	100 mg	Biocon		14
		Bevacirel	Injection	400 mg	Reliance		12
		Versavo	Injection	100 mg	DRL		23
		Versavo	Injection	400 mg			28
12.	Adalimumab	Adfrar	Injection	20 mg, 40 mg	Torrent	Inflammation of the joints (rheumatoid arthritis)	
		Adlumab	Injection	40 mg	RPG		
13.	Nivolumab (POI-Inhibitor)	Opdyta	Injection	40 mg	Bristol Myers	Treat unresectable or metastatic melanoma, melanoma as adjuvant treatment	7
		Opdyta	Injection	100 mg			22
14.	Pembrolizumab (POLI-Inhibitor)	Keytruda	Injection	100 mg	MSD	Nonsmall-cell lung cancer, cervical cancer	50
15.	Denosumab	Xgeva	Injection	120 mg	DRL	To treat osteoporosis (thinning of the bones)	30
		Olimab	PFS	60 mg	Intas		
		Prolia	Injection	60 mg	DRL		6
		Denoci	Injection	120 mg	Cipla		

■ SUGGESTED READING

1. Abramson A, Kirtane AR, Shi Y, Zhong G, Collins JE, Tamang S, et al. Oral mRNA delivery using capsule-mediated gastrointestinal tissue injections. Matter. 2022;5(3):975-87.
2. Brownlee C. (2021). Gene therapy for Duchenne muscular dystrophy. Available from: https://www.hopkinsmedicine.org/news/articles/gene-therapy-for-duchenne-muscular-dystrophy [Last accessed April, 2024].
3. Center for Cancer Research. Jennifer Brudno, who is involved in several trials of CAR T-cell therapies in NCI's Center for Cancer Research. Available from: https://ccr.cancer.gov/staff-directory/jennifer-n-brudno#:~:text=Brudno%20researches%20the%20use%20of,of%20phase%20I%20clinical%20trials [Last accessed April, 2024].
4. Chandramohan D, Zongo I, Sagara I, Cairns M, Yerbanga RS, Diarra M, et al. Seasonal malaria vaccination with or without Seasonal Malaria Chemoprevention. N Engl J Med. 2021;385(11):1005-17.
5. Chen W, Hu Y, Ju D. Gene therapy for neurodegenerative disorders: advances, insights, and prospects Acta pharmaceutica sinica b. 2020;10(8):1347-59.
6. Chiesa R, Georgiadis C, Syed F, Zhan H, Etuk A, Gkazi SA, et al. Base-Edited CAR T Group. Base-Edited CAR7 T Cells for Relapsed T-Cell Acute Lymphoblastic Leukemia. N Engl J Med . 2023;389(10):899-910.
7. Dec 2023 American Society of Hematology (ASH) annual meeting Program: Oral and Poster Abstracts presentation
8. Jin KT, Chen B, Liu YY, Lan HU, Yan JP. mAbs and CAR T cells in the treatment of colorectal cancer. Cancer Cell Int. 2021;21(1):83.
9. Khurana A, Allawadhi P, Khurana I, Allwadhi S, Weiskirchen R, Banothu AK, et al. Role of nanotechnology behind the success of mRNA vaccines for COVID-19. Nano Today. 2021;38:101142.
10. Longhurst HJ, Lindsay K, Petersen RS, Fijen LM, Gurugama P, Maag D, et al. CRISPR-Cas9 In Vivo Gene Editing of KLKB1 for Hereditary Angioedema. N Engl J Med. 2024;390(5):432-41.

11. Müller F, Taubmann J, Bucci L, Wilhelm A, Bergmann C, Völkl S, et al. CD19 CAR T-cell therapy in autoimmune disease: a case series with follow-up. N Engl J Med. 2024; 390:687-700
12. NEJM January 24, 2024
13. Patricia Inácio. January 23, 2024, Department of Microbiology & Immunology, Columbia University, New York, USA.
14. Rocha LFM, Braga LAM, Mota FB. Gene editing for treatment and prevention of human diseases: a global survey of gene editing-related researchers. Hum Gene Ther. 2020;31(15-16):852-62.
15. Schofield D. (2020). Types of monoclonal antibodies. Available from: https://www.evitria.com/journal/monoclonal-antibodies/types-monoclonal-antibodies/ [Last accessed April, 2024].
16. Strikas RA, Orenstein WA. (2018). Active Immunization. Available from: https://www.sciencedirect.com/topics/immunology-and-microbiology/active-immunization [Last accessed April, 2024].
17. Wikipedia. (2024). Monoclonal antibody therapy. Available from: https://en.wikipedia.org/wiki/Monoclonal_antibody_therapy [Last accessed April, 2024].

Immunization in Special Clinical Circumstances Including Solid Organ Transplant (Immunocompromised and Immunosuppressed SOT and HSCT Recipients)

Jr Uduman, AK Uduman

INTRODUCTION

Solid organ transplantation (SOT) of the kidney, liver, heart, lung, pancreas, or intestine (including the esophagus, stomach, small or large intestine, or any portion of the gastrointestinal tract) means the damaged or diseased organ of a recipient is replaced by a healthy one. The donor and recipient may be at the same location or the same family or organs may be transported from a donor site to another location. The types of transplants are:

- *Autograft:* Organs and/or tissues that are transplanted within the same person's body are called autografts—the transplant of cells or tissue to the same person.
- *Allograft (allogeneic):* It is a tissue or an organ graft from a donor of the same species as the recipient but is not genetically identical.
- *Isograft (syngeneic):* Transplant of an organ or tissue from a genetically identical donor or from a donor to a genetically identical recipient such as from a sibling and/or from a genetically identical twin.
- *Xenogeneic–xenografts:* Transplantation of cells, tissues, or organs from one species to another. For example, from animal species to human.

Vaccination recommendations for individuals with special circumstances, including those who have undergone SOT may vary based on individual health conditions and specific medical needs. SOTs are common now—the kidney is the most commonly transplanted solid organ.

BACKGROUND

Immunization in special circumstances refers to specific situations where individuals may have unique immunization needs or considerations. Physicians need to assess individual circumstances, review medical history, and consult relevant guidelines to determine the appropriate immunization approach for individuals in special circumstances. Tailored immunization plans help ensure that individuals receive the necessary vaccines while considering their unique needs and health conditions.

Individuals with chronic conditions, such as diabetes, heart disease, chronic respiratory diseases, and chronic renal diseases (CRD) may be at higher risk for severe complications from vaccine-preventable diseases. They are often encouraged to stay up-to-date on vaccinations.

CONSIDERATION OF MESSENGER RIBONUCLEIC ACID VACCINES

Literature has evidence to suggest that the Food and Drug Administration- (FDA)-approved messenger ribonucleic acid (mRNA) vaccines may be more effective in producing an immune response in immunocompromised individuals compared to other vaccine types. However, individual circumstances vary and recommendations should be personalized based on medical history.

These special clinical circumstances follow guidelines provided by health authorities and organizations such as the World Health Organization (WHO), the Centers for Disease Control and Prevention (CDC), and the Advisory Committee on Immunization Practices (ACIP) to ensure that vaccines are administered safely and effectively in these situations. In some cases, consultation with specialists, i.e., infectious disease and vaccine experts may be necessary to make individualized recommendations.

Here are some examples of special circumstances that may require tailored immunization approaches include:

- *Age and immunization:* Special considerations apply to infants, young children, adults, and the elderly. Immunization recommendations may vary based on age-appropriate specific vaccines that are dependent on individual immunologic status and working backgrounds. Vaccine schedules need to be adjusted based on the gestational age of the pregnant mothers and potential exposure risk. This includes vaccines such as the rotavirus vaccine for infants, the human papillomavirus (HPV) vaccine for adolescents, and the shingles vaccine for older adults (Refer to Chapter 6: Adults and Elderly Vaccinations).

- *Pregnancy:* Vaccines are commonly recommended during pregnancy to provide maternal and fetal protection. Certain vaccines, such as the flu and tetanus, diphtheria, and acellular pertussis (Tdap), are recommended during pregnancy to protect both the mother and the developing fetus. Live vaccines, such as measles, mumps, and rubella (MMR) and varicella (VAR), are generally contraindicated during pregnancy (Refer to Chapter 7: Pregnancy and Lactation Immunization).
- *Immunocompromised individuals:* People with weakened immune systems, such as those with certain underlying medical conditions, those undergoing cancer treatment, or SOT and hematopoietic stem cell transplant (HSCT) recipients or may require modified immunization schedules and/or need additional vaccines.
- *Vaccinations and revaccination are less well-defined,* and they may not respond as effectively to vaccines and in some cases, modified or higher-dose vaccines may be necessary. This is to ensure optimal protection against vaccine-preventable diseases while considering their specific health status.
- *Occupational exposures:* Certain occupations, such as healthcare workers, laboratory personnel, or animal handlers, may have increased exposure to specific pathogens. As a result, they may require additional or specialized vaccines to protect against occupational hazards, such as hepatitis B (HepB), influenza, or rabies vaccines.

  Settings with close living conditions, for example, prison populations and homeless individuals may be at higher risk for infectious disease outbreaks and healthcare providers may need to adapt immunization strategies accordingly (Refer to Chapter 20: Vaccinations for Healthcare Staff).
- *Travelers:* Individuals traveling to certain regions or countries may require additional vaccines to protect against diseases that are more prevalent in those areas. Depending on the destination and specific travel itinerary, travelers may require vaccinations not routinely recommended in their home country, such as meningococcal disease, yellow fever, typhoid, or Japanese encephalitis vaccines (Refer to Chapter 14: Vaccinations for Travelers).
- *Allergies or adverse reactions:* Individuals with known allergies such as from eggs (in the case of some influenza vaccines) or gelatin need special considerations. Previous adverse reactions to specific vaccines or vaccine components may require alternative vaccine options or additional precautions. Allergists can help determine the best approach for such cases. This may involve conducting allergy testing or administering vaccines in a controlled setting under medical supervision.
- *History of severe allergic reactions (anaphylaxis):* Vaccines in the past should be evaluated by an allergist or immunologist to assess the risks and benefits of future vaccinations. In some cases, they may receive vaccines in a controlled medical setting (Refer to Chapter 15: Vaccinations Adverse Reaction).
- *Catch-up immunizations:* Individuals who have missed or delayed their routine immunizations may require catch-up immunization schedules to ensure they are adequately protected against vaccine-preventable diseases. This is particularly important for children, adolescents, and individuals entering certain educational or healthcare settings (Refer to Chapter 17: Catch-up Vaccination).

VACCINATION FOR IMMUNOCOMPROMISED AND IMMUNOSUPPRESSED INDIVIDUALS

Vaccination recommendations for immunocompromised and immunosuppressed (ICIS) individuals are crucial to provide them with protection against vaccine-preventable diseases.

For example, VAR (chicken pox) is generally regarded as a mild, self-limiting viral illness with occasional complications. However, ICIS people with primary (VAR) or reactivated (herpes zoster) infection are at increased risk of severe disease and death. Severe VAR and disseminated zoster are more likely to develop in children with congenital T-lymphocyte defects or acquired immunodeficiency syndrome than in people with B-lymphocyte abnormalities **(Fig. 1)**. Other groups of patients who may experience more severe or complicated VAR include infants, adolescents, adult patients with chronic cutaneous or pulmonary disorders, and patients receiving systemic corticosteroids or other immunosuppressive therapy or long-term salicylate therapy.

The specific recommendations may vary depending on the individual's underlying condition, treatment regimen, and immune status. Here are some general considerations for vaccination in ICIS individuals:

Immunocompromised individuals need to consult with their healthcare provider, who can assess their

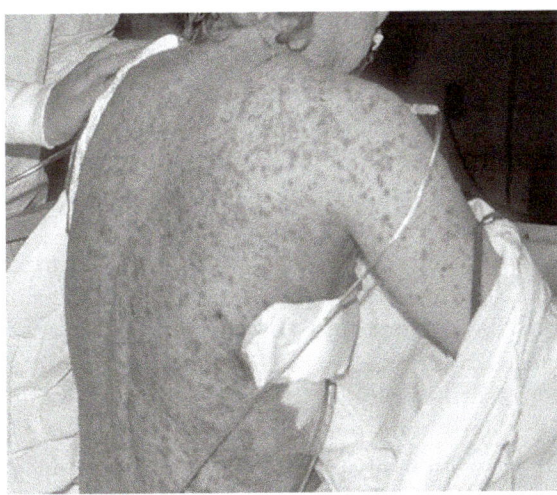

Fig. 1: Severe varicella with pneumonitis (varicella vaccinated) in a 17-year-old with Hodgkin's disease with failure to respond to intravenous acyclovir.
Courtesy: The Centers for Disease Control and Prevention (CDC) and Redbook, 2022.

specific medical condition, immune status, and treatment plan. They can then make tailored recommendations for vaccination based on individual circumstances.

Inactivated vaccines: Immunocompromised individuals can have inactivated vaccines, which contain killed or inactivated pathogens. These vaccines are generally safe because they do not contain live organisms that could cause infections. Examples of inactivated vaccines include severe acute respiratory syndrome coronavirus 2 (SARS-CoV-2), influenza (flu), HepB, and pneumococcal vaccines.

Live attenuated vaccines (LAV): Most immunocompromised individuals should avoid live vaccines, as these vaccines contain weakened live pathogens that could potentially cause illness in people with weakened immune systems. However, the decision to administer LAV should be made on a case-by-case basis, considering the individual's specific condition and treatment plan. Examples of LAV include the MMR, VAR, and yellow fever vaccines.

Household contacts and caregivers: It is often recommended that close contacts of immunocompromised individuals, such as family members and caregivers, be up-to-date with their vaccinations to reduce the risk of transmitting vaccine-preventable diseases. For example, ensuring that family members are vaccinated against the flu and whooping cough (pertussis) can help protect immunocompromised individuals.

Timing and scheduling: In some cases, the timing and scheduling of vaccinations for immunocompromised individuals may need to be adjusted. They may need to be timed carefully to ensure optimal immune response and this may involve administering vaccines during periods of relative immune stability or adjusting the timing of vaccination based on the individual's treatment schedule. For example, they may require additional booster shots or more frequent revaccination to maintain protection.

Serologic testing: This involves measuring antibody levels used to assess an individual's immune response to specific vaccines. This can help determine if additional doses or booster shots are needed to achieve adequate protection.

Herd immunity: Immunocompromised individuals may rely on herd immunity, which is the indirect protection from infectious diseases that occurs when a large proportion of the population is vaccinated. Encouraging vaccination among the general population helps protect immunocompromised individuals who may have a reduced ability to mount an immune response to vaccines.

Vaccine recommendations may vary for different types of immunocompromised states, such as those caused by cancer, organ transplantation, human immunodeficiency virus (HIV) infection, or autoimmune diseases. Additionally, recommendations can change over time as new research and vaccines become available. Therefore, it is crucial to have an ongoing dialogue with infectious disease (ID) specialists to ensure you receive the most up-to-date and appropriate vaccination guidance available to these.

Vaccine-preventable infections are common after pediatric transplant; therefore, maximal efforts must be made to ensure complete immunization of transplant candidates and recipients. Hospitalization for vaccine-preventable infections occurred in >15% of SOT recipients in the first 5 years after transplant at a rate of up to 87 times higher than in the general population. There was significant morbidity, mortality, and costs from these infections, demonstrating the importance of immunizing all transplant candidates and recipients. Further research on improving immunization delivery, preventing nosocomial infections, and monitoring response to vaccines in the transplant population is needed.

As new vaccines become available and recommendations evolve, it is essential to stay informed and discuss these options with your healthcare provider who is knowledgeable about immunizations and your specific medical condition. They can provide personalized recommendations based on your medical history and the specific vaccines you may need. Immunocompromised individuals may also be candidates for clinical trials or emerging treatments that can enhance their immune response to vaccines. These options should be discussed with a healthcare provider.

VACCINATION FOR SOLID ORGAN TRANSPLANT CANDIDATES AND RECIPIENTS

Solid organ transplant candidates and recipients should receive all vaccines indicated based on their ages, medical conditions, and other factors that apply to non-SOT candidates or recipients.

- Current guidelines recommend patients complete coronavirus disease 2019 (COVID-19) vaccination whenever possible and ideally complete all vaccination series a minimum of 2 weeks prior to the transplant.
- All SOTs receive their annual flu vaccine shots.
- All SOT candidates and recipients should be vaccinated against pneumococcus with pneumococcal conjugate vaccine 13 (PCV13), 15, or 20 and pneumococcal polysaccharide vaccine 23 (PPSV23).
- All SOT candidates and recipients should receive a HepB vaccine series with postvaccination titers unless they have a documented HepB surface antibody (anti-HBs) titer of ≥10 mIU/mL after a properly timed HepB series or unless they have known HepB virus (HBV) infection.
- All SOT candidates and recipients should receive a hepatitis A (HepA) vaccine series unless previously administered or unless they have a positive HepA virus immunoglobulin G (IgG)-positive titer.
- *LAV should not be administered to SOT recipients*, SOT candidates on immunosuppression, or SOT candidates who may undergo SOT within 4 weeks. The timing of inactivated, subunit or toxoid vaccines is discussed further **(Table 1)**.

TABLE 1: Vaccines and their utility guidelines for SOT.

Vaccine	Notes
SARS-CoV-2	Strongly recommended
Influenza	Should be given annually before the beginning of the influenza season for all SOTs. Can be given pre- and/or post-SOT
Tdap or Td	Can be given pre- and/or post-SOT
MMR	A LAV is to be given pre-SOT only; generally, those born before 1957 (among others) are considered immune
Varicella	A LAV is to be given pre-SOT only; generally, those born in the US before 1980 (among others) are considered immune
RZV, Shingrix	Only indicated for those ≥60 years old; has not been well studied in SOT recipients and is not routinely recommended after SOT, though is likely safe
HPV	Can be given pre- and/or post-SOT for patients aged 26 years or younger
PCV13, PPSV23	Can be given pre- and/or post-SOT
HepA, HepB, or HepA–HepB	Can be given pre- and/or post-SOT
MenACWY or MenB	Can be given pre- and/or post-SOT; only if asplenia or complement deficiencies
Hib	Can be given pre- or post-SOT; only if asplenia or complement deficiencies

(HepA: hepatitis A; HepB: hepatitis B; Hib: haemophilus influenzae type b; HPV: human papillomavirus; LAV: live attenuated vaccine; MenACWY: meningococcal conjugate vaccine; MenB: meningococcal B; MMR: measles, mumps, and rubella; PCV13: pneumococcal conjugate vaccine 13; PPSV23: pneumococcal polysaccharide vaccine 23; RZV: recombinant zoster vaccine; SARS-CoV-2: severe acute respiratory syndrome coronavirus 2; SOT: solid organ transplant; Td: tetanus and diphtheria; Tdap: tetanus, diphtheria, and acellular pertussis; US: United States)

Source: Adapted and modified from Stanford Health Care. (2018). Guidelines for Vaccination of Adult Solid Organ Transplant Candidates and Recipients. Available from: https://med.stanford.edu/content/dam/sm/bugsanddrugs/documents/clinicalpathways/SHC-Vaccination-SOT.pdf [Last accessed April, 2024].

Live Vaccines

Live vaccines (MMRV) have not been recommended after SOT due to concern for inciting vaccine strain infection in an immunocompromised host. However, the rates of measles, mumps, and VAR are rising nationally and internationally, leaving susceptible immunocompromised children and adults at risk for life-threatening conditions.

Individual SOT programs may adopt modified versions of these vaccine guidelines and mirror their respective SOT protocols. Primary care providers and other specialists, including SOT providers, should be encouraged to vaccinate SOT candidates and recipients.

Timing of Vaccination

The timing of vaccination for the transplant and immunosuppressive medications is critical because the response to vaccinations is decreased in patients with end-stage organ disease and in the first 6 months after transplantation. The efficacy, safety, and protocols of several vaccines in this patient population are poorly understood. In some cases, it may be recommended to delay vaccination until a certain period after the transplant surgery or adjust the immunosuppressive medications temporarily to enhance vaccine response.

- Vaccination timing for SOT recipients is a critical aspect of posttransplant care. Preferably, vaccinations should be given as early before SOT as possible when the patient is first seen and evaluated for SOT candidature.
- Inactivated, subunit, or toxoid vaccines should ideally be given 2 weeks or more prior to immunosuppression or SOT to achieve maximum immunogenicity.
- To maximize immunogenicity and effectiveness, inactivated, subunit, or toxoid vaccines should preferentially be given starting at 6 months post-SOT, though they can be given as early as 2 months based on patient-specific risk factors.
- Flu vaccination can begin as early as 1 month after SOT if there is significant local influenza activity. Similarly, to maximize vaccine effectiveness, vaccination should ideally be delayed during other periods of intensified immunosuppression.
  - Most vaccines appear to be safe in SOT recipients, but LAV should be avoided until further studies are available.
  - SOT recipients will benefit from consistent immunization practices.
  - The live vaccinations may be safe and immunogenic after SOT in select pediatric and adult recipients and can offer protection against circulating measles, mumps, and VAR.

Other Exceptional Medical Risk Factors

- Vaccinations should ideally be given 2 weeks or more before splenectomy, eculizumab administration, or other iatrogenic procedures, resulting in asplenia or complement component deficiencies. For further details involving both vaccinations and other considerations in caring for these patients.
- Given the risk of meningococcal infection with eculizumab use, even when vaccination is appropriately provided, patients should generally be prescribed penicillin V potassium 500 mg by mouth twice daily for the duration of eculizumab treatment and for 4 weeks after treatment finishes. Patients who report penicillin allergy should be prescribed azithromycin 250 mg by mouth daily and referred to the allergy division for consideration of skin testing, drug challenge, or desensitization.
- Patients with complex medical conditions not discussed in these recommendations and those with unique risk factors associated with travel or occupation (including contact with animals or work with pathogens) should be referred to the infectious diseases clinic to determine optimal immunization strategies.

Vaccination of Family Members and Household Contacts of Solid Organ Transplant Candidates and Recipients

Vaccination strategy should include vaccination of household contacts and healthcare workers at transplant centers unless contraindicated.

- To protect immunocompromised patients from transmissible diseases, immunocompetent family members, and household contacts should be encouraged to receive all age-appropriate vaccinations, particularly an annual flu shot and LAVs such as MMR and VAR, with these exceptions or additions:
  - *Live attenuated influenza vaccine (LAIV):* Household contacts of SOT candidates and recipients should avoid LAIV or, if obtained, avoid contact with the immunocompromised patient for 7 days after vaccination.

- *VAR/zoster vaccine live (ZVL) (for ZVL called Zostavax):* Recipients may develop rarely localized or generalized VAR-like rash within 1 month after vaccination. Nonimmune SOT candidates and recipients should avoid contact with those having rash illness until their skin lesions clear. Except in those rare individuals who develop a VAR-like rash, recipients of VAR or ZVL vaccines are not capable of transmitting the virus and can interact with SOT candidates and recipients without restriction. This issue is not relevant with recombinant zoster vaccine (RZV) (Shingrex) when the SOT candidate or recipient is already immune to varicella zoster virus (VZV).

Rotavirus: SOT candidates and recipients should avoid handling diapers of infants who have been vaccinated with rotavirus vaccine for 4 weeks after vaccination.

Other concerns: Chronic hepatitis E virus (HEV) infection is rare and, to date, has only been reported in more developed countries, mostly among SOT recipients with immunosuppression. Approximately, 60% of recipients of SOTs fail to clear the virus and develop chronic hepatitis and 10% will develop cirrhosis.

CORONAVIRUS DISEASE 2019 VACCINE FOR SOLID ORGAN TRANSPLANT

(American Society of Transplantations (AST) updated 1/12/2023 Key Recommendations):

As of the last knowledge update in February, 2024, the guidance provided by health authorities such as the CDC and the WHO included recommendations for COVID-19 vaccination in special populations are included in this section. This recommendation is subject to change and will be updated as new information or data becomes available.

- Recommended in individuals aged 6 months and older, including all SOT candidates, recipients, and living donors, as well as vaccination of their household members and caregivers to reduce infection risk for these vulnerable patients.
- A three-dose series of mRNA vaccines for primary vaccination in SOT recipients who are 6 months and older. Patients 6 months to 4 years who received Pfizer BioNTech mRNA for their first two doses may receive a bivalent Pfizer BioNTech mRNA dose as the third dose of their primary series. Patients 6 months to 4 years who received a Moderna mRNA series and patients 5 years of age and older who have received all doses of either mRNA primary series are eligible for an additional mRNA bivalent booster dose of their vaccine 2 months after completion of the initial series.
- For those who have received a dose of the Johnson & Johnson/Janssen vaccine, a second dose of mRNA SARS-CoV-2 vaccine, followed by a bivalent booster 2 months following the completion of the primary series. Data from immunocompetent patients shows a higher antibody response when the second dose is one of the mRNA vaccines.
- For those who have received the two-dose series of Novavax vaccine, a bivalent booster can be administered 2 months after completion of the series.
- A bivalent booster can be given after completion of any primary series for patients. See qualifications for those under 5.
- Continued adherence of all transplant recipients to protective measures such as masking and social distancing should be considered based on the risk of transmission and local infection rates and vaccination status.
- At this time, there is no recommendation for pre-exposure prophylaxis with any monoclonal antibody (mAb), including tixagevimab and cilgavimab (Evusheld).
- Recommend vaccination for SARS-CoV-2 in patients who have recovered from COVID-19, after symptoms have resolved and the period of isolation has ended. For persons with current or recent COVID-19, the appropriate timing of booster vaccination is unknown and the decision to receive a booster should be individualized. Depending on patient and clinician preference and the individual risk of reinfection, up to a 3-month delay from SARS-CoV-2 infection may be considered.
- Whenever possible, vaccination should occur prior to transplantation (ideally with completion of the primary vaccine series at a minimum of 2 weeks prior to transplant).
- For posttransplant patients, we recommend administering vaccination beginning as early as 1–3 months after transplantation. This can be individualized based on the type and degree of immunosuppression and local circulation of SARS-CoV-2.
- AST does not recommend routinely checking antibody responses to the vaccine and does not recommend routine adjustment of immunosuppressive medications prior to vaccination outside of clinical trials.

- Each center develops approaches to educate patients on the importance of vaccination and consider tracking vaccination rates.
- AST supports the development of institutional policies regarding pretransplant vaccination as we believe that this is in the best interest of the transplant candidate, optimizing their chances of being safely transplanted, especially at times of continued virus circulation.

There are currently several vaccine candidates in use or under development. In the United States (US), there are currently four vaccines available for use as the primary series.

The types of vaccines are as follows (January, 2023)—vaccines under development or available in the US and other countries:

- *US FDA approved:* mRNA-1273 (SpikeVax) (Moderna) and BNT162b2 (Tozinameran; Comirnaty) (Pfizer-BioNTech)
- *United Kingdom (UK), Euro, India, etc. approved:* Replication—defective adenoviral vector—AZD1222 (Covishield) (Oxford–AstraZeneca) and JNJ-78326735/Ad26.COV2.S (Janssen/Johnson Johnson)
- *USA approved: Nanoparticle*—saponin-based Matrix-M adjuvant—NVX-CoV2373 (Nuvaxovid) (Novavax)
- *USA not approved but India, China, Middle-east approved inactivated vaccine:* BBV152 (Covaxin) (Bharat Biotech) and BBIBP-CorV (CoronaVac) (Sinopharm).

What vaccines are available to transplant recipients?

The Pfizer and Moderna mRNA vaccines, Janssen/Johnson & Johnson Adenovirus—vector vaccine and Novavax protein subunit vaccine are available for administration in the US.

The Moderna vaccine is FDA approved for ages 18 years and older. The Pfizer vaccine is FDA approved for ages 12 years and older and both have emergency use authorization (EUA) for ages 6 months and older.

The Janssen vaccine has received emergency use authorization for 18 years and older, but mRNA vaccines are recommended over J&J due to the risk of serious adverse events such as thrombosis. Novavax is available as a two-shot primary series.

What is known about the safety of these vaccines?

mRNA vaccines: Not observed significant side effects reported beyond the early postvaccination. The rare serious side effects are noted in the first few days after vaccination. The potential for anaphylaxis to either mRNA vaccine may range from 2.5 to 4.7/million doses; this continues to be closely monitored in the US and other countries. Since April 2021, increased cases of myocarditis and pericarditis have been reported in the US after mRNA vaccines (both Pfizer-BioNTech and Moderna), particularly in young adults and adolescents under 40 years of age.

J&J/Janssen COVID-19 vaccine: Rare events of vaccine-induced thrombotic thrombocytopenia (VITT) were observed at a rate of 7 per 1 million doses administered in women between 18 and 49 years. Also, around 100 episodes of Guillain–Barré syndrome (GBS) have also been reported after the administration of the J&J/Janssen vaccine. Most cases were in older men and presentations were similar to GBS from other causes with a rate of 16 cases per 1 million doses administered in males 50 through 64 years. There was no association with immunosuppression.

To date, there have been no reports of rejection triggered by adenovirus vector vaccines. The safety of other candidate vaccines will be updated as further information is available.

How effective are COVID-19 vaccines in transplant recipients?

Coronavirus disease 2019 vaccination is generally recommended for individuals with SOT. However, the effectiveness of the immune response may be lower in immunocompromised individuals, including transplant recipients. In some cases, additional doses (booster shots) may be recommended to enhance protection.

- Existing data suggest that transplant patients have better antibody responses with mRNA vaccines than the adenovirus vectored vaccines.

Although transplant recipients have low antibody responses (approximately, 30–54% antibody positivity), some patients despite not developing antibodies still generate virus-specific T-cell responses suggesting that protection may be dependent on multiple arms of the immune system. Lastly, patients vaccinated pretransplant may have reduced protection posttransplant, particularly if therapies that reduce B-cell function (e.g., rituximab) are used. The impact of specific therapies, such as Belatacept, also warrants specific study.

Should transplant patients receive a fourth dose (booster) of mRNA vaccine?

At this time, the optimal number of doses of the SARS-CoV-2 vaccine is unknown, but the current CDC guidelines (updated December 22, 2022) recommend bivalent booster dosing in transplant recipients at least 2 months following completion of the initial three-dose series of mRNA vaccines or 2 months after their last booster dose. The original mRNA monovalent vaccines are no longer approved for booster doses.

Can a transplant recipient still receive the vaccine even if they have had COVID-19?

Yes, the current guidance is that everyone should receive the vaccine, irrespective of past COVID-19 or prior evidence of humoral immunity.

Immunosuppressed patients can develop SARS-CoV-2 reinfection, suggesting a lack of appropriate immune response especially against variants or waning immunity after the first infection. In addition, emerging data highlight that after COVID-19, vaccinated individuals are less likely to acquire a new infection compared to unvaccinated people.

If a transplant recipient has had COVID-19, they should wait until all symptoms are resolved and the period of isolation has ended before receiving the vaccine. The ideal period for vaccination after infection is still being investigated.

Can the COVID-19 vaccine be given at the same time as other vaccines?

There is limited data on the safety or efficacy of the mRNA COVID-19 vaccines when administered with other vaccines. Although ACIP initially recommended that the COVID-19 vaccine series should be administered alone and with a minimum of 14 days before or after giving any other vaccines, this recommendation has been discontinued and *coadministration of vaccines is now allowed including coadministration with influenza vaccine*. If multiple vaccines are being given concurrently, they should be given at different sites.

Should we check for antibody response after vaccination in SOT recipients?

Currently, AST does not recommend routinely checking antibody responses after any dose and does not recommend its use to determine the need for additional vaccine doses. Further, there is not a well-established protective threshold to target. Lastly, it may be difficult to interpret antibody levels in patients who already received either pre-exposure tixagevimab–cilgavimab (Evusheld) or mAb therapy for prior COVID-19 episodes. Assessment of responses should be done in the context of trials with experts who can interpret results and provide data on titers of neutralizing antibodies.

Should we hold mycophenolate mofetil or other immunosuppressants around the time patients are vaccinated?

Mycophenolate appears to significantly decrease antibody response to the COVID-19 mRNA vaccine. This is consistent with previous data on the impact of mycophenolate on influenza vaccine responses. However, mycophenolate is a critical part of the overall immunosuppression regimen. These data are observational and insufficient to support the reduction or cessation of any immunosuppression to improve vaccine efficacy. Therefore, the adjustment of mycophenolate or other immunosuppression for the sole purpose of increasing the antibody response is *not* routinely recommended outside of a trial setting.

Can patients stop wearing a mask after vaccination?

No, patients should be counseled to continue to practice COVID-19 safety measures including wearing masks around others, hand hygiene, and physical distancing in public places. It is likely that the efficacy and immunogenicity of the vaccine in transplant recipients will be lower than shown in the vaccine clinical trials.

Although masking requirements have been removed for the general public in many locations, adherence to masking, etc. should be strictly followed until more is known about the immune response and clinical effectiveness of the vaccine in the transplant population.

VACCINES FOR SOLID ORGAN TRANSPLANT—KIDNEY, LIVER, INTESTINES, HEART, LUNG, AND PANCREAS

End-stage Renal Disease and Kidney Transplant Patients' Vaccines

Key points:

- Patients with CRD and ESRD have diminished vaccination responses owing to renal diseases associated with premature aging of the immune system and chronic systemic low-grade inflammation.
- Vaccine responses in patients with kidney failure might also be increased through the use of higher vaccine doses, adjuvants, or temporary reduction of immunosuppressive drugs before vaccination might also be feasible.
- Both humoral (B-cell driven) and cellular (T-cell driven) immunity are generally required to control infections.

Antibodies are particularly efficient in preventing viral infections, whereas T-cells have a key role in viral clearance and help to prevent severe disease. The T-cell responses against the SARS-CoV-2 spike protein can be detected even in patients who are not able to produce antibodies owing to primary or secondary immune deficiency.

- For hemodialysis or chronic kidney disease (CKD) patients who do not respond to the primary vaccination, a new schedule with four doses of 40 µg is recommended.
- In general, there are mandatory vaccine requirements for all waitlisted SOT patients. Except for the flu vaccine and the COVID vaccine and unless instructed otherwise by the transplant team, the SOT recipient should wait until 6 months, to get posttransplant vaccines. If planning on traveling after the SOT, one may need additional vaccines.

Worldwide, the kidneys are the most transplanted organ. Organ donors may be living or brain-dead with a beating heart. For a transplant to succeed, the immunological barrier must be better understood to avoid graft rejection and clinical management.

Infection is the second leading cause of death in patients with CKD [chronic renal failure (CRF)]. Adequate humoral IgG antibody and cellular (T-cell driven) immunity are required to minimize pathogen entry and promote pathogen clearance to enable infection control. Vaccination can generate cellular and humoral immunity against specific pathogens and is used to prevent many life-threatening infectious diseases. However, vaccination efficacy is diminished in patients with CKD. Premature aging of the immune system and chronic systemic low-grade inflammation are the main causes of immune alteration in these patients.

Individuals with CRF or ESRD who are treated with maintenance dialysis might not respond as effectively to vaccines as compared with the general population. In many countries, the dialysis population is prioritized in vaccination programs. Serious obstacles that could inhibit the expected protective effects of the vaccines are the aberrations in the immune system in ESRD, consisting of immunodepression and immune activation.

Kidney Transplantation has been shown to Improve Survival as Compared to Patients on Dialysis

Impaired antibody response after different vaccines (e.g., those protecting against tetanus, influenza, HepB, diphtheria, and pneumococcal and Tdap diseases) in hemodialysis patients is well known. Depending on individual immune status, the physician might recommend additional or booster doses if needed. It is crucial for patients with kidney failure who are undergoing dialysis to follow their healthcare provider's guidance and consult with their nephrologist team for personalized recommendations.

Vaccines that are recommended for people on dialysis include COVID-19, influenza, HepB, pneumococcus, Tdap, and others **(Table 2)**.

TABLE 2: Recommended vaccines in chronic kidney disease patients including SARS-CoV-2.

Vaccine	Age	Dose	Vaccination schedule/route of administration	Booster doses
Hepatitis B, Engerix-B	≥20 years	40 µg	0, 1, 2, and 6 months/IM	Yes, when anti-HBs <10 mIU/mL
	<20 years	10 µg	0, 1, and 6 months/IM	Yes, when anti-HBs <10 mIU/mL
Pneumococcal				
Influenza	3–8 years	15 µg	Each year/IM	No
	9–12 years	15 µg	Each year/IM	No
	>12 years	15 µg	Each year/IM	No
Varicella	1–12 years	0.5 mL	Single dose/SC	No
Hepatitis A, Havrix®	>17 years	1,440 U	0, 6–12 months/IM	No
Measles, mumps, and rubella	>18 years	0.5 mL	Single dose/SC	No
Inactivated poliovirus	<18 years	0.5 mL	Three doses with an interval of 1–2 months	No (revaccination 1 year after the third dose)
Diphtheria and tetanus toxoids	7 years	0.5 mL	Three doses/IM	No

(anti-HBs: HepB surface antibody; IM: intramuscularly; SARS-CoV-2: severe acute respiratory syndrome coronavirus 2; SC: subcutaneously)

COVID-19 vaccination: This is highly recommended for dialysis patients including all transplant recipients. COVID-19 infection in transplanted patients carries a ~30% risk of mortality in the unvaccinated.

As of an update in May 2023, The National Kidney Foundation, American Society of Nephrology, and AST—all recommend COVID-19 vaccine for people living with kidney disease or who have had a kidney transplant.

Correlates of protection against SARS-CoV-2 have not been established for patients with kidney failure, but they are urgently needed to enable personalized vaccination regimens. The glomerular filtration rate correlates with the severity of COVID-19—among patients with kidney disease, the worst COVID-19 outcomes are observed in patients with kidney failure. Patients with absent or low responses should be identified for targeted additional booster doses or preemptive therapy with mAbs.

Correlates of protection against SARS-CoV-2 have not been established for patients with kidney failure, but they are urgently needed to enable personalized vaccination regimens. COVID-19 can have considerable detrimental effects in patients with CKD, especially in those with kidney failure. COVID-19 prevention through successful vaccination is therefore paramount in this vulnerable population. Although patients receiving dialysis have seroconversion rates comparable to those of patients with normal kidney function, most kidney transplant recipients could not generate humoral immunity after two doses of the COVID-19 vaccine. Importantly, some patients who were not able to produce antibodies still had a detectable vaccine-specific T-cell response, which might be sufficient to prevent severe COVID-19.

While more research is needed to learn more about the effectiveness in people with advanced renal disease (ESRD), those on dialysis, and transplant recipients, mRNA vaccines have been demonstrated to be safe in this population. Renal experts further should urge these patients to continue masking and practicing social distancing, after being fully vaccinated.

Vaccine Second Booster for Immune Suppressed

Booster doses are recommended for certain populations, including those with compromised immune systems. Transplant recipients may be considered a priority group for booster shots to enhance and prolong protection against COVID-19.

The US FDA has authorized the use of a second booster of the COVID-19 mRNA vaccine from either Pfizer-BioNTech or Moderna in patients who are immunocompromised (have a weak immune system). Patients with organ transplants, and others who are immunocompromised, should get a dose of mRNA booster of the COVID-19 vaccine after having received three doses and the first booster. Using a different brand of mRNA vaccine is allowed for the booster if the brand previously received is not available **(Table 3)**.

Influenza (Flu) Vaccine

The annual influenza vaccine is usually recommended for dialysis patients. Influenza can be especially severe in individuals with CKD. Dialysis patients are at increased risk of influenza-related mortality.

Influenza vaccine should be given annually before the beginning of the influenza season for persons 6 months of age or older on dialysis. Household contacts and healthcare workers should also be vaccinated annually to decrease the transmission to high-risk CKD patients.

The vaccine dose is 0.25 mL by intramuscular route for those between the ages of 6 and 35 months and 0.5 mL thereafter. To those <9 years of age, two doses of influenza vaccine are administered at least 1 month apart and at 9–12 years, one dose of split virus vaccine should be given.

TABLE 3: COVID-19 vaccination schedule for people with moderate or severe immunocompromise.

Primary vaccination	Age group in years	Primary vaccine dose	Number of booster doses	Interval between first and second dose	Interval between second and third dose	Interval between third and fourth dose
mRNA Pfizer	5–11	3	N/A	3 weeks	4 weeks or more	N/A
mRNA Pfizer	12 and older	3	1	3 weeks	4 weeks or more	3 months or more
Moderna mRNA	18 and older	3	1	4 weeks	4 weeks or more	3 months or more
Janssen	18 and older	1 mRNA	1	4 weeks	2 weeks or more	N/A

(COVID-19: coronavirus disease 2019; mRNA: messenger ribonucleic acid)

After the age of 12 years, one dose of whole or split virus vaccine should be given.

A fourfold increase in serum antibody titer against influenza antigens has been observed in 50% of dialysis patients compared to 40% of healthy controls and no systemic reactions have been reported following influenza vaccination in dialysis patients.

Hepatitis B Virus Vaccine

Individuals with CRF/ESRDs including those receiving hemodialysis are highly recommended to receive the HepB vaccine. The vaccine is generally considered safe and effective for this group and is particularly important for this population because they are at an increased risk of contracting and experiencing potentially life-threatening infectious complications from HBV.

The prevalence and incidence of HepB infections are high, at about 7.6% and 3.2%, respectively, among dialysis patients in India. The vaccine provides effective protection against the infection. Vaccination in the early stages of CKD has a better seroconversion rate than late vaccination.

- HepB vaccination is recommended for all CRF and ESRD patients. Patients with uremia who were vaccinated before they required dialysis have higher seroprotection rates and antibody titers. The response to vaccination is also better in children.
- Dialysis patients if they have not already been immunized are at a higher risk of HBV infection due to the frequent medical procedures involving blood. HepB vaccination is recommended for all individuals on dialysis. They may need an accelerated vaccination schedule to achieve protection more rapidly, such as receiving the second dose 1 month after the first and the third dose 2 months after the second.
- The timing and dosage of the HepB vaccine may vary depending on individual circumstances. Additionally, postvaccination blood tests to check for antibody levels (serologic testing) may be performed to ensure an adequate immune response. Some cases may require personalized recommendations based on their specific health status, treatment, and immune function.

Dosage and schedule: Higher vaccine dosages or an increased number of doses are recommended for subjects with CKD [estimated glomerular filtration rate (eGFR) <30 mL/min].

- Should receive four doses of the HepB vaccine as early in the course of the disease as possible. Recombinant HepB vaccine is recommended.
- Use special formulations of vaccine (40 μg/mL) or two 1 mL 20 μg doses given at one site. The dose schedule should be 0, 1, 2, and 6 months.
- Vaccine should be given intramuscularly in deltoid regions.
- Assess antibody titer (anti-HBs). The first titer should be done 1–2 months after the primary course is completed and annually thereafter.
- Booster dose should be given if anti-HBs titer falls below 10 mU/mL.
- Revaccination with full doses is recommended for persons who do not develop protective antibody titer after the primary course.

If an adult patient begins the vaccine series with a standard dose before beginning hemodialysis treatment and then moves to hemodialysis treatment before completing the series, completing the series using the higher dose is recommended for hemodialysis patients (with four doses of 40 μg is recommended).

No specific recommendations have been made for higher doses for pediatric hemodialysis patients. If a lower-than-recommended vaccine dose is administered to adults or children, the dose should be repeated.

- There is no difference in seroconversion rate in recombinant and plasma-derived vaccine, but recombinant vaccine is preferred due to fear of disease communication with plasma.
- Double dose (40 μg) and four doses give a better seroprotection rate (73–92%) compared to 45–67% with a conventional three-dose schedule.
- Antibody titer falls with time in patients on dialysis, necessitating annual monitoring.
- The deltoid region is preferred to ensure intramuscular administration. Intradermal administration has no advantage over intramuscular administration.

An increase in anti-HBs response with coadministration of zinc, erythropoietin, or immunomodulators such as alpha and gamma interferon, thymopentin, interleukin-2, and granulocyte–macrophage colony-stimulating factor have been reported. Such approaches should be reserved for patients in whom it is difficult to achieve seroconversion with at least two courses of the vaccine.

Adverse reactions: Vaccine has been shown to be safe for patients on dialysis with only minor local reactions including pain, redness, or swelling at the vaccination site.

Pneumococcal Vaccines

The ACIP recommends that all adults with CRD, regardless of age, receive the conjugated PCV13 vaccine followed by the PPSV23 vaccine at least 8 weeks later. This sequential vaccination strategy provides optimal protection against pneumococcal infections in CRD individuals. With the recent availability of the newer version of PCV15 and PCV20, the initial dose of this higher could be used instead of PCV13.

Other vaccines: Your healthcare provider may also recommend other vaccines, depending on your specific health conditions and risk factors. These may include vaccines such as the shingles vaccine (if age appropriate) and the Tdap vaccine.

Timing and frequency: The timing and frequency of vaccinations may vary based on your medical history and the specific recommendations of your healthcare provider. Some vaccines may need boosters or may be administered on a different schedule for dialysis patients.

Always remember that individual health conditions can vary and recommendations may change over time. Therefore, it is essential to consult with your nephrologist and healthcare team for personalized advice regarding vaccinations and other aspects of your healthcare. They will consider your unique medical history and any new developments in medical guidelines.

The Recommendations for administering PCV13 and PPSV23 in patients with CKD are shown in **Table 4**.

Pre- and Post-Liver Transplant Vaccination

A surgical procedure is typically performed in cases of end-stage liver disease, where the liver can no longer function adequately. This can be due to various causes, including cirrhosis, hepatitis, fatty liver disease, or genetic conditions. The damaged or diseased liver is replaced with a healthy liver from a living or deceased donor.

Cirrhosis is a common reason for liver transplantation and this can result from various factors, such as chronic alcohol abuse, viral hepatitis (A, B, C, D, and E), nonalcoholic fatty liver disease (NAFLD), and autoimmune conditions, for example, primary biliary cholangitis (PBC) and primary sclerosing cholangitis (PSC). Liver transplanted recipients are at an increased risk for liver failure when infected with HepA virus (HAV) and HBV. Therefore, it is important to vaccinate these individuals.

Also, inherited disorders such as Wilson disease, hemochromatosis, alpha-1 antitrypsin deficiency, and glycogen storage diseases can cause liver problems that may necessitate a transplant. Liver cancer, both primary hepatocellular carcinoma and secondary liver tumors (metastases from other cancers), may require liver transplantation in certain cases.

Individuals who are candidates for a liver transplant may need vaccinations as part of their pretransplant evaluation and posttransplant care.

Pretransplant vaccinations: It is essential to ensure that the recipient of the liver transplant is up-to-date on all recommended vaccinations before the transplant procedure. This helps protect the individual from vaccine-preventable diseases, which can be particularly important for people with compromised immune systems due to liver disease.

Posttransplant vaccinations: After a liver transplant, recipients often need to continue receiving vaccinations as part of their ongoing medical care. This is because they are prescribed immunosuppressive medications to prevent rejection of the transplanted organ. These medications suppress the immune system, making it more difficult for the body to fight off infections. Therefore, maintaining immunity through vaccinations is crucial for preventing serious illnesses.

Specific vaccination recommendations are based on the types of vaccines and the timing of vaccination; they can vary from person to person their medical history, age, and other factors.

- LAV are generally contraindicated after transplantation. It is preferred that close contacts be vaccinated against MMR and VAR *4 weeks before the transplant* so as to prevent the transplanted patient from having contact with wild-type viruses.
- Other recommended vaccines for liver patients before transplantation include influenza, pneumococcus, HepA and HepB, and DTaP, as well as HPV, especially among younger women.
- HepB vaccination is recommended for all patients with chronic liver disease (CLD) with and without cirrhosis. Currently, both single antigen vaccines such as Engerix-B, Heplisav-B, and Recombivax-HB, and combination vaccines such as Twinrix (combined HepA and HepB vaccines) are available.
- Ideally, you should receive all necessary vaccines before your transplant. However, if you did not have time to receive all the recommended vaccines before your transplant, vaccines can be given 3-6 months after transplantation.

TABLE 4: Recommendations for administering PCV13 and PPSV23 in patients with CKD.

Infants and children (ages 0–18 months)

Vaccine history	Recommended regimen		Notes
Never vaccinated with PCV7 or PCV13 up to age	Routine vaccination for PCV13 (four-dose series)	Administer one dose of PPSV23 at age ≥2 years and ≥8 weeks after last indicated dose of PCV13	Administer one dose of PPSV23 after 5 years
Completed all recommended doses of PCV7	Administer one dose of PCV13 ≥8 weeks later	Administer one dose of PPSV23 at age ≥2 years and ≥8 weeks after last indicated dose of PCV13	Administer one dose of PPSV23 after 5 years
Children aged 24–71 months who received <3 doses of PCV7 before age 24 months	Administer two doses of PCV13 now	Administer one dose of PPSV23 ≥8 weeks later after last indicated dose of PCV13	Administer one dose of PPSV23 after 5 years
Children aged 24–71 months who received any incomplete schedule of three doses of PCV7 before age 24 months	Administer one dose of PCV13 now	Administer one dose of PPSV23 ≥8 weeks later	Administer one dose of PPSV23 5 year after
Completed all recommended doses of PCV13	Administer one dose of PPSV23 at age ≥2 years and ≥8 weeks after last indicated dose of PCV13	Administer one dose of PPSV23 after 5 years	
Children aged 6–18 years who have not received PCV13	Administer one dose of PCV13 now		

Age 19–64 years

Vaccine history	Recommended regimen		Notes
Never vaccinated with PCV13 or PPSV23	Administer one dose of PCV13 now	Administer one dose of PPSV23 ≥8 weeks later	Administer one dose of PPSV23 ≥5 years later
Previously vaccinated with one dose PPSV23 ≥1 year ago; never vaccinated with PCV13	Administer one dose of PCV13 now	Administer one dose of PPSV23 ≥8 weeks after PCV13, which must be ≥5 years after first dose of PPSV23	
Previously vaccinated with two doses of PPSV23 (last dose was ≥1 year ago); never vaccinated with PCV13	Administer one dose of PCV13 now		
Previously vaccinated with ≥1 dose PCV13 (≥8 weeks ago); never vaccinated with PPSV23	Administer one dose of PCV13 now	Administer one dose of PPSV23 ≥5 years later	
Previously vaccinated with ≥1 dose PCV13 (≥8 weeks ago) and 1 dose PPSV23	Administer one dose of PPSV23 now ≥5 years after first PPSV23 dose		

Age 65 years and over

Vaccine history	Recommended regimen	
Never vaccinated with PCV13	Administer one dose of PCV13 now	Administer one dose of PPSV23 ≥8 weeks after PCV13, which must be ≥5 years after last dose of PPSV23
Previously vaccinated with ≥1 dose PCV13 (≥8 weeks ago)	Administer one dose of PPSV23 now	

(CKD: chronic kidney disease; PCV13: pneumococcal conjugate vaccine 13; PPSV23: pneumococcal polysaccharide vaccine 23)

(Personal communication with J Uduman, Medical Director—Inpatient Dialysis and CRRT, Division of Nephrology and Hypertension, Division of Hospital Medicine, Henry Ford Hospital, Detroit, MI, USA.)

MONOCLONAL ANTIBODIES IN SOLID ORGAN TRANSPLANT

Monoclonal antibodies given following transplantation are used to treat allograft rejection and more recently as maintenance immunosuppressants. Administration of these agents is mainly reserved for severe allograft rejection in which the immunologic insult must be controlled quickly.

The ultimate goal of posttransplant immunosuppression is tolerance, a state in which the host immune system recognizes the foreign tissue but does not react to it. This goal is yet to be achieved under modern immunosuppression secondary to immune system redundancy as well as the toxicity of currently available agents. Therefore, mAbs are used to provide targeted, immediate immunomodulation aimed at attenuating the overall immune response.

Specifically, mAbs have been used to:
- Spare exposure for maintenance of immunosuppressive agents
- Decrease the inherent immunoreactivity of the potential transplant recipient before engraftment
- Induce global immunosuppression at the time of transplantation allowing for modified introduction of other immunosuppressive agents (calcineurin inhibitors or corticosteroids)
- Treat acute allograft rejection. mAb selection, as well as the dose, is based on patient-specific factors, such as indication for transplantation, type of organ being transplanted, and the long-term immunosuppression objective.

Vaccine Schedule Recommendations and Updates for Patients with Hematologic Malignancy Posthematopoietic Stem Cell Transplant or Chimeric Antigen Receptor T-cell Therapy

Revaccination after receipt of a hematopoietic cell transplant (HCT) or chimeric antigen receptor T-cell (CAR T-cellular) therapy *is less well-defined.*

Infection remains a significant cause of morbidity and mortality among patients with hematological malignancies, including those experiencing enduring remission after transplant or cellular therapies. Vaccination strategy represents a pillar of supportive care that can help augment protection against infection.

Between 50,000 and 100,000 HCT are performed annually worldwide. *Over 20,000 people globally have received FDA-approved cellular therapy,* particularly CAR-T) products for the treatment of lymphoma, myeloma, or leukemia.

Together with antimicrobial prophylaxis, intravenous immunoglobulin (IVIg), and early antimicrobial therapy, vaccination aims to reduce the burden of infection in patients post-HCT transplant and cellular therapies.

Chimeric antigen receptor T-cell therapy is a type of cancer immunotherapy treatment that uses patients' T-cells that are genetically altered in a laboratory to enable them in locating and destroying cancer cells more effectively. CAR T treatment can be very effective against some types of cancer, even when other treatments are not working.

Chimeric antigen receptor T-cells have a new receptor so they can bind to cancer cells and kill them. Different types of cancer have different antigens. Each kind of CAR T-cell therapy is made to fight a specific kind of cancer antigen. So, a CAR T-cell therapy made for one type of cancer will not work against another type of cancer.

Since 2017, six CAR T-cell therapies have been approved by the FDA. All are approved for the treatment of several types of hematological malignancies, including lymphomas, some forms of leukemia, and most recently, multiple myeloma.

In 2023, CD19-directed CAR T-cell therapy, which has transformed the treatment landscape for B-cell malignancies, is now showing great promise in at least three distinct autoantibody-dependent autoimmune diseases. Now with substantially longer follow-up, the investigators have gained a greater understanding of "the B-cell biology behind our treatment."

- A serious complication of CAR T-cell therapy is cytokine release syndrome (CRS). CAR T-cells may release chemicals called cytokines, which causes a reaction from the immune system. Most cancer care centers have specialized treatments to manage this complication. Signs and symptoms may include:

- *Infusing the CAR T-cells:* As an outpatient department (OPD) procedure and recommended chemotherapy before the CAR T-cell infusion to help boost the treatment's effectiveness.

Regarding vaccine-preventable infections, late viral reactivations, such as VAR zoster, are common among both HCT recipients and CAR T cellular therapy patients, with reports of severe disseminated disease. Similarly, instances of overwhelming sepsis secondary to encapsulated organisms, such as *Streptococcus pneumoniae* or *Haemophilus influenzae*, have been reported.

The COVID-19 pandemic demonstrated how hematology patients, especially those treated with cellular therapies and HCT, are disproportionately affected by infectious diseases that lack adequate prevention strategies, leading to more severe disease, more frequent reinfections, and poorer vaccine response.

Vaccination following Cellular Therapies

- Less is known about the burden of vaccine-preventable infections and the role of revaccination in patients treated with cellular therapies.
- The field is currently aiming to determine the extent to which antibody immunity is preserved following cellular therapies, optimize timing of revaccination following treatment, and identify key predictors of vaccine response from hematological markers of immune reconstitution.

Late-infection data are still emerging and the long-term effects of sustained B-cell depletion on infection are unclear. Prolonged B-cell aplasia, loss of memory B-cells, and subsequent hypogammaglobulinemia may impair humoral protection against various infections, including vaccine-preventable diseases.

Preservation of Immunity: The Retention of Pathogen-specific Antibodies following Cellular Therapies

- Few studies have systematically explored the persistence of pathogen-specific IgG after CAR T-cell therapy.
- Available seroprevalence data is often adjunctive and exploratory; for example, comparing the prevalence of existing antibodies to vaccine-preventable infections between CAR-T treated patients and healthy controls to explore reasons for poor humoral response following SARS-CoV-2 vaccination.

Role and Recommended Monoclonal Antibody Therapies for Solid Organ Transplant Recipients

Monoclonal antibody has been increasingly utilized for individuals who have undergone solid SOT. Transplant recipients often require immunosuppressive medications to prevent rejection of the transplanted organ. This suppression of the immune system can make them more vulnerable to infections, including viral infections such as COVID-19.

Monoclonal antibody therapy has shown promise in preventing severe illness and hospitalization in individuals infected with certain viruses, including SARS-CoV-2. However, the decision to administer mAb therapy to SOT recipients should be made carefully, considering factors such as their specific immunosuppressive regimen, the potential for drug interactions, and the underlying condition for which they received the organ transplant. Some immunosuppressive medications may interact with mAb therapies or alter their effectiveness, but the overall benefit must be weighed against potential risks. Dosages and administration schedules should be determined by healthcare professionals familiar with the patient's case.

The commonly used mAbs in transplant medicine to prevent organ rejection and manage complications post-transplantation include:

Basiliximab (Simulect): It is a chimeric mAb that targets the interleukin-2 receptor (IL-2R) on activated T lymphocytes. It is used as induction therapy to prevent acute rejection in kidney transplant recipients.

Rituximab (Rituxan): It is a chimeric mAb that targets the CD20 antigen present on B lymphocytes. It is used to treat antibody-mediated rejection and in the management of various autoimmune diseases that may affect transplant recipients.

Alemtuzumab (Campath): It is a mAb that targets CD52, which is present on the surface of B and T lymphocytes. It is used for induction therapy in kidney and liver transplant recipients, particularly in patients at high risk of rejection.

Muromonab-CD3 (Orthoclone OKT3): It is a murine mAb that targets the CD3 antigen on T lymphocytes. It is used to treat acute rejection episodes in various types of SOT recipients.

Eculizumab (Soliris): It is a humanized mAb inhibits the complement protein C5. It is used in the management of atypical hemolytic uremic syndrome (aHUS), which may occur in kidney transplant recipients.

Belatacept (Nulojix): It is a fusion protein that acts as a selective T-cell costimulation blocker by binding to CD80 and CD86, thereby inhibiting T-cell activation. It is used as maintenance immunosuppression in kidney transplant recipients.

Infliximab (Remicade): It targets tumor necrosis factor alpha (TNF-α). It is used in the management of inflammatory conditions such as graft-versus-host disease (GVHD) and autoimmune disorders that may affect transplant recipients.

CONCLUSION

There are well-recognized vaccine schedules for the HCT population, with new vaccine formulations including PCV20, adjuvanted RZV (aRZV), and bivalent booster COVID-19 vaccines that require ongoing assessment. Revaccination postcellular therapies at present mostly follow the HCT schedule, but further research is required to optimize the timing of vaccine delivery and clarify which vaccines would be of most benefit to cellular therapy patients.

It is important that guidance and recommendations may evolve and new information may have emerged since this last update. Therefore, individuals with special circumstances, including SOTs, should regularly review and update guidelines based on emerging data and research.

SUGGESTED READING

1. Babel N, Hugo C, Westhoff TH. Vaccination in patients with kidney failure: lessons from COVID-19. Nat Rev Nephrol. 2022;18:708-23.
2. Feldman AG, Beaty BL, Curtis D, Juarez-Colunga E, Kempe A. Incidence of Hospitalization for Vaccine-Preventable Infections in Children Following Solid Organ Transplant and Associated Morbidity, Mortality, and Costs. JAMA Pediatr. 2019;173(3):260-8.
3. Feldman AG, Beaty BL, Ferrolino JA, Maron G, Weidner HK, Ali SA, et al. Safety and Immunogenicity of Live Viral Vaccines in a Multicenter Cohort of Pediatric Transplant Recipients. JAMA Netw Open. 2023;6(10):e2337602.
4. Gautreaux MD. An Introduction to Transplant Immunology. Available from: https://www.afdt.org/pdf/Histo-Specialist-2021/Introduction%20to%20TP%20Immunology%20(Gautreaux).pdf [Last accessed April, 2024].
5. Laserson U, Vigneault F, Gadala-Maria D, Yaari G, Uduman M, Vander Heiden JA, et al. High-resolution antibody dynamics of vaccine-induced immune responses. Proc Natl Acad Sci USA. 2014;111(13):4928-33.
6. Reynolds G, Hall VG, Teh BW. Vaccine schedule recommendations and updates for patients with hematologic malignancy post-hematopoietic cell transplant or CAR T-cell therapy. Transpl Infect Dis. 2023;25(Suppl 1): e14109.

CHAPTER 11: Cancer Vaccines: Preventive and Therapeutics

Mohd Uduman, Jr Uduman, AK Uduman

■ INTRODUCTION

Global cancer burden is growing amid mounting need for services. *Three major cancer types in 2022:* Lung, breast, and colorectal cancers.

Is cancer hereditary?

Yes, cancer can be hereditary, although not all cancers are inherited, in about 5–10% of cases, wherein an individual will inherit a faulty gene from their parents which will be again transmitted down to his or her kids. Genes play an important role in determining our susceptibility to cancer. Certain genetic mutations can significantly elevate the risk of developing specific types of cancer. These mutations can be inherited from our parents, creating a familial link to the disease. In these cases, the presence of a mutated gene may act as a proverbial loaded gun, increasing the likelihood of cancer.

Breast and ovarian cancers, for instance, have well-established genetic connections. Mutations in the *BRCA1* and *BRCA2* genes are responsible for substantially raising the risk of these cancers. Individuals inheriting these mutations face a higher-than-average probability of developing breast or ovarian cancer at some point in their lives. Identifying the faulty gene by blood test in a person with high risk for genetic cancer and then treating him by prophylactic surgery are recommended. For example, a person with BRCA mutation can undergo a prophylactic mastectomy to prevent the development of breast cancer.

In 2022, there were an estimated 20 million new cancer cases and 9.7 million deaths. The estimated number of people who were alive within 5 years following a cancer diagnosis was 53.5 million. About 1 in 5 people develop cancer in their lifetime; approximately 1 in 9 men and 1 in 12 women die from the disease.

The estimated number of incident cases of cancer *in India for the year 2022* was found to be 1,461,427 (crude rate: 100.4 per 100,000). In India, one in nine people is likely to develop cancer in his/her lifetime. Lung and breast cancers were the leading sites of cancer in males and females, respectively.

Lung cancer was the most commonly occurring cancer worldwide with 2.5 million new cases, accounting for 12.4% of the total new cases. *Female breast cancer* ranked second (2.3 million cases, 11.6%), followed by colorectal cancer (CRC) (1.9 million cases, 9.6%), prostate cancer (1.5 million cases, 7.3%), and stomach cancer (970,000 cases, 4.9%).

As part of its normal function, the immune system detects and destroys abnormal cells and most likely prevents or curbs the growth of many cancers. Even though the immune system can prevent or slow cancer growth, cancer cells have ways to avoid destruction by the immune system. For example, cancer cells may:

- Have genetic changes that make them less visible to the immune system
- Have proteins on their surface that turn off immune cells
- Change the normal cells around the tumor so they interfere with how the immune system responds to the cancer cells
- Immunotherapy helps the immune system to better act against cancer.

These vaccines are a type of cancer treatment called immunotherapy to boost the body's immune system to fight cancer. Given to people who already have either existing cancer (therapeutic cancer vaccine) or prophylactic to prevent the development of a cancer. Most cancer vaccines are only offered through clinical trials, which are research studies that use volunteers. As of this date (February, 2024), there are about 369 cancer vaccine studies ongoing all around the world.

- Basically, examples of *preventive cancer vaccines* are human papillomavirus (HPV) and hepatitis B (HepB) virus (HBV) vaccines to prevent cervix cancer and hepatocellular cancer (HCC).
- Examples of *therapeutic cancer vaccines*—prostate, melanoma, bladder cancers, etc. are often used in combination with other cancer treatments.

- *Personalized vaccines*—strategy can be a potent approach to trigger a broad-based antitumor response that is both beneficial and relevant to individual cancer patients. Also, a cancer vaccination strategy can be designed to help elicit immunological memory for long-lasting tumor control. Prepared from individual patient's tumor cells and tumor-derived cellular products (i.e., *neoantigens*).
- *New human type 2 innate lymphoid cells (ILC2s)*—to attack and eliminate cancers, coronavirus disease 2019 (COVID-19), etc. Researchers have discovered a type of immune cell in the human body known to be important for allergy and other immune responses that can also attack and eliminate cancer and fight viruses such as severe acute respiratory syndrome coronavirus 2 (SARS-CoV-2), which causes COVID-19 infection.

■ BACKGROUNDS—CLINICAL TRIALS

Researchers are testing vaccines against (in an alphabetic order) as follows:
- *Solid organ cancers:* (1) Bladder, (2) brain, (3) breast, (4) cervix, (5) ovarian, (6) uterine, (7) colorectal, (8) esophageal, (9) gastric, (10) kidney, (11) liver, (12) lymphomas and leukemia, (13) lung, (14) melanoma, (15) myeloma, (16) pancreatic, (17) prostate, (18) primary bone, and (19) testicular germ cell tumors (GCTs)
- *Vaccines against pediatrics malignancy*: Retinoblastoma (RB), Wilms tumor (WT), leukemia and lymphomas, and central nervous system (CNS) tumors
- *Human gut—microbiome in cancer prevention*

■ CANCER VACCINES' BACKGROUND

Cancer vaccines mainly use tumor-associated antigens (TAAs) and tumor-specific antigens (TSAs) to "educate" and activate the patient's immune system against the cancer cells. These vaccines have the potential to trigger both specific cellular immunity and humoral immune response to prevent tumor growth and ultimately eradicate tumor cells. *These treatments fall under a category of cancer therapy known as immunotherapy,* which boosts the body's natural immune defenses against cancer.

After many years of limited advancements, cancer treatment vaccines are now showing potential. Several vaccines have been formulated to prevent particular types of cancer. Among them, the HPV vaccine and the HepB vaccine stand out for their proven efficacy in preventing specific cancers.

Designing a cancer treatment that very specifically targets and kills tumor cells with minimal side effects is often regarded as the "holy grail" of oncology. This approach aligns with the principles of precision medicine, which seeks to tailor treatments to individual patients based on their unique genetic and molecular profiles **(Fig. 1)**.

In the last 20 years, the field of cancer immunotherapy has seen significant advancements, particularly with the identification of numerous TAAs. While a range of cancer immunotherapy approaches have been devised and subjected to clinical trials, the complexity and diversity of tumor cell characteristics and host immune cell responses seem to limit the therapeutic efficacy of this treatment modality.

Today, most cancer vaccine research is focused on specifically targeting known or unknown TAAs. The first therapeutic cancer vaccine to be approved by the United States (US) Food and Drug Administration (FDA) is sipuleucel-T (Provenge®), a vaccine composed of patients' own stimulated dendritic cells (DCs), approved for prostate cancer. Sipuleucel-T was approved in 2010 to treat asymptomatic or minimally symptomatic metastatic

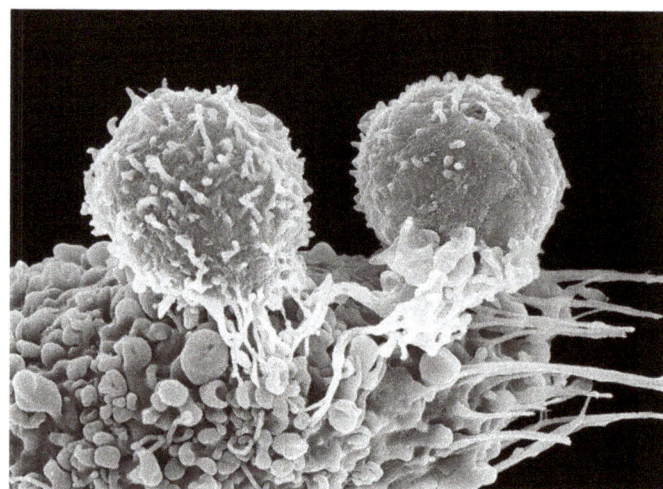

Fig. 1: Interaction of immune cells with cancer cells. T cells (depicted in white) recognize and bind to cancer cells (depicted in gray). This cytotoxic engagement signifies the immune system's active response in recognizing and targeting cancerous cells, a natural defense against tumor progression. Innovative drugs pioneered by researchers stimulate the ability of T cells to recognize and destroy cancer cells.

castration-resistant prostate cancer (CRPC). It consists of antigen-presenting cells (APCs) derived from the patient's peripheral blood mononuclear cells obtained by leukapheresis and cultured with a recombinant fusion protein consisting of human prostatic acid phosphatase (PAP) linked to granulocyte–macrophage colony-stimulating factor (GM-CSF). Up to 95% of prostate cancer overexpresses PAP which is a nonessential protein. The PAP expression is largely limited to the prostate making it a near-ideal target antigen. By culturing the APCs with the PAP-GM-CSF fusion protein, they are matured. The mature PAP-specific APCs are reinfused into the patient and can generate PAP-specific immunity and thereby tumor-specific immune responses.

- *To date, sipuleucel-T is the only therapeutic vaccine approved to treat established tumors. A number of other vaccines are being tested in late-stage clinical trials.*

The remarkable success of messenger ribonucleic acid (mRNA) COVID-19 vaccines has spotlighted mRNA's potential for other diseases and therapeutic applications. Scientists, especially at Pfizer-BioNTech and Moderna, have been exploring mRNA for cancer long before COVID-19. This global attention could speed up the development of *mRNA cancer vaccines*. While the US does not have any approved yet, many are in clinical trials, hinting at a promising future.

There are other different types of cancer vaccines, including:

Preventive or Prophylactic Vaccines

Preventive or prophylactic vaccines are designed to prevent certain types of cancer caused by infectious agents. For example, the HPV vaccine can help prevent cervical, anal, and other HPV-related cancers.

Human papillomavirus vaccination prevents new HPV infection. It does not treat existing HPV infections or diseases. It is highly effective for the prevention of HPV serotypes (STs) 16 and 18, which cause 70% of cervical cancer. HPV also causes most precancerous changes found with Pap testing. Research continues on vaccines that help treat each stage of cervical cancer.

Gardasil 9 is an HPV vaccine against STs 6, 11, 16, 18, 31, 33, 45, 52, and 58, approved by the US FDA and can be used for both girls and boys. This vaccine can prevent most cases of cervical cancer if the vaccine is given before girls or women are exposed to the virus; ideally given before an individual becomes sexually active and is likely to be exposed to HPV. This vaccine can also prevent vaginal and vulvar cancer.

The Centers for Disease Control and Prevention (CDC) estimates the HPV vaccine could prevent over 31,000 HPV-related cancers per year. That does not include all the abnormal Pap results it can prevent.

Side effects: They may vary according to the type of cancer vaccine—and what exactly it targets—and may also be influenced by the location and type of cancer as well as a patient's overall health.

Hepatitis B vaccine can help prevent the development of HBV-related liver cancer (three-dose and two-dose regimen strategies).

Treatment or Therapeutic Vaccines

Treatment or therapeutic vaccines are used to treat existing cancer.

These vaccines are a type of cancer treatment called immunotherapy. These vaccines are used to treat existing cancer by stimulating the immune system to recognize and attack cancer cells. Therapeutic cancer vaccines can be made from cancer cells, tumor antigens, or specific proteins found on cancer cells.

Therapeutic cancer vaccines that have been approved include:

- Sipuleucel-T (Provenge®) for people whose *prostate cancer* has metastasized
- Bacillus Calmette–Guerin (TheraCys) is a live attenuated vaccine which makes use of mycobacterium bovis strain *for invasive bladder cancer.*
- Talimogene laherparepvec (T-VEC or Imlygic) is a vaccine for advanced oncolytic *melanoma.*
- The human immunodeficiency virus (HIV) treatment vaccine has struggled against obstacles as of February, 2024.

These treatment vaccines are used to treat existing cancers and to boost the immune system's ability to find and destroy antigens. Most cancer vaccines are only offered through clinical trials. In 2010, the FDA approved sipuleucel-T (Provenge) for people with metastatic prostate cancer, which is prostate cancer that has spread. Sipuleucel-T is tailored to each person through a series of steps—they are often used in combination with other cancer treatments, such as chemotherapy or radiation therapy.

Therapeutic vaccines can be categorized into several subtypes:
- *Tumor cell vaccines:* These vaccines are made from cancer cells that have been removed from a patient's body and modified in the laboratory to enhance their immune-stimulating properties. Once injected back into the patient, they can provoke an immune response against the cancer cells.
- *Antigen vaccines:* These vaccines use specific tumor antigens (proteins found on cancer cells) to stimulate an immune response. The antigens may be obtained from cancer cells or produced synthetically.
- *Deoxyribonucleic acid (DNA) vaccines:* DNA vaccines involve injecting genetic material (DNA) encoding specific tumor antigens into the body. This genetic material instructs the cells to produce the tumor antigens, triggering an immune response.
- *Vector-based vaccines:* These vaccines use modified viruses or bacteria (vectors) to deliver tumor antigens into the body. The vector serves as a carrier to transport the antigens, stimulating the immune system.

Cancer vaccines are not available for all types of cancer. Even though cancer vaccines show promise, they are still an area of active research and their *effectiveness* can vary depending on the type and stage of cancer. However, many cancer vaccines are still in clinical trials and more research is needed to fully understand their potential efficacy, with the goal of improving treatment outcomes and providing new options for cancer patients.

Personalized Vaccines

Personalized vaccines, also known as individualized vaccines, are tailored to an individual's specific tumor based on their unique genetic and immunological characteristics. The concept behind personalized vaccines is to create a vaccine that is highly effective for a particular person or a subset of the population by taking into account their specific needs and responses to immunization. Personalized cancer vaccines are still in the early stages of development and are being studied in clinical trials.

There are two types of therapeutic vaccines, namely autologous and allogeneic vaccines:
1. Autologous means "derived from oneself"—is a personalized vaccine which is made from an individual's own cells which could be either cancer cells or immune system cells.
2. Allogeneic vaccines (allo means "other"—which are made from a different individual's cancer cells which are grown in a laboratory).

Creating a cancer vaccine is often a tailored approach, focusing on identifying and choosing antigens specific to an individual's cancer. It involves:
- *Genomic and immunological analysis:* The individual's genetic makeup and immune system are analyzed to identify specific antigens or proteins that are likely to trigger a robust immune response. This analysis can involve techniques such as DNA sequencing and immune profiling.
- *Antigen selection:* Based on the analysis, researchers select antigens that are most likely to be recognized by the individual's immune system and stimulate a strong response. These antigens can be derived from the pathogen the vaccine aims to protect against.
- *Vaccine formulation:* A custom vaccine is formulated using the selected antigens. This may involve combining these antigens with adjuvants or other compounds to enhance the immune response.
- *Administration:* The personalized vaccine is administered to the individual.

Given that cancer is notably heterogeneous and can be distinct at the molecular level for each individual, the concept is to customize and personalize the vaccine to a person's unique cancer and immune system profile. This could enhance its effectiveness and induce a more potent, enduring immune response. Such a strategy might prove especially valuable for conditions where conventional vaccines fall short, including specific cancers or swiftly mutating viruses.

Personalized vaccines are still an area of active research and development and their use is not yet widespread. They are most commonly associated with cancer immunotherapy, where treatments such as DC vaccines and neoantigen vaccines are designed to target cancer cells based on the specific mutations found in a patient's tumor. However, the concept of personalized vaccines is also being explored for infectious diseases and other health conditions.

What are the different types of antigens used for cancer vaccines?

Choosing which antigen or antigens to target is one of the biggest challenges in the development of cancer vaccines. Generally, strong target antigens should be unique to the cancer (so that the immune system does not attack any healthy cells) and readily recognized by the immune system. The types of antigens that have been used in cancer vaccines fall into three categories:
1. Cancer-associated antigens

2. Neoantigens—tumor antigens that arise when a mutation in the DNA of cancer cells causes them to produce a mutated protein that is entirely new to the body and looks unfamiliar to the immune system. Unlike cancer-associated antigens, these proteins are not produced in any normal, healthy cells in the body, so they stand out to the immune system as "non-self."
3. Undefined antigens—the whole cancer cell

Cancer researchers believe that therapeutic cancer vaccines may work better for smaller tumors or cancer in its early stages.

■ VACCINES AND CLINICAL TRIALS

Clinical trials are typically the last phase of testing before a new treatment or vaccine is approved for broader use.

New Human Type-2 Innate Lymphoid Cells

Recent research promises that these cells called human type-2 ILC2s can be expanded outside of the body and applied in larger numbers to overpower a tumor's defenses and eliminate malignant cells in mouse models with cancer.

In the future, these ILC2s do not need to come from the cancer patient's own cells, meaning that there may be the possibility of harvesting and freezing ILC2s from healthy donors for ILC2s treatment options in the future.

Unlike T-cell-based therapies such as chimeric antigen receptor (CAR) T cells, which necessitate using the patient's own cells due to their specific characteristics, ILC2s may be sourced from any healthy donors.

Researchers have discovered these ILC2s types of immune cells in the human body are known to be important for all allergy and for other immune response that can also attack and eliminate cancer and fight viruses such as SARS-CoV-2, which causes COVID-19 diseases.

■ BLADDER CANCER

The most common type of bladder cancer is urothelial bladder cancer. This is also called transitional cell bladder cancer (TCC). There are some rarer types. These include squamous cell bladder cancer, adenocarcinoma, sarcoma, and small cell bladder cancer. *In the Indian population, bladder cancer is predominantly TCC* and >95% of the patients present with painless hematuria. Male preponderance is much more frequent in Indians than in other races.

Intravesical Bacillus Calmette-Guerin (BCG) is a vaccine that is used to treat early-stage bladder cancer. It is a type of immunotherapy medicine. The initial BCG induction therapy occurs weekly for 6 weeks. If the treatment is working, BCG maintenance therapy is given once a week for 3 weeks at the 3-, 6- and 12-month marks.

Up to 35% of patients have long-term, sustained remissions with intravesical BCG. However, as many as 60% of patients will have a recurrence of cancer within 2 years. With intravesical BCG treatment, the oncologist delivers immunotherapy drugs directly into the bladder through a catheter. Unlike oral or injectable drugs, BCG treatment targets bladder cancer cells without having a negative systemic impact on the rest of the body.

April 23rd, 2024, the US FDA approved the first-in-class interleukin (IL)-15 superagonist nogapendekin alfa inbakicept-pmln (Anktiva), plus bacillus Calmette-Guérin (BCG), for the treatment of certain non–muscle-invasive bladder cancers that fail to respond to BCG alone.

The recommended dose is 400 mcg administered intravesically with BCG once a week for 6 weeks as induction therapy, with an option for a second induction course if patients don't achieve a complete response at 3 months. The recommended maintenance therapy dose is 400 mcg with BCG once a week for 3 weeks at months 4, 7, 10, 13, and 19. Patients who achieve a complete response at 25 months and beyond may receive maintenance instillations with BCG once a week for 3 weeks at months 25, 31, and 37. The maximum treatment duration is 37 months.

Metastatic bladder cancer—these are stage 4 disease patients and the disease is not curable. Patients are treated with platinum-based chemotherapy. If they do well, they are given maintenance avelumab therapy. However, if cancer progresses, either second-line chemotherapy or *immunotherapy with nivolumab or pembrolizumab are given*. Sometimes, palliative therapy is offered.

Researchers are testing how well a vaccine made from a virus altered with the human epidermal growth factor receptor 2 (HER2)* antigen works. These antigens

---

Human epidermal growth factor receptor 2: Amplification or overexpression of HER2 occurs in approximately 15–30% of breast cancers and 10–30% of gastric/gastroesophageal cancers and serves as a prognostic and predictive biomarker. HER2 overexpression has also been seen in other cancers such as the ovary, endometrium, bladder, lung, colon, and head and neck. The introduction of HER2-directed therapies has dramatically influenced the outcome of patients with HER2-positive breast and gastric/gastroesophageal cancers; however, results have been proved disappointing in other HER2 overexpressing cancer.

or molecules live on the surface of some bladder cancer tumors. The virus may help teach the immune system to find and destroy these tumor cells. Researchers also want to know which works better: Standard bladder cancer treatment or standard treatment with a vaccine.

- *HER2 testing and HER2-directed therapies are recommended in only breast and gastric/gastroesophageal cancers.*

Currently, there is no bladder cancer-specific vaccine that targets the HER2 antigen specifically in bladder cancer. HER2 is a protein that is often overexpressed in certain types of cancer, including breast cancer and some gastric and esophageal cancers. While targeted therapies such as trastuzumab (Herceptin) have been developed to treat HER2-positive breast cancer, these drugs are not vaccines but rather antibodies that target HER2.

The development of cancer vaccines, including those targeting specific antigens such as HER2, is an active area of research. It is important to note that the development and approval of cancer vaccines and targeted therapies are complex processes that require extensive research, clinical trials, and regulatory approval.

■ BRAIN TUMOR

Glioblastoma (GBM) is the most common and aggressive primary malignant brain tumor. Due to the lack of effective treatment options, Cancer Research, United Kingdom (UK) has included GBM in the category of "cancers of substantial unmet need." *The blood–brain barrier (BBB) obstructs passage and complicates treatments within the brain. Only 2% of current drugs and nanoparticles can cross the BBB.* The goal is to improve clinical outcomes for patients with GBM, from preclinical development of novel therapies to early and later phase clinical trials.

The current standard treatment for GBM involves 6 weeks of radiotherapy followed by 6 months of chemotherapy. In contrast, the new immunotherapy treatment, which was tested in a clinical trial proved to be highly effective. Patient experienced a headache after taking the drug, to which doctors explained that it was a positive sign indicating the activation of his immune system.

Unfortunately, there has been less success in monoclonal antibody (mAb) immunotherapy for brain tumors than in other cancer types. When it comes to the brain, immune-based treatments face a number of obstacles before they can even reach the tumors.

Chimeric antigen receptor T-based immunotherapy represents a promising therapeutic approach, but antigenic heterogeneity and restoration of immunosuppressive milieu post-therapy may limit the durability of responses to CAR T therapy. Identification of stably expressed and sufficiently TSAs and agents that target immunosuppressive molecules is required to overcome the barrier.

Oncolytic viruses (OVs) might exert proinflammatory responses, thus providing the potential to overcome the immunosuppression of GBM. The future direction of OVs seems to be focused on combinations with other immunotherapy strategies, in the hope of exploiting the potentially durable anticancer immune responses initiated by the viral infection to elicit prolonged clinical responses. Based on this, a combination of CAR T and OVs may benefit mutually. OV infection induces local inflammation and attracts T cells to tumors, which can reinforce the attraction of CAR T cells in tumor microenvironment (TME). Despite the promise of this combination approach, the main impediment to this strategy is the rapid clearance of OVs, presenting a challenge to clinical practice in future.

The UK Cancer Research now set up a national program of immunotherapy clinical trials for patients with GBM. In a phase II, open-label, randomized clinical study of ipilimumab [anticytotoxic T lymphocyte antigen (CTLA)] and temozolomide (TMZ) versus TMZ alone after surgery and chemoradiotherapy in patients with recently diagnosed GBM. We are currently actively developing new clinical trials with miraculous success results (March 9, 2024).

Miracles of immunotherapy for cancer curing: Intraventricular CARv3-T-cell-engaging antibody molecule (TEAM)-E T cells in recurrent GBM.

Brief summary: In this first-in-human, investigator-initiated, open-label study, three participants with recurrent GBM were treated with CARv3-TEAM-E T cells, which are CAR T-cells engineered to target the epidermal growth factor (EGF) receptor (EGFR) variant III TSA, as well as the wild-type EGFR protein, through secretion of a TEAM.

Chimeric antigen receptor-v3-TEAM-E T cells are a form of CAR T-cell therapy that involves taking a person's own immune cells (T cells), genetically modifying them, and then reintroducing them back into the body to target and kill cancer cells. This innovative approach is part of the broader category of CAR T-cell therapies, which are designed to harness the body's immune system to fight cancer more effectively.

Specifically, CARv3-TEAM-E T cells are engineered to express a CAR targeting EGFRvIII, a mutation associated with certain cancers and a TEAM comprising a bispecific T-cell engager (BiTE) that targets EGFR and CD3. This design aims to induce the killing of tumor cells expressing both the mutated EGFRvIII and the wild-type EGFR, offering a potential therapeutic strategy for conditions such as GBM, where these mutations are prevalent.

Treatment with CARv3-TEAM-E T cells did not result in adverse events (AEs) greater than grade 3 or dose-limiting toxic effects. Radiographic tumor regression was dramatic and rapid, occurring within days after receipt of a single intraventricular infusion, but the responses were transient in two of the three participants.

There are currently no approved vaccines for brain tumors. However, there are few experimental vaccines in clinical trial. Vaccine therapy has been considered one of the most promising approaches to improve the outcomes of patients with GBM, but data from the clinical trials are disappointing. Given that the lack of high expression of GBM-specific antigens are limiting factors in the development of peptide vaccine-based strategies. The personalized neoantigen-based vaccines have attracted much attention in GBM vaccine therapy, although its clinical efficacy requires further investigation.

A vaccine to treat GBM: GBM is the most aggressive primary brain tumor in adults, with >10,000 new cases diagnosed in the US each year. Standard treatment involves surgery, radiation, and chemotherapy and the median overall survival (OS) rate is only 15–17 months from diagnosis. A personalized vaccine developed by University of California, Los Angeles (UCLA) Health scientists has been shown to potentially extend the life of patients with GBM, the most aggressive form of brain cancer.

A vaccine to treat GBM called DCVax-L has been in development for several years. A team of UCLA researchers was the first to investigate whether a patient's own DCs (a specialized type of immune cell) could be used to create a personalized treatment for the deadly cancer.

The vaccine consists of two components: A patient's DCs, which are special types of immune cells and proteins prepared from a patient's tumor. To create the vaccine, which is individualized for each patient, medical staff first perform a procedure called leukapheresis, in which a patient's blood is drawn and their white blood cells are collected. Then, the patient's tumor is removed and sent to a laboratory where researchers obtain proteins from the specimen, called *tumor lysate*. The white blood cells are cultured to differentiate into DCs and then combined with the tumor lysate to make the vaccine.

Rindopepimut (also known as CDX-110), a peptide vaccine targeting EGFRvIII, has been tested in several clinical trials. In three uncontrolled phase II studies, Rindopepimut vaccination in GBM patients with gross total resection and chemoradiotherapy have provided evidence of improved median survival of 24 months compared with historical controls. Following these encouraging findings, an international phase III trial (NCT01480479), ACT IV was conducted to further assess the efficacy of Rindopepimut in newly diagnosed patients with EGFRvIII-positive GBM. Despite the strong anti-EGFRvIII immune response generated in patients, the primary study analysis did not show a survival benefit for patients with minimal residual disease (MRD) who received Rindopepimut with TMZ versus those who received TMZ alone. Of note, the spontaneous loss of antigen was seen in both the treatment and control arm, questioning the utility of immunotherapy targeting a single tumor antigen with heterogeneous tumor expression. Recent evidence from a double-blind, randomized, phase II study (NCT01498328) in a smaller cohort of patients with recurrent EGFRvIII-positive GBM suggested favorable outcomes for Rindopepimut when combined with standard bevacizumab versus bevacizumab alone. Taken together, the positive results with Rindopepimut in recurrent GBM in ReACT and the negative results of ACT IV in newly diagnosed GBM lend support to further clinical trials that use combination strategies such as immunotherapy with angiogenesis inhibition.

Recently, advances in next-generation sequencing and novel bioinformatics tools have enabled the systematic discovery of tumor neoantigens, which are derived from somatic mutations of the tumor and are therefore tumor specific.

Neoantigens are highly specific for individual patients and hence, tumor vaccines targeting neoantigens can effectively trigger de novo T-cell responses against neoantigens, thereby achieving personalized precision treatment. Initial studies of personalized neoantigen-based vaccines have demonstrated robust tumor-specific immunogenicity and preliminary evidence of antitumor activity in patients with high-risk melanoma and other cancers. Based on the encouraging findings, a phase I/

Ib study of personalized neoantigen vaccines has been tested in 10 patients with newly diagnosed methylguanine DNA methyltransferase (MGMT)-unmethylated GBM following surgical resection and conventional radiotherapy. Patients who did not receive dexamethasone generated circulating polyfunctional neoantigen-specific CD4+ and CD8+ T-cell responses that were enriched in a memory phenotype and showed an increase in the number of tumor-infiltrating T cells. Despite generating systemic and intertumoral neoantigen-specific immune responses postvaccination, all patients showed tumor recurrence and ultimately died of progressive disease, indicating that the induced T-cell responses must still overcome considerable challenges to produce clinically relevant antitumor activity, including tumor-intrinsic defects and immunosuppressive factors in the microenvironment. Given that neoantigen-targeting vaccines have the potential to favorably alter the immune milieu of GBM, thus combining vaccination with other regimens such as immune checkpoint inhibition may be beneficial.

Also, there is emerging evidence that DNA organization is critical in mediating responses to cancer treatment including chemotherapy and immunotherapy. Researchers are now characterizing the DNA architecture in GBM and how it can be modified to enhance treatment efficacy.

■ BREAST CANCER VACCINES

Breast cancer, the most frequently detected cancer globally, had over 2.3 million new cases and resulted in approximately 685,000 deaths in the year 2020. In the US alone, in 2022, approximately 287,850 new cases of invasive breast cancer and 51,400 cases of ductal carcinoma in situ (DCIS) were diagnosed among women, leading to 43,250 female deaths from breast cancer.

There has been a disturbing increase in the incidence of breast cancer in young women aged 15–40 years worldwide. More younger women from India are suffering from breast cancer than younger women from the West. Younger women are often diagnosed at advanced stages than in older women, as they do not undergo routine screening mammograms. Most of the screening programs are suggested for women >40 years of age with the benefit of diagnosis at early stages, thus helping in better prognosis and cure rates. In recent years, breast cancer in India accounts for 25–32% of all female cancers and more than one fourth of all female cancer. As of 2024, 1 in every 8 women (13%) will be diagnosed with breast cancer at some point in their life, according to the American Cancer Society (ACS).

Recent research has demonstrated the presence of the Epstein–Barr virus (EBV) genome in a subset of breast cancer cases. The virus has been found restricted to tumor cells, suggesting a possible role in the tumorigenesis process. One systematic review found an overall prevalence of EBV in breast cancer cases to be around 26.37%, indicating a significant presence of the virus in breast cancer samples. Despite these findings, the role of EBV in breast cancer remains a subject of ongoing research. Scientists are exploring how the virus might contribute to the initiation and progression of breast cancer, including its interaction with other risk factors. However, the causal relationship and mechanisms behind this association are still under investigation and further research is needed to fully understand the potential role of EBV in breast cancer development.

Treatment for breast cancer depends on the subtype of cancer and how much it has spread outside of the breast to lymph nodes (stages II or III) or to other parts of the body (stage IV).

Treatment for breast cancer is based on the individual, cancer type, stage, and its spread. 50% of breast cancer cases are not linked to usual risks like specific genes or habits.

Rapid diagnosis needs to be linked to effective cancer treatment that in many settings requires some level of specialized cancer care. By establishing centralized services in a cancer facility or hospital, using breast cancer as a model, treatment for breast cancer may be optimized while improving management of other cancers.

To reduce the global burden of breast cancer, there is an urgent need for more cost-effective treatments and strategies. Conventional treatments, such as surgical ablation, radiotherapy, chemotherapy, and hormone therapy, are often associated with side effects, resistance, and recurrence.

Immunotherapy has revolutionized cancer treatment, offering specific tumor targeting with minimal cytotoxicity. This field of medicine seeks to stimulate an antitumor immune response, leading to tumor shrinkage and improved clinical outcomes. Recent advances have included several distinct classes of drugs, such as cytokines, immune checkpoint blockade (ICB), adoptive T-cell treatments, and vaccinations.

- Despite being the most prevalent malignant disease for women worldwide, breast cancer patients have limited access to immunotherapy benefits.

Monoclonal antibodies work by recognizing and finding specific proteins on cancer cells. Each mAb recognizes one particular protein. So different mAbs have to be made to target different types of cancer. Depending on the protein they are targeting, they work in different ways to kill the cancer cell.

Trastuzumab, pertuzumab, and margetuximab are approved for therapeutic use; the oncogene-targeted treatment with proven survival benefit in women with HER2-positive metastatic breast cancer.

CDK4/6 inhibitors are a class of medicines used to treat certain types of hormone receptor-positive, HER2-negative breast cancer. These medicines interrupt the process through which breast cancer cells divide and multiply by targeting specific proteins known as the cyclin-dependent kinases 4 and 6, abbreviated as CDK4/6. *Currently, three CDK4/6 inhibitors are approved and available to treat breast cancer: Palbociclib, ribociclib, and abemaciclib.* CDK4/6 inhibitors are pills and are used in combination with hormone therapy to treat some breast cancers.

There are not any breast cancer vaccines available yet, but a few are in clinical—a vaccine called NeuVax is furthest along in the research.

- The simplest way to breast cancer prevention is by being able to do a self-breast examination. Women should be doing this on a regular basis after they turn 30 years old.

Currently, there is no approved vaccine available for the prevention of breast cancer. However, *therapeutic vaccination* has many key advantages over other immunological therapies such as creating and amplifying a highly specific adaptive immune response and setting up immunologic memory with the potential to manage and remove residual disease.

Breast cancer is a complex disease with multiple factors involved in its development, including genetic, hormonal, and environmental factors. Efforts to develop a therapeutic vaccine for breast cancer are ongoing, but it is a challenging task due to the complexity of the disease and the various subtypes of breast cancer.

- Vaccination is an active immunotherapy strategy designed to stimulate the patient's immune system and help recognize and destroy tumor.

Messenger RNA vaccination has the potential to convert cold breast cancer into hot and expand the responders. Effective mRNA vaccine design for in vivo function requires consideration of vaccine targets, mRNA structures, transport vectors, and injection routes.

Researchers are exploring different approaches, such as targeting specific proteins or antigens associated with breast cancer cells, to stimulate an immune response against the cancer cells.

Many studies are testing treatment vaccines for breast cancer, given alone or with other treatments. Other researchers are working to get vaccines that prevent breast cancer into clinical trials. There are vaccines still in the testing phase. It still requires the FDA approval and there is a long way to go before it is available to the public. If the vaccine is successful, it will move on to phases 2 and 3 trials.

Triple negative breast cancer (TNBC) is a kind of cancer that is likely to come back and is harder to treat. It has receptors that are not usually found in breast cancer. TNBC does not have estrogen or progesterone receptors and makes less or none of the HER2 protein. This vaccine is still in the testing phase.

Breast cancer is a cancer that has a very high probability of being cured if diagnosed at an early stage. New methods of risk-based screening are beginning to garner attention, where screening would be tailored to each individual based on their level of risk. Currently, national breast cancer screening programs are nonpersonalized and individual risks are not taken into account. Saliva DNA contains 30% leukocytes, making it comparable to blood in terms of DNA quality; it is a noninvasive method of collection and can introduce genetic testing in a large scale for breast cancer screening. Saliva samples confirm the identical BRAC1 and BRAC2 mutations in DNA from saliva and from blood from the same individual. Therefore, saliva DNA was sufficient enough for the detection of the mutations, for high throughput genotyping and starting appropriate breast cancer managements.

Artificial Intelligence System Utility in Breast Cancer

By using artificial intelligence (AI) technology for cancer screening, one can maintain the accuracy of diagnosis and reduce the burden on radiologists, even if many people undergo medical checkup. The AI system is trained on thousands of deidentified mammograms. The AI-powered system integrates into breast cancer screening workflows to help radiologists identify breast cancer earlier and more consistently. Our published research shows that our technology can identify signs of breast cancer as well as trained radiologists.

■ CERVICAL CANCER

Cancer is uncommon in women under the age of 25 years across the world. However, the frequency rises between the ages of 35 and 40 years, peaking in the women in their 50s and 60s.

The current estimates indicate approximately 132,000 new cases diagnosed and 74,000 deaths annually in India, accounting to nearly one third of the global cervical cancer deaths. One woman dies of cervical cancer every 8 minutes in India. The country also accounts for the highest number of cervical cancer cases in Asia (followed by China), according to a 2022 Lancet study.

Despite this burden, action against cervical cancer has been slow in India. In January 2023, the Indian Ministry of Health and Family Welfare requested state governments to start preparations for the roll out of the HPV preventive vaccine for girls aged 9–14 years. The only way to protect women is to vaccinate them against HPV at an early age.

- *Yes, these are preventive vaccines and no therapeutic vaccines available yet.*

Cervical Cancer Screening

Several professional organizations offer guidance on cervical cancer screening, including the American College of Obstetricians and Gynecologists (ACOG), the American Cancer Society (ACS), the American Society for Colposcopy and Cervical Pathology (ASCEP), and the US Preventive Services Task Force (USPSTF). These organizations, with one exception, all recommend that cervical cytologic testing begin at 21 years of age for all healthy female individuals, regardless of sexual history (the ACS recommends testing begin at 25 years of age).

HIV-infected female adolescents who have initiated sexual intercourse should have cervical cytologic screening (liquid-based or Pap smear) performed twice at 6-month intervals during the first year after diagnosis of HIV infection, and if the results are normal, annually thereafter (https://clinicalinfo.hiv.gov/en/guidelines).

Sexually active female adolescents who have had an organ transplant or are receiving long-term corticosteroid therapy also should undergo similar cervical cytologic screening.

Now, a new AI-assisted screening tool developed by the Thiruvananthapuram-based Regional Cancer Centre (RCC), patented and ready for use, has come as a genuine breakthrough for early detection and vaccine prevention. Urine-based HPV-DNA testing with "CerviScan" is a reliable tool to detect high-risk HPV subtypes. CerviScan is a polymerase chain reaction (PCR)-based diagnostic kit for early detection of HPV that is the cause of cervical cancer. It could become an alternative that will substantially cut down detection time for cervical cancers compared to the traditional Pap test.

The US FDA approved HPV vaccines that prevent cervical cancer. Research continues on vaccines that help treat each stage of cervical cancer.

Preventive vaccines: Cervical cancer is primarily caused by persistent infection with certain types of HPV and vaccines such as Gardasil and Cervarix have been successful in preventing HPV infection and subsequently, reducing the risk of cervical cancer.

Therapeutic HPV vaccines deliver tumor antigens to stimulate an immune response to eliminate tumor cells. Vaccine antigen delivery platforms are diverse and include DNA, RNA, peptides, proteins, viral vectors, microbial vectors, and APCs.

Therapeutic HPV vaccine candidates *targeting TSAs* associated with cancer cervix include *HPV E6 and E7 oncoprotein vaccines.*

The E6 and E7 oncoproteins of high-risk HPV types are responsible for the transformation of normal cervical cells into cancerous ones. By targeting these oncoproteins, the vaccine aimed to stimulate the immune system to recognize and attack cells infected with HPV precancerous or cancerous cells.

- *The development of therapeutic vaccines can be a lengthy and complex process,* including preclinical studies, clinical trials, and regulatory approval.

Randomized, controlled trials have demonstrated that therapeutic HPV vaccines are efficacious in patients with cervical intraepithelial neoplasia.

DNA-based vaccine: Approaches to deliver genetic material encoding specific HPV antigens to stimulate an immune response.

Peptide-based vaccines: Use short pieces of HPV-specific proteins (peptides) to trigger an immune response against the cancer cells.

Virus-like particle (VLP) vaccines: Similar to preventive HPV vaccines, VLPs can be engineered to present HPV antigens and stimulate an immune response against HPV-associated cancer.

DC-based vaccines: They are a type of immune cell that can be modified and used in vaccines to target HPV-infected cells more effectively.

The US FDA has only approved one therapeutic cancer vaccine, Sipuleucel-T, is an autologous "peripheral blood mononuclear cell" (PBMC)-based vaccines. In patients with HPV-mediated malignancies, evidence of efficacy is limited. However, numerous ongoing studies evaluating updated therapeutic HPV vaccines in combination with immune checkpoint inhibition and other therapies exhibit significant promise.

Monoclonal Antibodies in Cervical Cancer

The usage of mAbs is one of the most promising ways of improving patient outcomes. The rationale behind the use of mAbs in the treatment of cancer is to selectively target tumor cells that express TAAs, with the goal of particularly antagonizing receptor signaling pathways that are required for tumor cell migration, proliferation, and survival.

Bevacizumab (Avastin®) is an angiogenesis inhibitor that can be used to treat advanced cervical cancer. It is a mAb (a man-made version of a specific immune system protein) that targets vascular endothelial growth factor (VEGF). This drug is often used with chemotherapy in metastatic or in a recurrent advanced cervical cancers.

Pembrolizumab is a mAb drug therapy used to treat certain patients whose cervical cancer has the biomarker programmed death-ligand 1 (PD-L1). Checkpoint proteins are found on the surface of cells. Pembrolizumab targets and blocks a checkpoint protein called programmed death receptor 1 (PD-1) on the surface of T cells. PD-1 is found on the body's T cells and PD-L1 on normal and often cancer cells.

Tisotumab vedotin has an accelerated FDA approval for second-line therapy in the recurrent setting for patients with cervical cancer (July, 2023).

Thus, by attacking selected tumor cells, mAbs provide more customized results based on the targeting of several particular pathways critical for cancer metastasis and development. Moreover, the great specificity of the target reduces harmful side effects in normal tissue, which are common with standard chemotherapeutic drugs, allowing patients to maintain a quality lifestyle.

■ OVARIAN CANCER IMMUNOTHERAPY

Ovarian cancer occurs when cells in the ovaries grow at an unrestricted and accelerated rate. There is currently no vaccine for ovarian cancer. According to the ACS, approximately 20,000 females in the US will receive a new diagnosis of ovarian cancer in 2024.

In India, ovarian cancer has emerged as one of the most common malignancies affecting women and has shown an increase in the incidence rates over the years. Although cervical cancer is on a declining trend, it remains the second most common cancer in women in India.

The FDA has not approved any vaccines for ovarian cancer. Specifically, researchers have been investigating the effectiveness of immunotherapy to prevent ovarian cancer.

Immunotherapy involves several interventions, such as vaccines, boosting the immune system, and cell therapy. The primary goal of immunotherapy is to train the body's immune cells to identify and attack cancer cells. These immune cells include cytotoxic T cells and tumor-infiltrating lymphocytes (TILs).

Bevacizumab (Avastin®) is often used to treat recurrent ovarian cancer, which refers to cancer that returns after a disease-free period of at least 6 months. Other types of immunotherapy drugs for ovarian cancer include *durvalumab, avelumab, and nivolumab.*

T-cell Therapies

- *Based on DC-mediated presentation of neoantigens* derived from malignant ovarian cancer cells to T cells through major histocompatibility (MHC) class I T-cell receptors (TCRs). However, clinical trials with more participants are required to determine the benefits of DC vaccines.
- *Immune checkpoint inhibitors* (ICPIs) could effectively prevent this effect. Antibody-mediated blockade of CTLA-4, an inhibitory immune checkpoint molecule that binds CD80 and CD86 and prevents their interaction with CD28, which can promote T-cell priming by DCs.
- *Similarly, anti-B7–H3 antibody-mediated blockade* could neutralize T-cell exhaustion in patients with ovarian cancer.
- *Neoantigens*, including HER2, cancer antigen 125 [mucin 16 (MUC16)], and mesothelin, are also presented on tumor cell surfaces independent of MHC

class I receptors and these neoantigens are specific targets of CAR T-cell therapies.

Genetic engineering is also applied to produce viruses that selectively infect or replicate in tumor cells and finally destroy tumor cells. Cell destruction can also promote immunogenic tumor cell death, which can activate antigen presentation and an adaptive antitumor immune response.

Ovarian cancer vaccine targets—some researchers are investigating the potential of protein-based vaccines and recombinant viral vaccines.

Protein-based vaccine targets have included the protein p53, a tumor suppressor protein that is in many cancers, including ovarian cancer. However, these have shown a lack of clinical benefits.

Recombinant viral vaccines use modified viruses (viral vectors) to deliver the genetic material needed to code for an antigen. This triggers an immune response that primes the immune system to fight cancers. A recent study utilizing a recombinant viral vaccine along with chemotherapy drugs found that there was an increase in participants' immune response, as well as a subsequent longer progression-free survival (PFS). However, this was a very small study and some participants had poor tolerance to the chemotherapy drug.

While many of these potential vaccines are in clinical trial stages, the FDA is yet to approve a vaccine for ovarian cancer.

■ UTERINE CANCER IMMUNOTHERAPIES
Endometrial Cancer

Endometrial cancer (EC) includes two types—EC cancer (more common) accounts for about 95% of all cases and uterine sarcoma (rare). EC is common in western women and the rates are very high and estimated that more than 3,300 females were diagnosed in the USA in 2023. The average age at diagnosis is 65 years old.

As per the population-based cancer register, it is the fourth common cancer in India, particularly Chennai, Tamil Nadu. The morbidity and mortality rates of EC are increasing yearly.

Human papillomavirus does not cause uterine cancer. Having a family history of cancer increases the risk of developing uterine cancer. This is especially true if your family has a pattern of uterine cancer or a specific type of CRC known as Lynch syndrome. Lynch syndrome is a hereditary type of cancer that can also increase the risk of EC.

Early-stage EC can be effectively treated through surgery or surgery combined with radiotherapy and chemotherapy. Advanced and recurrent EC is treated with chemotherapy and comprehensive treatment; however, the prognosis for patients at this disease stage is poor. Consequently, novel and effective treatment strategies are urgently required for these patients. Breakthrough progress has been made with the use of immunotherapies in the treatment of EC.

Immunotherapy—while chemotherapy works to kill cancer cells, immunotherapy aims to boost the body's immune system to fight cancer.

Monoclonal antibody therapy for uterine EC is an emerging area of research and treatment. mAbs are laboratory-produced molecules engineered to mimic the immune system's ability to fight off harmful pathogens or abnormal cells, such as cancer cells.

One of the mAbs that has shown promise in the treatment of uterine EC is *pembrolizumab*. Pembrolizumab is a checkpoint inhibitor that targets the programmed cell death protein 1 (PD-1) receptor on T cells, which helps to unleash the body's immune system to attack cancer cells. Clinical trials have demonstrated the efficacy of pembrolizumab in certain patients with advanced or recurrent uterine endometrial carcinoma, particularly those with microsatellite instability-high (MSI-H) or mismatch repair deficient (dMMR) tumors.

Other mAbs and targeted therapies are also being investigated, including bevacizumab which targets VEGF to inhibit tumor angiogenesis and trastuzumab which targets HER2 in tumors that overexpress this protein.

Use of mAb therapy for EC may depend on various factors, including the specific characteristics of the tumor, the patient's overall health, and previous treatments received. Treatment decisions should be made in consultation with a healthcare provider who can assess the individual patient's situation and recommend the most appropriate therapy based on current evidence and guidelines.

Other types of mAbs boost our immune system by inhibiting or stopping immune checkpoints. These are called 'immune checkpoint inhibitors (ICPIs) proteins used by the body to naturally stop an immune system response and prevent the immune system from attacking healthy cells. Cancer cells can find ways to hide from the immune system by activating these checkpoints. Drugs that target these checkpoints (called ICPIs) can be used to treat some ECs.

PD-1 inhibitors pembrolizumab (Keytruda) and dostarlimab (Jemperli) are drugs that target PD-1, a protein on immune system cells called T cells. PD-1 normally helps keep T cells from attacking other cells in the body (including some cancer cells). By blocking PD-1, these drugs boost the immune response against cancer cells. This can shrink some tumors or slow their growth.

Checkpoint immunotherapy is currently available; an immunotherapy drug called *pembrolizumab* (used in combination with the targeted therapy drug lenvatinib) may be an option for some people with EC that has spread or are no longer responding to treatment with chemotherapy. Pembrolizumab is given as an intravenous (IV) infusion, typically once every 3 or 6 weeks.

Pembrolizumab can be used by itself to treat advanced ECs, typically after other treatments have been tried, if surgery or radiation are not good options and if the cancer cells have any of the following:
- A high level of *MSI-H* or a *defect in a mismatch repair gene (dMMR)*
- A *high tumor mutational burden (TMB-H)*—meaning the cells have many gene mutations

Tumor cells can be tested for these changes.

Pembrolizumab can also be used along with the targeted drug lenvatinib (Lenvima) to treat advanced ECs that are not dMMR or MSI-H, typically after at least one other drug treatment has been tried.

Dostarlimab can be used to treat advanced or recurrent EC either:
- Along with chemotherapy as the first treatment (and then afterward by itself), if the cancer cells have a dMMR or a high level of MSI-H
- By itself, after chemotherapy has been tried (and if surgery and radiation are not good options), if the cancer cells have a dMMR

Tumor cells can be tested for these changes. This drug is given as an IV infusion, typically once every 3 weeks at first and then every 6 weeks.

Bevacizumab, a mAb targeting VEGF-A, has been studied in a phase II trial of recurrent EC and had favorable response.

Monoclonal antibodies, such as nivolumab and ipilimumab, may help the body's immune system attack the cancer and may interfere with the ability of tumor cells to grow and spread.

What is the best immunotherapy for EC?
Pembrolizumab can be used by itself to treat advanced ECs, typically after other treatments have been tried if surgery or radiation are not good options and if the cancer cells have any of the following: A high level of MSI-H or a dMMR. Tumor cells can be tested for these changes. This drug is given as an IV infusion, typically once every 3 weeks at first and then every 6 weeks.

Vaccine Directed Against Uterine Endometrial Cancer

As of our last update in February, 2024, there is not a specific vaccine directed against uterine EC available for widespread use. Vaccines are typically developed to prevent infectious diseases, such as those caused by viruses or bacteria. Uterine EC is a type of cancer that originates in the lining of the uterus and is not caused by infectious agents like viruses or bacteria.

A personalized neoantigen vaccine in combination with platinum-based chemotherapy to treat an inoperable EC demonstrated the safety and immunogenicity of the personalized DC vaccine. Interestingly, a complete oncological response was obtained concerning both radiological assessment and the tumor marker CA-125.

Furthermore, this association between chemotherapy and therapeutic vaccine elicited immune response as demonstrated by polyfunctional and durable T-cell responses. Moreover, this combination leads to a long-lasting oncological complete response in this otherwise challenging recurrent metastatic setting. Thus, this treatment association is promising and should be further investigated in the current and other potential settings.

■ COLORECTAL CANCER

Colorectal cancer is the third most common cancer worldwide and is often diagnosed at advanced stages, limiting treatment options. With a majority of cases occurring in the developed countries, India has a low prevalence of CRC—estimated 5-year prevalence is 87 per 100,000 population. Several dietary factors may contribute to the low overall rate of cancer in India. Among them are a "relatively low intake of meat and a mostly plant-based diet, in addition to the high intake of spices." 40% of Indians are vegetarians and even the ones who do eat meat do not eat a lot.

Colon cancer, particularly in young individuals, has been on the rise, with the ACS reporting it as the leading cause of cancer deaths in men under 50. The reasons for the increase in CRC cases among young people remain unclear to experts. The ACS' estimates for the number of CRCs in the US for 2023 are: 106,970 new cases of colon cancer and 46,050 new cases of rectal cancer.

Colorectal cancer is typically not caused by infectious agents like some other types of cancer, which can be prevented through vaccination (e.g., HepB vaccine for liver cancer caused by the HBV and cervical cancers caused by HPV). Instead, CRC is often associated with genetic and lifestyle factors, such as family history, diet, and physical activity.

Surgery is the most preferred treatment for CRC, where the tumor and its surrounding tissues are surgically removed and results in a cure in approximately 50% of patients. Cure is not possible for most patients with metastatic CRC. Surgeons could also choose laparoscopic surgery as it is a less risky process and the recovery time for the same is also short.

Prevention and early detection of CRC typically involve measures such as regular screening, lifestyle changes (such as maintaining a healthy diet and weight), and managing risk factors.

Current therapies such as surgery, chemotherapy, and radiotherapy encounter obstacles in preventing metastasis of CRC even when applied in combination. ICPIs depict limited effects due to the limited cases of CRC patients with MSI-H.

Immunotherapy in Gastrointestinal Oncology: A New Dawn for Cancer Treatment

Over the last decade, new wave of treatments known as immunotherapy is revolutionizing the landscape of gastrointestinal (GI) oncology, offering improved outcomes and increased hope for patients in downstaging the disease and aiding more patients to become operable.

Unlike traditional treatments that directly target cancer cells, immunotherapy harnesses the power of the body's own immune system to fight cancer. It does this by removing the "brakes" that cancer cells use to evade immune attack, allowing immune cells to recognize and destroy cancer cells effectively.

Types of Immunotherapy in Gastrointestinal Oncology

- *ICPIs:* These antibodies target specific proteins on immune cells, such as PD-1 and CTLA-4, allowing them to become more active against cancer cells. These are the most well-established immunotherapies, approved for various GI cancers including colorectal, gastric, and esophageal cancers.
- *T-cell therapies (CAR T-cell therapy):* These involve extracting T cells, a type of immune cell, from the patient, genetically modifying them to recognize and attack cancer cells and then reinfusing them back into the patient. CAR T-cell therapy has shown promising results in certain GI cancers, particularly those with specific genetic mutations.
- *OVs:* These genetically engineered viruses selectively infect and destroy cancer cells while leaving healthy cells unharmed. They can also stimulate the immune system to attack tumors.
- *Cancer vaccines:* These vaccines teach the immune system to recognize and attack specific cancer antigens. While still under development, cancer vaccines hold promise for preventing GI cancers and treating early-stage disease.

mAbs and CAR T Cells in the Treatment of CRC

Monoclonal antibodies demonstrate the great ability to completely recognize cancer cell surface receptors and obstruct proliferative or inhibitory pathways. On the other hand, T-cell activation by genetically engineered CAR receptor via the TCR/CD3 and costimulatory domains can induce potent immune responses against specific TAAs. Both of these approaches have beneficial antitumor effects on CRC.

Colorectal and pancreatic cancers are often KRAS mutated and are incurable when tumor DNA or protein persists or recurs after curative intent therapy. Cancer vaccine ELI-002 2P enhances lymph node delivery and immune response using amphiphile (Amph) modification of G12D and G12R mutant KRAS (mKRAS) peptides (Amph-Peptides-2P) together with CpG oligonucleotide adjuvant (Amph-CpG-7909).

Cancer vaccines are designed to trigger the elevation of tumor-infiltrated lymphocytes, resulting in the intense response of the immune system to tumor antigens. Vaccines targeted at a transmembrane MUC1 antigen that were proven safe and elicited tumor-specific long-term memory in clinical trials are under consideration for preventative purposes. However, how strong this immunity will be and how long it will persist are crucial points that deserve further investigation. Future clinical trials will be urged to carry out in stratified patient populations.

Several trials are exploring the safety and effect of prophylactic vaccines in patients diagnosed with Lynch syndrome.* Rapid development of neoantigens and nanovaccines also sheds new light into the field, making CRC vaccines a proud member of the immunotherapy family.

There are no approved treatment vaccines for CRC. However, researchers are developing treatment vaccines that tell the body to attack cells with antigens thought to cause CRC. These antigens include carcinoembryonic antigen (CEA), MUC1, guanylyl cyclase C, and NY-ESO-1.

Cancer vaccines are designed to trigger the elevation of tumor-infiltrated lymphocytes, resulting in the intense response of the immune system to tumor antigens.

Recently "PD1-Vaxx"—immunotherapy expert biotech firm Imugene is seeking to put its potentially ground-breaking bowel cancer vaccine known as *"PD1-Vaxx"* to the test with around 44 patients set to be enrolled in a phase 2 trial over the next 18 months. The trial will take place across six sites in Australia and another four in the UK.

Three doses of the vaccine will be given 2 weeks apart before surgery to activate the immune system to kill the cancer. This research is still in its early stages and could take years before becoming available for patients. However, the new trial was laying crucial groundwork that could help develop less toxic and more precise new anticancer therapies—a desperately needed trial to turn the tide against cancers.

The KIMS Health Vaccinology book authors anticipate that when patients go to operation, there will not be much cancer left and with some people, it might go completely. We need to do the trials to prove that and that is what happening now.

Highlights

- Immunotherapy brings hope to tumor therapy and it is also a new direction of tumor therapy.
- Facing all these challenges, there is still a long way to go in tumor vaccination in CRC. However, combinations containing tumor vaccines, other immune therapies, and traditional therapies are a potential strategy to resolve some of these challenges and may become the future.

ESOPHAGEAL CANCER

Esophageal cancer is the fourth common cause of cancer-related deaths in India. It is prevalent among both men and women and the risk of esophageal cancer increases with age, with most cases occurring in people over the age of 50 years. Squamous cell carcinoma (SCC) accounts for up to 80% of these cancers, although adenocarcinoma is on the increase due to changing lifestyles. Asian countries with a high human development index such as China have also reported an increased incidence of esophageal adenocarcinoma. Data on the epidemiology of esophageal cancer in India are limited.

The midesophagus is the most common site (42%). There is no evidence of an epidemiological shift or an increase in the occurrence of adenocarcinoma or of lower esophageal/gastroesophageal junction (GEJ) malignancy over the past two decades. esophageal cancer is a serious and often fatal disease with a 5-year survival rate of around 20%. The exact cause of esophageal cancer is unknown, but certain factors can increase the risk of developing it. The most common risk factors for esophageal cancer are smoking, heavy alcohol drinkers, and gastroesophageal reflux disease (GERD).

The treatment options vary depending on the stage of the cancer and the overall health of the patient. Surgery, radiation therapy, and chemotherapy are the most common treatments and they can be used alone or in combination to achieve the best results. Patients need to work closely with their healthcare team to determine the best treatment plan for their individual needs.

Immunotherapy drugs for esophageal cancer are ICPIs. They essentially take the brakes off the immune system. Our body has built-in checkpoint proteins on immune system cells that help stop them from attacking normal cells. Cancer cells sometimes take advantage of these blocks to grow without being destroyed by the body.

These checkpoint proteins act as switches that can turn an immune system reaction on or off. ICPIs turn these switches off to allow the immune system to fight cancer cells. Specifically, ICPIs for esophageal cancer work on two different switches, as follows:

National Cancer Institute. Esophageal cancer treatment. They block PD-1, a protein on T-cells (a type of immune cell) that usually keeps them from attacking other cells in the body. PD-1 binds to PD-L1 on some

---

*An inherited genetic condition which increases the risk of developing cancers such as colon cancer, EC, and other cancers.

cancer cells, stopping the T-cell from killing the cancer cell. By blocking this binding, PD-1 inhibitors allow the T-cell to kill the cancer.

They block CTLA-4, another protein on T-cells that helps keep them in check. CTLA-4 binds to a protein called B7 on cancer cells, stopping the T-cell from killing the cancer. By blocking this binding, CTLA-4 inhibitors allow the T-cells to kill the tumor cells.

In 2022, the FDA approved the use of nivolumab (Opdivo®) in combination with fluoropyrimidine- or platinum-based chemotherapy as a first-line treatment for some patients with advanced or metastatic esophageal SCC.

Pembrolizumab (Keytruda) and nivolumab (Opdivo) are drugs that target PD-1, a protein on T-cells (a type of immune system cell). The PD-1 protein normally helps keep T-cells from attacking other cells in the body. By blocking PD-1, these drugs boost the immune response against cancer cells.

■ GASTRIC CANCER

In India, stomach cancer, sometimes referred to as gastric cancer, is fifth in incidence among men and seventh in incidence among women. It ranks as the second most frequent cause of cancer-related deaths worldwide. In India, the prevalence of gastric cancer has gradually increased within the last 10 years, with comparatively high incidence of stomach cancer when compared to many western countries.

There are a number of factors that can raise one's risk of stomach cancer, yet the actual cause of the illness is still unknown. Infection with *Helicobacter pylori* (*H. pylori*) is a major risk factor that can cause chronic inflammation of the stomach lining and raise the chance of stomach cancer over time.

In addition, EBV infection is an important risk factor in the development of gastric cancer. A previous study showed that EBV and *H. pylori* coinfection may synergistically induce severe inflammatory responses in the stomach tissue and increase the risk of developing gastric cancer.

An increased risk of stomach cancer may result from certain lifestyle choices, including smoking, drinking too much alcohol, and eating a diet high in pickled, smoked, or salty foods.

Older age, male gender, obesity, and radiation or chemical exposure are additional risk factors. Although stomach cancer is not a common occurrence in people with these risk factors, living a healthy lifestyle and limiting exposure to recognized risk factors can help lower the chance of contracting this possibly fatal illness.

Immunotherapies approved for use in untreated gastric cancer patients include monotherapy and chemotherapy–immunotherapy combinations.

For advanced stomach cancer, treatment aims to stabilize disease progression and improve patients' prognosis. Immunotherapy uses a person's own immune system to help kill cancer cells. There are currently six FDA-approved immunotherapy options for stomach cancer.

Gastric cancer treatments are evolving rapidly. For example, ICPIs, especially those that target PD-1 or PD-L1, have long-term efficacy in a subset of gastric cancer patients and are currently the first-line therapy demonstrated clinical benefit for HER2-negative advanced gastric cancer. For HER2-positive advanced gastric cancer in upfront settings, a combination of pembrolizumab with trastuzumab plus chemotherapy showed promising efficacy and other combinations of anti-HER2 therapy and ICPIs have indicated promising effects.

Epstein–Barr virus—positive gastric cancer is associated with high CD8-positive T-cell infiltration and PD-L1/L2 expression, indicating its sensitivity to ICPIs. Several retrospective cohort studies reported that PD-L1 expression on tumor cells was associated with EBV positivity.

Targeted CAR T-cell therapy, a novel immunotherapy approach different from ICPIs, is expected to become a personalized treatment strategy for advanced gastric cancer in the future. A novel immunotherapy approach using CAR T-cell therapies might be used as a personalized treatment for advanced gastric cancer. Despite these breakthroughs, there is still an urgent need to establish novel biomarkers for immune therapy and to develop new immunotherapies.

Regardless, it remains unclear whether the malignancy results from accumulated tissue damage caused by the EBV and HPV coinfection or whether it is due to the close interaction between EBV and HPV genes. Although the coinfection of two pathogens has been known to be related to carcinogenesis, it was not associated with the prognosis of gastric cancer after diagnosis. Although several studies found an association between the coinfection and gastric cancer pathogenesis, few studies have focused on the effect of an EBV and HP coinfection on the clinical outcomes and prognosis of gastric cancer.

ONCOLYTIC VIRUSES

The OVs recognize, infect, and lyse the tumor cells, thereby reducing their burden. The engineered OVs exhibit several mechanisms that direct the infected host cells to a lytic phase, leading to the apoptosis of the host's tumor cell. The lysis releases antigens into the surrounding TME that activate the host's immune system and results in an antitumor/antiviral response. Therefore, OVs modify the TME from an unrecognizable to an antigenic state. It enables the host immune system to identify the abnormal cells that otherwise remain hidden and maintain a state of anticancer immunity.

KIDNEY CANCER

Kidney cancer is usually found by chance during an abdominal imaging test for other vague abdominal complaints. Renal cell carcinoma (RCC) constitutes almost 3% of all cancers. RCC is the most frequent solid tumor in kidney which accounts for almost 90% of all kidney malignancies with clear-cell RCC (ccRCC) being the most common type.

According to the Indian Council of Medical Research (ICMR), kidney cancer is among the top 10 cancers in India accounting for approximately 2–3% of all the cases and is mostly diagnosed in people aged between 50 and 70 years.

Globally, there are an estimated 400,000 cases of kidney cancer diagnosed each year, along with 175,000 deaths. The ACS' most recent estimates for kidney cancer in the US for 2024 are: About 81,610 new cases (52,380 in men and 29,230 in women) will be diagnosed which is up from 76,090 in 2021. About 14,390 people (9,450 men and 4,940 women) will die from this disease. The yearly incidence of kidney cancer in India is 16,861 with a 5-year prevalence of 2.84/100,000 population. The cumulative risk of developing kidney cancer in males is 1 in 442 and 1 in 620 in females.

- Like most cancers, kidney cancer is difficult to treat once it has spread to other parts of the body. Metastatic kidney cancer has a 5-year survival rate of 12%.
- The 5-year survival rate is 93%, while the cancer diagnosed is still local (has not spread beyond the kidney).

The incorporation of nivolumab, an ICPIs, into the treatment framework for treatment-refractory metastatic clear-cell RCC has been crucial in improving outcomes for patients. In the CheckMate-214 study, ipilimumab, the first approved ICPI, was combined with nivolumab, which prolonged OS in treatment-naive patients. Disruption of cancer-induced immune tolerance with these drugs substantially improved all meaningful endpoints when compared with previous standards of care.

Kidney cancer therapeutic treatment options depend on individual factors, including the exact location of the tumor, stage of the tumor, and the person's general health.

- Treatments for early kidney cancer stages (1–3) include complete and partial nephrectomy.
- A section of patients with high-risk features might be eligible to receive immunotherapy after surgery.
- Advanced or metastatic kidney cancer is treated with systemic therapy that includes targeted therapy and immunotherapy.

Even early kidney cancer tends to be resistant to chemotherapy. However, some preliminary studies highlight the potential role of stereotactic body radiotherapy (SBRT) in kidney cancer.

Immunotherapy takes advantage of a person's own immune system to help kill cancer cells. The first indication that kidney cancer might be a good target for immunotherapy came from the observation that patients with metastatic kidney cancer occasionally experienced spontaneous regressions after surgical removal of the primary tumor.

In the past, cytokines were a common first-line therapy for advanced kidney cancer, but today, they are used only for cancers unresponsive to targeted therapies because of the risk of serious side effects. [The cytokines interleukin-2 (IL-2) and interferon-alpha cause kidney cancers to shrink in approximately 10–20% of patients and provide durable remissions in a subset of these patients.]

Several newer immunotherapies, in particular PD-1/PD-L1 and CTLA-4 checkpoint inhibitors, have become an integral part of the management of advanced or metastatic kidney cancer. There are currently seven FDA-approved immunotherapy options for kidney cancer either as a single agent or in combination with another immunotherapy or targeted therapy.

Targeted Antibodies

Bevacizumab (Avastin®): A mAb that targets the VEGF/VEGF receptor (VEGFR) pathway and inhibits tumor blood vessel growth; approved for subsets of patients with advanced kidney cancer

Immunomodulators:

- *Aldesleukin (Proleukin®):* A cytokine that targets the IL-2/IL-2R pathway; approved for subsets of patients with advanced kidney cancer
- *Avelumab (Bavencio®):* A checkpoint inhibitor that targets the PD-1/PD-L1 pathway; approved for subsets of patients with advanced kidney cancer, including as a first-line therapy in combination with chemotherapy
- *Dostarlimab (Jemperli):* A checkpoint inhibitor that targets the PD-1/PD-L1 pathway; approved for subsets of patients with advanced kidney cancer that has DNA dMMR
- *Ipilimumab (Yervoy®):* A checkpoint inhibitor that targets the CTLA-4 pathway; approved in combination with nivolumab, for subsets of patients with advanced kidney cancer
- *Nivolumab (Opdivo®):* A checkpoint inhibitor that targets the PD-1/PD-L1 pathway; approved for subsets of patients with advanced kidney cancer, including as a first-line therapy in combination with chemotherapy
- *Pembrolizumab (Keytruda®):* A checkpoint inhibitor that targets the PD-1/PD-L1 pathway; approved for subsets of patients with kidney cancer, including as a first-line therapy

Several ongoing trials are testing the feasibility of using immunotherapy in early-stage kidney cancer alone and in combination with surgery.

Immunotherapy with mAbs, such as Pembrolizumab (Keytruda) and Nivolumab (Opdivo) and ipilimumab that target PD-I T-cells. These may help the body's immune system attack the cancer and may interfere with the ability of tumor cells to grow and spread. Cabozantinib may stop the growth of tumor cells by blocking some of the enzymes needed for cell growth.

Adjuvant pembrolizumab was associated with a significant and clinically meaningful improvement in overall survival, as compared with placebo, among participants with clear-cell renal-cell carcinoma at increased risk for recurrence after surgery. [April 17, 2024, N Engl J Med 2024;390:1359-1371]

There is currently *no vaccine* that is approved for kidney cancer—it is a complex disease with various subtypes and genetic mutations involved in its development. Modified cytokines, IL-2 is a proven treatment for metastatic kidney in development.

Several potential vaccines have been evaluated for the treatment of patients with RCC. They include:

- DCs pulsed with tumor lysate—a DC tumor cell hybrid, irradiated tumor cells admixed with adjuvants, and a heat shock protein peptide complex
- Targeting specific antigens or proteins expressed by kidney cancer cells, to stimulate an immune response against the cancer cells

Adjuvant and neoadjuvant therapies that reduce the risk of RCC recurrence remain an area of unmet need. Advances have been made in metastatic RCC recently by leveraging PD-1/PD-L1 ICPIs. These agents are currently being investigated in the adjuvant and neoadjuvant settings to determine if intervention early in the disease trajectory offers a clinically meaningful benefit.

The current literature provides support for the use of pembrolizumab in the adjuvant setting postnephrectomy for those at high risk of RCC recurrence based on tumor stage, grade, and histology. ICPIs hold great promise in the adjuvant treatment of RCC both as monotherapy and in combination with other agents such as tyrosine kinase inhibitors (TKIs), hypoxia-inducible factor-2 alpha (HIF-2α) inhibitors, and personalized vaccines. At present, an individualized approach that takes into consideration an assessment of disease recurrence risk, other comorbidities, and patient preferences would be important in determining candidacy for adjuvant ICPIs.

While there is no vaccine for the prevention of kidney cancer, there are other important strategies for reducing the risk of kidney cancer. These include:

- Maintaining a healthy lifestyle, such as avoiding tobacco use
- Maintaining a healthy weight and managing conditions such as high blood pressure and diabetes, which are known risk factors for kidney cancer.

LIVER CANCER

Liver cancer or HCC is one of the most common cancers in the world, especially in countries such as India which have a high incidence of HBV infection. Apart from HBV, it may be caused by other diseases that lead to cirrhosis of the liver such as hepatitis C virus (HCV) infection and alcohol abuse.

Hepatitis B virus occurs at birth (around 90%) if not vaccinated soon after birth when the virus passes from an infected mother to the chronic HBV and leading on to developing cancer. In contrast, unvaccinated adults infected with the HBV can clear the virus spontaneously in cirrhosis in 90% of cases, even without medications.

The Indian government introduced HBV vaccination into its Universal Immunization Programme (UIP) in 2002. This single measure has prevented numerous infections already and complications resulting from it, India harbors 10–15% of the global pool of HBV and has 40 million HBV carriers of which 15–25% develop cirrhosis and complications leading to healthcare costs and premature death. Prevention of liver cancer is possible at two levels. The first level of prevention is to avoid alcohol abuse and to prevent the occurrence of HBV or HCV infection.

Liver cancer treatment: Conventionally, considered to be a high risk surgery until 10 years ago, a hepatectomy can now be performed with high degree of success in India, thanks to the bloodless liver-splitting techniques devised by surgeons. In some suitable cases, especially those where the liver has cirrhosis along with cancer, liver transplantation is also possible. This procedure can treat both liver cirrhosis and cancer at the same time.

VACCINES FOR LEUKEMIA, LYMPHOMA, MYELOMA, ETC.

Vaccines for leukemia, lymphoma, and myeloma are still in development and available only in clinical trials. The goal of vaccine therapy is to recognize cancer cell antigens and attack any cancer cells that make them immune.

Acute myeloid leukemia (AML) is most common leukemia among adults. The morphology, cytogenetics and molecular abnormalities of leukemic cells (blasts) are currently used to classify AML into various risk categories. The projected number of newly diagnosed lymphomas in India in 2020 was 11,230 and 41,607 for Hodgkin lymphoma (HL) and non-Hodgkin lymphoma (NHL), respectively. Large number of cancers (>70%) are diagnosed in the low- and middle-income countries.

Currently, there are no licensed blood cancer vaccines for leukemia, e.g., AML, chronic lymphocytic leukemia (CLL), lymphoma, and myeloma which are types of blood cancers that arise from abnormal growth and proliferation of certain cells in the blood or bone marrow. These are still in development and available only in clinical trials.

Hematopoietic stem cell transplantation is an option in the younger patients who are at higher risk of relapse and improves the survival further. Some are meant to help other treatments, such as a bone marrow/stem cell transplant, work better. Other vaccines made from a person's cancer cells and other cells may help the immune system destroy any cancer cells.

In hematological malignancies, *rituximab*, a chimeric murine/human anti-CD20 monoclonal immunoglobulin G, subclass 1, κ light chain (IgG1κ) antibody or ofatumumab, a humanized anti-CD20 monoclonal IgG1κ antibody, targeting CD20 on B-cells, is currently indicated for the treatment of B-cell NHL and CLL.

The development of vaccines for these types of cancers is complex due to the diverse nature of these diseases and the challenges in targeting cancer cells specifically. However, there are ongoing research efforts to explore immunotherapies and vaccines as potential treatment options for these cancers. These approaches typically involve using the patient's immune system to target and attack cancer cells.

Some of the notable strategies and treatments being explored include—there are several types of vaccine therapies, which are distinguished by how they are made. Basically, there are four vaccine types considered, including autologous patient-derived immune cell vaccines, tumor antigen-expressing recombinant virus vaccines, peptide vaccines, DNA vaccines, and heterologous whole-cell vaccines derived from established human tumor cell lines.

Most cancer vaccine studies involve administering chemotherapy, radiation, or other standard cancer therapy to reduce the amount of disease in the body before giving the vaccine. Immunotherapy is changing the therapeutic landscape of many hematologic diseases, with ICPIs, bispecific antibodies, and CAR T-cell therapies being its greatest expression.

Chimeric antigen receptor T-cell therapy involves genetically modifying a patient's T-cells to express receptors that can target specific proteins found on the surface of cancer cells. CAR T-cell therapies have shown promise in treating certain types of lymphoma and leukemia.

Checkpoint inhibitors: ICPIs, such as pembrolizumab and nivolumab, are used in the treatment of some lymphomas. These drugs can block certain proteins that inhibit the immune system's ability to recognize and attack cancer cells.

Peptide-based vaccines: Some research has focused on developing peptide-based vaccines to stimulate the immune system to target cancer-specific antigens found on leukemia, lymphoma, and myeloma cells. These vaccines aim to train the immune system to recognize and attack these cancer cells.

DC vaccines: They involve isolating a patient's DCs, which are a type of immune cell, and exposing them to cancer cell antigens before reintroducing them into the patient's body. This approach aims to activate the immune system to target cancer cells.

Immune-stimulating antibodies: Monoclonal antibodies, like rituximab, have been used to treat certain types of lymphoma by targeting specific proteins on cancer cells and marking them for destruction by the immune system.

Acute myeloid leukemia vaccine—immunotherapy is changing the therapeutic landscape of many hematologic diseases. Nevertheless, in AML, the anti-CD33 antibody drug conjugate gemtuzumab ozogamicin is the only approved drug.

A promising field of research in AML therapy relies on antileukemic vaccination to induce remission or prevent disease relapse. Compared to other immunotherapeutic strategies, anti-AML vaccines have the advantage of being a less toxic and a more manageable approach, applicable also to elderly patients with poorer performance status and may be used in combination with currently available therapies.

Lymphoma vaccine (March 24, 2023): Currently, no vaccines have been approved for the treatment of lymphoma. However, lymphoma vaccines are being tested in clinical trials.

It is important to note that the treatment of leukemia, lymphoma, and myeloma typically involves a combination of chemotherapy, radiation therapy, targeted therapies, and stem cell transplantation, depending on the specific type and stage of the cancer.

Vaccine for Multiple Myeloma

Myeloma is a type of blood cancer that develops in the bone marrow. The bone marrow is home to various type of cells like red blood cells, neutrophils, lymphocytes, plasma cells, and platelets. Plasma cells are a type of white blood cells that help antibodies fight infections. When their natural way of functioning gets affected, there will be an unregulated production of plasma cells. A cancerous plasma cell is called a myeloma cell. Myeloma is also referred to as "multiple myeloma" because in most cases, there are multiple patches or areas in the bone where it grows.

There are many clinical trials looking at vaccines for people with multiple myeloma who are near remission. Researchers are also testing vaccines in people with smoldering myeloma or who need to have an autologous bone marrow/stem cell transplant.

Monoclonal antibody is a standard treatment for CLL.

Targeting CD20—CD20 is a protein found on the surface of B lymphocytes (the cells from which CLL starts). A number of mAbs used to treat CLL target the CD20 antigen. These drugs include:

- Rituximab (Rituxan, other names) has become one of the main treatments for CLL. It is most often used along with chemotherapy or a targeted drug, either as part of the initial treatment or as part of a second-line treatment, but it may also be used by itself for people too sick to get chemotherapy.
- *Obinutuzumab (Gazyva)* can be used along with the chemotherapy drug chlorambucil or the targeted drug ibrutinib (Imbruvica) as a part of the initial treatment for CLL. It can also be used alone for CLL that comes back after treatment or does not respond to other treatments.
- *Ofatumumab (Arzerra)* is used mainly if CLL is no longer responding to other treatments such as chemotherapy or other mAbs such as alemtuzumab (discussed below). It can be given by itself.

All of these drugs can cause HepB infections that were dormant (inactive) to become active again, which can lead to severe liver problems or even death. These drugs may also increase a person's risk of certain serious infections for many months after the drug is stopped. For example, rituximab has been linked to a rare brain disease known as progressive multifocal leukoencephalopathy (PML) that is caused by a virus. It can lead to headache, high blood pressure, seizures, confusion, loss of vision, and even death.

AML mAb—the genetically engineered, humanized anti-CD33 antibody HuM195 has demonstrated modest activity against overt relapsed AML and more substantial activity against MRD in acute promyelocytic leukemia.

Lymphomas—rituximab (Rituxan) is the mAb most often used to treat lymphoma. This drug targets the CD20 antigen, which many types of lymphoma make too much of. CD20 is found on a type of white blood cell called a B-cell.

Non-Hodgkin lymphoma—several mAbs that target CD20 antigen, a protein on the surface of B lymphocytes, are now used to treat NHL. Rituximab (Rituxan, other brand names) is often used along with chemotherapy for some types of NHL, but it may also be used by itself. Obinutuzumab (Gazyva) is often used along with chemotherapy as a part of the treatment for small lymphocytic lymphoma (SLL)/CLL. It can also be used along with chemotherapy in treating follicular lymphoma. Ofatumumab (Arzerra) is used mainly in patients with

SLL/CLL that is no longer responding to other treatments. Ibritumomab tiuxetan (Zevalin) is made up of a mAb.

T-cell-engaging bispecific antibodies: They are designed so they can attach to two different targets. These are known as bispecific antibodies. An example is T-cell-engaging bispecific antibodies. Once in the body, one part of these antibodies attaches to the CD3 protein on immune cells called T-cells. Another part attaches to a target on lymphoma cells, such as the CD20 protein. This brings the two cells together, which helps the immune system attack the lymphoma cells.

Multiple myeloma: There are three mAb drugs for multiple myeloma: Daratumumab (Darzalex)—attaches to the CD38 antigen on myeloma cells. Isatuximab (Sarclisa)—attaches to the CD38 antigen on myeloma cells. Elotuzumab (Empliciti)—attaches to the SLAM7 antigen on myeloma cells.

■ CELL THERAPIES

One of the most promising treatments for blood cancer is CAR T-cell therapy. These therapies use body's own immune system to help fight cancer. CAR T-cell therapy is a type of cancer immunotherapy treatment that uses immune cells called T-cells that are genetically altered in a laboratory to enable them in locating in destroying cancer cells more effectively.

Currently, CAR T-cell therapy is FDA approved to treat several types of hematological malignancies, including leukemia, lymphoma, and multiple myeloma.

Personalized Chimeric Antigen Receptor T-cell Therapy Process

The process takes a few weeks and the steps generally include:

Collecting the T-cells: We draw blood from a vein in your arm. The blood flows through a tube into an apheresis machine, which removes T-cells. The machine returns the rest of the blood back into your body through a different tube.

Engineering the T-cells: In a laboratory, scientists engineer the T-cells by adding a manufactured CAR. Then the laboratory lets the CAR T-cells multiply and grow.

Infusing the CAR T-cells: Once the laboratory has enough CAR T-cells, the cells are injected back (mostly IV) to patient. Your healthcare team might recommend chemotherapy before the CAR T-cell infusion to help boost the treatment's effectiveness. CAR T-cells circulate throughout the body as per their programming, recognize, and attack cancer cells. This recognition is independent of MHC complex, allowing CAR T-cells to target cancer cells more effectively than the body's natural T-cells.

- When CAR T-cells bind to cancer cells, they release cytotoxic substances that destroy cancer cells.

The process may take place in an outpatient infusion center or in the hospital. Several CAR T-cell therapies are approved by the US FDA and more are being developed **(Table 1)**.

TABLE 1: FDA-approved CAR T-cell therapies.

Generic name	Brand name	Target antigen	Targeted disease	Patient population
Tisagenlecleucel	Kymriah	CD19	B-cell ALL	Children and young adults with refractory or relapsed B-cell ALL
			B-cell NHL	Adults with relapsed or refractory B-cell NHL
Axicabtagene ciloleucel	Yescarta	CD19	B-cell NHL	Adults with relapsed or refractory B-cell NHL
			Follicular lymphoma	Adults with relapsed or refractory follicular lymphoma
Brexucabtagene autoleucel	Tecartus	CD19	MCL	Adults with relapsed or refractory MCL
			B-cell ALL	Adults with refractory or relapsed B-cell ALL
Lisocabtagene maraleucel	Breyanzi	CD19	B-cell NHL	Adults with relapsed or refractory B-cell NHL
Idecabtagene vicleucel	Abecma	BCMA	Multiple myeloma	Adults with relapsed or refractory multiple myeloma
Ciltacabtagene autoleucel	Carvykti	BCMA	Multiple myeloma	Adults with relapsed or refractory multiple myeloma

(ALL: acute lymphoblastic leukemia; BCMA: B-cell maturation antigen; CAR: chimeric antigen receptor; FDA: Food and Drug Administration; MCL: mantle cell lymphoma; NHL: non-Hodgkin lymphoma)

Different types of cancer have different antigens. Each kind of CAR T-cell therapy is made to fight a specific kind of cancer antigen. So a CAR T-cell therapy made for one type of cancer will not work against another type of cancer.

CAR T-cell therapy side effects: CAR T-cell therapy may cause some side effects or complications. A serious complication of CAR T-cell therapy is cytokine release syndrome (CRS). CAR T-cells may release chemicals called cytokines, which cause a reaction from the immune system.

Addendums

Novel chemotherapy-free regimens and optimal use of combination therapy are among the advances in acute lymphoblastic leukemia (ALL).

First is a phase 2 trial of a chemotherapy-free combination of blinatumomab and ponatinib as consolidation therapy in adults with newly diagnosed disease. The combination proved to be safe and effective, achieving high rates of residual disease (MRD) negativity. Newly diagnosed B-cell ALL comes under the spotlight in the next study, which indicated that hyper-CVAD [cyclophosphamide, vincristine sulfate, doxorubicin hydrochloride (Adriamycin), and dexamethasone] chemotherapy with or without inotuzumab ozogamicin followed by blinatumomab achieved excellent outcomes.

The use of consolidation blinatumomab after chemotherapy in B-lineage ALL. An analysis of phase 3 trial data suggested that achieving a survival benefit may require four cycles of the BiTE.

■ LUNG CANCER

Lung cancer is the third most common cancer affecting adults in the US and the leading cause of cancer death. There are two primary types of lung cancer: Non-small cell lung cancer (NSCLC) and small cell lung cancer (SCLC), each with its own subtypes and specialized treatment.

NSCLC: It constitutes about 85% of the total cases of lung cancer reported. This form of lung cancer consists of several subtypes. Adenocarcinoma often originates in the outer regions of the lung and is the most common type of NSCLC. Smoking has been linked to the development of SCC, which often starts in the bigger airways. A less frequent variant of lung cancer called large cell carcinoma can appear anywhere in the lungs.

SCLC: It is also known as "oat cell carcinoma" and combined small cell carcinoma and is more aggressive and difficult to treat, unlike NSCLC. This form of lung cancer begins as a small tumor in the lungs and spreads rapidly to other parts of the body during its initial stages of development.

This form of lung cancer has two distinct stages, namely limited and extensive. While the limited stage SCLC is confined to one lung and nearby lymph nodes, the extensive stage SCLC spreads to other parts of the lung and distant sites.

NSCLC and SCLC diagnosis: It is done by biopsies, molecular testing, and imaging studies. Cancer staging establishes the extent of the disease's spread and directs medical decisions. The selection of treatment depends on the stage, which ranges from stages I (localized) to IV (advanced).

Tissue biopsies, while reliable, can be challenging to obtain, especially in advanced cases or when the tumor is hard to reach. However, there is hope on the horizon with emerging biomarkers. These are measurable molecular indicators found in body fluids or tissues that reveal the presence or progression of cancer. Ongoing research has uncovered some promising biomarkers that offer a less invasive and more accurate alternative to traditional diagnostic approaches.

The promise of liquid biopsies: This is a tool in cancer detection and monitoring. By analyzing circulating tumor components in blood or other body fluids, liquid biopsies can provide real-time information on cancer status, allowing for early detection and monitoring of treatment response.

Detecting early stage lung cancer: One of the most promising types of emerging biomarkers for lung cancer is circulating tumor DNA (ctDNA). When cancer cells die, they release DNA into the bloodstream and ctDNA can be detected and analyzed to identify specific genetic changes associated with lung cancer. This approach has shown encouraging results in detecting early-stage lung cancer and tracking treatment response, allowing doctors to adjust therapies as needed.

MicroRNAs (miRNAs)—small but powerful indicators—are tiny RNA molecules that play a crucial role in regulating gene expression. They have been linked to various diseases, including cancer. In lung cancer, specific miRNAs have shown potential as diagnostic and prognostic biomarkers. Researchers have identified miRNA signatures associated with different lung cancer subtypes and stages. These miRNA profiles could be used to create more accurate and personalized diagnostic tools. Furthermore, miRNAs might serve as indicators of treatment response and disease progression, helping doctors tailor therapies for individual patients to achieve better outcomes.

Several emerging biomarkers are being studied for their potential to predict immunotherapy response. TILs and PD-L1 expression have shown promise in guiding treatment decisions. Additionally, the TMB—the number of mutations in a tumor's DNA—has emerged as a potential predictor of immunotherapy response. These biomarkers could help identify patients who are most likely to benefit from immunotherapy, sparing others from potential side effects and enabling alternative treatment strategies.

Immune System and Immunotherapy Biomarkers

Traditional treatment approaches, such as surgery, chemotherapy, and radiation therapy, have made strides in improving patient outcomes. The emergence of immunotherapy has revolutionized the landscape of lung cancer treatment. Joining the body's immune system to combat cancer cells, immunotherapy has shown remarkable promise in extending survival and improving the quality of life for lung cancer patients.

Monoclonal antibody—amivantamab is a new bispecific antibody that targets NSCLC by two different pathways, by bindings to epithelial growth factor receptor and mesenchymal epithelial transition factor. The use of amivantamab in chemotherapy resulted in superior efficacy as compared with chemotherapy alone as first-line treatment of patients with advanced NSCLC with EGFR exon 20 insertions.

Immune Checkpoint Inhibitors Immunotherapy

Unlike traditional treatments that directly attack cancer cells, immunotherapy enhances the body's immune system to recognize and destroy cancer cells. One of the most significant breakthroughs in immunotherapy for lung cancer is the development of ICPIs. These inhibitors block specific proteins in cancer cells, which prevent the immune system from attacking cancer cells effectively. By inhibiting these checkpoints, the immune system can regain its ability to identify and eliminate cancer cells.

Immune Checkpoint Inhibitors in Lung Cancer Treatment

The ICPIs have shown exceptional promise in the treatment of lung cancer, especially in patients with advanced stages of the disease. Pembrolizumab, nivolumab, and atezolizumab are well-known ICPIs that have demonstrated remarkable efficacy in clinical trials. These drugs have been approved for first-line and second-line therapy in advanced NSCLC patients and have improved OS rates compared to conventional chemotherapy. Additionally, ICPIs have exhibited a more favorable side effect profile, with fewer severe AEs compared to traditional treatments.

Combination therapies: Researchers are now exploring combination therapies to maximize the benefits of immunotherapy. Combining ICPIs with other immunotherapeutic agents, targeted therapies, or even chemotherapy has demonstrated synergistic effects in lung cancer treatment.

Furthermore, novel approaches such as *personalized neoantigen vaccines* are being developed, wherein a vaccine is created using the patient's unique tumor profile to stimulate their immune system to target cancer cells specifically. These approaches are transforming lung cancer treatment into a more precise and personalized endeavor, improving the chances of successful outcomes.

Despite its unprecedented success, immunotherapy is not without challenges.

The future of immunotherapy in lung cancer treatment appears promising. Some patients do not respond to immunotherapy and in others, resistance may develop over time. Researchers are actively investigating biomarkers and other predictive tools to identify patients who are most likely to benefit from immunotherapy, enhancing treatment selection and individualizing therapy.

Additionally, efforts are underway to understand the resistance mechanisms and develop strategies to overcome them. Combination therapies, as mentioned earlier, are one avenue being explored to tackle resistance and enhance treatment efficacy.

Vaccines that researchers have studied or are studying for lung cancer include:
- Cancer vaccine for advanced NSCLC beats chemotherapy on survival, and it has been found to be safe in phase III trial.
- T-cell vaccination with OSE2101 prolongs OS and is associated with fewer AEs compared with

chemotherapy in select patients with HLA-A2-positive advanced NSCLC, according to the results of the phase III ATALANTE-1 trial.

"The mechanism of action of OSE2101 that enhances a new specific CD8+ T-cell effector function, and which maintains antigen presentation and avoids immune escape leading to decreased T-cell recognition of the tumor, is a mechanistically plausible explanation of the clinical benefit observed in our study and in emerging new studies with cancer vaccines."

- *Belagenpumatucel-L vaccine (Lucanix):* This causes the body to produce more of a protein called transforming growth factor beta-2 (TGF-β2), which can kill cancer cells. Phase 2 trial results were reported in 2019 and were generally positive.
- *Stimuvax or tecemotide:* This generates an immune response against a protein called MUC1. In NSCLC, there is too much of this protein. A 2011 study showed positive results but not strongly positive.
- *Melanoma-associated antigen 3 (MAGE-A3):* This targets an antigen made by cancer genes called melanoma-associated antigen. This vaccine did not work well in a 2016 and researchers are no longer studying it.
- *CIMAvax-EGF:* This targets a protein called EGFR which is overexpressed on lung cancer cells. The vaccine stops EGF from binding to the receptor, which stops a tumor from growing. This vaccine is currently being used in Cuba, where multiple clinical trials found it to be safe and effective. A US trial is underway.
- Osimertinib plus chemotherapy bumps up PFS in advanced EGFR-mutated NSCLC.

In the first-line treatment of patients with advanced NSCLC harboring EGFR mutation, the combination of osimertinib plus pemetrexed and platinum-based chemotherapy outperformed osimertinib alone in terms of extending PFS, according to the interim results of the phase III FLAURA2 trial presented at World Conference on Lung Cancer (WCLC) in October, 2023.

- *Racotumomab:* This helps the body develop antigens against a type of lipid called NeuGcGM3. A phases 2 and 3 study found that this vaccine led to significantly longer OS rates compared with the placebo.
- *TG4010:* This expresses a protein called IL-2, which activates T-cells and natural killer cells to attack cancer cells. A phase 2 study of this vaccine showed it led to longer survival times.

Historically, vaccination approaches against lung cancer have been disappointing. However, over the past decade, a greater understanding of the immune system and of the antigens expressed by tumors, coupled with advances in immunoadjuvants and improved delivery systems, has led to advances in the use of immunotherapy including vaccines to target lung cancer.

Path Ahead

The future of lung cancer management lies in harnessing the potential of emerging biomarkers. With ongoing research, collaboration between scientists, and advancements in technology, we are moving closer to a new era of personalized lung cancer care.

Early detection through liquid biopsies, tailored treatments based on miRNA signatures, and improved immunotherapy selection could soon become a reality, offering new hope to patients and their families in the fight against lung cancer. Vaccines for lung cancer show promise, but they are likely still years away. The most promising NSCLC vaccine results is plausible explanation of the clinical benefit observed in emerging new studies with cancer vaccines, hopefully.

■ MELANOMA

An estimated 325,000 new cases of malignant melanoma were diagnosed worldwide in 2020.

Malignant melanoma is an extremely rare malignancy in the Indian subcontinent and Southeast Asia. It is known that Asian countries have different clinical presentation of melanoma. Reportedly, India witnesses more than a million cases of melanoma per year (September 30, 2021).The frequency of melanoma is increasing, particularly in lighter-skinned people and for the minority of patients diagnosed with metastatic disease, the 5-year survival rate is 35%, although the introduction of immunotherapy has doubled the median survival time for these patients.

In a groundbreaking advance in March, 2022, led by Hopkins' scientists and oncologists, the FDA approved the combination of anti-PD-1 with another checkpoint blocker, antilymphocyte-activation gene 3 (LAG-3), as the first systemic treatment a patient might receive for advanced melanoma.

Another approved (October 27, 2023) "Talimogene laherparepvec" (T-VEC) is designed to replicate inside melanoma cells to kill those cells. It works by causing cancer cells to burst, releasing cancer antigens. These antigens can then stimulate immune responses that can seek out and eliminate any remaining tumor cells. T-VEC is an OV therapy that is used to treat some patients with metastatic melanoma that cannot be surgically removed.

The best mAb immunotherapy for melanoma: Nivolumab (Opdivo®) and pembrolizumab (Keytruda®) belong to a class of drugs called PD-1 blockers. Both of these medications work by inhibiting the molecule PD-1. These drugs have proven very effective against metastatic melanoma and stage III melanoma that cannot be removed completely with surgery. Also, the FDA has granted breakthrough therapy designation to the investigational vaccine mRNA-4157-P201 in combination with pembrolizumab (Keytruda) as an adjuvant treatment for patients with high-risk melanoma following complete resection (February 23, 2023).

Melanoma is an aggressive cancer that can spread quickly. Immunotherapy is cancer treatment that enhances your immune system's ability to destroy melanoma cells and prevent their spread. These therapies are key in treating advanced melanoma to help prevent its spread—and even provide a cure, in some cases.

Now, there is new hope for patients undergoing therapy to help stop the melanoma from coming back. A clinical trial focusing *on a personalized vaccine* is now releasing results, showing the new option reduced the risk of recurrence by nearly half.

Cell therapy—(February 15, 2024): The US FDA grants accelerated approval for Iovance Biotherapeutics' skin cancer cell therapy:

Lifileucel, branded as Amtagvi, is a tumor-derived immunotherapy composed of a patient's own disease-fighting white blood cells known as T-cells, with a specific type called tumor-infiltrating lymphocytes. Also, late-stage trial is being conducted to confirm clinical benefits of the therapy. *Amtagvi will be sold in the US at a list price of $515,000 per patient.*

"Tumor-infiltrating lymphocyte therapy offers a promising option for patients with solid tumors." "CAR T or other cell therapies have so far not shown great success in treating these cancer types."

■ PANCREATIC CANCER VACCINE

The most common cancer is pancreatic ductal adenocarcinoma (PDAC) that accounts for 90% of cases and arises from a part of the pancreas that makes digestive enzymes. About 1–2% cases of pancreatic cancer are neuroendocrine tumors that arise from hormone-producing cells of the pancreas which are generally less aggressive. Despite modern therapies, only about 12% of people diagnosed with this cancer will be alive 5 years after treatment.

- Pancreatic cancer is often referred to as a "silent killer" because it tends to exhibit minimal or vague symptoms in its early stages, making it challenging to detect.

Pancreatic cancer is usually not found until advanced stages because it takes long for symptoms to appear. Usually, no symptoms are seen in the early stages and symptoms that are specific enough to suggest pancreatic cancer typically do not develop until the disease has reached an advanced stage. By the time of diagnosis, pancreatic cancer has often spread to other parts of the body.

Surgical resection offers the best chance of cure, but many patients are ineligible due to late-stage diagnosis. Chemotherapy and radiation therapy aim to control the disease and lessen symptoms, yet outcomes remain modest. Patients who have undergone surgery for pancreatic cancer are still at risk for relapse of the disease, even after they finish chemotherapy. This is especially true for patients who are positive for ctDNA, which puts them at a higher risk for relapse. Vaccine could become a crucial new tool against one of the deadliest common cancers.

Current treatments include precision oncology and immunotherapy. Precision oncology tailors treatment strategies to the specific molecular characteristics of a patient's tumor. Immunotherapy harnesses the body's immune system to recognize and attack cancer cells.

Researchers are working on many treatment vaccines designed to boost the immune system's response to pancreatic cancer cells. The vaccine may be given as the only treatment or along with mAb to stimulate a person's own immune system to recognize and destroy cancer cells more effectively. Certain types of immunotherapy pembrolizumab can be used to treat pancreatic cancer.

Pembrolizumab (Keytruda) is a mAb drug that targets PD-1, a checkpoint protein T-cells, that normally helps keep these cells from attacking normal cells in the body. By blocking PD-1, this drug boosts the immune response against pancreatic cancer cells and can often shrink tumors. Pembrolizumab is given as an IV infusion every 2 or 3 weeks.

The pancreatic cancer vaccine is a form of immunotherapy. The vaccine uses pancreatic cancer cells that have been treated with radiation to inhibit their ability to grow. These cells have also been genetically altered to secrete a molecule called granulocyte-macrophage colony-stimulating factor (GM-CSF).

Personalized Messenger Ribonucleic Acid (mRNA) Vaccines Against Pancreatic Cancer

A new experimental approach to treating pancreatic cancer is progressing to the next step in making it available to more patients. The mRNA vaccines are custom-made for every person. They use proteins in the pancreatic tumors, called neoantigens, to alert the immune system that the cancer cells are foreign. In this way, the mRNA vaccine trains the body to protect itself against cancer cells. After results from a small study, a phase 2 clinical trial has now opened to test the effectiveness of using an mRNA vaccine to fight one of the deadliest cancers.

The phase 2 trial follows results from a phase 1 trial involving 16 Memorial Sloan Kettering (MSK) patients, shown that the vaccines were well tolerated for most patients and the phase 2 study will provide more clarity on the vaccine and its potential benefits, if any, for patients with the most common type of pancreatic cancer.

Personalized vaccines while promising also have challenges. They take time to make and are costly. By contrast, an off-the-shelf vaccine manufactured in batches could be given to patients with minimal delay and would be cheaper to produce.

At a glance,
- A personalized mRNA vaccine against pancreatic cancer created a strong antitumor immune response in half the participants in a small study.
- The vaccine will soon be tested in a larger clinical trial. The approach may also have the potential for treating other deadly cancer types.

The trial of new mRNA pancreatic cancer vaccine will start its next phase.

A new vaccine shows encouraging early results as a potential off-the-shelf treatment for certain patients with pancreatic cancer or CRC, according to a study coled by researchers at MSK Cancer Center and nearly 80 sites around the world. The vaccine targets tumors with mutations (or changes) in the KRAS gene, a driving force in many cancers.

This cancer vaccine is different from another type of pancreatic cancer vaccine, which is custom-made for each patient using mRNA. Both are therapeutic vaccines given after surgery to prevent or delay the cancer from coming back in high-risk patients.

In practice: AI model could mitigate the inadequacies of imaging and the diagnostic errors in interpretation, which often contribute to delayed diagnosis of pancreatic cancer. In combination with emerging blood-based biomarkers, such a model could be evaluated to screen for sporadic cancer in ongoing trials of high-risk cohorts such as the early detection initiative.

■ PROSTATE CANCER VACCINES

In 2010, the FDA approved sipuleucel-T (Provenge) for people with metastatic prostate cancer. Provenge is an autologous vaccine which is *a personalized, therapeutic vaccine* made from a patient's own cell-derived immune cell vaccine.

Prostate cancer is a leading cause of death in men worldwide. Prostate cancer incidence in India, like in many other countries, has been increasing over the years and is one of the top 10 leading cancers in India. It usually affects men in the age group of 65+ years. It is generally lower than in western countries, but it has been on the rise due to changes in lifestyle, increased life expectancy, and improved access to healthcare and diagnostic services.

Colorectal cancer and PDAC are the second and third leading causes of cancer death, respectively, with standard locoregional treatment for resectable disease, resulting in <20% 5-year survival and few effective treatments for relapse.

According to the ICMR, prostate cancer is the third most common cancer in Indian men (June, 2023). The underlying factor linking diet and prostate cancer is probably hormonal. Fats stimulate increased production of testosterone and other hormones and testosterone acts to speed the growth of prostate cancer. High testosterone levels may stimulate dormant prostate cancer cells into activity.

Why is prostate cancer low in Japan?
The quasi-vegan nature of the Japanese diet may have contributed importantly to their protection from

prostate cancer. But there is reason to suspect that heavy consumption of green tea and regular consumption of soy products rich in isoflavones may have contributed to this protection as well.

Prostate Health Index (PHI) is a blood test that measures the level of prostate-specific antigen (PSA) and other prostate-related proteins to determine the risk of prostate cancer. This test is highly recommended for men over 50 years of age or those with a family history of prostate cancer.

- "Serum PSA is not recommended for routine screening without urinary symptoms" (ICMR, 2023).

Current therapies for prostate cancer: Essentially, it is important to have a good early diagnosis and assess the risk of the disease. The prostate cancer stage of the disease and the patient's profile must be clearly understood to choose the best treatment for each patient. After this, there exists a variety of approaches to be considered, which include watchful waiting, surgery, radiation, chemotherapy, hormone therapy, and immunotherapy. All these approaches can be used alone or in combination. As with hormone therapy and chemotherapy, this type of treatment has not been shown to cure prostate cancer **(Fig. 2)**.

Monoclonal antibody—immunotherapy is a promising prostate cancer therapy that uses patients' own immune cells stimulated to target the antigen PAP to recognize and kill cancer cells.

Provenge (Sipuleucel-T), a cell-based vaccine, is the only first FDA-approved therapeutic cancer vaccine (2010) that utilizes the power of the patient's own immune cells stimulated to identify and target prostate cancer cells. This vaccine is used to treat advanced prostate cancer that is no longer responding to hormone therapy, but that is causing few or no symptoms.

The process of making Provenge involves collecting a patient's immune cells by a procedure (leukapheresis). The cells are then at the laboratory, where they are mixed

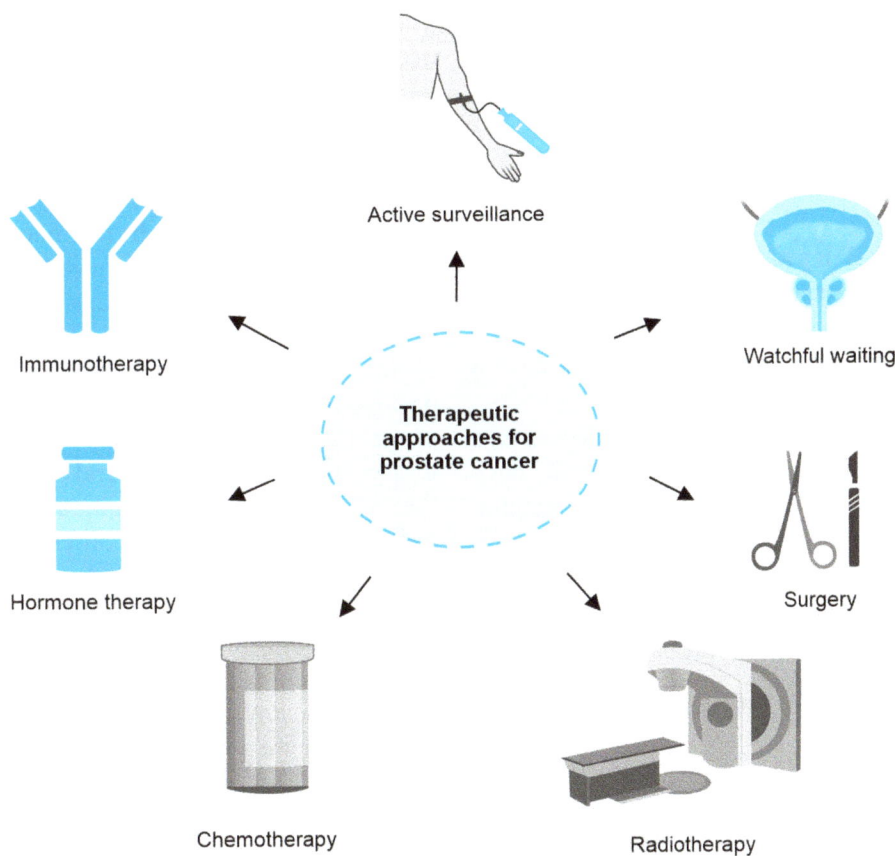

Fig. 2: Therapeutic approaches for prostate cancer.

with a protein from prostate cancer cells called PAP. These PAP-mixed cells are then given back to patient by IV infusions. This vaccine is made specifically for each man.

This process is repeated two more times, 2 weeks apart, so that you get three doses of cells. The cells help your other immune system cells attack prostate cancer. This process activates the patient's immune cells to help the immune system better fight the disease. Provenge has allowed men to live longer with minimal side effects and reducing the risk of death by 22.5%.

Other immunotherapies are being tested in clinical trials, such as: *Prostvac*: PSA is a molecule found on the surface of many prostate cancer cells. Upon administration, Prostvac is designed to "teach" the immune system (T-lymphocytes and other type of immune cells) to identify and kill tumor cells that express PSA.

But drugs that target these checkpoints, known as checkpoint inhibitors, hold a lot of promise as cancer treatments.

For example, pembrolizumab (Keytruda) and dostarlimab (Jemperli) are drugs that target PD-1, a checkpoint protein on immune system cells called T-cells. By blocking PD-1, these drugs boost the immune response.

Pembrolizumab can be used if the cancer cells have any of the following:
- A high level of MSI-H or a *dMMR* gene
- A TMB-H—meaning the cancer cells have many gene mutations.
- Dostarlimab can be used if the cancer cells have a *dMMR* gene.

Unfortunately, these types of changes are not common in prostate cancer. But for men whose cancer cells have one of these changes, one of these drugs might be helpful. These drugs are given as an IV infusion, typically every 3–6 weeks.

There are more ongoing studies and clinical trials with these ICPIs drugs but whose results still do not allow their approval by the competent authorities and their commercialization.

■ PRIMARY BONE CANCERS (SARCOMAS)

Primary bone cancers include chondrosarcoma, Ewing sarcoma, osteosarcoma, and chordoma.

Bone cancer is a group of diseases that affects bones, cartilage, and cells that form bones. Most cases of the bone cancer are metastatic in origin. It occurs when a primary cancer somewhere else in the body spreads to the bones. The outlook for people with metastatic bone cancer is poor.

Primary bone cancer that starts in bones, is a very rare. The types of primary bone cancer include:
- *Chondrosarcoma:* It begins in the cartilage and the risk of developing it increases with age.
- *Ewing sarcoma (ES):* It is the second most common form of bone cancer and is most common in people under the age of 30 years. However, ES is a rare type of bone cancer that typically strikes teenagers and young adults between 10 and 20 years old.
- *Osteosarcoma (OS):* It begins in young bone cells and most often occurs in people aged 10–30 years.
- *Chordoma:* This cancer begins in the spine's bones. It occurs most frequently in adults over 30 years.

In general, treatment options include surgery to remove as much of the cancer as possible, chemotherapy, and radiation. Targeted drugs are especially important in treating types of bone cancer where chemotherapy has not been very useful, such as chordomas. Other types of nonchemotherapy drugs that can be used to treat some types of bone cancers include bone-directed drugs and immunotherapy drugs.

Active and adoptive immunotherapies are used in the treatment of OS. Although treatment strategies involving surgery and chemotherapy have improved outcomes for patients with OS, the prognosis of recurrent OS is quite unsatisfactory.

Immunotherapy, however, has been shown to be a promising therapeutic strategy against OS. As research progresses, immunotherapy is gradually becoming irreplaceable. There are several therapeutic strategies for OS including immunomodulation, vaccine therapy, and immunologic checkpoint blockade. Active immunotherapies using DCs, pulsed vaccines, and cytokines influence immune responses toward tumor cells. Adoptive immunotherapy involves administering ex vivo-expanded tumor-specific cytotoxic immune cells.

Chimeric antigen receptor T-cells belong to the latter strategy and are an impressive application of both insights into T-cell biology and advances in genetic engineering. Generally, immunotherapy shows promising data for treating OS; however. further research is needed to determine more precise curative effects.

Spleen Cancer

Primary spleen Ca that first starts in the spleen is rare and uncommon. It is unusual, in that it only rarely develops within the organ itself. Typically develops as secondary metastasis from another body site Ca. Researchers believe it happens in less than 2 percent of all lymphomas and 1 percent of all non-Hodgkin lymphomas

A form of cancer that does develop in the spleen is called splenic marginal zone lymphoma or SMZL, which is considered a kind of non-Hodgkin lymphoma. Researchers believe it happens in less than 2 percent of all lymphomas and 1 percent of all non-Hodgkin lymphomas.

Common treatments for spleen cancer include surgery (splenectomy), chemotherapy, radiation, and immunotherapies.

Historically, splenectomy was often the first treatment used, and studies have shown that most who had splenectomy did not need any further treatment for 5 years. However, treatment with a human-made mAb (rituximab) is almost as effective as surgery at reducing symptoms in people with SMZL. Also, it may be easier to use than surgery.

■ TESTICULAR GERM CELL TUMORS

Germ cell tumors represent a heterogeneous neoplasm family, affecting gonads and rarely occurring in extragonadal areas. Most of patients have a good prognosis, often even in the presence of metastatic disease; however, in almost 15% of cases, tumor relapse and platinum resistance are the main challenges.

Among solid tumors, GCTs represent an example of neoplasm without any significant mutational burden, as confirmed by The Cancer Genome Atlas (TCGA). Most of the studies testing immunotherapeutic strategies against GCTs are based on PD-L1 checkpoint inhibitor, which maintain the activity of T-cells through the linkage with CTLA4 or PD-1/PD-L1 molecules. CAR T-cell therapy is a novel fascinating strategy for nonresponders to ICPIs and for less immunogenic neoplasms. Should the role of CAR T-cell therapy in GCTs be confirmed with a larger sample size clinical trials, this would represent a significant step forward in this category of patients who are so young, for whom only chemotherapy is currently approved. A better understanding of the mechanisms of activation of the immune system, including epigenetic influence in immune checkpoint expression, could also lead to a reconsideration of therapy with ICPIs against GCTs.

VACCINES FOR PEDIATRIC MALIGNANCY AND IMMUNOTHERAPY: ADVANCES, OPPORTUNITIES, AND CHALLENGES

Traditionally administered pediatric immunizations to prevent childhood infections can work as lifetime cancer prevention vaccines, down the road that occur later in life. Examples are the HBV vaccine preventing HCC, or HPV, against male and female orogenital cancers.

Although survival for many pediatric cancers has improved with advances in conventional chemotherapeutic regimens and surgical techniques in the last several decades, it remains a leading cause of disease-related death in children. Outcomes in patients with recurrent, refractory, or metastatic disease are especially poor.

Approximately, 400,000 children and adolescents (0–19 years) across the globe develop cancer every year. Most common childhood cancers include leukemias, brain cancers, lymphomas, and solid tumors such as neuroblastomas and WT.

Wilms tumor is the common type of cancer seen in children beside hepatoblastomas and the tumors of the nervous system in the abdomen are called neuroblastoma and lymphomas. The most common cancer found in the child is a blood cancer which is called leukemia and lymphoma.

■ RETINOBLASTOMA

Retinoblastoma is a highly curable neoplasm in high-income countries, where patient survival exceeds 99%, making it the most curable of all pediatric cancers. Most common presenting symptom was white pupillary reflex in 60% of children.

Ocular palliative approaches have made great strides during the last few decades, making it the most treatable pediatric cancer for intraocular RB in a high-income country. In striking contrast, in many lower-income countries, most patients present with disseminated and metastatic disease, which is almost always fatal.

- The incidence of RB is 1 in 20,000 live births, with about 1,500 children being diagnosed in India each year. It is the most common intraocular cancer in India.

Patients can be cured by enucleation, but it can lead to vision loss. Chemotherapy is the main method of treatment for RB currently. Unfortunately, children suffering from disseminated RB have virtually no options for treatment. New therapeutic strategies are expected to be highly effective for both intraocular and extraocular diseases, provided that the risk of toxicity is lower. In addition, the availability of more new nonchemotherapy therapies gives patients more options, such as targeted therapies, immunotherapy, and lysing viruses.

Targeting not only tumor cells but also the active TME is a novel strategy for RB treatment. Several potential targets for RB immunotherapy, including gangliosides GD2, programmed cell death 1 (PD-1) and programmed cell death ligand 1 (PD-L1), B7 family checkpoint molecules, (CD276) B7H3, epithelial cell adhesion molecule (EpCAM), and spleen tyrosine kinase (SYK).

Also, the techniques for CAR T, bispecific antibodies and genetically modified DCs are according to the characteristics of different targets.

In developing countries, RB is mostly detected in advanced stages, resulting in poor outcomes. Increased awareness and accessibility to dedicated centers for treating childhood malignancy can lead to early diagnosis, better prognosis, and increased vision salvage.

In summary, RB treatment has evolved over the last century, resulting in a striking change in the treatment paradigm of this ocular tumor. Advances in the knowledge of its tumor biology and drug response and the development of new routes of drug delivery promise to lead to additional new, more effective, and less toxic therapies in RB.

GENERAL INFORMATION ABOUT CHILDHOOD KIDNEY TUMORS

Wilms tumor is the most common renal malignancy in children, accounting for >90% of all pediatric renal cancers. Dramatic improvements in survival have been achieved for children and adolescents with cancer. Between 1975 and 2020, childhood cancer mortality decreased by >50%. For children younger than 20 years with WT (also known as nephroblastoma), the 5-year relative survival rate is 93%. Childhood and adolescent cancer survivors require close monitoring because cancer therapy side effects may persist or develop months or years after treatment. For information about the incidence, type, and monitoring of late effects in childhood and adolescent cancer survivors.

Childhood kidney cancers account for about 7% of all childhood cancers. Most childhood kidney cancers are WT, but in the 15–19-year age group, most tumors are RCC. The 5-year relative survival rate for patients with RCC in this age group is 76% (National Cancer Institute, Bethesda, MD, USA, December 15, 2023).

Wilms tumor affects approximately 1 in 10,000 children with the median age of onset being 3.5 years. Girls are slightly more likely than boys to develop WT and African Americans are also at a higher risk. Cure rates of childhood malignancies are inferior in India compared with upper middle-income countries. There is paucity of quality data addressing outcome of childhood WT from India.

Approximately, one third of WT cases involve mutations. Elevated rates of WT are observed in patients with a number of genetic disorders, including WAGR (WT, aniridia, genitourinary abnormalities, and range of developmental delays) syndrome (WAGR spectrum), Beckwith–Wiedemann syndrome, hemihypertrophy, Denys–Drash syndrome, and Perlman syndrome. Other genetic causes that have been observed in familial WT cases include germline mutations in REST and CTR9.

There are limitations of conventional therapies, including surgery, chemotherapy, and radiotherapy, in preventing recurrence in WT patients. Also, their potential for exerting long-term side effects necessitate the application of novel therapeutic strategies, like immunotherapy, in this disease. Immunotherapy is an emerging treatment approach based on the concept of harnessing the patient's immune system to fight tumor cells.

This approach has demonstrated promising results in various types of cancers due to its relatively high specificity, efficacy, and tolerability. The potential implication of different immunotherapy approaches, like mAbs; adoptive cell therapy, e.g., CAR T-cell therapy; and ICPIs, in patients with WT, with a particular emphasis on the tumor's genetic and histological features.

- The precise effects of immunotherapy in WT remain to be explored. Moreover, the potential beneficiary roles of the combination of immunotherapy and conventional treatments should be investigated in future research.

CHILDHOOD LEUKEMIA AND LYMPHOMAS

As the technology of genomic testing has advanced, its routine use for diagnosis, risk stratification, and the modification of treatment of childhood cancers has increased. Childhood cancer research now more frequently incorporates the range of testing in children with cancer spans from a targeted test that identifies a single genetic variant in a tumor to next-generation sequencing becoming more common for children with cancer.

This is not unique to pediatrics because such testing is also becoming increasingly incorporated into standard practice in adult oncology.

Early successes in ICPIs and CAR T-cell therapy have shown remarkable outcomes in pediatric patients, particularly in certain types of leukemia and lymphoma.

Novel chemotherapy-free regimens and optimal use of combination therapy are among the advances in ALL.

By harnessing the power of the immune system, immunotherapy offers new hope for children battling cancer, minimizing long-term side effects, and improving the overall prognosis. Continued advancements in immunotherapy hold the key to unlocking the full potential of treating pediatric cancers and improving the quality of life for young patients.

Immunotherapy is changing the treatment landscape for specific subsets of pediatric cancer patients. It has been employed in the treatment of neuroblastoma and OS.

To date, cancer vaccination has remained largely understudied in the pediatric population. Though there are no current ongoing clinical trials, there are promising preclinical data to suggest that viral-based vaccines may be effective in Pediatric cancer. There are different types of tumor antigens and vaccine technologies (DCs, peptides, nucleic acids, and viral vectors) evaluated in clinical trials with a focus on those used in children.

- *Vaccines and oncolytic virotherapy* are still being studied to determine their usefulness for pediatric cancer patients.

Cancer vaccines (Ca Vaxes) work by stimulating T-cells with tumor neoantigens, thus leading to a greater antitumor response. Ca vaxes alone have been shown to activate antigen-specific T-cells; however, these T-cells eventually become dampened by the suppressive TME. These T-cells have been shown to have an increased expression of "PD-1 on T-cells, thus suggesting a role for PD-1 blockade. Preclinical murine models of the prostate, neuroblastoma, and pancreatic cancers have demonstrated increased immunogenicity by increasing TILs with subsequent greater antitumor effect when combining, i.e., CTLA-4 blockade with cancer vaccines. Metastatic melanoma and OS models in particular are vulnerable to cancer vaccine and immune checkpoint combination therapy.

The etiology of many of these neoplasms remains poorly understood, but it is likely a combination of genetic and environmental factors which makes vaccine development to prevent these neoplasms challenging. Currently, several types of neoantigen vaccines are being evaluated, both alone and in combination with other treatments, in a variety of cancer types in clinical trials. Most of the efforts are geared toward immunotherapy, which involves using the body's immune system to fight cancer. CAR T-cell therapy, e.g., has shown promise for certain types of leukemia in children.

Highly targeted agents with more favorable toxicity profiles and improved therapeutic efficacy are urgently needed to improve the quality of life and long-term outcomes of children's cancer. Immunotherapy harnesses the ability of the immune system to combat infection and neoplasia and has emerged as a promising treatment modality for many pediatric and adult malignancies. Examples of successful immunotherapies include antibodies that block immunosuppressive pathways, such as pembrolizumab, a PD-1 ICPI that has gained approval for treating a myriad of solid tumors.

CENTRAL NERVOUS SYSTEM MALIGNANCIES

Central nervous system malignancies are among the most aggressive of pediatric cancers and are notoriously difficult to manage. Brain tumors account for over 20% of childhood cancers and are the biggest cancer killer in children and young adults. Several initiatives over the past 40 years have tried to identify more effective drug treatments but with very limited success. This is largely due to the BBB which restricts the entry of many drugs into the brain.

The challenges of treating CNS tumors in young children are many. These include age-specific tumor characteristics, limited treatment options, and susceptibility of the developing CNS to cytotoxic therapy. Most new cancer drugs in clinical trials do not cross the BBB. Techniques to enhance brain tumor drug delivery are explored in this review and cover those that augment penetration of the BBB and those that bypass the BBB. Developing appropriate delivery techniques could improve patient outcomes by ensuring efficacious drug exposure to tumors (including those that are drug resistant), reducing systemic toxicities, and targeting leptomeningeal metastases. Together, this drug delivery strategy seeks to enhance the efficacy of new drugs and enable reevaluation of existing drugs that might have previously failed because of inadequate delivery.

Oncolytic viruses have been explored as therapeutic cancer vaccines for quite a few decades. Pioneering work done by Lindenmann and Klein in 1967 demonstrated

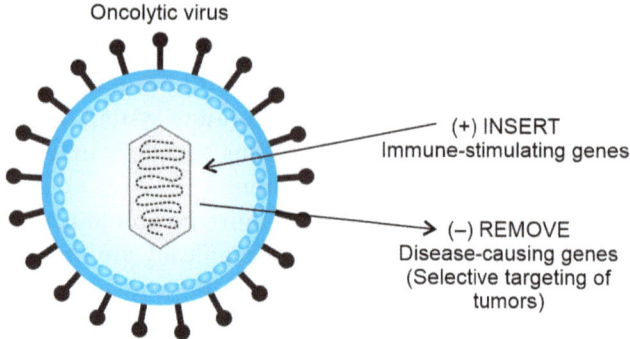

Fig. 3: Oncolytic virus therapy.

that viral oncolysis of tumor cells by influenza virus increases immunogenicity of tumor cell antigens.

Oncolytic viruses are a form of immunotherapy that uses viruses to infect and destroy cancer cells. Viruses are particles that infect or enter our cells and then use the cell's genetic machinery to make copies of themselves and subsequently spread to surrounding uninfected cells.

Oncolytic virus therapy uses modified viruses that infect and destroy tumor cells (Fig. 3). T-VEC, an OV, is approved for treating melanoma. T-VEC is a weakened and modified form of the herpes simplex virus type I (HSV-1). It is also known as Imlygic. T-VEC is an OV therapy that is used to treat some patients with metastatic melanoma that cannot be surgically removed.

Other examples of oncolytic DNA viruses include adenoviruses, parvoviruses, and poxviruses such as vaccinia virus (VACV) and myxoma virus (MYXV).

ONCOLYTIC VIRUS THERAPY WITH ENGINEERED VIRUSES TO FIGHT CANCER

More recently, viruses have been used to target and attack tumors that have already formed. These viruses—some, but not all, of which have been modified are known as OVs and they represent a promising approach to treating cancer for several reasons:
- Cancer cells often have weakened antiviral defenses that make them susceptible to infection.
- Natural viruses can be engineered to give them advantageous properties, including decreasing their ability to infect healthy cells as well as yielding them the ability to deliver therapeutic payloads specifically to tumors and produce immune-boosting molecules once they infect tumor cells.

After infection, these OVs can cause cancer cells to "burst"—killing the cancer cells and releasing cancer antigens. These antigens can then stimulate immune responses that can seek out and eliminate any remaining tumor cells nearby and potentially anywhere else in the body.

In 2015, the US FDA approved the first OV immunotherapy for the treatment of cancer T-VEC for melanoma. This treatment involves a herpes virus that has been engineered to be less likely to infect healthy cells as well as cause infected cancer cells to produce the immune-stimulating GM-CSF protein.

Common side effects associated with the currently approved OV may include but are not limited to chills, fatigue, flu-like symptoms, injection site pain, nausea, and fever. Side effects may vary according to the type of OV and what exactly it targets and may also be influenced by the location and type of cancer as well as a patient's overall health. Due to their potential to infect healthy cells as well as stimulate overall immune activity, sometimes OVs may cause the immune system to attack healthy cells and their use may carry some risk of infection.

Oncolytic virus clinical trial platforms under evaluation include:
- *Adenovirus:* A family of common viruses that can cause a wide range of typically mild effects including sore throat, fatigue, and cold-like symptoms
- *HSV:* Commonly occurring recurrent oral blisters lesions
- *Maraba virus:* A virus found exclusively in insects
- *Measles:* A highly contagious human virus
- *Newcastle disease virus:* Primarily found in birds; can cause mild conjunctivitis and flu-like symptoms in humans
- *Picornavirus:* A family of viruses that can cause a range of diseases in mammals and birds; the coxsackie virus is an example from this family.
- *Reovirus:* A family of viruses that can affect the GI and respiratory tracts in a range of animal species
- *VACV:* The virus that was used to help vaccinate against and eliminate smallpox; rarely causes illness in humans
- *Vesicular stomatitis virus:* The virus that belongs to the same family as the Maraba virus; can cause flu-like symptoms in humans

To conclude
The development of cancer vaccines holds significant promise in the field of oncology. However, it is essential to understand that cancer is a complex disease with various

types and subtypes, each presenting unique challenges. Many ongoing clinical trials being systematically analyzed, have shown encouraging results in early-stage clinical trials.

Research expertise and medical oncology support teams are internationally recognized for the use of vaccines to stimulate the immune system in the treatment of cancer. One should always consult with an Infectious Disease (ID) specialists and/or oncologist for evolving information about specific cancer vaccines, their availability, and their potential benefits in the context of individual cancer treatment plans.

SCOPE AND CURRENT STATUS

Cancer prevention vaccines can potentially prevent the development of cancer by targeting specific viruses known to cause certain types of cancers, such as the HPV vaccine for cervical cancer, have been developed and are in widespread use. Efforts continue to expand preventive vaccines for other virus-related cancers, such as HBV vaccine to prevent liver cancer.

Cancer treatment (therapeutic) vaccines aim to stimulate the immune system, so that it recognizes the cancer cells as foreign and attacks the cells. Cancer treatment vaccines are sometimes made with cells from the patient's own tumor, which are modified in the laboratory and then returned to stop, destroy, or delay the growth of the cancer.

Several therapeutic cancer vaccines have been developed and tested in clinical trials. While some have shown promise in stimulating immune responses against cancer cells, their efficacy in terms of improving patient outcomes, such as survival rates, remains a subject of ongoing research.

Recently, therapeutic cancer vaccines have shown promise by eliciting de novo T-cell responses targeting tumor antigens, including TTAs and TSAs. The objective was to amplify and diversify the intrinsic repertoire of tumor-specific T-cells.

Personalized cancer vaccine: Advancements in technology and understanding of cancer biology have paved the way for personalized cancer vaccines tailored to an individual's specific tumor profile, known as neoantigens. These personalized neoantigen vaccines are a highly specific cancer treatment designed to induce a robust cytotoxic T-cell attack against a patient's cancer antigens. These vaccines are designed to target mutations specific to an individual's tumor, potentially offering a more precise and effective treatment approach.

CHALLENGES AND FUTURE DIRECTIONS

- Cancer is characterized by genetic and phenotypic heterogeneity, posing challenges for developing vaccines that can effectively target all cancer cells within a tumor.
- Cancers employ various mechanisms to evade the immune system, including immune checkpoint pathways. Overcoming these immunosuppressive mechanisms is crucial for the success of cancer vaccines.
- Combining cancer vaccines with other treatment modalities, such as ICPIs or traditional therapies such as chemotherapy and radiation, may enhance their efficacy by synergistically targeting different aspects of the cancer.
- Moving from preclinical research to clinical application requires rigorous testing to ensure safety and efficacy.
- Large-scale clinical trials are needed to validate the effectiveness of cancer vaccines in diverse patient populations.

HUMAN GUT—MICROBIOME IN CANCER PREVENTION

Role of the gut microbiota in anticancer therapy: The gut microbiome is known to have an essential role in the regulation of the host's health and physiology. The gut microbiota and their metabolites may induce immunological and cellular pathways to eliminate invading pathogens and trigger an immune response to prevent cancer. By elucidating the intricate dynamics of the gut microbiome and its influence on cancer biology, we uncover promising avenues for preventive measures and therapeutic interventions. Evolving research studies suggest that a gut microbial has a profound influence on cancer development and treatment response.

The gut microbiota, comprising trillions of microbes, orchestrates critical functions in our bodies, including digestion, metabolism, and immune regulation **(Fig. 4)**. Through a delicate balance of beneficial and harmful microbes, the gut microbiome maintains homeostasis and contributes to overall health. Disruptions in this balance, known as dysbiosis, have been linked to various diseases, including cancer. Understanding the intricate interactions within the gut microbiome provides valuable insights into cancer biology and therapeutic strategies.

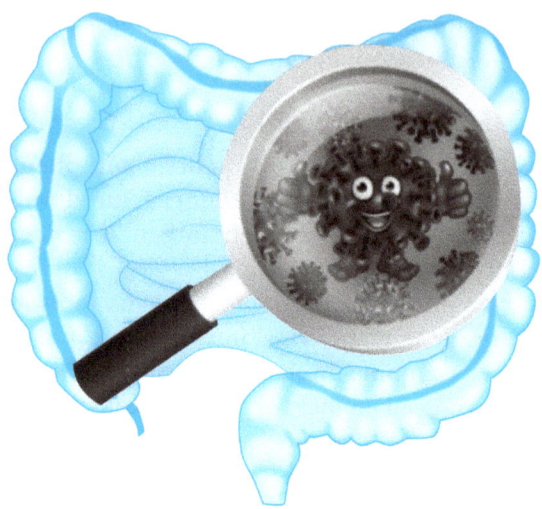

Fig. 4: Human gut residing bacterial, fungal, and viral microbes in trillions.

Research specifies that about 20% of the global cancer burden is due to pathogenic bacteria and viruses. Restoring gut health through dietary interventions, probiotics, or fecal microbiota transplantation can potentially reduce cancer risk and prevent tumorigenesis. Diet plays a crucial role in shaping the composition of the gut microbiome, with certain foods promoting the growth of beneficial gut bacteria.

Fiber-rich fruits and vegetables, fermented foods, and prebiotics nourish beneficial microbes, while minimizing the consumption of processed foods and antibiotics helps maintain microbial diversity. Probiotics, consisting of live beneficial bacteria, can also restore microbial balance and support overall gut health. Furthermore, fecal microbiota transplantation, a procedure where fecal matter containing healthy microbes is transferred to a patient's gut, has shown promise in treating certain GI conditions and may have implications for cancer prevention.

ENHANCING CANCER TREATMENT EFFICACY

While conventional treatments remain vital, emerging research points to the crucial role of the gut microbiome—our body's microbial ecosystem—in cancer therapy and prevention. Certain gut bacteria such as *Bifidobacterium* have shown the ability to augment the effectiveness of cancer treatments, such as immunotherapy and chemotherapy. By modulating the immune system and metabolizing drugs, these microbes can potentially enhance treatment outcomes while mitigating side effects. For example, research has revealed that specific bacterial strains can activate immune cells to target and destroy cancer cells more effectively. Harnessing these interactions may lead to personalized treatment approaches that optimize therapeutic benefits while minimizing chemotherapeutic adverse effects.

CHALLENGES AND CONSIDERATIONS— THE PROMISE AND CHALLENGE OF CANCER MICROBIOME RESEARCH

While the potential of the gut microbiome in cancer care is promising, there are significant challenges existing. Recent work has shed light on the multifaceted role that the community of organisms in and on the human body plays in cancer onset, development, detection, treatment, and outcome.

By elucidating the intricate dynamics of the gut microbiome and its influence on cancer biology, we uncover promising avenues for preventive measures and therapeutic interventions. From dietary modifications to innovative treatments such as fecal microbiota transplantation, the potential for leveraging the gut microbiome in cancer care is vast. Interdisciplinary collaboration, robust clinical studies, and stringent regulation are essential to ensure the safety, efficacy, and ethical implementation of microbiome-based therapies. The complex interactions within the gut microbiome pose challenges in deciphering its role in cancer development and treatment response. In addition, ensuring equitable access to microbiome-based interventions and addressing concerns regarding safety and long-term effects are critical considerations in advancing this field.

CONCLUSION

These advancements in cancer immunotherapy have transformed the landscape of cancer treatment, offering new hope for patients with previously untreatable or advanced malignancies. Ongoing research continues to refine existing therapies and develop novel approaches to harness the power of the immune system against cancer. Further research and clinical trials are needed to realize their full potential in preventing and treating cancer in humans. Collaborative efforts between researchers, clinicians, and pharmaceutical companies are essential to advance this promising area of cancer immunotherapy.

■ SUGGESTED READING

1. Adotévi O, Vernerey D, Jacoulet P, Meurisse A, Laheurte C, Almotlak H, et al. Safety, immunogenicity, and 1-year efficacy of universal cancer peptide-based vaccine in patients with refractory advanced non-small-cell lung cancer: A phase ib/phase iia de-escalation study. J Clin Oncol. 2023;41:373-84.
2. American Society of Clinical Oncology (ASCO). What are Cancer Vaccines? Available from: https://www.cancer.net/navigating-cancer-care/how-cancer-treated/immunotherapy-and-vaccines/what-are-cancer-vaccines [Last accessed May, 2024].
3. American Society of Hematology. (2023). ASH Annual Meeting and Exposition. Available from: https://www.hematology.org/meetings/annual-meeting [Last accessed May, 2024].
4. Cancer Council Australia. (2023). Understanding Cancer of the Uterus. Available from: https://www.cancer.org.au/assets/pdf/understanding-uterus-cancer-booklet [Last accessed May, 2024].
5. Castle JC, Uduman M, Pabla S, Stein RB, Buell JS. Mutation-Derived Neoantigens for Cancer Immunotherapy. Front Immunol. 2019;10:1856.
6. Dibajnia P, Cardenas LM, Lalani AA. The emerging landscape of neo/adjuvant immunotherapy in renal cell carcinoma. Hum Vaccin Immunother. 2023;19(1):2178217.
7. Faustino-Rocha AI, Jota-Baptista C, Nascimento-Gonçalves E, Oliveira PA. Evolution of Models of Prostate Cancer: Their Contribution to Current Therapies. Anticancer Res. 2023;43(1):323-33.
8. Gil-Gil M, Alba E, Gavilá J, de la Haba-Rodríguez J, Ciruelos E, Tolosa P, et al. The role of CDK4/6 inhibitors in early breast cancer. Breast. 2021;58:160-9.
9. Greene BL, Rosenberg AR, Marron JM. A Communication and Decision-Making Framework for Pediatric Precision Medicine. Pediatrics. 2024;153(4):e2023062850.
10. Harari A, Sarivalasis A, de Jonge K, Thierry AC, Huber F, Boudousquie C, et al. A personalized neoantigen vaccine in combination with platinum-based chemotherapy induces a T-cell response coinciding with a complete response in endometrial carcinoma. Cancers (Basel). 2021;13(22):5801.
11. Hui P, Gysler SM, Uduman M, Togun TA, Prado DE, Brambs CE, et al. MicroRNA signatures discriminate between uterine and ovarian serous carcinomas. Hum Pathol. 2018;76:133-40.
12. Hu Z, Leet DE, Allesøe RL, Oliveira G, Li S, Luoma AM, et al. Personal neoantigen vaccines induce persistent memory T cell responses and epitope spreading in patients with melanoma. Nat Med. 2021;27(3):515-25.
13. Iqbal N, Iqbal N. Human Epidermal Growth Factor Receptor 2 (HER2) in Cancers: Overexpression and Therapeutic Implications. Mol Biol Int. 2014;2014:852748.
14. Jiang XT, Liu Q. mRNA vaccination in breast cancer: current progress and future direction. J Cancer Res Clin Oncol. 2023:1-16.
15. Jia W, Zhang T, Huang H, Feng H, Wang S, Guo Z, et al. Colorectal cancer vaccines: The current scenario and future prospects. Front Immunol. 2022;13:942235.
16. Jin KT, Chen B, Liu YY, Lan HU, Yan JP. Monoclonal antibodies and chimeric antigen receptor (CAR) T cells in the treatment of colorectal cancer. Cancer Cell Int. 2021;21(1):83.
17. Mehrotra R and Yadav K. Cervical Cancer: Formulation and Implementation of Govt of India Guidelines for Screening and Management. Indian J Gynecol Oncol. 2022;20(1):4.
18. Narita Y, Muro K. Updated Immunotherapy for Gastric Cancer. J Clin Med. 2023;12(7):2636.
19. National Institutes of Health. (2023). An mRNA vaccine to treat pancreatic cancer. Available from: https://www.nih.gov/news-events/nih-research-matters/mrna-vaccine-treat-pancreatic-cancer [Last accessed May, 2024].
20. Noh JH, Shin JY, Lee JH, Park YS, Lee IS, Kim GH, et al. Clinical Significance of Epstein-Barr Virus and Helicobacter pylori Infection in Gastric Carcinoma. Gut Liver. 2023;17(1):69-77.
21. Pant S, Wainberg ZA, Weekes CD, Furqan M, Kasi PM, Devoe CE, et al. Lymph-node-targeted, mKRAS-specific amphiphile vaccine in pancreatic and colorectal cancer: the phase 1 AMPLIFY-201 trial. Nat Med. 2024;30:531-42.
22. Penn Medicine. CAR T Cell Therapy. Available from: https://www.pennmedicine.org/cancer/navigating-cancer-care/treatment-types/immunotherapy/what-is-car-t-therapy [Last accessed May, 2024].
23. Rojas LA, Sethna Z, Soares KC, Olcese C, Pang N, Patterson E, et al. Personalized RNA neoantigen vaccines stimulate T cells in pancreatic cancer. Nature. 2023;618(7963):144-50.
24. Schepisi G, Gianni C, Cursano MC, Gallà V, Menna C, Casadei C, et al. Immune checkpoint inhibitors and Chimeric Antigen Receptor (CAR)-T cell therapy: Potential treatment options against Testicular Germ Cell Tumors. Front Immunol. 2023;14:1118610.
25. Srinivasan S, Ramanathan S, Prasad M. Wilms Tumor in India: A Systematic Review. South Asian J Cancer. 2023;12(2):206-12.
26. Stallard J. (2024). Investigational mRNA Vaccine Induced Persistent Immune Response in Phase 1 Trial of Patients With Pancreatic Cancer. Available from: https://www.mskcc.org/news/can-mrna-vaccines-fight-pancreatic-cancer-msk-clinical-researchers-are-trying-find-out [Last accessed May, 2024].
27. Supra R, Agrawal DK. Immunotherapeutic Strategies in the Management of Osteosarcoma. J Orthop Sports Med. 2023;5(1):32-40.
28. Talbot LJ, Lautz TB, Aldrink JH, Ehrlich PF, Dasgupta R, Mattei P, et al. Implications of Immunotherapy for

Pediatric Malignancies: A Summary from the APSA Cancer Committee. J Pediatr Surg. 2023;58(11):2119-27.
29. Verdun N, Marks P. Secondary Cancers after Chimeric Antigen Receptor T-Cell Therapy. NEJM; Published online 24 January 2024. DOI: 10.1056/NEJMp2400209
30. Wang L, Li S, Mei J, Ye L. Immunotherapies of retinoblastoma: Effective methods for preserving vision in the future. Front Oncol. 2022;12:949193.
31. Wan HH, Zhu H, Chiang CC, Li JS, Ren F, Tsai CT, et al. High sensitivity saliva-based biosensor in detection of breast cancer biomarkers: HER2 and CA15-3. J Vac Sci Technol B Nanotechnol Microelectron. 2024;42(2): 023202.
32. Yang C, Xia BR, Zhang ZC, Zhang YJ, Lou G, Jin WL. Immunotherapy for Ovarian Cancer: Adjuvant, Combination, and Neoadjuvant. Front Immunol. 2020;11: 577869.
33. Yin S, Biran A, Kretzmer H, Ten Hacken E, Parvin S, Lucas F, et al. B Cell-Restricted Depletion of Dnmt3a Activates Notch Signaling and Causes Chronic Lymphocytic Leukemia. Blood. 2021;138:249.
34. Zeng Z, Fu J, Cibulskis C, Jhaveri A, Gumbs C, Das B. Cross-site concordance evaluation of tumor DNA and RNA sequencing platforms for the CIMAC-CIDC network. Clin Cancer Res. 2021;27(18):5049-61.
35. Zhou C, Tang KJ, Cho BC, Liu B, Paz-Ares L, Cheng S, et al.; PAPILLON Investigators. Amivantamab plus Chemotherapy in NSCLC with EGFR Exon 20 Insertions. N Engl J Med. 2023;389:2039-51.

CHAPTER 12

Vaccines and Immunotherapies against Noncommunicable Diseases

Jr Uduman, AK Uduman

■ INTRODUCTION

Noncommunicable diseases (NCDs) are also known as chronic diseases that do not spread, nor are transmissible directly from one person to another person and are one of the major burdens on public health. According to the World Health Organization (WHO), NCDs kill 41 million people each year, which is 74% of all deaths globally. This is more than all communicable disease deaths combined.

Vaccines and immunotherapy represent innovative approaches to managing NCDs, which include a wide range of chronic conditions such as cardiovascular diseases (CVDs), cancers, chronic respiratory diseases, and degenerative neurologic disorders, and diabetes. Unlike infectious diseases (IDs), NCDs are not caused by pathogens and therefore present unique challenges for vaccine development and immunotherapy. However, recent advances have shown promise in these areas.

Currently, there are no vaccines available that can directly prevent NCDs such as cancer, heart disease, and diabetes. However, certain vaccines can indirectly reduce the risk of developing these diseases by targeting specific factors associated with them.

The predominant NCDs are multiple sclerosis (MS), Parkinson's disease (PD), autoimmune diseases, atherosclerosis, strokes, heart diseases, most cancers, diabetes, chronic kidney disease, osteoarthritis (OA), osteoporosis, Alzheimer's disease (AD), and others. Most are noninfectious, although there are some noncommunicable IDs, such as parasitic diseases in which the parasite's life cycle does not include direct host-to-host transmission.

The development of vaccines specifically targeting NCDs remains an area of ongoing research. Focusing on specific risk factors for heart disease, like high cholesterol and high blood pressure, is important. Vaccines that lower cholesterol could help prevent heart problems in people who are at higher risk.

■ BACKGROUND

Vaccines are primarily designed to prevent IDs, which are caused by pathogens such as bacteria and viruses that can be transmitted from person to person. Also allow people to live longer and healthier as their life expectancy has increased. NCDs, on the other hand, are generally not caused by infectious agents and are not transmissible from one person to another. Instead, they are typically associated with lifestyle factors, genetics, and environmental influences.

Noncommunicable diseases, mostly autoimmune disorders are characterized by the immune-mediated attack on healthy tissue, often due to a misdirected immune response to self-antigen. The regulatory T-cells (Tregs) play an important role in suppressing the activation of the immune system and maintaining immune homeostasis and self-antigen tolerance.

There are clinical situations where vaccines can indirectly help prevent some NCDs. For example, vaccines that protect against certain IDs can reduce the risk of complications that might contribute to the development of an NCD. Clinical evidence suggests that pneumococcal and influenza vaccinations can prevent community-acquired pneumonia and acute exacerbations in chronic obstructive pulmonary disease (COPD) patients, while pneumococcal vaccination early in the course of COPD could help maintain stable health status.

Also, the hepatitis B vaccine can help prevent chronic hepatitis B infection, which, if left untreated, can lead to liver disease and potentially liver cancer. This shifting burden of disease has heightened the already urgent need for therapies that treat or prevent NCDs, a need that is now being met with increased efforts to develop NCD vaccines.

- An active vaccine targeting "proprotein convertase subtilisin/kexin 9 (PCSK9)" or apolipoprotein CIII (APOC3) has the potential to reduce the progression of atherosclerosis, the underlying cause of heart attacks and strokes.

- Active research is underway in the field of creating a vaccine against AD, where the target proteins are amyloid β and tau proteins.
- A significant breakthrough has been made in the development of allergy vaccines based on recombinant allergens. Some of them are now in the final stages of clinical research.
- NCD vaccinations against cancers including vaccines against breast, ovarian, and prostate cancer are discussed in detail.

NEW WAVE OF VACCINES FOR NONCOMMUNICABLE DISEASES

Although NCDs are typically associated with lifestyle factors, genetics, and environmental influences, efforts are underway to develop NCD vaccines, especially against infectious agents that are linked with certain NCDs, e.g., MS versus Epstein–Barr virus (EBV), Crohn's disease (CD), rheumatic heart disease (RHD) versus group A *Streptococcus* (GAS), and type 1 diabetes versus enteroviruses (EVs).

Noncommunicable disease vaccines present an interesting challenge for the US Food and Drug Administration (FDA), which is tasked with approving new treatments based on efficacy and safety. This chapter explores the emerging class of NCD vaccines, explains how they differ from traditional vaccines, and describes some regulatory implications of this innovative type of therapeutic.

The impact of vaccines on NCDs is often indirect, as they reduce the risk factors or complications associated with NCDs. Preventing NCDs usually requires lifestyle modifications, such as a healthy diet, regular exercise, and not smoking, in addition to vaccination when applicable. Public health strategies often involve a combination of vaccinations and lifestyle interventions to address the burden of NCDs.

Scientists hope to offer new vaccines for cancer, heart disease, and other NCD conditions by 2030. Advancements in messenger ribonucleic acid (RNA) technology since the outset of the coronavirus disease (COVID) pandemic have ushered in a golden age for new preventive and therapeutic vaccines.

In India, NCDs are the leading cause of mortality, contributing to 66% of total deaths each year (WHO, 2019); further revealed that there was a 22% probability of death between the ages of 30 and 70 due to any type of NCD, including CVDs, cancer, diabetes, or COPD. Individuals with these diseases are more susceptible to vaccine-preventable diseases (VPDs) and have an increased risk of associated disease severity and complications. This poses a substantial burden on healthcare systems and economies, exemplified by the coronavirus disease-2019 (COVID-19) pandemic.

Also, monoclonal antibodies (mAbs) biologicals represent the largest class of therapeutic proteins in clinical use. The majority of currently marketed mAbs are used for the treatment of NCDs such as cancer or autoimmune disorders. Only a small number of mAbs have to date been licensed to treat or prevent IDs, the number of such products in development is growing.

TWO CASE-BASED CLINICAL SCENARIOS

Authors have dealt with vaccinations' role in "NCDs" in recent years in Question and Answer format. These are our introductory messages for readers of this chapter.

1. *Case scenario question and answer:*

    Answered query from a senior physician, in Tamil Nadu (requested not to quote his identity): A 71-year-old Tamil Nadu medical practitioners asking us how to diagnose AD as he gets easy forgetfulness, these days. States that, has been taking daily vitamins, and his recent executive blood screening tests are all OK. He is not diabetic nor has BP issues. Sir, what test you can suggest to confirm or exclude Alzheimer's, please"?

    The author's suggested advice is as follows:
    - You may discuss with your neuro and/or geriatric physicians. They may recommend one or more of these diagnostic tests and procedures as part of an evaluation for AD.
    - Brain MRI to ensure no gross neuronal or space-occupying abnormalities. The positron emission tomography (PET) scan certainly identifies amyloid proteins that are associated with AD.
    - Can get a blood test called a "Precivity AD test" that measures the amounts of proteins such as beta-amyloid and ApoE in blood.
    - Recently shown simple urine spot test for *formic acid excretion* by colorimetry. This test may not yet be available commercially, I guess nor have the FDA approval yet.
    - One of the greatest medical advances in history is soon coming. *"Beta-amyloid vaccines"* for the treatment and prevention of AD could be 2 or 3 years away from learning whether it works!!!

To conclude: The *"beta-amyloid vaccine"* strategy is now being applied to the treatment and prevention of Alzheimer's. It is designed to train the immune system to recognize beta-amyloid plaques, leading to the production of beta-amyloid antibodies.

2. *Case scenario question and answer:*
   A senior Indian philanthropist wrote to us about the news flash that appeared on "The Hindu" newspaper; "The Cuban developed Alzheimer's vaccines, is this news really, true? Please tell me sir"?

   Author's response: As of January 6, 2023, at least nine Alzheimer's vaccines are in clinical trials.
   - Vaccines are one of the greatest medical advances in history. This strategy is now being applied to treating and preventing Alzheimer's. We could be 4 years away from learning whether it works.
   - Nose drop vaccine for AD (Nasal Vax). This is a "remarkable milestone".
     Alzheimer's vaccine (called "Vaxxinity") has received the FDA's fast-track designation for its candidate Alzheimer's vaccine, UB-311 this past May 2022.
   - UB-311 is an immunotherapeutic vaccine candidate. It targets one of Alzheimer's main biomarkers: Toxic forms of aggregated amyloid protein in the brain. Its phase 1, phase 2a, and phase 2a long-term extension trials have shown it to be well tolerated in people living with mild-to-moderate Alzheimer's over 3 years of repeat dosing.

■ ALZHEIMER'S DISEASE VACCINES

Alzheimer's disease is the most common cause of dementia that normally starts in late life. Despite decades of intensive research on AD, there is still a lack of effective strategies to prevent and treat AD. Dementia is a broad terminology referring to a range of disorders that affect how a person's brain works, causing symptoms including memory loss, behavior changes, and difficulty speaking and walking. The most common form of dementia is AD, which accounts for 60–80% of dementia cases. Phosphorylated tau (p-tau) is a specific blood biomarker of AD pathology, with p-tau217 considered to have the most utility.

Vaccines and immunotherapies for diseases like Alzheimer's are being researched, with some approaches aiming to clear amyloid-beta plaques from the brain or to target tau proteins, both of which are hallmarks of AD pathology.

More than 55 million people around the world have dementia, with about 10 million cases added each year.

The diagnosis of AD, which is rapidly increasing in prevalence and incidence worldwide, can lead to a sense of "hopelessness" among patients, their caregivers, and their doctors.

There is currently no cure for AD. However, there is medicine available that can temporarily reduce the symptoms. Support is also available to help someone with the condition, and their family, cope with everyday life.

There are approved drugs and early diagnostic accuracy for Alzheimer's aimed at either changing disease progression or helping lower some symptoms of the condition in advance. The wider availability of high-performing assays may expedite the use of blood biomarkers in clinical settings and benefit the research community.

Approved drugs to treat AD are as follows:
- *Donepezil (Aricept®):* Approved to treat all stages of AD
- *Rivastigmine (Exelon®):* Approved for mild-to-moderate AD as well as mild-to-moderate dementia associated with PD
- *Galantamine (Razadyne®):* Approved for mild-to-moderate stages of AD

It is an exciting time in AD research, with over 100 potential therapies being tested at various stages of the research process, and many more being developed. However, there is currently no cure nor a preventative vaccine for AD or most cases of dementia.

The FDA has granted "accelerated approval" for the amyloid-targeting mAb drug lecanemab, which has been shown to moderately slow cognitive decline.

The novel vaccine that targets inflamed brain cells associated with AD may hold the key to potentially preventing or modifying the course of the disease, according to preliminary research presented at the American Heart Association's Basic Cardiovascular Sciences Scientific.

Alzheimer's Vaccine: That After Nearly 20 Years of Research

The first human clinical trial of a nasal candidate vaccine to slow the progression of AD is set to begin and has just received the FDA's fast-track designation! This is a "remarkable milestone" and amazed to have preclinical evidence suggesting the potential of this nasal vaccine for AD!

The vaccine features an experimental agent called Protollin that stimulates the immune system. It is designed to prompt white blood cells in the lymph nodes on the sides and back of the neck to migrate to the brain and clear beta-amyloid plaques, a hallmark of AD.

Currently, at least nine Alzheimer's vaccines are in trials right now.

Vaccines are one of the greatest medical advances in history. This strategy is now being applied to the treatment and prevention of Alzheimer's. We could be 4 years away from learning whether it works.

Beta-Amyloid Vaccines

Some of the vaccines in trials right now are designed to train the immune system to recognize beta-amyloid plaques, leading to the production of beta-amyloid antibodies.

All the Alzheimer's vaccines in clinical trials right now are given in **Table 1**.

The Institute for Molecular Medicine (IMM) developing a vaccine platform for Alzheimer's that expects to stimulate memory and naive T helper cells, which in turn activate B-cells to produce antibodies at a much higher rate up to 10 times than vaccines currently used in clinical trials. With a large number of produced antibodies, the goal is to prevent/suppress the aggregation of (beta-amyloid) and/or tau and stop or at least delay the onset of the disease.

Monoclonal Antibody Therapy for Alzheimer's

Two antiamyloid monoclonal antibodies (mAbs) lecanemab (Leqembi®) and aducanumab (Aduhelm®) mAbs have been approved in the USA for the treatment of AD.

Antiamyloid mAbs are the first disease-modifying therapies for AD that achieve slowing of clinical decline by intervening in the basic biological processes of the disease. These are breakthrough agents that can slow the inevitable progression of AD into more severe cognitive impairment. The results of trials of antiamyloid mAbs support the amyloid hypothesis and amyloid as a target for AD drug development.

The success of mAbs reflects a relentless application of neuroscience knowledge to solving major challenges facing humankind. The success of these transformative agents will foster the development of more antiamyloid mAbs, other types of antiamyloid therapies, treatments of other targets of AD biology, and new approaches to therapies for an array of neurodegenerative disorders.

In essence, at present, two mAbs against beta-amyloid showed efficacy in the early stages of AD. In terms of everyday clinical practice, setting up the infrastructure for the diagnosis and treatment of these patients, and for follow-up, will be expensive and will be a major problem for most healthcare systems.

Cell-based Immunotherapy

The innate immune system and the adaptive immune system are both involved in the pathology of AD. Postmortem AD patients' brain parenchyma has revealed the presence of T-cells, and T-cell abnormalities have been detected in the blood and cerebral spinal fluid of AD patients. In comparison to the non-AD control group, the majority of AD patients exhibit a higher occurrence of T-cells in the brain parenchyma.

There is remarkable evidence indicating that the innate immune mechanism and adaptive immune response play significant roles in the pathogenesis of AD. Several studies have reported changes in CD8+ and CD4+ T-cells and cytokines in AD pathogenesis.

TABLE 1: Alzheimer's vaccines in clinical trials.

Name	Phase	Company	Target
AADvac1	2	Axon Neuroscience SE	Tau
UB-311	2B	Vaxxinity	Beta-amyloid
ACI-35	2	AC Immune SA, Janssen	Tau
Bacillus Calmette–Guérin	1	Massachusetts General Hospital	Immune system
ABvac40	2	Araclon Biotech	Beta-amyloid
ACI-24	2	AC Immune SA	Beta-amyloid
GV1001	2	GemVax & KAEL Bio	Immune system
ALZ-101	1	Alzinova AB	Beta-amyloid
Protollin	1	Brigham and Women's Hospital	Immune system

Enhanced natural killer cell therapy has shown promise in Alzheimer's. Emerging cell-based immunotherapy is highly specific to the cells responsible for Alzheimer's, avoids drug resistance, has long-lasting results, and has fewer side effects than drug counterparts.

The use of antigen-specific regulatory T-cells (Tregs) targeting β-amyloid through adoptive transfer has shown promise for the treatment of many AD patients.

■ MULTIPLE SCLEROSIS VACCINE

The global incidence of MS appears to be increasing. Although it may not be associated with a high mortality rate, this disease has a high morbidity which affects the quality of life of patients and reduces their ability to do their activities of daily living.

Multiple sclerosis is a long-lasting condition that affects the central nervous system (CNS), which includes the brain and spinal cord and can be severely debilitating. It is typified by the immune system targeting the myelin sheath that surrounds nerve fibers for protection, which causes communication issues between the brain and the body as a whole. The immune system going awry might eventually lead to irreversible nerve injury or degeneration **(Fig. 1)**.

The exact cause is unknown but mainly occurs between the ages of 20 and 40. Women are two to three times more likely than men to develop it. Individuals with a family history of the disease are at a higher risk. Infection with EBV has long been postulated to trigger MS and nearly everyone is infected with EBV during childhood, but only a small fraction develops MS. Other risk factors, such as genetic susceptibility, low levels of vitamin D, and smoking have been linked and are important in MS pathogenesis. It is more prevalent in people living in temperate climates.

The EBV seropositivity was nearly ubiquitous at the time of MS development, with only one of 801 MS cases being EBV seronegative at the time of MS onset. These findings provide compelling data that implicate EBV as the trigger for the development of MS. Further, multiple studies have identified EBV-infected B-cells in the brains of MS patients.

Model for Multiple Sclerosis Development

In at-risk individuals, EBV infection of B-cells promotes the development of MS through several possible mechanisms. These include molecular mimicry by EBV nuclear antigen 1 (EBNA-1), B-cell transformation through latent membrane protein 1 (LMP1) and LMP2A, induction of B-cell trafficking to the CNS, and/or other unknown mechanisms.

Multiple sclerosis is a chronic autoimmune disease of the CNS in which the immune system attacks the protective covering of nerve fibers, leading to a range of neurological symptoms. While there are treatments available to help manage the symptoms and slow the progression of the disease, there is no known cure for MS at this time. Research into potential MS therapies, including vaccines, is ongoing; however, no vaccine has been developed to cure MS.

Epstein–Barr Virus Role in Multiple Sclerosis

Experts believe that in susceptible individuals, EBV-infected B-cells travel to the brain and cause inflammation and damage. By preventing this at an early stage of infection, the infected B-cells cannot go on to cause the development of secondary diseases like MS.

A recent paper in Science about MS in the US military demonstrated that there was a 32-fold increased risk for MS among 955 members of the military, who unfortunately developed MS. Almost all who developed MS had evidence in their smaller cohort, where they had samples longitudinally to assess for EBV, that they developed MS only after EBV infection. This was, on average, 10 years after acquiring the virus.

Given that EBV is a major risk factor for developing MS, an effective vaccine that prevents EBV infection in humans may also have an important role in preventing the onset of MS. Although the extent of EBV's involvement in ongoing disease activity in MS remains unclear, the pursuit of therapeutic vaccines to treat MS is an area of active investigation.

Epstein–Barr virus (HHV-4) is one of the most common human viruses in the world. It is the first identified oncogenic virus, which establishes permanent infection in humans. It spreads primarily through saliva. EBV can cause infectious mononucleosis, also called mono. Also associated with several other distinct disorders, including nasopharyngeal carcinoma, Burkitt lymphoma, undifferentiated B- or T-lymphocyte lymphomas, X-linked lymphoproliferative syndrome, posttransplantation lymphoproliferative disorders, etc. A variety of clinical manifestations have also been associated with EBV reactivation.

Although rare; EBV reactivation has also been associated with symptoms of long-term COVID even in immunologically normal individuals. These are:

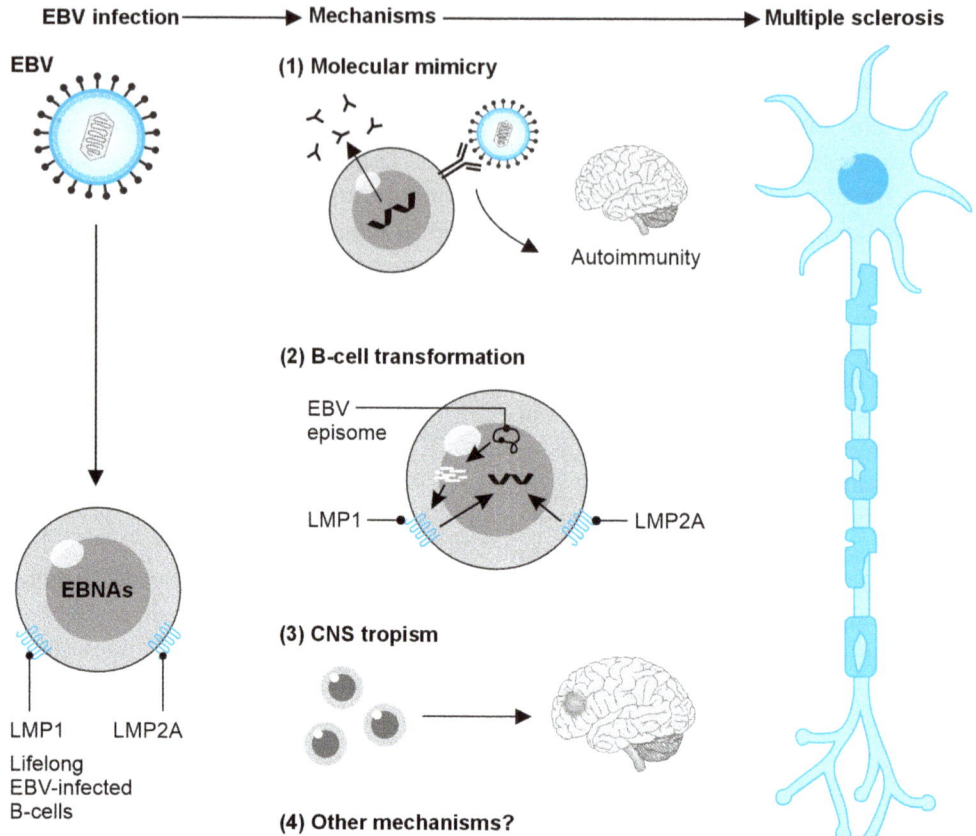

Fig. 1: Part of the Epstein–Barr virus (EBV) mimics a protein made in the brain and spinal cord, leading the immune system to mistakenly attack the body's nerve cells. Risk of multiple sclerosis (MS) increased 32-fold after infection with EBV but was not increased after infection with other viruses, including the similarly transmitted cytomegalovirus. Serum levels of neurofilament light chain, a biomarker of neuroaxonal degeneration, increased only after EBV seroconversion. These findings cannot be explained by any known risk factor for MS and suggest EBV as the leading cause of MS.

- Multifaceted neurologic, hematological, and cardiovascular complications
- EBV-associated multisystem failure has been documented to also result in acute liver injury, kidney injury, respiratory failure, and hemolytic anemia
- EBV reactivation has been reported to play a role in the pathogenesis of myocarditis, inflammatory cardiomyopathy, etc.
- EBV is also associated with several lymphoid and epithelial tumors

Therefore, EBV vaccine development has been an elusive goal for many years and may cut the risk of MS, but also many various cancers and autoimmune disorders.

Inverse Vaccine

Scientists hope this new type of inverse vaccine could help treat autoimmune diseases, such as MS, type 1 diabetes, allergic asthma, or CD.

In autoimmune diseases, the body's immune system—our defense against illness—cannot tell the difference between good cells and bad cells and ends up attacking them all. So people get sick either way. In a study published October 2023 in Nature Biomedical Engineering, the scientists say a so-called "inverse vaccine" helped them stop an immune response from attacking healthy cells when it was faced with a laboratory model of an autoimmune disease.

What is an Inverse Vaccine?

Conventional vaccines train the immune system to spot IDs and stop them from multiplying and spreading. Take the COVID-19 vaccine, for example, it contains elements that represent the coronavirus (CoV)—severe acute respiratory syndrome coronavirus 2 (SARS CoV-2) spike protein; the thing that attaches itself to cells and infects them and makes people sick of COVID-19. For people who had a COVID-19 vaccine, their body should be able to recognize that spikey shape of the virus attached to a cell and kill it.

An inverse vaccine, on the other hand, stops the immune system from attacking cells specifically, good and healthy cells. Instead, it retrains the immune system to save healthy cells, essentially by adding a "do not attack" flag.

The inverse vaccine is still in development and has not been tested on humans. Inverse vaccines are "a whole new concept of vaccination" that may one day treat many autoimmune diseases. The concept of an inverse vaccine is not new. It was pioneered by Stanford researcher Lawrence Steinman in the early 2000s.

Now that the initial trigger for MS has been identified, perhaps MS could be eradicated. Thus, given these additional gating factors in MS pathogenesis, infection with EBV is likely to be necessary, but not sufficient, to trigger the development of MS. Infection with EBV is the initial pathogenic step in MS, but additional fuses must be ignited for the full pathophysiology.

To conclude, as most MS cases appear to be caused by EBV, a suitable vaccine could, in theory, prevent infection and prevent MS. Also, antivirals that target EBV early in the course of the disease may be an effective therapy.

Monoclonal Antibody Used in Multiple Sclerosis

Monoclonal antibodies are one of the preferred treatments for MS due to their target specificity and usually high efficacy. These have usually targeted the immune system, which plays a key role in the pathogenesis of MS, especially during the early inflammatory stages.

Monoclonal antibodies bind very specifically to epitopes or parts of larger proteins (antigens) that allow them to mediate their effects on very specific pathways. In MS, mAbs can more specifically neutralize key immune players that negatively impact the CNS.

Natalizumab was the first mAb approved by the US-FDA for the treatment of MS in 2004, heralding the age of mAbs for the treatment of MS. Other mAbs have followed including alemtuzumab and ocrelizumab.

Rituximab and *ofatumumab* have been used off-label in the treatment of MS and *ofatumumab* are undergoing phase 3 studies for approval in MS.

Frexalimab

The CD40-CD40L costimulatory pathway regulates adaptive and innate immune responses and has been implicated in the pathogenesis of MS. Frexalimab is a second-generation anti-CD40L mAb being evaluated for the treatment of MS. Inhibitors of the CD40 pathway could downregulate innate immunity in the CNS, a major contributor to progressive MS.

In a phase 2 trial involving participants with MS, inhibition of CD40L with frexalimab had an effect that generally favored a greater reduction in the number of new gadolinium-enhancing T1-weighted lesions at week 12 as compared with placebo. Larger and longer trials are needed to determine the long-term efficacy and safety of frexalimab in persons with MS.

New Horizons and Future Trends for Therapeutic MS mAbs

Monoclonal antibodies have become a mainstay of MS treatment and they are likely to continue to be developed and optimized for the treatment of this disease, such as analyzing the safety of faster infusion times and administration by subcutaneous routes.

Monoclonal antibodies are some of the most effective therapies for relapsing MS without the side effects associated with chemotherapeutic agents. Additionally, new mAbs are being developed to help repair the damage/disability that has already occurred, which is promising.

New advancements in bioengineering are being incorporated into antibodies that are more humanized to help optimize their effectiveness and improve their tolerability and safety. Overall, it is expected that mAbs will continue to be a preferred therapy for MS in the foreseeable future.

Cell-based Therapies for Multiple Sclerosis

According to an announcement, the FDA has cleared Kyverna Therapeutics' investigational new drug application to test KYV-101, a CAR T-cell therapy, in patients with refractory progressive MS, a disease for which there are limited available therapies.

Stem Cell Therapy

There is convincing evidence that autologous hematopoietic stem cell transplantation (aHSCT) is effective in stopping inflammatory MS activity and improving neurological disability in people with MS. In aHSCT, wiping out a person's immune system and then regrowing it using the person's hematopoietic stem cells. These are stem cells that can develop into all types of bone marrow (BM) cells.

■ MYASTHENIA GRAVIS VACCINE

This autoimmune disorder is characterized by weakness and rapid fatigue of any of the muscles under voluntary control due to a defect in the transmission of nerve impulses to muscles. The treatment typically focuses on managing symptoms and may include medications such as acetylcholinesterase inhibitors, immunosuppressant drugs, and therapies like plasmapheresis or intravenous immunoglobulin (IVIG). In some cases, surgical removal of the thymus gland may improve symptoms. It is crucial to note that each patient's case is unique, and the course of the disease and response to treatment can vary widely.

Immunotherapies are crucial for any treatment options because the long-term success of myasthena gravies therapy ultimately depends on limiting the underlying autoimmune process.

Monoclonal antibodies (mAb) therapy: RYSTIGGO (rozanolixizumab-noli) is indicated for the treatment of generalized myasthenia gravis (gMG) in adult patients who are anti-acetylcholine receptor (AChR) or anti-muscle-specific tyrosine kinase (MuSK) antibody positive.

As of this date, there is no anti-myasthenia gravis (MG) specific vaccine; also the risk of exacerbation after vaccines is debated. The issue of vaccinations in patients affected by immune-mediated diseases has frequently raised concerns and speculations of possible causal relationships between certain vaccines and disease onset or exacerbation. For example, there are by now many articles and reviews reporting the risk of Guillain–Barré syndrome (GBS) following influenza vaccination; in particular, a meta-analysis has confirmed the evidence of such a slight, yet significant risk.

Regarding MS, several case reports and articles have been published; however, a review published in 2017 highlights the absence of an association between many vaccines and MS onset or exacerbation, except H1N1 and yellow fever vaccinations, where further studies are needed to establish a potential causal relationship.

Myasthenia gravis is a disease caused by a type-II hypersensitivity reaction and, as such, the production of pathogenic antibodies might precede clinical manifestations by years. For such diseases, it has been postulated that vaccines might respectively exacerbate or "unveil" manifest and subclinical preexisting diseases, through nonspecific systemic immune stimulation, rather than triggering a de novo disease. Regarding the relationships between vaccines and MG, there are also various experimental studies investigating the potential use of therapeutic vaccines or peptides against MG.

Vaccines for Myasthenia Gravis

T-cell Receptor Vaccines

A pathogenic T-cell population expressing the Vβ5.1 has been defined in patients with MG expressing the HLA-DR3 haplotype. In experimental autoimmune MG, Vβ5.1 T-cell receptor (TCR) vaccination proved to be efficient and associated with an increase of anti-TCR antibodies. The TCR vaccine may boost innate regulatory T-cells and antibodies directed against the TCR of pathogenic T-cells and reverse clinical deficits after the onset of the disease. Therefore, the TCR vaccination approach is effective in MG, which has the potential to improve the type and quality of care available to these patients and reduce the considerable cost of their clinical care over the long term.

Peptide-based Vaccines

Therapeutic vaccines are developed with an algorithm for the design of peptides that assume complementary contours to proteinaceous autoantigenic determinants. These peptides, termed complementary peptides, can bind the target determinant and in a sense appear as antigen receptor mimetics (ARM). Thus, when used as vaccines, they elicit anti-idiotypic (Id) responses against the combining sites of antigen receptors on certain autoreactive T- and B-lymphocytes. By targeting ARM vaccines to the AChR T- or B-cell epitope, antibody can be induced that specifically recognized and bound antigen receptors on AChR α100–116 reactive T-cells and AChR α61–76 reactive B-cells, respectively. The resulting anti-ARM antibody/antigen receptor interactions interfere with autoreactive T-cells and autoreactive B-cells, thereby significantly reducing the level of AChR-reactive auto-antibody. This, in turn, leads to significant clinical improvements in reducing muscle fatigue, reducing mortality and maintaining muscle AChR levels.

Inactivated and subunit vaccines are safe and effective in MG. Although some of them, such as the anti-SARS-CoV-2 vaccine, might uncommonly cause MG exacerbations, data from the literature review suggest that the benefits still outweigh by far the potential risks, thus they should be recommended to these patients. Nevertheless, large prospective studies are needed for further investigations.

The review of the MG literature suggests that inactivated and subunit vaccines are safe in myasthenic patients. Remarkably, increasing vaccination rates against respiratory pathogens might reduce the burden of disease exacerbation at the population level.

Regarding anti-SARS-CoV-2 vaccination, results from available literature suggest that it might rarely lead to disease worsening. However, the evidence has shown that the combination of MG and COVID-19 might trigger the exacerbation of either of the two. Thus, given the entity of the current pandemic, the benefits of anti-SARS-CoV-2 vaccination in myasthenic patients still outweigh by far the potential risks. In addition, the reported cases of new-onset post-vaccine MG seem to be mostly anecdotal, except those putatively related to the Japanese encephalitis vaccination, which is indeed worth investigating.

Beneficial Monoclonal Antibody Therapies

Natalizumab (NTZ, Tysabri®), a humanized monoclonal antibody targeting the alpha chain of the α4β1 adhesion molecule, is approved for the treatment of relapsing-remitting multiple sclerosis (RR-MS). It has been shown to reduce the relapse rate by 68% and the risk of disability progression by 42%.

Most recently, in November 2023, the FDA approved the first biosimilar for MS, Tyruko (natalizumab-site), which is a biosimilar to Tysabri (natalizumab).

VACCINES AND PARKINSON PLUS SYNDROMES

Parkinson Plus Syndrome versus Parkinson's Disease versus Parkinsonism

Generally, there is a lot of confusion about Parkinson plus syndrome (PPS) versus PD and parkinsonism.
- *Parkinsonism* is not technically a diagnosis, but rather a set of symptoms including slowness, stiffness, tremor, and problems with walking and balance. There is a list of diseases that manifest with these parkinsonism symptoms and they include PD, drug-induced parkinsonism, vascular parkinsonism, multiple system atrophy (MSA), dementia with Lewy bodies (DLB), progressive supranuclear palsy (PSP), and corticobasal ganglionic degeneration (CBGD).
- *PD* fundamentally for the vast majority of people, is entirely preventable. We are not taking action to prevent people from getting this very disabling and very deadly disease.
- *PPS* is a group of neurodegenerative conditions in which PD symptoms are present along with other signs of neurologic impairment.
- Because there is no available biomarker (being researched) or specific test that can be performed to easily distinguish these conditions from each other, the diagnosis can sometimes be unclear and often is in fluidity.
- Patients with PD are at higher risk of vaccine-preventable respiratory infections. However, advanced, home-bound individuals may have less access to vaccinations.

Because the cause of Parkinson's is unknown, there are no proven ways to prevent the disease.

Parkinson's disease is associated with protein deposits in the brain called Lewy bodies, which are composed of an accumulation of alpha-synuclein. In Parkinson's, alpha-synuclein misfolds and aggregates into Lewy bodies. For that reason, it is thought that preventing alpha-synuclein aggregation and removing existing clumps could be an effective way to treat Parkinson's.

Parkinson's disease vaccines are currently being explored. Introducing antibodies to alpha-synuclein or inducing the body to produce its own antibodies to alpha-synuclein are strategies that are being developed by multiple pharmaceutical companies as potential treatments for PD.

The immune response triggered by UB-312, an experimental vaccine by Vaxxinity, effectively targeted alpha-synuclein protein aggregates and slowed their toxic buildup in the cerebrospinal fluid (CSF) of PD patients in a phase 1 trial, compared with those given a placebo.

The current approach to PD vaccines is the introduction of a molecule that induces the body to produce its antibodies against alpha-synuclein, leading to active immunity. In doing this, the antibodies will bind to clumped alpha-synuclein and help to break them down.

Challenges of Developing a Vaccine for Parkinson's

First, neurodegeneration evolves for many years before diagnosis, thus identifying patients at early stages of the disease is important. A vaccine might eventually be well-suited for the prevention of neurodegeneration, but we are still lacking diagnostic biomarkers that would help identify patients at the very early stages of the disease (i.e., before symptoms occur). Moreover, symptoms are generally slow progressing and heterogeneous, meaning that assessing a beneficial effect of an investigational drug needs to be conducted over long periods and in a large patient population.

There are no tools yet to diagnose people correctly to include the correct patients in the clinical trial, and then obviously follow the impact of the treatment. With the great progress in potential cancer vaccines where molecular targets have been identified, "but in neurological conditions like Parkinson's, our understanding is probably 10–15 years behind that.

Although a Parkinson's vaccine might one day be possible, particularly considering the initial promising results from the recent trials of AC Immune's ACI-7104 and Vaxxinity's UB-312. It is difficult to say whether we will see the successful development of an effective vaccine anytime soon. However, there is reason to be hopeful that a cure for the disorder might be within touching distance, with a variety of investigational treatments currently being developed for it.

Monoclonal Antibody Therapy for Parkinson's Disease

Two mAbs, prasinezumab and cinpanemab, directed at aggregated alpha-synuclein (α-synuclein) were investigated as PD-modifying therapies with a similar primary endpoin.

Genome-wide association study-linked variants of α-synuclein also contribute to the risk of sporadic PD. The introduction of emerging technologies may help address the challenges in α-synuclein-based immunotherapy. Despite the disappointing results, it may be premature to abandon exploring the potential of such therapeutic approaches.

■ HUNTINGTON'S DISEASE

Huntington's disease (HD) is a rare neurodegenerative, inherited autosomal disorder that causes the progressive breakdown of nerve cells in the brain. Symptoms first occur in people in their thirties and forties, though children are also known to develop the disease. HD patients can present with a variety of symptoms including chorea, behavioral and psychiatric abnormalities, and cognitive decline. HD is a progressive age-dependent neuropathological disorder in which immune activation is seen to be predominant in both the CNS and the periphery. The mutant Htt aggregates appear to trigger neurodegeneration and chronic neuroinflammation, which correlates well with HD clinical syndromes.

Huntington's Disease versus Parkinson's Disease

Both conditions involve involuntary motor symptoms. In PD, people may experience rigidity and slowed movements, while in HD, people may experience cognitive and psychological symptoms. HD affects both the brain and the muscles.

There is currently no cure for Huntington's, and it is usually fatal after a period of up to 20 years. However, there are measures in place to lessen the impact of HD on those stricken by the disease, and medicines are available to help manage the symptoms.

Treatment includes chorea medication, antipsychotic medication, antidepressants, mood-stabilizing medication as well as nondrug therapies. Fortunately, there are also many new HD therapeutics currently undergoing clinical trials that target the disease at its origin; lowering the levels of mutant huntingtin protein (mtHTT).

In HD, the mtHTT is the principal cause of pathological changes that initiate primarily along the corticostriatal axis. mtHTT is ubiquitously expressed and there is, accordingly, growing recognition that HD is a systemic disorder with the functional interplay between the brain and the periphery.

Reducing Huntingtin by immunotherapy delays disease progression in a mouse model of HD. Currently, much attention is being directed to antisense oligonucleotide (ASO) therapies, which bind to pre-RNA or messenger RNA (mRNA) and can alter protein expression via RNA degradation, blocking translation or splice modulation. Other potential therapies in clinical development include RNA interference (RNAi) therapies, RNA-targeting small molecule therapies, stem cell therapies, antibody therapies, non-RNA targeting small molecule therapies, and neuroinflammation-targeted therapies.

Potential therapies in preclinical development include zinc finger protein (ZFP) therapies, transcription activator-like effector nuclease (TALEN) therapies, and clustered regularly interspaced short palindromic repeats (CRISPR)/CRISPR-associated system (Cas) therapies.

IMMUNOTHERAPY FOR AUTISM SPECTRUM DISORDERS

Authors have dealt with vaccinations' role in childhood Autism in recent years in a Question and Answer format. These are our introductory messages for readers of this chapter.

Question: Sir, I have a 6-year-old child with autism spectrum disorder (ASD); is it due to my child's vaccination at an early age? What is the best latest treatment available now for autism? Your earlier response is anticipated.

Answer: Author's response:
- Early childhood immunization saves lives, they do not cause autism. Numerous studies have failed to show a causal link between vaccines and autism.
- Research suggests that autism develops from a combination of genetic and nongenetic, or environmental stimuli; has no known established cause of autism.
- The most effective treatments available today are occupational therapy/physical therapy (OT/PT), speech therapy, applied behavioral analysis (ABA), and pharmacological therapy supervised by an expert in developmental and behavioral pediatrics.
- There is currently no cure for ASD. However, research shows that early diagnosis and early intervention are critical; to helping people with autism and ASD, but educational, vocational, and support services must be applied across the lifespan.
  Recent research aims to enhance the quality of life for children and adults: Novel Stem cell therapy (BM transplant) to replace the damaged cells of the body to improve the quality of life of people affected by autism.
- How effective is stem cell therapy for autism/ASD? The answer to this is unknown. Not FDA approved.

Autism spectrum disorders are lifelong neurobiological conditions and less prevalent in females. Usually manifest in the first 3 years of a child's life and each child presents differently. These children show differences in three main areas of development:
1. *Communication:* The child may present verbal or nonverbal.
2. *Social interaction:* The child may not make eye contact or respond to their name when called.
3. *Imagination:* Very often, a repetitive play pattern is noticed during leisure activities.

Vaccines and vaccine ingredients do not cause autism. Some people have had concerns that ASD might be linked to the vaccines children receive, but studies have shown that there is no link between receiving vaccines and developing ASD. The National Academy of Medicine, formerly known as the Institute of Medicine, reviewed the safety of eight vaccines for children and adults. The review found that with rare exceptions, these vaccines are very safe.

Many different factors have been identified that may make a child more likely to have ASD, including environmental, biological, and genetic factors. For the most part, ASD is an inherited disorder: Scientists estimate that up to 80% of a child's risk of developing it is determined by DNA. Although the exact cause of autism is still unknown, there is evidence to suggest that autism genes are usually inherited from the father.

This is a novel way to think about treating neurological symptoms:

Based on the immunological abnormalities, various treatment modalities have been applied to children with ASD. One immunomodulatory treatment that has been studied in ASD is IVIG.

Intranasal oxytocin in children and adolescents did not improve social interaction or other measures of social function related to ASD.

In 2020, researchers at Harvard Medical School showed that the immune system "cytokine" molecule IL-17a, when applied to a particular brain region in mice modeling autism, improved social behavior and reduced repetitive behaviors. The study left open questions that, if answered, could enable the development of an immunotherapy for brain disorders.

Recent research hypothesizes that circulating maternal immunoglobulin G (IgG) autoantibodies (1) as a potential target for prevention, as a decrease could either possibly prevent ASD or lessen its severity, and (2) as biomarkers for screening, diagnosis, and treatment of ASD in infants and children. This research on ASD has the potential to affect healthcare policies concerning women who are pregnant or planning to become pregnant and lead to novel treatment of ASD.

Monoclonal Antibody and Cell Therapy
Monoclonal Antibody

As of this date in February 2022, there are no mAbs specifically approved for the treatment of ASD. However, research into the underlying biology of ASD is ongoing, and there have been investigations into various potential treatment approaches, including those involving mAbs targeting specific pathways or molecules implicated in ASD. These studies are still in the early stages, and no mAb therapy has been established as a standard treatment for ASD.

Stem Cell Therapy

Stem cell therapy is an area of research that holds promise for various neurological conditions, including ASD. Stem cell therapy for autism is still largely experimental and not yet a standard treatment.

Researchers speculate that stem cells could help repair or regenerate damaged neural circuits, modulate inflammation and immune responses, or enhance neuroplasticity. While some preclinical studies in animal models and a few small-scale clinical trials in humans have shown promising results, larger and more rigorous studies are needed to establish safety, efficacy, and long-term outcomes.

Types of stem cells: Different types of stem cells are being investigated for their potential in treating autism, including mesenchymal stem cells (MSCs) derived from sources such as BM, adipose tissue, or umbilical cord tissue. Induced pluripotent stem cells (iPSCs), which are generated from adult cells and can differentiate into various cell types, are also being studied.

Challenges and risks: There are significant challenges and risks associated with stem cell therapy for autism, including the potential for adverse effects, ethical considerations, and the need for careful patient selection and monitoring. Additionally, there is a lack of standardized protocols for stem cell treatment in autism, leading to variability in approaches and outcomes. Researchers and clinicians need to adhere to ethical and regulatory guidelines to ensure the safety and efficacy of stem cell treatments for ASD.

In conclusion, while stem cell therapy holds promise as a potential treatment for ASDs, much more research is needed to fully understand its safety, efficacy, and long-term effects.

Currently, there is no vaccine for ASD. However, despite extensive scientific research, no vaccine or specific medical treatment has been found to prevent or cure autism.

■ SPINAL CORD INJURY

One of the most serious diseases in neurology is paraplegia or tetraplegia due to spinal cord injury (SCI) which can be divided into three phases, e.g., acute (within 2 weeks), subacute (2 weeks to 6 months), and chronic (over 6 months).

The pathological process of SCI includes primary injury (initial traumatic insult) and a progressive secondary injury cascade characterized by ischemia, proapoptotic signaling, peripheral inflammatory cell infiltration, and the release of proinflammatory cytokines.

Secondary injury plays a key role in the loss of spinal cord function after trauma. Therefore, early treatment to prevent secondary injury is the key to improving prognosis.

Tumor necrosis factor-α (TNF-α) mAb is a TNF-α inhibitor that could control the inflammatory response and is now widely used in the treatment of ankylosing spondylitis, rheumatoid arthritis (RA), and other autoimmune diseases. In this study, the investigators will treat patients with acute SCI with TNF-α mAb and compare them with the control group.

From animal experiments; there are mechanisms behind possible repair and degeneration in these conditions. Biological factors and neurotransmitters that can promote repair and axonal neurogrowth. Then there are also biological factors that inhibit these repair mechanisms. Accidental SCI causes neural disconnection and persistent neurological deficits, so axon sprouting and plasticity might promote recovery. Now there is a new molecule, soluble Nogo-Receptor-Fc decoy, (AXER-204) blocks inhibitors of axon growth and promotes recovery of motor function after SCI in animals.

For the first time, as described in Lancet Neurology, this drug was given to patients with cervical SCIs. The first group received the drug intrathecally as a proof of concept to show pharmacokinetics (PK). In the second part of the study, 24 patients were treated in a placebo-controlled design. Very importantly, this drug was well tolerated and the levels in the CSF were achieved that were needed to show a positive biological result.

This first-in-human and randomized trial sought to determine primarily the safety and PK of AXER-204 in individuals with chronic SCI, and secondarily its effect on recovery, which blocks the inhibitors of axonal growth and improves motor function after spinal lesions. Further, a larger phase 2 trial soon could investigate efficacy in patients with moderately severe SCI.

Immunotherapy is a rapidly advancing field in the treatment of various medical conditions, including SCI. While immunotherapy has shown promise in preclinical studies, its application in clinical settings for SCI is still in the early stages. Here are some potential approaches and developments in immunotherapy for SCIs:

- *Immunomodulatory drugs:* Drugs that target immune cells or signaling pathways involved in inflammation and tissue repair are being investigated for their potential to improve outcomes in SCI. For example, drugs that target microglia, macrophages, or T-cells may help modulate the immune response and promote tissue repair.
- *Inflammatory modulation:* SCI often leads to inflammation at the injury site, contributing to secondary tissue damage. Immunotherapies aimed at modulating the inflammatory response, such as targeting specific cytokines or immune cells, may help reduce secondary injury and promote tissue repair.
- *Cell-based (stem cell-based) therapies:* Certain cell-based immunotherapies, such as MSCs or neural stem cells, have shown potential for promoting tissue repair and functional recovery in SCI. These cells can modulate the immune response, reduce inflammation, and promote regeneration of damaged tissue.
- *Vaccines:* Targeting specific antigens associated with SCI or neuroinflammation may help promote tissue repair and functional recovery. These vaccines could potentially modulate the immune response to reduce inflammation and promote regeneration of damaged tissue.
- *Gene therapy:* Approaches aimed at modulating immune responses or promoting tissue repair are being explored for their potential in SCI. For example, gene therapy techniques can be used to deliver genes encoding anti-inflammatory cytokines or growth factors to the injury site to promote tissue repair.

A combination of immunotherapies and well-coordinated approaches with traditional treatments such as surgery or rehabilitation may enhance their effectiveness in promoting tissue repair and functional recovery in SCI. While these approaches show promise in preclinical studies, more research is needed to evaluate their safety and efficacy in clinical trials involving spinal cord-injured individuals. Additionally, personalized approaches considering the heterogeneity of SCI and individual patient characteristics may be necessary for optimizing treatment outcomes.

GUILLAIN–BARRÉ SYNDROME AND CHRONIC INFLAMMATORY DEMYELINATING POLYRADICULONEUROPATHY

Inflammatory neuropathies are a heterogeneous group of rare diseases of the peripheral nervous system that include acute and chronic diseases, such as GBS and chronic inflammatory demyelinating polyradiculoneuropathy (CIDP). The etiology and pathophysiological mechanisms of inflammatory neuropathies are only partly known but are considered autoimmune disorders in which an aberrant immune response, including cellular and humoral components, is directed toward components of the peripheral nerve causing demyelination and axonal damage.

Guillain–Barré syndrome is an acute autoimmune disorder where the immune system attacks the nerves, leading to an acute, immune-mediated polyradiculoneuropathy that can lead to significant weakness and paralysis. It can be triggered by various factors, including certain infections; however, as GBS is not caused by an infectious agent that a vaccine could target. The management of GBS primarily involves immunotherapies rather than preventive vaccines.

The pathophysiologic mechanism of an antecedent illness and of GBS can be typified by *Campylobacter jejuni* infections. The virulence of *C. jejuni* is thought to be based on the presence of specific antigens in its capsule that are shared with nerve sheath. Immune responses directed against lipopolysaccharide (LPS) antigens in the capsule of *C. jejuni* result in antibodies that cross-react with ganglioside GM1 in myelin, resulting in immunologic damage to the peripheral nervous system. This process has been termed molecular mimicry.

Literature has reported a small association between certain vaccinations (notably, the influenza vaccine) and an increased risk of developing GBS. Although, the risk is very low, and the benefits of vaccination in preventing serious disease are far outweigh this small risk. The pathology is not clear. Both cellular and humoral immunity are involved in the occurrence of the disease, and molecular mimicry is currently the most widely recognized pathogenesis.

Traditional treatment for GBS typically involves supportive care and interventions to manage symptoms and reduce the immune system's attack on the nerves. This may include therapies such as plasma exchange (PE) (plasmapheresis = PE) and IVIG to help modulate the immune response and alleviate symptoms.

Research into potential therapies for GBS continues, but as of now, there is no definitive vaccine or immunotherapy specifically targeting GBS prevention or treatment.

Immunotherapies that aim to reduce the immune system's attack on the peripheral nerves include:
- *IVIG:* It is thought to modify the immune response. It is widely used in the treatment of GBS and is considered effective in hastening recovery.
- *Plasmapheresis (PE):* It involves removing and treating the plasma from the blood, which may contain factors that contribute to the immune attack on the nervous system. It is another effective treatment for GBS, particularly in the early stages of the disease.

Ten years after the first report of PE, immunoglobulin was first reported in the treatment of GBS. Patients treated with IVIG showed more improvement after 4 weeks than those with PE. Currently, clinical trials have shown that PE and IVIG have equal effects. IVIG has become the most popular therapy in most countries unless the costs limit its use.

There is no vaccine against GBS, as this is not caused by an infectious agent that a vaccine could target. New treatment strategies for GBS are mostly immunotherapies, including treatment against antibodies, complement pathways, immune cells, and cytokines. Some of the new strategies are being investigated in clinical trials, but none of them have been approved for the treatment of GBS.

Miller Fisher syndrome (MFS) is a variation of GBS, and the clinical features of MFS are facial muscle weakness and ataxia. Most MFS patients have anti-GQ1b antibodies, implying a potential role for ganglioside antibodies in disease pathogenesis or as reliable diagnostic biomarkers. Anti-GQ1b antibodies have been proven to activate complement at the neuromuscular junction in vitro, and complement activation is thought to be the primary pathogenic mechanism of MFS.

Acute motor axonal neuropathy (AMAN) is the second most common subtype of GBS. AMAN presents as a primary axonal injury with antibody and membrane attack complex (MAC) deposition in nodes of Ranvier without obvious inflammatory cell infiltration or demyelination. Antibodies related to AMAN include anti-GM1 and anti-GD1a antibodies. In AMAN patients related to *C. jejuni*, the gangliosides of the peripheral nerves are similar in structure to the lipo-oligosaccharides of *C. jejuni*. This suggests that the pathogenic mechanism of AMAN may be the cross-reaction of homologous epitopes between bacterial lipo-oligosaccharides and peripheral motor axon ganglioside.

Anti-inflammatory cytokines, such as interleukin-4 (IL-4) and interleukin-10 (IL-10), inhibit disease progression or promote myelin repair by exerting anti-inflammatory effects.

In conclusion, IVIG and PE are still the most effective therapies for GBS. Additionally, immunotherapies are still the most popular methods for GBS treatment **(Box 1)**. Further clinical and basic studies are needed to prove the role of these methods in the treatment of GBS and provide more possibilities for treatment.

The combination of new therapies with classical therapies could help to improve the prognosis in patients with poor outcomes after treatment with classical therapies alone. Immunotherapies are still the most popular methods for GBS treatment. Further clinical and basic studies are needed to prove the role of these methods in the treatment of GBS and provide more possibilities for treatment.

Campylobacter Jejuni-mediated GBS (The Molecular Mimicry and Vaccine Development Approaches)

Molecular mimicry between *C. jejuni* LPS and peripheral nerve gangliosides may play a significant role in the development of GBS vaccine. Although LPS was recognized as a potent antigen by different studies, nevertheless, the antigenic diversity and the lack of clearly defined protective epitopes are major constraints in developing vaccines against *C. jejuni*.

BOX 1: The second course of IVIG immune regulations.
- Eculizumab-complement pathway
- Rituximab is an antibody that targets CD20 on B-cells, resulting in B-cell depletion. It has been reported to be effective in patients not responding to conventional treatment, particularly in autoimmune nodopathy patients. Some authors, including ourselves, have observed reductions in IgG4 autoantibody levels in CIDP patients treated with rituximab

(CIDP: chronic inflammatory demyelinating polyradiculoneuropathy; IVIG: intravenous immunoglobulin)
Source: Querol L, Lleixà C. Novel Immunological and Therapeutic Insights in Guillain-Barré Syndrome and CIDP. Neurotherapeutics. 2021;18(4):2222-35.

MUSCLE DISORDERS INCLUDING AMYOTROPHIC LATERAL SCLEROSIS

Amyotrophic lateral sclerosis (ALS) is a rare disease that affects the motor neurons that control voluntary muscles. While the exact cause is unknown, genetic factors can play a role in some cases. Predicting who will develop ALS is challenging as it does not strictly follow familial patterns. Typically, ALS onset occurs in mid to late adulthood, often beginning with weakness in one part of the body such as the hands or legs. Eventually, ALS affects the control of the muscles needed to move, speak, eat, and breathe. There is no cure for this fatal disease.

Amyotrophic lateral sclerosis can be hard to diagnose early because it can have symptoms similar to other diseases. Tests to rule out other conditions or help diagnose neuromuscular degeneration in patients with ALS pathology cause the loss of motor neurons and paralysis of skeletal muscles, and currently, there is no cure or effective treatment.

A possible combined therapy of treatments targeting motor neuron inflammation together with treatments targeting muscle regeneration could have a greater chance of success in extending and improving the quality of life of patients suffering from this terrible disease. Drugs such as talampanel, beta-lactam antibiotics, pramipexole, dexpramipexole, and arimoclomol are currently considered as potential therapeutic compounds in the treatment of ALS. Alternatively, studies are testing the uses of stem cell therapy and immunotherapy for the potential treatment of ALS.

Several promising results obtained in ALS animal models have shown not to be effective in humans. Crossing the human blood-brain barrier is crucial for a drug to reach its target; thus, activating the appropriate site of action to produce the expected drug effects. Moreover, ALS biomarkers would be crucial in identifying an effective therapy that impacts disease progression of ALS patients.

Stem cell therapy is promising in the treatment of ALS since stem cells have the potential to be grown to slow the progression of motor neuron disease or even replace motor neurons. MSCs are derived from adult stem cells. These cells are BM cells that are differentiated into mesodermal cell derivatives. It has been indicated that MSCs lead to the release of trophic factors, anti-inflammatory cytokines, and immunomodulatory chemokines to delay disease progression. A clinical trial was performed, in which the intravenous (IV) administration of MSCs in ALS patients was shown to be safe and induced immediate immunomodulatory activity.

Immunotherapy

One of the factors that contribute to the progression of ALS includes oxidative stress or the accumulation of free radicals as a consequence of the mutation of the SOD1 enzyme. The acquisition of a cytotoxic activity is associated with protein misfolding/aggregation. The identification of this pathogenic process has led to a focus on immunotherapy in ALS. Specifically, mouse mAbs against misfolded forms of mutant SOD1 (mSOD1) were produced to determine its effectiveness as a passive immunization for ALS. It was shown that infusing D3H5 antibody through the intracerebroventricular (ICV) route for 42 days reduced levels of toxic SOD1 species in the spinal cord.

Furthermore, ALS biomarkers would be crucial in identifying an effective therapy that impacts the disease progression of ALS patients. It is noteworthy that a combination of drugs or methods might provide effective therapy for patients with ALS.

VACCINE FOR DIABETES

As per the International Diabetes Federation (IDF) Atlas, 2021, India accounts for one in seven adults with diabetes globally. From 61.3 million in India to an increase of 74.2 million in 2021, diabetes prevalence has been exponentially increasing in the country. India is often referred to as the "Diabetes Capital of the World" due to its high prevalence of diabetes.

Where Do We Stand?

Current developments in our understanding related to autoimmune responses leading to diabetes have developed a cause for concern in the prospective usage of immunomodulatory agents to prevent diabetes. The mechanism of action of vaccines varies greatly, such as removing autoreactive T-cells and inhibiting the interactions between immune cells. Currently, most developed diabetes vaccines have been tested in animal models, while only a few human trials have been completed with positive outcomes.

Diabetes vaccines attempt to stop the T-cells from attacking the human body's cells. Studies have been able to treat diabetes in mice, but a working vaccine in humans has yet to receive pharmaceutical approval.

While there is no vaccine for diabetes, vaccines can prevent infections such as rubella and mumps. These infections can sometimes lead to complications like pancreatitis, which can increase the risk of type 1 diabetes. Historically, mumps and rubella viral infections are well known to be associated with the onset of type 1 diabetes apart from other environmental factors that may operate over populations with different genetic susceptibility. Research into potential vaccines or cures for type 2 diabetes is ongoing, but no such vaccine has been developed and approved for clinical use. Instead, treatment typically focuses on controlling blood sugar levels, preventing complications, and improving overall health.

Currently, most developed diabetes vaccines have been tested in animal models, while only a few human trials have been completed with positive outcomes.

- Type 1 diabetes is an autoimmune condition in which the immune system mistakenly attacks and destroys insulin-producing beta cells in the pancreas.
- Type 2 diabetes is typically associated with insulin resistance and a relative insulin deficiency. Both types of diabetes are managed through lifestyle changes, medications, and insulin therapy as needed.

Interestingly, previous research elucidated evidence for EVs being a causative factor for the onset of type 1 diabetes. Hence, an ongoing effort to develop and synthesize an EV vaccine is currently in progress with the aid of technological advances. Yet, various issues are still under discussion, such as diabetogenic EV serotypes and safety concerns before this novel vaccine can be tested in clinical trials.

However, a noteworthy accomplishment was achieved in a recent preclinical study involving the invention of the first multivalent formalin-inactivated CVB1 vaccine, where the vaccine proved to be effective with no adverse effects. Apart from the usage of vaccines indicated for viral infections, the tuberculosis DNA vaccine known as DNA-HSP65 exemplifies a high possibility of becoming the latest immunotherapeutic agent for the management of diabetes. A list of new vaccine products in the pipeline that could be employed for diabetes can be found in **Table 2**.

The urgent need for more effective prophylaxis in addition to conventional dietary modification advice to patients has prompted various attempts in developing vaccines to delay or prevent the onset of this chronic disease.

As seen in recent approaches protein-based, self-antigen, and non-antigen-specific interventions have exhibited promising potential for use as vaccines against diabetes shortly. However, a deeper understanding is still required to ameliorate and invent potent therapies with minimal side effects regardless of the cause-related factors, especially for chronic diseases, such as type 2 diabetes.

Monoclonal Antibody Role in Diabetes

The US-FDA has approved the anti-CD3 mAb teplizumab-mzwv (Tzield, Prevention Bio) to delay the onset of clinical type 1 diabetes in people aged 8 years and older who are at high risk for developing the condition. The anti-CD3 mAb treatment increases endogenous insulin production and improves the lifestyle of patients by reducing insulin dosage. Future studies should consider the limitations, including sample size, heterogeneity, and duration of follow-up, to validate the generalizability of these findings further.

TABLE 2: List of vaccine products for diabetes.

Type of vaccine	Vaccine name	Indication	Mechanism of action
Adjuvant-based vaccines	Alum adjuvant-based vaccine	T1DM and T2DM	Activation of immune response and promoting humoral immunity
Protein-based vaccines	• IL-1β-targeted epitope peptide (1βEPP)	T2DM	• Alters the level of glucose tolerance and provides a hyperglycemia shield
	• Dipeptidyl peptidase-4 inhibitor (DPP4- based vaccine)	T2DM	• Inhibition of dipeptidyl peptidase-4 inhibitor (DPP4) enzyme
	• CTB-InsB vaccination product	T1DM	• Downregulation response in the onset of T1DM and induction of immune tolerance
Specific self-antigen-based approach in vaccine production	IA-2 as a vaccine product	T1DM	Islet autoantigen mechanism and delaying the onset and the late stages of autoimmune diabetes

(CTB: B-subunit of cholera toxin; InsB: B-chain of human insulin; T1DM: type 1 diabetes mellitus; T2DM: type 2 diabetes mellitus)

In clinical trials, the use of teplizumab-mzwv has delayed the development of stage 3 type 1 diabetes by approximately 2 years, on average. However, to identify eligible candidates to receive it, broader autoantibody screening would be needed because most people who develop type 1 diabetes do not have first-degree family members with the condition.

The agent, which interferes with T-cell mediated autoimmune destruction of pancreatic beta cells, is the first disease-modifying therapy for impeding the progression of type 1 diabetes. It is administered by IV infusion once daily for 14 consecutive days.

CARDIOVASCULAR DISEASES VACCINE

Numerous observational studies have reported higher incidences of myocardial infarction, heart failure (HF), and stroke with influenza infection, naturally spurring an interest in the influenza vaccine as a preventive measure against adverse cardiovascular events.

Influenza and pneumococcal infections have been suggested to be potential risk factors for causing adverse cardiovascular events, especially in high-risk patients. Vaccination against respiratory infections in patients with established CVD could serve as a potentially cost-effective intervention to improve their clinical outcomes and cardiac societies have encouraged it.

Previous studies have shown that influenza vaccination reduces mortality, acute coronary syndromes, and hospitalization in patients with coronary heart disease (CHD) and/or HF. However, there is a paucity of randomized prospective clinical trials in the field of pneumococcal vaccination, and additional higher-quality evidence is needed. Furthermore, questions around the role of vaccination in the primary prevention of CVD, the optimal dose, and timing are largely unanswered.

The pathophysiologic mechanism in which vaccination provides cardiovascular protection may be related to the modification of the immune-inflammatory model of atherogenesis. While traditional vaccines for CVDs are not yet available, research into immunotherapy approaches to reduce risk factors, such as high cholesterol, is ongoing. For instance, vaccines targeting PCSK9, a protein that regulates cholesterol levels in the blood, are under investigation. Although vaccines do not directly prevent CVDs, they can indirectly reduce the risk by preventing infections that are associated with these diseases.

Group A *Streptococcus* Vaccines to Control Acute Rheumatic Fever, RHD, and Other Renal and CNS Disorders

Attempts to develop a GAS vaccine have been underway since the early 1920s and a number have progressed to early human trials. Progress toward a safe, effective, affordable, and practical GAS vaccine has accelerated in recent years. Several vaccine candidates are in early human trials, funded by the Governments of Australia and New Zealand began in 2013.

In recent years, preclinical antigen discovery, vaccine formulation, and efficacy studies in animal models have progressed significantly. There is now a need to move promising candidates through the clinical development pathway to establish their efficacy in preventing GAS infections and their complications.

Group A *Streptococcus* and Monoclonal Antibodies

Group A *Streptococcus* has evolved multiple strategies to evade human antibodies, making it challenging to create effective vaccines or mAb treatments.

The streptococcal M protein is a major virulence factor that mediates bacterial adhesion and immune evasion. No human antibodies have been generated against the M protein, partly due to its inherent antibody-binding ability.

The existence of dual-Fab binding as an antibody–antigen interaction modality and its influential role in mediating immune function was until this report unknown. This is particularly important since the antibody response against the M protein is not always opsonic and can lack immune function. The prevalence of this phenomenon and how it influences immune outcomes upon vaccination or infection is an important factor to consider in the future development of anti-streptococcal therapeutics.

KAWASAKI DISEASES—ACQUIRED HEART DISEASE (CORONARY ARTERY ABNORMALITIES) PREVENTIONS

Kawasaki Disease and Kawasaki Disease—Septic Shock Syndrome

Immunotherapies and Perspective of Immunopathogenesis

Kawasaki disease (KD), mostly occurs in children aged under 5, with some rare cases affecting older children or adults. The cause is unknown and there is no evidence that vaccination can lead to KD. Whilst a diagnosis of KD may be made following immunization, this association is temporal and research has not identified a causal association.

Epidemiologic and clinical features suggest an infectious and/or environmental cause or trigger in genetically susceptible individuals. As of this date in February 2024, there is no vaccine specifically designed to prevent KD and Kawasaki disease shock syndrome (KDSS) which is an inflammatory, autoimmune vasculitis that primarily affects children under the age of 5. The incubation period is unknown.

The disease was first described in 1967 by Dr Tomi Saku Kawasaki in a landmark paper entitled "Acute Febrile Mucocutaneous Lymph Node Syndrome" with specific desquamation of the fingers and toes in children in the Japanese journal Arerugi ("Allergy"). This is now known universally as KD, although he did not use that term himself. Dr Kawasaki died on June 5, 2020, at age 95 years.

Kawasaki disease is the most common cause of acquired heart disease in developed countries, e.g., coronary artery abnormalities (CAAs).

The management of KD remains centered on early diagnosis and treatment typically involving polyclonal IVIG and aspirin to mitigate the risk of CAAs. KD shares clinical symptoms with the multisystem inflammatory syndrome in children (MIS-C) which is related to COVID-19.

Incidence rates as high as 60–150 per 100,000 children below 5 years of age have been reported from several countries. In India (as also perhaps in many other developing countries), however, the majority of children with KD continue to remain undiagnosed probably because of the lack of awareness among pediatricians. A significant proportion of infants with KD had cardiac involvement. Infants were more likely to have IVIG-resistant disease. Around 10–20% of patients are IVIG resistant. Prolonged fever and unresponsiveness to the first dose of IVIG are significant risk factors for CAAs. Valvular regurgitation constitutes an important cardiac association and may be due to pancarditis in the acute stage or aortic root dilation or valvulitis in case of late-onset involvement. Hence, once a diagnosis of KD is made, a thorough echocardiographic study is warranted to evaluate for signs of myocarditis, besides evaluation for coronary artery aneurysms.

It is debatable whether KD is a postinfectious hyperinflammation reaction, an autoinflammatory syndrome, or an autoimmune disorder. Inflammation-inducing substances may play an important role in KD, such as those originating from pathogens, pathogen-associated molecular patterns (PAMPs), toxins (superantigens), and antigens from injured or infected-host cells that behaved as damage-associated molecular patterns (DAMPs) that are causing the hyperinflammatory response of KD.

Based on the understanding of the immunopathogenesis of KD and the resistance to IVIG, the literature suggests a stepwise approach to IVIG resistance and KDSS, as described in **Figure 2**.

The development of different types of immunotherapies, including vaccines (prophylactic and therapeutic), and the use of pathogens, mAbs, recombinant proteins, cytokines, and cellular immunotherapies, have been proposed as adjunct therapies, and some of these are currently in different phases of clinical trials.

There is no directly acting vaccine against KD and/or against KD-acquired heart diseases. However, research into the cause and potential preventive measures, such as vaccines, is ongoing.

Directly Preventing Acquired Heart Diseases in Children

There is no direct vaccine against all forms of acquired heart disease in children, vaccinations against pneumococcal disease, influenza, and COVID-19 are crucial in preventing infections that can lead to serious cardiac complications in children with existing heart conditions or vulnerabilities.

Pneumococcal Vaccination

Children with chronic heart conditions, including congenital heart defects, are at increased risk of invasive pneumococcal disease. The pneumococcal conjugate vaccine (PCV) can significantly reduce this risk. The Centers for Disease Control and Prevention (CDC) recommends pneumococcal vaccination for children with chronic heart disease to prevent pneumococcal disease, direct prevention of acquired heart diseases in children through vaccination primarily focuses on preventing infections that can lead to complications affecting the heart. While there is no specific vaccine that directly prevents all forms of acquired heart disease in children, vaccinations can play a crucial role in preventing certain

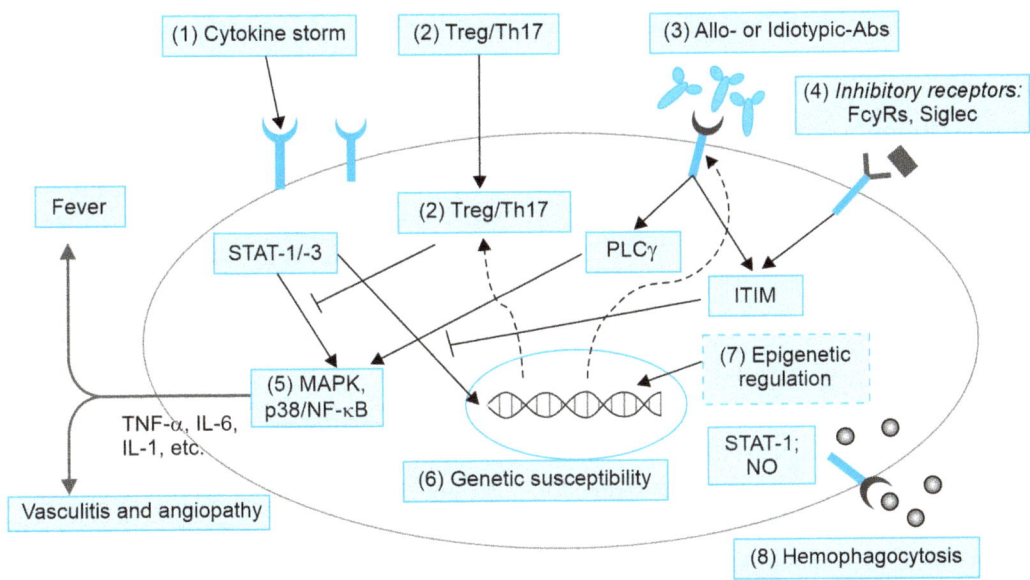

Fig. 2: The perspective of immunotherapies for Kawasaki disease (KD) refractory to conventional treatment. (1) Targeting the cytokine storm: Anti-TNF-α and anti-IL-1 have been used to rescue intravenous immunoglobulin (IVIG) resistance. In addition, other Th17 and Th1 cytokines are also candidates for therapeutic targets. (2) Addressing the Th17/Treg imbalance can be achieved by augmentation of Th2 or Treg polarization, including the enhancement of FoxP3 expression. (3) Blockade or immunoregulation by allotypic and idiotypic IgG provides immunoregulation of KD. (4) Enhancement of immunoinhibitory receptors transduces the immunoreceptor tyrosine-based inhibitory motif (ITIM) to inhibit cytokine production. (5) Targeting the signal transduction of mitogen-activated protein kinases (MAPK) including p38 phosphorylation to suppress cytokine (TNF-α, IL-6, IL-1, etc.) production. (6) Screening genetic variants related to KD with IVIG resistance protects KD patients from coronary complications. (7) Epigenetic regulation of Treg immune responses reverses the Th17/Treg imbalance in KD with IVIG resistance. (8) Anti-hemophagocytosis can be achieved by targeting IFN-γ and TNF-α as well as the inhibition of their downstream effector STAT-1 (signal transducer and activator of transcription 1) or nitric oxide (NO) synthase activation (→ indicates activation; ⊥ indicates inhibitory regulation; - - -> indicates epigenetic regulation).

IDs that may have serious cardiac complications. Here are some relevant points based on the information available, which can lead to severe cardiac complications.

Influenza Vaccination

Children with cardiac diseases are also recommended to receive the influenza vaccine. Influenza can be particularly severe in children with heart conditions, leading to increased hospitalizations and complications. Vaccination against influenza is a key preventive measure to protect these children from potential heart complications related to the flu.

COVID-19 Vaccination

Given the risk of COVID-19 infection in children, including those with congenital heart disease, vaccines against COVID-19 have been approved for use in children aged 6 months and older. COVID-19 can have serious implications for children with heart conditions, making vaccination an important preventive strategy.

Kawasaki Disease and Vaccination

Kawasaki disease is a leading cause of acquired heart disease in children in the United States. While there is no vaccine against KD itself, research into the safety and effects of vaccines, such as the 13-valent PCV, in children with a history of KD is ongoing. The focus is on ensuring vaccination safety and preventing infections that could complicate the condition.

In summary, while there is no direct vaccine against all forms of acquired heart disease in children, vaccinations against pneumococcal disease, influenza, and COVID-19 are crucial in preventing infections that can lead to serious cardiac complications in children with existing heart conditions or vulnerabilities.

RNA THERAPEUTICS TO CONTROL BP (SMALL INHIBITORY RNAS)

A single injection of the investigational antihypertensive agent zilebesiran (Alnylam Pharmaceuticals) effectively lowered BP in adults with mild to moderate hypertension for up to 6 months, with what appeared to be an encouraging side-effect profile, in phase 2 dose-ranging KARDIA-1 clinical trial study.

Zilebesiran is a subcutaneous RNA interference therapeutic that targets hepatic angiotensinogen synthesis, the sole precursor of all angiotensin peptides. Study results showed sustained reductions in serum angiotensinogen (between 88 and 98%) over the 6-month follow-up period.

Zilebesiran is being further evaluated as an add-on therapy for the treatment of hypertension in the ongoing KARDIA-2 phase 2 study. No drug-related severe adverse events were seen.

These preliminary data further support the potential for quarterly or biannual dosing of subcutaneous zilebesiran in achieving a consistent pharmacodynamic effect and effective BP reduction through 6 months.

Monoclonal Antibody to Angiotensin II, Controlling Hypertension

Monoclonal antibodies to angiotensin II are useful in the diagnosis and treatment of angiotensin II-induced hypertension.

■ VACCINE FOR HYPERCHOLESTEROLEMIA

High levels of low-density lipoprotein (LDL) cholesterol can cause artery blockages and diseases such as heart attacks and strokes. Further, it raises the risk of arteriosclerotic cardiovascular disease (ASCVD). The quantity of LDL receptors, which are proteins on the surface of cells, is regulated by the *PCSK9* gene protein. These receptors are essential for controlling the amount of cholesterol in the circulation. Vaccines targeting PCSK9, an important regulator of LDL receptors, can be highly beneficial.

According to the results of the phase 1b HEART-1 trial, a single dose of a CRISPR-based gene-editing therapy resulted in substantial reductions in LDL-cholesterol (LDL-C) and PCSK9 levels in patients with heterozygous familial hypercholesterolemia (HeFH) and ASCVD *[presented at the 2023 Scientific Sessions of the American Heart Association (AHA) held in Philadelphia, Pennsylvania from November 11-13, 2023.1-3]*.

Further, a small interfering RNA (siRNA) called INCLISIRAN prevents PCSK9 from being synthesized inside cells. When given to people taking the highest dosage of a statin, inclisiran cuts LDL cholesterol by 50%.

Monoclonal Antibody in Hypercholesterolemia

Proprotein convertase subtilisin/kexin 9 (PCSK9) mAbs, as an attractive therapy for lowering LDL-C levels, can bind the LDL-receptor (LDL-R) on the surface of hepatocytes, interfering with LDL clearance in circulation, hence playing a pivotal role in regulating cholesterol homeostasis.

Inhibition of PCSK9 prevents degradation of LDLRs, permitting more LDL-C to be removed from circulation. These mAbs (evolocumab, alirocumab, and bococizumab) inhibit the interaction between PCSK9 and the LDLRs.

These results are promising and lead the way for a groundbreaking novel treatment option, "a single-course therapy that may lead to deep LDL-C lowering for decades" instead of the large number of daily medications, which the patients are required to take and therefore may not comply with.

■ RESPIRATORY DISEASES VACCINE

Vaccination is an important part of medical care in childhood. Adults also should keep up with vaccinations. They are important for respiratory illnesses as well as other serious conditions. Respiratory infection happens when the pathogen gets into the mucosa, or inner lining, of the upper airway (nasal and oropharyngeal mucosal linings). Clinical symptoms occur after an incubation period and the length of this period depends on the type of virus or bacteria. For the common cold, the time between the pathogen entering the body and symptoms starting can be as little as 10–12 hours, and for influenza, it is 3–4 days.

Exacerbations of COPD are a major cause of hospital admission, readmission, and mortality. Thus, exacerbation prevention is a priority to improve the quality of life and reduce healthcare costs. Vaccines such as the influenza vaccine and the pneumococcal vaccine can reduce the risk of respiratory diseases such as pneumonia and bronchitis, which can contribute to the development and exacerbation of NCDs like COPD.

Common pathogens that lead to respiratory infections include:
- *Viruses:*
  - Adenovirus
  - *Enterovirus*
  - Influenza virus
  - Rhinovirus
  - Respiratory syncytial virus (RSV)
  - SARS-CoV-2

- *Bacteria:*
  - *Streptococcus pneumoniae*
  - *Mycoplasma pneumoniae*

Types of vaccines include:
- *Inactivated vaccine:* Uses a dead version of the germ.
- *Live vaccine:* Uses a weak but live version of the germ.
- *mRNA vaccine:* Makes proteins to activate a specific immune response.
- *Subunit, recombinant, polysaccharide, and conjugate vaccines:* Use pieces of the germ, such as a protein or casing
- *Toxoid vaccine:* Uses the toxins caused by a germ to fight the illness the toxin causes.
- *Viral vector vaccine:* Uses a harmless virus to deliver instructions to the immune system to fight a harmful germ
- Depending on the type of vaccine, you may need to get more than one dose or a booster shot for optimal effectiveness.

Respiratory diseases that have vaccines include:
- COVID-19
- Diphtheria
- *Haemophilus influenzae* type B (Hib)
- Influenza
- Measles
- Pneumococcal disease
- Polio
- RSV
- Rubella
- Typhoid fever
- Whooping cough
- Pertussis

BRONCHIAL ASTHMA VACCINE

Asthma is a common noncommunicable respiratory disease affecting children, adults, and the elderly all over the world, with high morbidity and mortality in severe cases.

Asthma is a long-term inflammatory disease of the airways of the lungs. It is characterized by variable and recurring symptoms, reversible airflow obstruction, and easily triggered bronchospasms. Patients with severe refractory asthma represent a small subset of the asthmatic population (between 5 and 10% of all patients) but are the greatest burden to the healthcare system.

In allergic asthma, the most common type, antigen-specific Th2 cells and the cytokines secreted by them, i.e., IL-4, IL-5, IL-9, and IL-13, are primary mediators of the pathological consequences leading to airway eosinophilic inflammation, high-serum IgE concentrations, and airway hyperresponsiveness (AHR).

- Th2 and Th17 cells and their cytokines are pathogenic, while Th1 and Treg cells and their cytokines protect against asthma.
- Mycobacterial antigens protect against asthma by shifting the immune responses from Th2 and Th17 to Th1 and/or Treg types.
- The immunomodulatory property of mycobacterial antigens suggests their potential as a vaccine against asthma.

Monoclonal antibodies are biological drugs that work in a targeted manner on inflammation in people with severe asthma. Currently, around six mAbs are FDA-approved to treat severe eosinophilic asthma.

1. *Humanized mAbs, Omalizumab, (Xolair), Subcutaneous use:* That bind to Ig E are approved for the treatment of allergic asthma, blocking IL-5 will also provide benefits in patients with severe asthma with persistent eosinophilia. This mAb is for people with severe allergic asthma caused by exposure to allergens such as dust mites, pollen, and dander. Further, it emphasizes the importance of careful phenotyping of patients with severe refractory asthma before embarking on treatment with humanized mAb, omalizumab.
2. *Mepolizumab (Nucala) Sc use:* To treat eosinophilic asthma called eosinophilic granulomatosis with polyangiitis (EGPA). People with EGPA experience eosinophilic asthma, a high number of white blood cells, and swelling of the blood vessels.
3. *Reslizumab (Cinqair):* It is for people with severe eosinophilic asthma. It is different from other mAbs for asthma because you receive it by IV injection once every 4 weeks. Each dose usually takes about 20–50 minutes.
4. *Benralizumab (Fasenra):* Therapies have revolutionized severe asthma care in many ways. Patients with severe asthma controlled on benralizumab can safely minimize high-dose inhaled corticosteroid (ICS) exposure.
5. *Dupilumab (Dupixent)*

CYSTIC FIBROSIS IMMUNOTHERAPY

As of this date, there is no available vaccine ot gene therapy specifically designed for cystic fibrosis (CF). CF is a genetic disorder caused by mutations in the *cystic fibrosis transmembrane conductance regulator (CFTR)* gene, which leads to the production of a defective protein involved in regulating the flow of salt and water in and out of cells that lead to respiratory and digestive problems.

While there has been significant progress in understanding CF and developing potential treatments, a definitive cure has not yet been discovered. Current treatment approaches focus on managing symptoms, preventing complications, and improving the quality of life for individuals with CF. This typically involves a combination of medications, therapies, and lifestyle adjustments to maintain lung function and prevent infections.

The *CFTR* gene contains the instructions for making the CFTR protein. When there is a mutation or alteration in the genetic instructions, the production of the CFTR protein may be affected. In people with CF, mutations in the *CFTR* gene can result in no protein, not enough protein, or the protein being made incorrectly. Each of these defects leads to a cascade of problems that affect the lungs and other organs.

The *mRNA therapy* is one way to deliver the correct genetic instructions to cells, which would allow them to make functional CFTR proteins regardless of an individual's CF mutation. This treatment would not affect a person's DNA or CFTR mutations. mRNA therapy is not permanent and would need to be re-dosed regularly to be effective.

Messenger Ribonucleic Acid Vaccine against Cystic Fibrosis

Technology that enabled the highly successful COVID-19 vaccines has now set a path for a whole new class of mRNA vaccines with the potential to eradicate countless NCDs including CF, and even cancer. mRNA vaccines are being developed, e.g., delivering mRNA into the lungs where it will instruct cells to create healthy CFTR and/or alter the DNA to fix the defective CFTR protein and several potential mRNA therapies for CF are currently in R & D and D & D pipeline.

Monoclonal Antibody Therapeutic Utility in Cystic Fibrosis

Some mAbs such as mepolizumab and omalizumab are already being used in the treatment of asthma and constitute an invaluable therapeutic option for patients who tolerate corticosteroid treatment poorly. Other biologics such as depemokimab can be administered highly infrequently, even once per 6 months, significantly reducing the risk of adverse effects.

As evidenced by the large number of ongoing clinical trials, biological drugs are a category of therapeutic that is likely to see a surge in importance and prevalence. In the treatment of chronic lung inflammation, biologics offer meaningful advantages over currently used small-molecule drugs.

IMMUNOTHERAPY AGAINST NONALCOHOLIC FATTY LIVER DISEASE AND NONALCOHOLIC STEATOHEPATITIS NASH-RELATED HEPATOCELLULAR CARCINOMA

According to a study published in the National Library of Medicine, nonalcoholic fatty liver disease (NAFLD) is the major cause of hepatocellular carcinoma (HCC) in many developed nations and is a rapidly expanding cause of chronic liver disease. In comparison to HCC from other etiologies, NAFLD-HCC patients also typically have more comorbidities and tend to get older. The most prevalent primary liver cancer, HCC, typically develops in conjunction with liver cirrhosis. The nomenclature of nonalcoholic steatohepatitis (NASH) and NAFLD has recently been changed to metabolic dysfunction-associated steatohepatitis (MASH) and metabolic dysfunction-associated steatotic liver disease (MASLD).

The MASH patients are overweight and obese and those who are taking over the counter, allopathic drugs, and those who have underlying diabetes and hypothyroidism. Fatty liver is more common in women than males. It is also more common in the age group of 40–50 years.

The MASH could develop into advanced liver fibrosis, cirrhosis, or HCC. Growing shreds of evidence support that the pathogenesis and progression of MASLD are closely related to immune system dysfunction and the prospect of using immunotherapy for MASLD.

Researchers found that the protein, called TEAD1, was found to play a role in regulating how liver cells absorb fat. Blocking TEAD1 protected liver cells from the harmful accumulation of fat. Since the activity of TEAD proteins is elevated in cancer, blocking TEAD at an early stage can also be positive from a cancer point of view. Notably, over the past 10 years, there has been a ten-fold increase in the number of patients with MASLD-related cirrhosis who require a liver transplant, and Bayesian modeling forecasts a staggering global prevalence rate of 55.7% by 2040.

The US-FDA has approved resmetirom (Rezdiffra, Madrigal Pharmaceuticals), the first drug to treat patients with MASH and moderate to advanced liver fibrosis (consistent with stage F2 and F3 disease), along with diet and exercise. Resmetirom is a once-daily, oral thyroid hormone receptor beta-selective agonist. The FDA granted the drug breakthrough therapy designation and priority review.

Also, a recent study published in the journal Molecular Systems Biology shows how a new medicine that is under development can become a future treatment for fatty liver disease and liver cancer. "Patients suffering from liver cancer are currently diagnosed very late. If the patient is given this drug early in the process to protect against fatty liver, it can hopefully also prevent the development of liver cancer."

ANTI-ALLERGEN MONOCLONAL ANTIBODIES FOR ALLERGIC REACTIONS TO FOOD AND ALLERGENS

Omalizumab, a humanized mAb against IgE was originally approved in 2003 for the treatment of moderate-to-severe persistent allergic asthma in certain patients. The drug is also approved to treat chronic spontaneous urticaria and chronic rhinosinusitis with nasal polyps in certain patients. A recently approved medication called omalizumab (Xolair) helps lessen the severity of an accidental allergic reaction in people who are allergic to multiple foods.

February 20, 2024, the US-FDA has approved omalizumab (Xolair) injection for IgE-mediated food allergy in certain adults and children aged ≥1 year for the reduction of allergic reactions, including reducing the risk of anaphylaxis, that may occur with accidental exposure to one or more foods. However, Xolair is not approved for the immediate emergency treatment of allergic reactions, including anaphylaxis. Anaphylaxis is a serious and sometimes life-threatening allergic reaction that requires immediate medical treatment, including an epinephrine injection.

The drug omalizumab is composed of antibodies that bind and deactivate IgE molecules in the blood, which otherwise trigger the immune system when certain allergens are present. In trials, patients not only withstood exposures—two-thirds reported being able to ingest small amounts of food that would typically trigger a reaction.

Allergic diseases are a growing global health concern, with food allergies leading the way. Roughly 19 million people in the US (around 5.5 million children) have food allergies, resulting in about 30,000 emergency room visits annually. The drug meant to be injected regularly, not taken after a reaction begins, and has already been approved for use in those older than 1 year by the health officials.

Alternate antibody approaches have been employed, but until recently no naturally occurring allergen-specific human IgE mAbs have existed. Thanks to advances in human hybridoma technology, IgE mAb can now be generated from patients with allergies. The specificities of the IgE mAb generated using this technology reflect the IgE sensitizations and allergic diseases of the patient from which they were derived. These unique antibody tools can be used to obtain highly detailed insights into their specific interactions with their disease-causing allergen.

The ability to now study human IgE mAb hereby marks a major milestone in the allergy field, where authentic epitopes can be determined, and structure-based design of hypo-allergens can be pursued. These human IgE mAb will contribute to analyzing the human IgE antibody repertoire and associated epitopes, and lead to the development of new molecules for diagnosis and therapy of allergic diseases.

VACCINE AGAINST HEMOGLOBINOPATHIES (SICKLE CELL DISEASE AND THALASSEMIA'S) SCD AND β-THALASSEMIA

Sickle cell disease (SCD) and β-thalassemia are two inherited rare diseases caused by genetic mutations that affect the production or function of hemoglobin (Hb), the protein found in red blood cells that carries oxygen around the body. Both diseases are life-long debilitating genetic disorders caused by errors in the genes for Hb, a substance composed of a protein ("globin") plus an iron molecule ("heme") that is responsible for carrying oxygen within the red blood cell.

While β-thalassemia is caused by a defect in the beta-globin gene, controlling the production of the beta-globin chains of Hb, SCD is caused by a defect in Hb itself with the presence of abnormal hemoglobin S (HbS). New gene therapy may free patients from the burden of frequent transfusions and painful vaso-occlusive crises (VOCs) that occur when sickled red blood cells block small blood vessels, and has the potential to significantly improve their quality of life. A gene-editing treatment called Casgevy, which in trials has been found to restore healthy Hb production in the majority of participants with SCD and transfusion-dependent β-thalassemia, relieving the symptoms.

The only FDA-approved gene therapy works by putting functional copies of the abnormal gene into a patient's blood stem cells. The red blood cells are then able to make normal or near-normal levels of Hb. At present, there is no specific vaccine for hemoglobinopathies.

Gene Therapy Background

Gene therapy has been studied for various genetic diseases since the 1980s. More than 1,800 gene therapy trials have been conducted since then. Extended gene therapy clinical trials in β-thalassemia were approved in 2012. It is an approach, as previously mentioned, that aims to cure genetic diseases by replacing or correcting (editing) the defective or nonfunctional gene in the patient's DNA. In the case of β-thalassemia, a defect (mutation) in the β-globin gene results in the decrease or absence of Hb the vital oxygen-carrying protein of the body. If this gene is replaced by a functional one, then it is anticipated that Hb production will be restored and consequently the patient's red blood cells will have normal function.

Currently, the primary approaches for managing SCD include supportive care, medications, blood transfusions, and, in some cases, BM or stem cell transplantation. There are ongoing studies exploring gene therapy as a potential cure for SCD. These studies are still in the experimental stages, but initial results have shown promise. These new therapies aim to correct the genetic mutation that causes SCD or to compensate for the dysfunctional gene.

The first cell-based gene therapies for SCD in adolescents and adults received FDA approval on Friday, December 8, 2023, demonstrating the continued momentum of this promising new area of medicine. The potential that these two products (gene therapies) can have to transform the lives of patients living with SCD is enormous, bringing hope to thousands with the disease.

The medicines, called Casgevy (exa-cel) and Lyfgenia, are potential cures for people with sickle cell, a debilitating and life-shortening inherited red blood cell disorder that disproportionately affects African Americans.

Casgevy (exa-cel) from Vertex Pharmaceuticals Inc. and Lyfgenia (lovo-cel) from Bluebird Bio Inc. were approved for patients 12 years and older who have experienced VOCs or vaso-occlusive events (VOEs).

Casgevy is a cell-based gene therapy medicinal product using CRISPR/Cas9 technology to edit the patient's blood stem cells. It is a personalized one-off treatment that involves mobilizing BM stem cells from a patient's blood. *CRISPR* gene editing finds a specific sequence of DNA inside a cell. Using "molecular scissors" to make precise cuts, enables adding, removing, or altering genetic material at that specific location of the genome of the cells. With Casgevy, stem cells are edited at the erythroid-specific enhancer region of the *BCL11A* gene which usually prevents the production of fetal hemoglobin (HbF). These modified cells are then infused back into the patient, and the reduction of *BCL11A* gene transcription leads to an increase in HbF production thus providing functioning Hb.

These two gene therapies use different ways to change the expression of an individual's genes but both therapies result in an individual *making more HbF*, a type of oxygen-carrying blood protein present at birth. When increased in adults with SCD, HbF can reduce complications associated with the disease, including VOCs or VOEs, a condition in which the blood vessels become clogged and cause severe pain and organ damage.

The US-FDA approved a pair of gene editing therapy treatments for SCD:
- *Exa-cel:* Casgevy is the CRISPR-based treatment
- *Lovo-cel:* Lyfgenia, uses an older gene therapy approach

These are approved two gene-editing treatments for patients aged 12 years or older with severe SCD. These "milestone treatments" mark the first cell-based gene therapies for this debilitating and potentially life-threatening blood disorder that affects about 100,000 people in the US.

Exa-cel uses *CRISPR* gene-editing technology. Before the infusion, patients undergo myeloablative conditioning, which removes cells from the BM. These cells are genetically modified to produce HbF. Patients then receive an infusion of the edited cells, which can help restore normal Hb production. Exa-cel could "provide a one-time functional cure" for patients with severe SCD.

Lovo-cel, a cell-based gene therapy, uses a different technology a lentiviral vector, or gene delivery vehicle that can also genetically modify a patient's blood stem cells.
- Like exa-cel, lovo-cel (Lyfgenia), is a one-time, single-dose infusion that contains the patient's modified cells. It also involves removing the patient's cells and then returning them. It is an older technology, using

a virus to deliver a healthy copy of the gene that produces adult Hb to make up for the one producing the sickled form. Before the infusion, patients undergo myeloablative conditioning. The patient's stem cells are then genetically modified to allow them to produce the most common form of Hb and HbA.

Both these two gene therapies have shown similarly encouraging results and bring tremendous benefits to the patients.

Cost concerns: Casgevy will cost $2.2 million for the one-time treatment, while Lyfgenia will cost $3.1 million.

The most common side effects included stomatitis; febrile neutropenia; and low platelet, white blood cell, and red blood cell counts. People with SCD are immuno-compromised, which means they have an increased risk of infection. For this reason, immunizations are an important part of these individuals.

Routine, immunization can help protect people with sickle cell from developing serious infections. Children with SCD should receive all recommended childhood vaccines as well as an annual flu shot. Adults should make sure their vaccinations are up to date. Special vaccine schedules are recommended for certain vaccines, including annual flu shots, Hib, pneumococcal vaccines, and meningococcal vaccines.

Adults age 19 and older with SCD who have not received a PCV should receive a single dose of either Vaxneuvance (PCV15) or Prevnar 20 (PCV20). Those who get PCV15 should get one dose of PPSV23 at least 1 year later.

Concerns about these immunizations should be discussed with healthcare providers.

Monoclonal Antibody Therapeutic Role in Sickle Cell Disease

Crizanlizumab is an anti-P-selectin mAb indicated to reduce the frequency/prevent recurrence of VOCs in patients with SCD aged ≥16 years.

The anti-P-selectin humanized mAb crizanlizumab functions through selective inhibition of P-selectin. At a dose of 5 mg/kg in a clinical trial, it led to a 45.3% decline in the median annual crisis rate in individuals with SCD.

Immunogenicity of IV *inclacumab*, a fully human IgG4 anti-P-selectin mAb in development for the treatment of SCD, at doses up to and exceeding those previously tested in healthy individuals. Inclacumab was well tolerated, with PK as expected for a mAb against a membrane-bound target and a long duration of PD effects after both single IV doses, supporting a prolonged dosing interval.

■ CROHN'S DISEASE VACCINE

Crohn's disease is a debilitating and aggressive form of inflammatory bowel disease (IBD). It affects an estimated 4 million worldwide, including 1.2 million in the USA and around 250,000 in the UK and numbers are increasing, especially in children. Treatment for CD has typically focused on alleviating symptoms to achieve clinical remission using corticosteroids or immunomodulators, but a need for more effective treatment remains.

There is no cure for CD and no cause is officially recognized. However, there is compelling evidence pointing to *Mycobacterium avium* subspecies paratuber-culosis (MAP) as the cause of CD. MAP belongs to a family of bacteria called "mycobacteria", which also includes tuberculosis and leprosy.

The MAP is the well-established cause of Johne's disease—a form of IBD very like CD which affects animals, including domestic livestock. Data from the US suggest 91% of dairy herds are infected (although most will not show outward signs of disease). Milk from infected animals often contains MAP and not all of it is killed by pasteurization because MAP is a very tough bug.

Almost everyone with Crohn's has a MAP infection. Historically, MAP in humans has been difficult to study as it cannot be seen under an ordinary microscope and is very difficult to grow. Testing for MAP by the presence of its DNA [using polymerase chain reaction (PCR)] has found MAP in up to 92% of Crohn's patients but until now no one has developed a test to show MAP in situ in the tissues of people with CD (Professor Hermon-Taylor).

The CD-MAP vaccine is an experimental viral vector vaccine intended to prevent or treat CD, by provoking an immune response to one possible causative agent of the disease, MAP. The vaccine is currently about to begin phase 2 of its development.

The test is an essential "companion diagnostic" for the vaccine trial; a simple blood test allowing doctors to confirm MAP infection prior to vaccination and monitor patients' responses to the vaccine. Validation of the new test is almost complete.

Because the commercial inactivated vaccines are not completely protective and interfere with bovine tuberculosis diagnostics, recent study results demonstrate that one of the fusion proteins (recombinant protein 66NC) is an efficient candidate for further development into a protective vaccine in terms of inducing specific protection against MAP.

Monoclonal Antibodies Benefits Crohn's Disease

There is no doubt that the advent of biological therapy with mAbs has provided significant benefits for patients with ulcerative colitis (UC) and CD. Their use has resulted in improvement in clinical symptoms, endoscopic evidence of inflammation, and quality of life.

Recently, several biologic agents have been approved for use. Adalimumab is a mAb that reduces inflammatory cytokines by inhibiting TNF-alpha. Ustekinumab is another, fully human IgG1 mAb against the p40 subunit of IL-12 and IL-23. Both treatment regimens resulted in clinical remission with similar toxicity profiles.

■ VACCINE FOR RHEUMATOID ARTHRITIS

Immunotherapy for RA involves the use of nonbiological medications that modulate the immune system to reduce inflammation and halt the progression of the disease. Also improve physical function, and slow down joint damage. However, like any medication, immunotherapy for RA can have side effects, including an increased risk of infections and other potential adverse effects related to immunosuppression. Therefore, individuals with RA need to work closely with their healthcare providers to determine the most appropriate treatment plan based on their specific condition and medical history.

Nonbiologic *disease-modifying antirheumatic drugs (DMARDs)* include traditional *DMARDs* that are not biologically derived. Methotrexate and sulfasalazine are pivotal in the long-term management of RA, slowing disease progression by modulating the immune system.

Here are some common types of biological DMARDs (bDMARDs) drugs made from living organisms. bDMARDs target specific components of the immune system involved in the inflammation process. They include drugs such as biologics, including TNF inhibitors (TNFIs) and interleukin-6 inhibitors (IL-6 Is) or blockers, target-specific immune system components to address inflammation, typically prescribed when DMARDs alone are inadequate. Examples of TNFIs include etanercept, infliximab, adalimumab, certolizumab, and golimumab. Examples of IL-6 Is include tocilizumab and sarilumab.

Janus kinase (JK) inhibitors (JKIs): These are small molecule drugs that inhibit the JK enzymes, involved in the signaling pathways of various cytokines. Examples include tofacitinib, baricitinib, and upadacitinib.

B-cell depleting agents: Rituximab is an example of a drug that targets B-cells.

T-cell costimulation blockers: Abatacept is an example that inhibits T-cell activation.

Interleukin-1 inhibitors (IL-1 Is): Anakinra is an example of a drug that blocks IL-1.

A RA vaccine and other mAb immune system drugs are likely years away from approval for use in humans. However, several types are in clinical trials or earlier phases of research. So far, they show real promise. mAbs have become a cornerstone in the treatment of RA, offering targeted therapies that can significantly improve patient outcomes. These biological agents are designed to target specific components of the immune system that play a key role in the inflammatory process of RA.

Monoclonal antibodies are part of a class of medications known as bDMARDs. They are typically used when conventional synthetic DMARDs (csDMARDs) have not provided adequate relief of symptoms or when rapid control of inflammation is needed. The choice of a specific mAb depends on various factors, including disease severity, patient history, comorbidities, and potential side effects.

Some of the mAbs that are used in the treatment of RA are as follow:
- *Infliximab (Remicade):* It is a chimeric mAb against TNF-α, a cytokine that plays a central role in inflammation. Infliximab is used in combination with methotrexate for the treatment of moderate-to-severe RA in patients who have not responded adequately to other DMARDs.
- *Adalimumab (Humira):* It is a fully human mAb against TNF-α. Like infliximab, it is used in patients with moderate to severe RA who have had an inadequate response to one or more DMARDs.
- *Sarilumab (Kevzara):* It is a human mAb against the interleukin-6 receptor (IL-6R). IL-6 is another cytokine implicated in the pathogenesis of RA. Sarilumab is approved for the treatment of adult patients with moderate to severe RA who have not responded adequately or are intolerant to one or more DMARDs.

- *Olokizumab:* It targets IL-6, used in combination with methotrexate in patients with RA who have not responded adequately to other treatments. It has shown significant improvement in the signs, symptoms, and physical function of RA patients.
- *Rituximab (Rituxan):* It is a chimeric mAb against CD20, a protein primarily found on the surface of B-cells. By targeting CD20, rituximab depletes B-cells, which are involved in the pathogenesis of RA. It is used in patients with moderate-to-severe RA who have had an inadequate response to one or more TNF inhibitors.

In short:
- Conventional mAbs (e.g., infliximab or adalimumab), Fc fusion proteins (etanercept and abatacept), and one antibody-derived molecule, a PEGylated anti-TNF Fab fragment (certolizumab pegol), are widely used for the treatment of patients with RA.
- Rituxan (rituximab), one of the first mAbs on the market, it is used to treat autoimmune conditions including RA and lupus in addition to blood cancers.

Roll of Rheumatoid Arthritis Vaccines

Unlike those for other serious conditions, an RA vaccine would not prevent you from getting the disease. Instead, it would control RA in a different way than biologics or DMARDs like methotrexate.

Targeting T-cells

Scientists are working on a vaccine that targets T-cells. These are cells that make several substances involved in RA inflammation. That means this vaccine may be able to attack RA on more than one front. Researchers are studying different types of vaccines for RA, along with other immune treatments.

Scientists at several US institutions have collaborated on research that transforms stem cells into RA fighters. Using the gene-editing tool CRISPR/Cas9, they created smart cells that could fight inflammation, deliver biologic drug therapy, and turn on and off as needed. To do this, they removed a gene involved in RA's inflammatory process. Then, they added a gene that releases a biological drug. The modified cells could even create cartilage tissue. Researchers call this a regenerative medicine approach. They say it could one day provide an effective vaccine for a range of diseases, not just RA.

Cellular Immunotherapies

Cellular immunotherapies involve modifying or manipulating immune cells to regulate the immune response. Currently, cellular immunotherapies are not as common as biologic or nonbiologic DMARDs in the treatment of RA, but they represent a growing area of research.

■ VACCINE FOR OSTEOARTHRITIS

Osteoarthritis is primarily a degenerative joint disease characterized by the breakdown of cartilage and other joint structures. Traditional treatments for OA focus on managing symptoms such as pain and inflammation through medications, PT, lifestyle modifications, and in severe cases, surgery.

Although OA can damage any joint, the disorder most commonly affects knee, hip, spine, and hand joints. OA affecting around 500 million people worldwide, or around 7% of the global population. In the United States, over 32 million have OA with a prevalence rate of 22–39% in India. Affects each person differently and for some people, relatively mild and does not affect day-to-day activities. For others, it causes significant pain and disability. Joint damage usually develops gradually over years, although it could worsen quickly in some people.

Researchers have been exploring the role of immunotherapy in treating OA, particularly targeting inflammatory pathways involved in the disease process. Immunotherapy, typically involves biological agents that target specific molecules or cells involved in the inflammatory response. These agents may include:

- *Anti-inflammatory cytokines:* Cytokines are signaling molecules involved in inflammation. Some research has focused on using cytokines with anti-inflammatory properties, such as interleukin-1 receptor antagonist (IL-1Ra), to reduce inflammation and slow down cartilage degradation in OA.
- *Do mAb therapies have a role in OA?* Several cytokine proteins have been identified as contributing to the inflammatory process involved in arthritic and other autoimmune conditions. mAbs have been developed to target these cytokine proteins.
- *mAbs:* These can target specific molecules involved in the inflammatory cascade. For example, antibodies targeting TNF-α or IL-6 have been investigated for their potential in reducing inflammation and symptoms in OA.

- *Cell-based therapies:* Stem cell therapy and platelet-rich plasma (PRP) therapy are examples of cell-based treatments that aim to promote tissue repair and regeneration in OA joints. These therapies may modulate the immune response and promote healing processes within the joint.
- *Tolerance-inducing therapies:* Some experimental approaches aim to induce immune tolerance to cartilage-specific antigens, thereby preventing the immune system from attacking the joint tissues. These therapies are still in the early stages of development and may hold promise for preventing or slowing down OA progression.

While these approaches show potential in preclinical and early clinical studies, more research is needed to establish their safety and efficacy in larger patient populations. Additionally, challenges such as delivery methods, treatment protocols, and long-term effects need to be addressed before immunotherapy becomes a standard treatment option for OA. As research progresses, immunotherapy may offer new avenues for managing OA and improving patient outcomes.

Osteoarthritis Pain Vaccine

Too many people living with pain do not get effective relief from the treatments that are currently available, and that is why the development of more effective painkillers, with fewer side effects, is vital for people living with arthritis.

The University of Oxford, researchers developed a *virus-like particle vaccine* able to trigger the immune system to produce antibodies to block naturally-occurring nerve growth factor (NGF), which causes pain in patients with OA. Scientists have developed and tested a vaccine that they say could be used to treat chronic pain caused by OA.

"This is the first successful vaccination to target pain in OA, one of the biggest healthcare challenges of our generation". Whilst there are still safety issues that need to be considered before these types of approaches can be used in patients, experts say that this vaccine design allows to "control antibody levels and thus tailor treatment to individual cases according to need".

■ OBESITY VACCINE

Obesity is considered as a NCD, and vaccines do not directly target it. There is no vaccine specifically designed or approved for the treatment or prevention of obesity. Obesity is a multifactorial condition influenced by genetic, environmental, and behavioral factors. Therefore, its management typically involves lifestyle modifications such as dietary changes, increased physical activity, and behavioral interventions. However, vaccines can prevent certain infections that might indirectly impact weight. For example, some studies suggest that certain gut bacteria related to obesity may be influenced by the gut microbiome, which can be influenced by vaccinations that affect the gut.

There have been some efforts to develop vaccines that target hormones or proteins involved in appetite regulation or fat metabolism. However, these investigational vaccines are still in the early stages of development and have not been approved for clinical use.

India, struggling with malnutrition and poverty, is also now a land of obesity. But obesity is not just affecting the urban well-to-do. Indian researchers have found it is also an issue in India's villages, where three out of four Indians still live. Increased automation, better transportation, and improved standards of living have resulted in less active lifestyles and access to processed foods. A study in the Indian Journal of Endocrinology and Metabolism says the percentage of rural Indians who were overweight grew from 2% in 1989 to 17.1% in 2012.

While there has been ongoing research into the causes and treatment of obesity, including the development of potential medications, vaccines specifically for obesity are not part of current medical practices.

■ VACCINE AGAINST ADDICTION

Like shots against disease, these vaccines would work by spurring the immune system to produce antibodies that would shut down the narcotic before it could take root in the body, or in the brain.

Drug abuse or over drug use [opioid use disorder (OUD)] is a worldwide problem that is detrimental to public health and extends to both legal and illicit drugs. Drawbacks associated with current treatments include limited effectiveness, potential side effects, and, in some instances, the absence of or concerns with approved therapy options. A significant amount of clinical research has been conducted investigating immunotherapy as a treatment option against drug abuse. Current treatments for OUD are methadone, buprenorphine, and naltrexone, and their effectiveness depends upon formulation, compliance, access to medications, and the specific misused opioid.

Unlike the COVID-19 vaccine, the best practice for an addiction vaccine would not be to receive the immunization in advance of coming into contact with the thing being immunized against (in this case, illegal drugs). Rather, subjects would be given the vaccine after they have already used the drug and developed a dependency.

A research team led by the University of Houston has developed a vaccine targeting the dangerous synthetic opioid fentanyl that could block its ability to enter the brain. This vaccine can generate antifentanyl antibodies that bind to the consumed fentanyl and prevent it from entering the brain, allowing it to be eliminated from the body via the kidneys.

The breakthrough discovery could have major implications for the nation's opioid epidemic by becoming a relapse prevention agent for people trying to quit using opioids. While research reveals OUD is treatable, an estimated 80% of those dependent on the drug suffer a relapse. The vaccine did not cause any adverse side effects in the immunized rats involved in laboratory studies. The team plans to start manufacturing clinical-grade vaccine in the coming months with clinical trials in humans planned soon.

Monoclonal Antibodies to Prevent Drug Addictions

Cessation Therapeutics, a North Carolina biotech company, touts its mAb as a way both to prevent overdoses and to treat overdoses and opioid addiction.

■ CONCLUSION

- Vaccines are an effective strategy to combat these challenges; however, utilization rates are inadequate immunization against NCDs has the potential to be a game-changer in reducing the burden of these diseases globally.
- With India running one of the world's largest COVID-19 vaccination programs, this presents an opportunity to improve vaccination coverage for all VPDs.
- The potential of immunization against NCDs could be a long haul. Would require research and development (R & D), investors/investments, a stronger healthcare system, and build public trust in vaccines.
- Raising awareness about the benefits of vaccinations, particularly for those with NCDs, and providing national guidelines with recommendations from medical societies, will increase vaccine acceptance. Adequate vaccine acceptance will reduce the VPD burden in this vulnerable population.
- Effective vaccination will have a significant impact on the disease burden of both VPDs and NCDs and beyond.

While there are no approved vaccines by licensing authorities available that can directly prevent NCDs and disorders. Vaccinations against IDs are particularly crucial for individuals with NCDs, as these individuals are at a higher risk of severe complications from infections. This underscores the importance of vaccination as a preventive measure to safeguard against additional health complications that could exacerbate NCDs.

The ongoing research and development in the field of vaccines offer hope for future advancements where vaccines may play a more direct role in the prevention or management of NCDs. Until then, the focus remains on utilizing available vaccines to protect vulnerable populations, including those with NCDs, from IDs and to maintain a high level of public health vigilance.

Authors have looked at the burden of VPDs in those with NCDs, the benefits of vaccinations, current challenges, and possible strategies that may simplify the accessibility of vaccination programs. Effective vaccination will have a significant impact on the disease burden of both VPDs and NCDs and beyond.

The integration of vaccination strategies into the management plans for individuals with chronic NCDs is essential. It not only helps in reducing the burden of IDs but also contributes to the overall well-being and quality of life of those living with NCDs. As the global health community continues to navigate the challenges posed by NCDs, the role of vaccinations remains a cornerstone of preventive health strategies, highlighting the need for continued research, education, and advocacy in this area.

Success in the fight against NCDs is challenging and requires the application of previously successful disease elimination approaches, including immunization. Currently, there are no vaccines available that can directly prevent NCDs. The development of vaccines specifically targeting NCDs remains an area of ongoing research. A significant breakthrough has now been made in the development of allergy vaccines based on recombinant allergens. Immunization against NCDs has the potential to be a game-changer in reducing the burden of these diseases globally.

■ SUGGESTED READING

1. Abou-Donia MB. Autism—a potential autoimmune disease: neurodegeneration-induced autoantibodies against neural proteins. J Cell Immunol. 2020;2(2):47-54.
2. Afsar A, Chen M, Xuan Z, Zhang L. A glance through the effects of CD4+ T cells, CD8+ T cells, and cytokines on Alzheimer's disease. Comput Struct Biotechnol J. 2023;21:5662-75.
3. Ashton NJ, Brum WS, Molfetta GD, Benedet AL, Arslan B, Jonaitis E, et al. Diagnostic Accuracy of a Plasma Phosphorylated Tau 217 Immunoassay Test for Alzheimer's Disease Pathology. JAMA Neurol. 2024;81(3):255-263.
4. Bakris GL. (2023). Sustained Blood Pressure Reduction With the RNA Interference Therapeutic Zilebesiran: Primary Results From KARDIA-1, a Phase 2 Study in Patients With Hypertension. Available from: https://www.abstractsonline.com/pp8/?_ga=2.252499981.569559676.1693429947-1069604919.1693247687#!/10871/presentation/16559. [Last accessed May, 2023].
5. Bartl S, Xie Y, Potluri N, Kesineni R, Hencak K, Cengio LD, et al. Reducing huntingtin by immunotherapy delays disease progression in a mouse model of Huntington disease. Neurobiol Dis. 2024;190: 106376.
6. Bhattad S, Gupta S, Israni N, Mohanty S. Profile of Kawasaki disease at a tertiary care center in India. Ann Pediatr Cardiol. 2021;14(2):187-97.
7. Bloom BT, Bushell MJ. Vaccines against Drug Abuse— Are We There Yet? Vaccines (Basel). 2022;10(6):860.
8. CBS News. (2021). Alzheimer's Disease Nasal Vaccine To Be Tested At Brigham And Women's Hospital. Available from: https://www.cbsnews.com/boston/news/alzheimers-disease-nasal-vaccine-trial-protollin-brigham-and-womens-hospital-boston/. [Last accessed May, 2024].
9. Chang L, Yang HW, Lin TY, Yang KD. Perspective of immunopathogenesis and immunotherapies for Kawasaki disease. Front Pediatr. 2021;9:697632.
10. Chellappan DK, Bhandare RR, Shaik AB, Prasad K, Suhaimi NAA, Yap WS, et al. Vaccine for diabetes: where do we stand? Int J Mol Sci. 2022;23(16):9470.
11. Chen XZ, Guo R, Zhao C, Xu J, Song H, Yu H, et al. A novel anti-cancer therapy: *CRISPR/Cas9* gene editing. Front Pharmacol. 2022;13:939090.
12. Cusi K. Selective agonists of thyroid hormone receptor beta for the treatment of NASH. N Engl J Med. 2024;390: 559-61.
13. Dale JB, Walker MJ. Update on Group A Streptococcal Vaccine Development. Curr Opin Infect Dis. 2020;33(3): 244-50.
14. Dotinga R. (2023). Epstein-Barr and MS: Just How Strong Is the Link? Available from: https://www.medscape.com/s/viewarticle/997749?ecd=wnl_tp10_daily_231029_MSCPEDIT_etid5998614&uac=48448CX&impID=5998614. [Last accessed May, 2024].
15. Fickman L. (2022). Fentanyl Vaccine Potential 'Game Changer' For Opioid Epidemic. Available from: https://uh.edu/news-events/stories/2022-news-articles/november-2022/11142022-fentanyl-vaccine-haile-kosten.php. [Last accessed May, 2024].
16. Healthline. (2023). How do vaccines help protect against respiratory diseases? Available from: https://www.healthline.com/health/vaccines-for-respiratory-diseases#adult-vaccines. [Last accessed May, 2024].
17. Jackson DJ, Heaney LG, Humbert M, Kent BD, Shavit A, Hiljemark L, et al. Reduction of daily maintenance inhaled corticosteroids in patients with severe eosinophilic asthma treated with benralizumab (SHAMAL): a randomised, multicentre, open-label, phase 4 study. Lancet. 2024; 403:271-81.
18. Jeong S, Shin WY, Oh YH. Immunotherapy for NAFLD and NAFLD-related hepatocellular carcinoma. Front Endocrinol (Lausanne). 2023;14:1150360.
19. Le MH, Yeo YH, Zou B, Barnet S, Henry L, Cheung R, et al. Forecasted 2040 global prevalence of nonalcoholic fatty liver disease using hierarchical bayesian approach. Clin Mol Hepatol. 2022;28:841-50.
20. Ludvigsson J. Immune Interventions at Onset of Type 1 Diabetes—Finally, a Bit of Hope. N Engl J Med. 2023; 389:2199-220.
21. Maynard G, Kannan R, Liu J, Wang W, Lam TKT, Wang X, et al. Soluble Nogo-Receptor-Fc decoy (AXER-204) in patients with chronic cervical spinal cord injury in the USA: a first-in-human and randomised clinical trial. Lancet Neurol. 2023;22(8):672-84.
22. Mustafa AS. Vaccine potential of mycobacterial antigens against asthma. Med Princ Pract. 2020;29(5):404-11.
23. NKGen Biotech. (2023). NKGen Biotech Presented Phase I Clinical Trial Data at the 16th Annual Clinical Trials on Alzheimer's Disease (CTAD) Conference. Available from: https://nkgenbiotech.com/nkgen-biotech-presented-phase-i-clinical-trial-data-at-the-16th-annual-clinical-trials-on-alzheimers-disease-ctad-conference/. [Last accessed May, 2024].
24. Ray KK, Wright RS, Kallend D, Koenig W, Leiter LA, Raal FJ, et al. Two Phase 3 trials of Inclisiran in patients with elevated LDL cholesterol. N Engl J Med. 2020;382(16): 1507-19.
25. Robinson WH, Steinman L. Epstein-Barr virus and multiple sclerosis. Science. 2022;375(6578):264-5.
26. Sahadulla MI, Uduman S. Compendium of the Pandemic Era, 1st edition. Kottayam, Kerala: DC Folio (An Imprint of DC Books); 2022.

27. Sansone G, Bonifati DM. Vaccines and myasthenia gravis: a comprehensive review and retrospective study of SARS-CoV-2 vaccination in a large cohort of myasthenic patients. J Neurol. 2022;269(8):3965-81.
28. Shao M, Cui N, Tang Y, Chen F, Cui F, Dang G, et al. A candidate subunit vaccine induces protective immunity against *Mycobacterium avium* subspecies paratuberculosis in mice. NPJ Vaccines. 2023;8(1):72.
29. Sikich L, Kolevzon A, King BH, McDougle CJ, Sanders KB, Kim SJ, et al. Intranasal oxytocin in children and adolescents with autism spectrum disorder. N Engl J Med. 2021;385:1462-73.
30. Smith SA, Chruszcz M, Chapman MD, Pomés A. Human monoclonal IgE antibodies: a major milestone in allergy. Curr Allergy Asthma Rep. 2023;23(1):53-65.
31. Smolen JS. (2022). Annals of Rheumatic Disease: The EULAR Journal. Available from: https://congress.eular.org/myUploadData/files/euroab_2022_book.pdf. [Last accessed May, 2024].
32. Spichak S. (2022). At Least 9 Alzheimer's Vaccines in Trials Right Now. Available from: https://www.beingpatient.com/there-are-9-alzheimers-vaccines-in-trials-right-now/. [Last accessed May, 2024].
33. David Andes, Carol Kauffman, and William Hope. End of an era in defining the optimal treatment of invasive candidiasis? The Lancet Respiratory. 2022;10(5):422-23.
34. van Dyck CH, Swanson CJ, Aisen P, Bateman RJ, Chen C, Gee M, et al. Lecanemab in early Alzheimer's disease. N Engl J Med. 2023;388:9-21.
35. Varadé J, Magadán S, González-Fernández Á. Human immunology and immunotherapy: main achievements and challenges. Cell Mol Immunol. 2021;18(4):805-28.
36. Vermersch P, Granziera C, Mao-Draayer Y, Cutter G, Kalbus O, Staikov I, et al. Inhibition of CD40L with Frexalimab in multiple sclerosis. N Engl J Med. 2024;390:589-600.
37. Vora A, Di Pasquale A, Kolhapure S, Agrawal A, Agrawal S. The need for vaccination in adults with chronic (noncommunicable) diseases in India: lessons from around the world. Hum Vaccin Immunother. 2022;18(5):2052544.
38. Wong GWK. Options for multiple food allergies: food avoidance or pharmacologic treatment? N Engl J Med. 2024;390(10):946-8.
39. Yao J, Zhou R, Liu Y, Lu Z. Progress in Guillain–Barré syndrome immunotherapy: a narrative review of new strategies in recent years. Hum Vaccin Immunother. 2023;19(2):2215153.

Innovative Infectious Diseases Vaccines (The Future of Vaccines)

Mohd Uduman

■ INTRODUCTION

The coronavirus disease-2019 (COVID-19) pandemic has also made possible scientific interests and quickened more for real innovation in terms of the technology, evaluation, and speed with which vaccines come to the market for human use. In their research and development (R&D), pharmaceutical companies are not just looking at new vaccines for diseases, but also looking at ways to make vaccines more effective and easier to use. That is especially important for infectious diseases (IDs) impacting parts of the world without developed healthcare systems. These include new advances in much-needed vaccines for malaria, respiratory syncytial virus (RSV), human immunodeficiency virus (HIV), tuberculosis (TB), *Shigella*, etc. As we are learning with COVID, breakthroughs in vaccines for one disease can lend knowledge and problem-solving to others.

■ A CASE-BASED FUTURISTIC CLINICAL SCENARIO

The authors have answered a query on "Vaccine for Tonsillitis": Mr Sankararaman, Ayikudy Amar Seva Developmental Disability Center, Tenkasi district Tamil Nadu, India:

Question: Is there any vaccine for tonsillectomy and adenoidectomy (T&A) Is there a shot for tonsillitis, i.e., vaccine against tonsillitis causing organisms?

Answer: Thanks Mr Sankararaman Sir; firstly; there is currently no vaccine available to prevent "tonsillitis-causing pathogens [group A *Streptococcus* (GAS)]" nor can we anticipate it in the near future.

Decades back; limited experiences of using "bacterial vaccination" in the treatment of recurrent tonsillitis; but these were not successful nor pursued further research, by the scientists. However, there is a pressing need for such a vaccine against "tonsillitis" at a global level.

The terms "tonsillitis" are also used interchangeably with "pharyngitis", "sore throat", "strep throat", etc., but they do not mean the same thing. In infants, toddlers, and preschoolers, the most frequent cause of sore throats is due to viruses and may develop a mild fever of 1–2 days self-limited, and the children will recover uneventfully.

In contrast; "strep throat" due to GAS is the commonly and frequently occurring bacterial tonsillitis in school-attending children; would require antibiotic therapy for strep throat fever illnesses. Failure to do that may result in dreaded complications such as acute rheumatic fever (ARF), rheumatic heart diseases (RHDs), skin, and kidney infections, which are still occurring in India and other developing countries.

Therefore, there is a place for a safe, effective, affordable, and practical GAS vaccine despite all the technical difficulties of making such a vaccine for these particular GAS bacteria, specifically. An effective GAS vaccine will prevent not only "tonsillitis", but also more serious invasive diseases (toxic shock syndrome) and post-infectious complications such as ARF, RHDs, and kidney and immunologic disorders.

There is an urgent need for preparatory GAS vaccine development on a global scale at an earlier date, hopefully! This could reduce the related burden on individuals, communities, health systems, and societies as a whole and, through a reduction of antibiotic use.

■ VACCINE INNOVATION FOR HUMANS

Background

Vaccines have been a part of the human fight against the disease for >200 years. While we can attribute many public health successes to vaccination, the future presents continued challenges. Despite the successes of vaccinations against many viruses, e.g., measles, mumps, and rubella (MMR), polio, and rotaviruses, a lot has yet to be achieved. Most potential new viral vaccines have an essential composition, sometimes characterized by low immunogenicity, with the inability to elicit powerful and long-lasting immune responses.

Beyond the well-recognized conjugated bacterial vaccines in recent years, many bacterial IDs remain for which researchers have been unable to find effective preventive bacterial vaccines. Vaccines are already important tools in reducing antimicrobial resistance (AMR) and future development will provide further opportunities to optimize the use of vaccines against bacterial resistance. Substantial diseases, such as HIV, dengue, TB, and malaria have spread all over the world and are still burdened by a high rate of morbidity and mortality, and are not yet protected by an effective vaccine.

Viruses that are capable of spreading by vector or airborne routes as one of the most important pandemic threats that will continue to emerge. New and reemerging pathogens, such as severe acute respiratory syndrome coronavirus 2 (SARS-CoV-2) variants and new influenza strains, will often pop up. More than 1.5 million as yet unknown viruses are estimated to exist in animals worldwide, and 38–50% of them are candidates to spread to humans.

Advances in our understanding of disease and leaps forward in science and technology are helping us design more effective vaccines, ones with a better immune response or vaccines that can be easier or quicker to manufacture. Development of futuristic ID vaccines is therefore important and often involves extensive research, global surveillance, rigorous testing, and governing policy.

The future of medicine is ribonucleic acid (RNA) vaccines and RNA therapeutics. Here are some key trends and technologies in futuristic ID vaccines research and development.

Messenger Ribonucleic Acid Vaccines

Like the Pfizer-BioNTech and Moderna COVID-19 vaccines represent a breakthrough in vaccine technology. This high-tech has the potential to revolutionize the way we respond to emerging IDs. The COVID-19 pandemic is a prime example of how rapidly new vaccines can now be developed and adapted for various IDs.

Certainly, the messenger ribonucleic acid (mRNA) platform disrupts the traditional vaccine-developing process because of its ability to develop candidate vaccines faster, combine vaccines, and target difficult viral antigenic sites. RNA vaccines are faster and cheaper to produce than traditional vaccines, and an RNA-based vaccine is also safer for the patient, as they are not produced using infectious elements.

Two forms of mRNA vaccines have been developed:
1. *Conventional mRNA vaccines:* The simplest type of RNA vaccine, a mRNA strand is packaged and delivered to the body, where it is taken up by the body's cells to make the antigen.
2. *Self-amplifying mRNA vaccines:* The pathogen-mRNA strand is packaged with additional RNA strands that ensure it will be copied once the vaccine is inside a cell. This means that greater quantities of the antigen are made from a smaller amount of vaccine, helping to ensure a more robust immune response.

The power of the mRNA vaccine technology (Pfizer/Moderna) is expected to bring much more safe and effective vaccines soon against the DNA latent virus vaccines including herpes simplex virus-1 (HSV-1), herpes simplex virus-2 (HSV-2), varicella zoster virus (VZV), Epstein–Barr virus (EBV), and cytomegalovirus (CMV).

Recombinant Deoxyribonucleic Acid Platforms

Recombinant deoxyribonucleic acid (DNA) platforms produce an exact genetic match to the proteins of a virus. The protein's DNA will be combined with DNA from a virus harmless to humans, and once injected, will rapidly produce large quantities of antigen which stimulate the immune system to protect against the virus.

Virus-like Particle Based Vaccines

Virus-like particles (VLPs) are molecules that closely resemble viruses but are noninfectious because they contain no viral genetic material. VLPs contain repetitive, high-density displays of viral surface proteins that present "conformational viral epitopes"—the part that causes an immune response.

Nonreplicating Viral Vectors

Viral vectors are tools commonly used to deliver genetic material into cells. A viral vector vaccine induces the expression of pathogen proteins within host cells similarly to other attenuated vaccines. However, since viral vector vaccines contain only a small fraction of pathogen genes, they are much safer, and infection by the pathogen is impossible.

Peptide vaccines are synthetic proteins that mimic naturally occurring proteins from viruses, causing an immune response.

- *Adjuvant technology:* This boosts the immune system's response to a vaccine, improving its efficacy and giving the potential for vaccines to be developed that are longer lasting and more effective in older populations.
- *Bioconjugation technology:* Developments in the process of joining a protein to an antigen could increase vaccine effectiveness.

Nanoparticle Vaccines

Nanoparticles (NPs) are extremely small particles, typically ranging in size from 1 to 100 nanometers, and they can be made from various materials such as lipids, proteins, polymers, or metals. In the context of vaccines, NPs are engineered to carry as a delivery system for antigens to the immune system in a controlled and targeted manner. The antigens can be derived from pathogens, tumor cells, or other disease-specific targets.

There are several advantages of encapsulating or attaching antigens to NP vaccines, e.g.,:
- NPs can mimic the size, shape, and surface properties of pathogens, which can help stimulate a stronger immune response. They can also be designed to release antigens slowly, leading to prolonged exposure to the immune system and potentially better immune memory.
- NPs can be engineered to specifically target certain cells or tissues, such as immune cells or tumor cells. This *targeted delivery system* can improve the efficiency of antigen presentation and enhance the immune response at the desired site.
- NPs have inherent *adjuvant properties* and enhance the immune response without the need for additional adjuvants. This can simplify the vaccine formulation and reduce the need for additional components.
- NPs can improve the *stability and shelf life of vaccines*, allowing for easier storage and transportation, especially in resource-limited settings.

In this context, nanotechnologies could represent one of the most modern and effective tools for vaccine production. New-generation vaccinology has already greatly benefited and will continue to benefit from the use of NPs as delivery vehicles and/or immune potentiators. Indeed, NPs can improve not only antigen uptake from antigen-presenting cells (APCs), but also immunogenicity and the slow release of antigens. Moreover, most NPs are biodegradable, biocompatible, and have minimal toxicity; therefore, they can offer a safe and effective alternative to traditional vaccines.

Recombinant Nanoparticles

Recombinant DNA is artificially created DNA. These types of vaccines use genetically engineered three-dimensional nanostructures that incorporate recombinant proteins critical to disease pathogenesis (the biological process that allows it to happen). In short, they support the production of the antigens that cause an immune response.

Multipathogen Vaccines

Rather than developing individual vaccines for each pathogen, scientists are exploring the development of multiple antigen-based vaccines (multivariant vaccines) on different platforms to tackle rapidly mutating infectious variants. This could be especially valuable in regions with limited healthcare infrastructure.

Advances in computational biology and bioinformatics are enabling the design of more effective antigens for vaccines. *Artificial intelligence (AI) and machine learning (ML)* are being used to analyze vast amounts of biological data, predict disease outbreaks, and optimize vaccine design. This precision in antigen design can lead to vaccines with improved efficacy and safety profiles.

Long-lasting Immunity

Research into vaccines that provide longer-lasting immunity without the need for frequent boosters is ongoing, as this could significantly improve disease control efforts.

The unprecedented scale and rapidity of dissemination of recent emerging IDs pose new challenges for vaccine developers, regulators, health authorities, and political constituencies. Therefore, there is the necessity to obtain modern and effective vaccines, by studying new antigens, adjuvants, and innovative delivery systems that will enhance their immunogenicity. This chapter on future vaccines is focused on clinically relevant selective old and new pathogens that are looked at in the context of technological innovations that help physicians and scientists with the new evolving vaccines that could reduce the burden of IDs.

Implementing the current vaccination strategies and focusing on new technologies to develop the vaccines of the future will certainly be the keystone in the endless fight against emerging IDs.

VACCINES TARGETING BACTERIA TO COMBAT ANTIMICROBIAL RESISTANCE (AMR)

Focusing on clinically significant gram-positive and gram-negative pathogens.

Role of Bacterial Vaccines Against Antimicrobial Resistance Bacteria

Globally, AMR has been rising at an alarming rate. Experts say in 2021, India alone reported 100,000 cases of AMR pathogens and India is among the notable countries that contribute significantly to global AMR due to extensive antibiotic abuse, both in healthcare and agriculture.

According to the World Health Organization (WHO), AMR causes an estimated 5 million deaths every year globally. This escalation is due to the spread of resistant organisms, leading to ineffective treatment of infections and increased mortality, more than HIV and malaria combined. These cases spanned across various bacterial infections, indicating widespread resistance, mostly among infants, the elderly, and those with comorbidities. AMR is threatening modern medicine beyond bacterial IDs; it also affects surgery, organ transplantation, and treatment for illnesses and ailments including HIV, liver and kidney disease, cancer, and physical trauma. Overuse and misuse of antibiotics are driving resistance to such an extent that we have entered the postantibiotic era, where some multidrug- and pan-drug-resistant bacterial infections are no longer treatable. If the situation is not reversed, 10 million people will die annually of drug-resistant infections by 2050. Vaccines can be highly effective tools in combating AMR.

Several vaccines against extracellular bacteria have been developed in the past and are still used successfully today, e.g., vaccines against tetanus, pertussis, and diphtheria. In bacterial cellular vaccines such as the Hib and PCVs, there is a broad spectrum of gram-positive/negative pathogens that are well expected to be highly effective tools in combating drug resistance-related deaths and morbidities.

Bacterial vaccines can help fight AMR by:
- Preventing and reducing AMR bacterial infections
- Reducing the need for antibiotics
- Minimizing the selective drug pressure that can result in resistant strains
- Reducing the emergence and spread of the AMR.

Apart from the diphtheria, tetanus, and pertussis (DTP) vaccines, there are other examples of successful bacterial vaccines that have noticeably reduced the antibiotic consumption IDs including:
- Hib vaccines in childhood against epiglottitis, meningitis, and invasive septicemia
- Pneumococcal vaccines against both pediatrics and adulthood sepsis, pneumonia, etc.
- Meningococcal septicemia and meningitis illnesses among travelers and college students
- Typhoid illnesses in many developing countries.

Despite the success of vaccination in greatly mitigating or eliminating the threat of diseases caused by pathogens, there are still known diseases and emerging pathogens for which the development of successful vaccines against them is inherently difficult. In addition, vaccine development for people with compromised immunity and other preexisting medical conditions has remained a major challenge.

Considerable advances have been made in vaccinology over the past four decades, which have been further accelerated by the response to the COVID-19 pandemic. These advances have opened up molecular targets and made it possible to vaccinate against more pathogens. Furthermore, vaccines present an opportunity to address increasingly difficult-to-treat infections caused by AMR bacteria.

There were 94 active preclinical vaccine candidates and 61 active development vaccine candidates, classified under four major bacterial groups.
- *Group A:* Bacterial pathogens with vaccines that are already licensed, such as the Hib, *Streptococcus pneumoniae*, *Mycobacterium tuberculosis* (Mtb) [Bacillus Calmette–Guérin (BCG)], and *Salmonella serotype typhi*.
- *Group B:* Pathogens with vaccines in late-stage clinical trials with high development feasibility, e.g., extraintestinal pathogenic *Escherichia coli* (ExPEC), *Neisseria gonorrhoeae*, and *Clostridium difficile* and *Salmonella serotype paratyphi*.
- *Group C:* Pathogens with vaccine candidates either in early clinical trials or with moderate to high feasibility of vaccine development. Enterotoxigenic *E. coli* (ETEC), *Klebsiella pneumoniae (Kpn)*, *Campylobacter* spp., *Shigella* spp., *Campylobacter* spp., and non-typhoidal *Salmonella* (NTS).
- *Group D:* Pathogens with either no candidates in clinical development or low development feasibility,

e.g., *Staphylococcus aureus (SA), Enterococcus faecium (Efe)*, and *Enterobacter* spp., *Pseudomonas aeruginosa, Acinetobacter baumannii*, and *Helicobacter pylori.*

Bacterial vaccines work by:
- Eliciting humoral antibodies against those particular bacteria
- Stimulating the immune system to produce a response against specific pathogens
- Preventing bacterial infection later.

These bacteria may infect humans and animals, and the infections they cause are harder to treat than those caused by nonresistant bacteria. Patients with drug-resistant infections alongside other health conditions require additional medical support, such as admission to intensive care units, admission to and longer stays in hospital, and the need for invasive treatment (such as mechanical ventilation). These lead to higher medical costs, prolonged hospital stays, and increased mortality.

This chapter will highlight selective bacterial pathogens that are associated with high clinical burden to all health care providers, globally. Group A: Pathogen vaccines that target *S. pneumoniae*, Hib, and *S. Typhi* are already licensed. Research to improve these vaccines continues and vaccine candidates in clinical development against *S. pneumoniae* outnumber any of the other pathogens considered.

Vaccine for Drug Resistance
Mycobacterium Tuberculosis

The only licensed BCG vaccine for Mtb was first used in 1921 but has variable effectiveness, and the immunity conferred wanes with age, leading to inadequate protection in adolescents and adults. BCG is rarely given to anyone over the age of 16 because there is little evidence it works well in adults. But it is given to adults aged 16–35 years who are at risk of TB through their work, such as some healthcare workers, veterinary staff, and abattoir workers.

Tuberculosis is one of the world's oldest and deadliest IDs. Every year, >10 million people fall ill, and more than a million die from TB disease, most of whom are adults and adolescents. With close to half a million people contracting drug-resistant forms of TB annually, AMR risks making the disease even more deadly and incurable. The rise of multidrug resistance (MDR) and extensively drug-resistant Mtb, together with the slow development of new drugs and vaccines, coinfection with HIV, and a partially effective vaccine, continue to impede the fight against this disease.

Neonatal BCG vaccination protects against disseminated infant disease, but efficacy against pulmonary disease declines to zero with time. Effective boosting for adolescents has great potential as a cost-effective intervention. Evidence suggesting protection against Mtb infection following BCG revaccination reopened the debate on revaccination in adolescents, and a more effective booster strategy might be needed for such settings.

At present, there are four vaccine candidates in phase 3 clinical trials targeting Mtb. VPM1002 is a prophylactic recombinant BCG (rBCG) vaccine, currently in phase 3 trial in newborn infants to assess its efficacy, safety, and immunogenicity against Mtb infection. The trial is scheduled to be completed in June 2025 (NCT04351685). A phase 2/3 trial of VPM1002 for preventing TB recurrence in treated patients is also underway in India. Also, Immuvac is a therapeutic vaccine that uses a heat-killed *Mycobacterium indicus pranii* and is in a phase 3 trial in India.

There is a subunit candidate, composed of an immunogenic fusion protein (M72) derived from two Mtb antigens (MTB32A and MTB39A), and the adjuvant AS01E. Few other preventive recombinant subunit vaccines studied in South Africa and Tanzania; also inactivated whole-cell approach prophylactic and therapeutic vaccine candidates are in late phase 2 clinical trials.

The COVID-19 served as a double-edged sword for the TB diseases. On one hand, it hampered the implementation of TB control, whereas on the other it showed that with adequate funding, vaccines and therapeutics can be developed rapidly. The COVID-19 pandemic highlighted priority areas in TB including the acceleration of new vaccines.

Leprosy Vaccine

Leprosy is endemic in several regions of the world. Over 200,000 new leprosy cases are reported globally every year. A vaccine for leprosy can eliminate the debilitating, biblical, and stigmatized disease in the twenty-first century and an estimated three to four million people are living with disabilities caused by leprosy.

Since the 1940s, many clinical studies have consistently shown that the BCG vaccine offers some level of protection but ranges between 18 and 90%. Throughout this time, different versions of BCG and new developments have resulted in new leprosy vaccine candidates and prevention strategies. *Mycobacterium leprae* remains a bacterium that requires animals for cultivation. Scientists still do not exactly know how *M. leprae* transmission occurs, how it induces immune responses, and what is the mechanism underlying the nerve damage.

The WHO officially recommended the BCG vaccine as a leprosy vaccine in 2018, a century after it was first used as a TB vaccine in 1921. It is important to note that the BCG vaccine is not specifically designed for leprosy prevention, and its effectiveness against leprosy may not be as high as for TB. Therefore, it is not routinely recommended as a standalone vaccine for leprosy prevention. However, a better leprosy vaccine and prevention strategy is still needed because we do not exactly know how *M. leprae* spreads and causes neurological damage in leprosy patients.

Strategies to increase BCG vaccine immunogenicity include mixed vaccine with the addition of killed *M. leprae* or killed *M. vaccae* (an environmental *Mycobacterium*) and rBCG that expresses foreign molecules. In three large clinical trial studies in Venezuela, Malawi, and India comparing the efficacy between BCG and BCG + killed *M. leprae*, no significant difference in protection was found in Venezuela (56% vs. 54%) after 5-year follow-up and in Malawi (49% vs. 49%) after 6- to 9-year follow-up. However, an improvement was found in the Indian study (34% vs. 64%), after 4- to 7-year follow-up.

The development of rBCGs, killed-related mycobacteria, and subunit recombinant vaccine candidates are showing promise in clinical trials for the future, with an improved and effective leprosy vaccine as immunoprophylaxis, a supplement to chemotherapy, and postexposure immunoprophylaxis.

Group A: Vaccines that are in our Clinical Use (PCV, Hib, and *S. Typhi*)

Pneumococcal Conjugate Vaccine

S. pneumonia (PCVs) prevents an estimated 23.8 million cases of antibiotic-treated illness among children younger than 5 years in low- and middle-income countries (LMICs) every year. Beyond PPSV23 valence (licensed 1983), four others PCVs have been on the market since 2009; these are PCV10, PCV13, PCV15, and PCV20-valent vaccines recommended by the WHO in childhood immunization use, also for adult and elderly age groups. These vaccines have reduced the incidence of infections caused by drug-susceptible and drug-resistant *S. pneumoniae*.

Haemophilus influenzae Type b

Effective vaccines against Hib have been available since the 1990s and the WHO recommends the inclusion of Hib vaccines in infant immunization programs. Through their use in children younger than 5 years, invasive disease caused by Hib is close to being eliminated in high-income countries. The Hib vaccines have also contributed to reducing the prevalence of some drug-resistant strains. Increasing the vaccine uptakes at a global level would reduce infections caused by drug-resistant Hib.

Salmonella Typhi

More than 20 vaccines have been authorized against *S. typhi*. The WHO-approved typhoid conjugate vaccine (TCV) is in favor of unconjugated Vi polysaccharide vaccine and live-attenuated Ty21a vaccine due to TCV's improved immune response, longer expected duration of protection, and its suitability for use in those younger than 2 years. Experts view that the introduction of routine immunization with TCV at age 9 months, with a catch-up campaign to age 15 years, would avert 21.2 million cases and 342,000 deaths from multidrug-resistant typhoid over the 10 years after introduction in the 73 countries eligible for Gavi, the Vaccine Alliance support.

Group B: Pathogens with Vaccines in Late-stage Clinical Trials with High Development Feasibility (ExiEPC, *C. difficile*, and Paratyphoid)

There are currently vaccine candidates in phase 3 of development targeting ExPEC, *Salmonella* paratyphi A, *Neisseria gonorrhoeae*, and *C. difficile*. Phase 3 is the most clinically advanced, and therefore most likely to be available shortly.

Extraintestinal Pathogenic *E. coli*

The ExPEC is a leading bacterial cause of sepsis, causing approximately 10 million cases of invasive ExPEC disease annually, worldwide. This is the most common gram-negative bacterial pathogen in humans, causes the vast majority of urinary tract infections (UTIs), is a leading cause of adult bacteremia, and is the second most common cause of neonatal meningitis. The AMR *E. coli* strains are an ongoing healthcare concern, with ExPEC a major driver behind the global AMR crisis.

Increasing MDR among ExPEC strains constitutes a major obstacle to treatment and is implicated in increasing numbers of hospitalizations and deaths and increasing healthcare costs associated with ExPEC infections. An effective vaccine against ExPEC infection is urgently needed. There are multiple challenges associated with developing vaccines against hospital-acquired infections, including the relatively low incidence of infections caused by ExPEC in vaccine target populations.

The O antigen, a component of the surface lipopolysaccharide, has been identified as a promising vaccine target. With the availability of a novel bioconjugation technology, it is expected that multivalent O antigen conjugate vaccines can be produced at an industrial scale. Clinical proof of concept of a 4-valent O antigen conjugate vaccine is ongoing.

An ExPEC vaccine effective against strains that are associated with major diseases and resistant to multiple drugs could be routinely delivered to individuals at risk of developing severe *E. coli* infection These high-risk individuals, e.g., such as elderly people, those undergoing abdominal surgery and prostatic biopsy procedures, and persons at risk of recurrent and/or complicated UTI.

Despite numerous anti-*E. coli* vaccine studies spanning more than five decades, no *E. coli* vaccine has been approved by the US Food and Drug Administration (FDA). ExPEC strains are comprised of many lineages, but only a subset is responsible for the vast majority of infections.

A 9-valent ExPEC experimental vaccine developed by Janssen is currently being tested against placebo in a phase 3 trial to evaluate its efficacy in preventing invasive *E. coli* disease (IED) caused by ExPEC9v O-serotypes in patients over 60 years of age. The study was started in 2021 by Janssen and continues to enroll patients.

As *E. coli* is a commensal pathogen, the effect on the broader microbiota and the potential consequence of disrupting it would also need to be assessed. There are four vaccine candidates in clinical development targeting ExPEC. The most advanced in development is ExPEC9V, a 9-valent-O-polysaccharide conjugate vaccine, currently in phase 3 clinical trial (NCT04899336) against invasive disease, which is expected to be completed in May 2027.

Clostridium difficile infection (CDI) most commonly affect people who have recently been treated with antibiotics but can spread easily to others. Untreated CDI can lead to life-threatening dehydration (from loss of fluids due to diarrhea), low blood pressure, a condition called toxic megacolon (an acutely distended colon that requires surgery), and colon perforation.

Clostridium difficile infections are unpleasant and can sometimes cause serious bowel problems but are often difficult to manage with repeated courses of antibiotics, and alternative strategies are greatly needed. Data from vaccine candidates that are currently in clinical development suggest that these agents could reduce symptomatic disease; however, *CDI* could continue to be shed by the host.

Further challenges to vaccine development include the recruitment of patients in appropriate target populations. Many of these patients are older, severely ill, or have other comorbidities, which creates difficulties in establishing and evaluating clinical endpoints.

There are currently three vaccine candidates against CDI in clinical trials. PF-06425090 is a recombinant toxin vaccine targeting CDI consisting of genetically and chemically detoxified TcdA and TcdB toxins.

Salmonella Paratyphi

The global mortality burden of drug-resistant *Salmonella paratyphi* was estimated to be 20,224 associated deaths in 2019, with 4,106 deaths directly attributed to it.

Paratyphoid fever is estimated to be responsible for approximately one-fifth of all enteric fever cases, but its overall relative burden compared to typhoid fever is highly variable depending on the geographic context and is reportedly increasing. There are observations that the increase may be associated with vaccination against typhoid, thus it is important to monitor the burden of paratyphoid fever, especially with the implementation of TCVs.

There is currently no vaccine available to prevent paratyphoid fever. Despite differences between *S. typhi* and *S. paratyphi A*, in particular, the absence of Vi capsular polysaccharide (CPS) in *S. paratyphi A*, the successful development of TCV suggests a vaccine against *S. paratyphi A* is also possible.

Three vaccines are in clinical development against *S. paratyphi*. A phase 3 trial of the O:2, 12-TT conjugate vaccine is currently being conducted in China. A vaccine would most likely be coadministered in combination with TCV, improving the value proposition of both vaccines.

Demonstration of vaccine efficacy against *S. paratyphi A* is considered difficult, as a low attack rate means that an efficacy study will need around 100,000–250,000 participant. Also, an oral vaccine is easy to administer and can stimulate "local" protective immune responses along the surface of the intestine, as well as systemic immunity. For more than a decade, the Oxford Vaccine Group has worked on projects to find improved ways to prevent typhoid and paratyphoid fevers.

Group C: The Pathogens in Group C Associated with Moderate Feasibility of Vaccine Development

These pathogens include NTS. *Kpn*, ETEC, *Campylobacter* spp., and *Shigella* spp. However, given the early stages of development of vaccines against these targets, no vaccine is likely to be available on the market soon.

Non-typhoidal Salmonella

Non-typhoidal Salmonella is a neglected group of enteric pathogens whose prevalence is increasing at alarming rates across India. The disease burden is being underestimated because of a lack of effective surveillance of NTS infections in the Indian population. NTS causes severe gastroenteritis and can even cause invasive infections, such as bacteremia, and focal infections, such as meningitis and septic arthritis, and is acquired through contaminated food and water sources.

Proper food and water treatment, better sanitary facilities, and public awareness campaigns are all part of prevention measures. The issue of AMR further emphasizes the necessity for prudent antibiotic usage. These actions will lessen the burden of NTS infections in India by assisting in their prevention and management.

The Global Burden of Disease (GBD) from invasive NTS (iNTS) in 2019 was 594,000 cases, 79,000 deaths, and 6.11 million global disability-adjusted life years (DALYs). The mean all-age case-fatality rate was 14.5%, with higher estimates (41.8%) among people living with HIV. NTS infections are a growing concern in India and becoming more common at worrisome rates, primarily because of inadequate surveillance. AMR is a growing concern and emphasizes the need for making a vaccine against NTS an important public health priority.

There are no currently licensed vaccines for iNTS although multiple candidates are in early phase development, including O-antigen (OAg) conjugates, oral attenuated vaccines, and multiple antigen display protein-polysaccharide conjugate vaccines.

K. pneumoniae has been identified by the WHO as a critical priority resistance threat with the highest mortality due to antibiotic-resistant infections including first-line therapy with ampicillin and gentamicin, second-line therapy with amikacin and ceftazidime, and meropenem. Multiple challenges are associated with the development of vaccines against highly resistant hospital-acquired infections. *Kpn* is associated with a high burden of neonatal sepsis in low-resource settings and a maternal vaccine has been suggested to combat this burden. Vaccination to prevent neonatal infection could reduce the burden of *Kpn* neonatal sepsis in LMICs, but the potential impact of vaccination remains poorly quantified.

Enterotoxigenic Escherichia coli Vaccines

Diarrheal disease attributable to ETEC causes substantial morbidity and mortality predominantly in pediatric populations in LMICs. In addition to acute illness, there is an increasing appreciation of the long-term consequences of enteric infections, including ETEC, on childhood growth and development.

Even when clinical care is accessible, increasing antibiotic resistance among ETEC strains has hampered the effectiveness of antibiotic treatment in both travelers and infants at high risk for ETEC diarrhea in endemic areas. Vaccines are needed to reduce the burden of ETEC. Although there are currently no licensed vaccines against this pathogen, rapid progress is being made with promising whole-cell and subunit candidates having entered clinical testing.

Three of the six vaccines in clinical trials against ETEC also target *Shigella* spp. and several candidates in preclinical development target even more combinations of pathogens. Such a multipronged approach would improve the value proposition of a vaccine. Evidence that the Dukoral cholera vaccine (Valneva, Solna, Sweden) provides 3 months' protection against some ETEC strains suggests that an ETEC vaccine is also possible.

Campylobacter jejuni and Triggers of Guillain–Barré Syndrome

Campylobacter jejuni (Cj) is the leading cause of human foodborne illness associated with poultry, beef, and pork consumption. Cj is highly prevalent in commercial poultry farms, where horizontal transmission from the environment is considered to be the primary source of infection. Cj is associated with several pathologic forms of Guillain–Barré syndrome (GBSy), including the demyelinating acute inflammatory demyelinating polyneuropathy (AIDP) and acute motor axonal neuropathy (AMAN) forms.

The 2019 GBD study estimated that over 500,000 children under 5 years of age died of diarrheal disease in that year alone.

The most common triggers of GBSy, in three-quarters of cases, are previous infections. The most common infectious agents that cause GBSy include Cj, *Mycoplasma pneumoniae*, and *CMV*. Cj is responsible for about a third of GBSy cases and is usually more severe than that due to other causes. Clinical presentation of GBSy is highly dependent on the structure of pathogenic lipo-oligosaccharides (LOS) that trigger the innate immune system via toll-like receptor (TLR)-4 signaling. AIDP is due to demyelination, whereas in AMAN, structures of the axolemma are affected in the nodal or internodal space.

Vaccination is considered a potential intervention strategy to control *Campylobacter*. There are no licensed vaccines against CJ although several have undergone preclinical and clinical development. Although GBSy has been causally related to several vaccinations, other studies do not confirm these findings. During the H1N1 influenza vaccination campaign in 1976, an increased risk was estimated, at roughly one additional case of GBS for every 100,000 people who had been vaccinated. However, with the use of the type B (H1N1) vaccine, the risk of developing GBSy declined to <1/1,000,000. Although some studies emphasize that the overall incidence of GBS has not increased since the introduction of SARS-CoV-2 vaccinations, several arguments support a causal relation.

Shigellosis Vaccine Prevention

Shigella is the main cause of diarrheal deaths in children over 1 year of age and the most common cause of bacterial diarrheal deaths globally. The most recent estimate from the Institute for Health Metrics and Evaluation (IHME) GBD study is 148,202 deaths due to shigellosis in 2019, with 93,831 in children under 5 years of age.

Levels of AMR are increasing globally among *Shigella* isolates making shigellosis increasingly difficult to treat. The growing appreciation of vaccines is a valuable tool for combatting AMR.

In recent years, there has been a resurgence of interest in the development of vaccines against *Shigella* driven by the growing awareness of the impact of this pathogen on global health.

The development of many *Shigella* vaccines has been described piecemeal over several years and in multiple papers, none providing the full story of the vaccine they relate to.

Despite over 100 years of development efforts, there has never been a widely licensed vaccine against shigellosis. There are several reasons for this, in addition to the lack of commercial incentives. Technically, it has proved difficult to develop an effective vaccine with many candidates proving to be either too reactogenic or insufficiently immunogenic to be efficacious.

Since there are over 50 serotypes of *Shigella*, a multivalent vaccine approach is likely to be required for a sufficiently effective vaccine, though most candidates to date have been in monovalent format. From the Global Enteric Multicenter Study (GEMS) it has been estimated that a 4-valent vaccine including *S. flexneri* 2a, 3a, 6, and *S. sonnei* would cover up to 75% of global strains and up to 93% through cross-protective epitopes.

In a recently published study, a *Shigella flexneri* 2a synthetic glycan-based vaccine induces a long-lasting immune response and was found safe and strongly immunogenic in adult volunteers.

Though *Shigella* vaccine development has proved a difficult path, there is much to be hopeful about with a range of promising technological platforms being applied to this challenge and several candidates already in the target population of young children in LMICs. In the next few years, we will find out which are successful.

Group D: Pathogens with a Small Number of or No Vaccine Candidates in the Pipeline or Low Vaccine Development Feasibility in the Near Future

ESKAPE pathogens (*Efe, SA, Kpn, Acinetobacter baumannii, Pseudomonas aeruginosa*, and *Enterobacter* spp.), are a serious challenge worldwide. Among ESKAPE pathogens, a group of multidrug-resistant bacteria that are the leading cause of hospital infections globally and "escape" the biocidal action of antibiotics. Both *P. aeruginosa* and enterococci are the leading causes of death worldwide.

Due to the lack of discovery of novel antibiotics, in the past two decades, it has become necessary to search for new antibiotics or to study synergy with the existing antibiotics to counter life-threatening infections.

Enterococcus Faecium

Enterococcus faecium causes hospital-acquired infections and has low incidence, morbidity, and mortality. It most commonly presents as a UTI or endocarditis. A potential vaccination strategy and target population have yet to be identified. AMR is of intermediate concern as resistance to last-line therapies has not been reported.

There are no vaccine candidates in preclinical or clinical development. A vaccine against Efe is unlikely to be cost-effective given the high cost of developing vaccines and the low incidence of infection. There is currently no pipeline for vaccines against Efe; neither commercial nor academic vaccine development programs are underway.

Staphylococcus Aureus

Staphylococcus aureus is becoming increasingly dangerous for its ability to rapidly develop antibiotic resistance and to acquire virulence factors encoding genes from the environment. SA is a gram-positive bacterium, belonging to the ESKAPE family, and is also responsible for persistent lung infections that affect patients with cystic fibrosis (CF).

Staphylococcus aureus can become resistant to many antibiotics, such as the well-known methicillin-resistant *S. aureus* (MRSA), but also the subsequent vancomycin-resistant *S. aureus* (VRSA), which is why new treatments different from antibiotics are needed.

There are multiple challenges to developing a successful vaccine against SA that do not have any vaccine candidates in preclinical or clinical development. Although multiple candidate monoclonal antibodies (mAbs) targeted against SA have been tested, these have also proven ineffective in clinical trials. Second, intermittent colonization with SA occurs in approximately two-thirds of the population; however, exposure does not appear to confer natural immunity. Finally, the diseases caused by SA are diverse, including bacteremia, skin infections, pneumonia, and others, and it is not clear whether a single vaccine would be protective against multiple clinical syndromes.

Klebsiella Pneumoniae Vaccine and Immunotherapy

There is no licensed vaccine for the prevention of Kpn infections and increasing levels of antibiotic resistance make this pathogen a high priority for vaccine and therapeutic development.

Although the design of Kpn K1 capsule polysaccharide (CPS) vaccine was first reported in 1985 and the designs of polyvalent Kpn CPS vaccines were then reported in 1986 (6-valent) and 1988 (24-valent), there is still no clinical Kpn vaccine available.

Immunotherapy against Acinetobacter Baumannii Infections

Infections caused by *A. baumannii* can be challenging to treat due to its ability to develop resistance to multiple antibiotics, including carbapenems, which are often used as a last resort for bacterial infections.

Efforts to develop vaccines have been ongoing, but as of this review, no licensed vaccine specifically targeting this bacterium was available. Vaccine development for bacterial infections can be challenging due to the complexity of the bacteria and the need to develop vaccines that are both effective and safe.

Immunotherapy, including the use of mAbs, has been explored as a potential treatment approach for *A. baumannii* infections with promising results in preclinical studies and early clinical trials. These antibodies could potentially be used either alone or in combination with antibiotics to enhance the immune response against the bacteria and improve treatment outcomes. However, it is essential to note that the development of vaccines and immunotherapies takes time and rigorous testing to ensure safety and efficacy.

Pseudomonas Aeruginosa

P. aeruginosa is a notorious pathogen in nosocomial infections, particularly ventilator-associated pneumonia, central line-associated bacteremia, and complicated catheter-associated UTIs. Preclinical and clinical studies have demonstrated the extremely challenging nature of developing a vaccine against *P. aeruginosa*. Most vaccines to date have used traditional methods of vaccine design involving the use of well-studied virulence factors such as vaccine antigens.

Due to its AMR, vaccines represent the sole valid alternative strategy to tackle the pathogen. However, although many advances have been made in this field in understanding the host immune response and the biology of *P. aeruginosa* over 50 years, no vaccine has yet been licensed. Emphasis is given to understanding the current state of pseudomonal vaccine development and the importance of incorporating appropriate adjuvants in the protective antigen to yield optimal protection.

Enterobacter Species

Enterobacteriaceae is a large, heterogeneous group of gram-negative rods that includes bacteria that naturally inhabit the mammalian gut but also can occur and multiply in other environments This group is characterized by the development of resistance to various antibiotics. In recent years, *Enterobacter cloacae* has emerged as a clinically important pathogen responsible for a wide range of healthcare-associated illnesses. Identifying *Enterobacter* species can be challenging due to their similar phenotypic characteristics. The emergence of multidrug-resistant *E. cloacae* is also a significant problem in healthcare settings.

Priority pathogens *S. aureus*, with one vaccine candidate in phase 2; *A. baumannii*, *P. aeruginosa*, and *H. pylori*, which have no vaccine candidates in clinical development; and *E. faecium* and *Enterobacter* spp.

INNOVATIVE VACCINES AGAINST ACQUIRED HEART DISEASES (RHD, ETC.)

Group A *Streptococcus* or Rheumatic Fever Prevention Vaccines

Group A *Streptococcus* is a bacterium that can cause a range of infections, including strep throat, skin infections, more serious invasive diseases, and nonsuppurative ARF resulting in cardiac value (RHD) complications.

Rheumatic heart disease primarily develops as a complication of untreated or inadequately treated GAS infections. Therefore, preventing GAS infections through measures like early diagnosis and treatment of strep throat with antibiotics is crucial in preventing ARF and subsequent RHDs. Additionally, there have been efforts to develop vaccines against GAS itself, primarily to prevent streptococcal infections and their complications.

As of this day in February 2024, there is no vaccine specifically available for the prevention of GAS or ARF. Efforts to develop a vaccine against GAS are ongoing, but it is a complex task due to the multiple strain variations of the bacteria, as well as the challenges in stimulating an effective immune response. Reasons why there is no vaccine for GAS include:

- Inadequate animal models and lack of defined human immune correlates of protection.
- Lack of commercial interests and uncertainty about the market for a GAS vaccine in high-income countries.
- Several vaccine candidates have been in various stages of development and clinical trials, but none have still reached widespread use.

Acute rheumatic fever is more common in school-age children (5 through 15 years old) and is very rare in children younger than 3 years old and adults. A vaccine that prevents GAS infections would also be expected to prevent ARF and debilitating RHDs now affecting mostly LMICs, especially in sub-Saharan Africa, the Middle East, Southeast Asia, and the Western Pacific. In India, the prevalence of RHD is estimated at around 0.9 cases per 1,000 children in the age group of 5–14 years. Presuming 20% of the country's total population is in 5–14 years age group, it is estimated that there are around 2.18 lakh cases of RHD in the country with debilitating illnesses for the rest of their life. Several vaccine candidates have been tested in clinical trials, but none have yet been approved for widespread use.

Prevention of GAS infections and rheumatic fever primarily relies on early diagnosis and appropriate treatment of streptococcal infections, such as prompt administration of antibiotics for strep throat. However, in about one-third of patients, ARF follows subclinical streptococcal infections or infections for which medical attention was not sought. Sometimes, people have such mild strep they do not realize they had an infection until rheumatic fever develops later on. Rheumatic fever causes many symptoms that look similar to other health issues.

It is also important to practice good hygiene, such as frequent handwashing, to reduce the spread of the bacteria.

Kawasaki Diseases–Acquired Hear Disease (CAAs) Preventions

Kawasaki Disease (KD) is more common in people of Asian or Pacific Island descent. Experts do not know exactly what causes KD. It is not contagious and might be the result of changes to certain genes or related to viral or bacterial infections. Infections may cause the immune system to attack the blood vessel walls and cause inflammation including coronary artery atherosclerosis (CAAs) mistake and cause inflammation.

After receiving traditional intravenous immunoglobulin (IVIG) and anti-inflammatory treatment for KD, most children recover fully. Long-term follow-up care usually is not necessary. However, children who have aneurysms or other complications related to the disease will need lifelong monitoring by a cardiologist.

The development of different types of immunotherapies, including vaccines (prophylactic and therapeutic) and the use of pathogens, mAbs, recombinant proteins, cytokines, and cellular immunotherapies, have been proposed as adjunct therapies, and some of these are currently in different phases of clinical trials. (Refer to Chapter 12 NCDs under Kawasaki Disease Acquired Heart Disease).

OTHER BACTERIAL VACCINES
Group B *Streptococcus* Vaccine

Group B *Streptococcus* (GBS) can cause potentially devastating diseases in infants, including sepsis, pneumonia, and meningitis. Annually, there are nearly 400,000 cases of infant disease and approximately 138,000 stillbirths and infant deaths worldwide due to GBS.

The development of GBS vaccines suitable for immunization during pregnancy has been identified as a priority by the WHO and key consensus documents presenting preferences for GBS vaccine development roadmap have been developed. Consensus-building about a preferred clinical development pathway and policy for vaccine use, once approved, has been highlighted as a priority activity.

GBS6 Vaccine

Hexavalent anti-CPS/genetically detoxified diphtheria toxin cross-reactive material (CRM) 197 glycoconjugate (GBS6) is being developed as an investigational maternal vaccine to help prevent invasive GBS in newborns. Polysaccharides conjugated to CRM have been successfully used by Pfizer in its pneumococcal vaccines, which have a proven track record of safety and effectiveness in millions of infants globally.

A phase 2 randomized placebo-controlled study from South Africa showed; "a vaccine given during pregnancy produced antibodies against GBS that were transferred to infants at immunoglobulin G (IgG) thresholds associated with a reduced risk of invasive GBS disease". Although these results apply only to a South African population with a high disease burden among infants, "the road to GBS vaccine licensure could occur through an accelerated pathway based on an established serologic correlate of protection followed by confirmation of effectiveness".

In pregnant women who received the GBS6 vaccine, antibody responses to all serotypes were induced, with maternal-to-infant antibody ratios of about 0.4–1.3, depending on the dose received, resulting in concentrations associated with a reduced risk of invasive disease.

For newborns, the primary risk factor for invasive GBS is exposure to maternal rectovaginal GBS colonization during delivery, and ascending GBS infection in mothers can also affect the fetus before delivery, with risks of intra-amniotic infection, premature labor, or stillbirth.

Group B *Streptococcus* vaccine could be beneficial because intrapartum antibiotic prophylaxis may contribute to AMR and disrupt the development of the infant microbiome. Also, the GBS vaccine would provide a much-needed measure in the prevention of GBS infection worldwide and to a substantial percentage of pregnant women living in resource-limited community settings where microbiologic screening and intrapartum antibiotic prophylaxis are unavailable.

Limitations

Pregnant women who test positive for colonization of GBS in their third trimester are treated with intrapartum antibiotic prophylaxis, which is >80% effective in the prevention of early-onset disease in infants during the first 6 days after birth, but is not effective against late-onset disease at 7–89 days.

Vaccine against other Gram-negatives, e.g., *Burkholderia Cepacia* Complex and *Helicobacter Pylori*

The *Burkholderia cepacia* complex (Bcc) encompasses >20 closely related species, including those most commonly found in patients with CF. Although the incidence of Bcc infections in CF is relatively low, about 3%, they are commonly associated with a severe decline in lung function, which can develop into a systemic infection. Moreover, Bcc members, and in particular *B. cenocepacia*, have a remarkable adaptability to environmental changes and are naturally resistant to several antibiotics commonly used in clinical practice, making their treatment very challenging. Therefore, the development of a vaccine could represent an important approach to preventing Bcc infections in CF patients, although relatively few studies have been conducted so far.

H. pylori infects >50% of the world's population and causes gastroduodenal diseases including gastritis, peptic ulcer, gastric adenocarcinoma, and gastric lymphoma; it has been classified as a type I carcinogen that causes gastric cancer.

Gastric cancer is still one of the leading causes of cancer-related death worldwide although the prevalence and incidence of this cancer have been decreasing since the last decade. Eradication of *H. pylori* is recommended to prevent gastric cancer, especially in developing countries where gastric cancer contributes to high economic morbidity and mortality.

H. pylori is treatable with antibiotics, proton pump inhibitors, and histamine H2 blockers. Once the bacteria are completely gone from the body, the chance of its return is low. However, the emergence of *H. pylori* strains that are resistant to multiple antibiotics has complicated the treatment strategy to eradicate this bacterium. Data on resistance are scarce. More research is needed to determine local, regional, and national patterns of *H. pylori* resistance to antibiotics to guide the choice of regimen.

Due to the limited immune response induced by monovalent vaccines, the development of multi-epitope vaccines is becoming the focus of immunotherapy against *H. pylori*. Current studies have shown that the multi-epitope vaccines could generate a broadly reactive antibody response against *H. pylori* antigens and significantly reduce *H. pylori* colonization in the stomach, indicating that the multi-epitope vaccine is a promising vaccine strategy.

In the construction of a multi-epitope vaccine, the B and T-cell epitopes with different permutations could produce different constructs. These different constructs make a difference in the stability of the recombinant vaccine and the exposure of the critical domains. The efficient immune response induced by the proper antigen is strongly dependent on the optimal structural stability of the vaccine protein. Therefore, the assembly and permutation of epitopes are the keys to the successful design of the multi-epitope vaccine.

Probiotics and natural products from plants show promising results to be harnessed as alternative therapies against *H. pylori* to combat the emergence of multidrug-resistant strains. *H. pylori* vaccines using new vaccine technologies show promising results in preclinical trials and should be explored further.

H. pylori vaccines currently in development are very early stage (phase 1 or preclinical). These vaccines are predominantly composed of purified or recombinant components of *H. pylori* antigens with an adjuvant.

Vaccination Against Lyme Disease

Borrelia Burgdorferi, the bacterium that causes Lyme disease is typically spread by the bite of an infected tick (*Ixodes, often called deer ticks or black-legged ticks*). However, fleas and mosquitos can also carry it.

It is estimated [Centers for Disease Control and Prevention (CDC), USA] that approximately 300,000 cases of Lyme disease occur each year, with possibly many more being underreported. Lyme disease is also common in many parts of Europe, yet it is believed to be underreported there as well.

Every year, only 3,000–5,000 Indians are diagnosed with Lyme disease, and again experts attribute this to a lack of awareness about the disease. In India, ophthalmologists and dermatologists tend to be most familiar with the disease, especially in more urban areas. Lyme often affects the vision, and a bulls-eye rash on the skin may appear in conjunction with the infection. Developing nations including India may miss many early onset stage-1 (skin lesion) that is always classical and stage 3, late one, e.g., post-treatment Lyme disease (PTLD), an analog of long COVID-19 that needs advanced laboratory technology of synovial Ag testing.

In areas where Lyme disease is more common, physicians may be able to diagnose early disseminated Lyme disease without doing any laboratory tests. A 4-week course of antibiotics is used to treat people who are diagnosed with Lyme disease, depending on the choice of drug (doxycycline). Treatment with antibiotics is effective only in the early stages of infection.

Although the first human Lyme disease vaccine (LYMErix by SmithKline Beecham, Pittsburgh, PA, USA) was marketed and distributed in the USA from 1998 until 2002, it was discontinued, and no vaccine is currently available.

Pfizer and French pharmaceutical peer Valneva have developed a Lyme disease vaccine candidate, VLA15, that is currently in phase 3 human trials. VLA15 is a multivalent, protein subunit vaccine that targets the outer surface protein A (OspA) of Borrelia.

A new global Lyme disease vaccine undergoing clinical trials showed a "strong immune response" in both children and adolescents a month after a booster shoot. "Pfizer and French pharmaceutical peer Valneva announced (*September, 2023*) that a phase 2 study for its VLA15 Lyme disease vaccine candidate as being "the most advanced Lyme disease vaccine candidate currently in clinical development" *[both the European Medicines Agency (EMA) and US FDA awaits the phase 3 clinical trial by 2026].*

Scrub Typhus Vaccine

Scrub typhus is a bacterial infection caused by the obligatory intracellular *Orientia tsutsugamushi* bacterium (formerly Rickettsia tsutsugamushi), sometimes known as bush typhus. It is transmitted through bites from infected chiggers, which are larval mites (adult mites does not bite) **(Fig. 1)**. It is a major cause of life-threatening acute undifferentiated febrile illness in Eastern Asia. Disease

The mite-borne scrub-bush typhus diagnosis is the tip of the iceberg due to poor awareness among the public as well as the medical fraternity. Because symptoms are similar to other fever-causing IDs, including the mosquito bite spreading dengue fever, malaria, chikungunya, and Zika virus fever. It is easily treatable with doxycycline or Chloromycetin if recognized early. Acute encephalitis syndrome (AES) happens in substantial numbers in both Japanese encephalitis (JE) and Indian typhus fever. Eschar is almost missed or is not there in 60% of typhus and conflicts with maculopapular skin eruption of the scrub's typhus and JE. Scrub disease is an antibiotic-treatable bacterial disease, but, clinically, it is difficult to diagnose.

Prevention

There is currently no vaccine to prevent scrub typhus, but you can reduce your risk by avoiding contact with infected chiggers. When visiting areas where scrub typhus is prevalent, it is advisable to stay away from densely forested and brushy areas where chiggers may be present.

Vaccination Against Scrub

In view of the concomitantly discovered heterogeneity of strain-dependent antigens, and the lack of cross-immunity among them, effective protection against scrub typhus has been difficult to achieve. Despite the wide range of preventative approaches that have been unsuccessfully attempted, currently, the selection of the proper antigens is one of the critical barriers to generating cross-protective immunity against antigenically variable strains of *O. tsutsugamushi*.

Vaccine against Bacterial STIs: Syphilis, Gonococcus, and Chlamydia

Syphilis: Vaccine, Challenges, Controversies, and Opportunities

Syphilis remains a widespread ID with a significant disease burden in many countries. Despite the absence of identified penicillin-resistant strains, challenges in syphilis treatment persist due to penicillin allergies, global supply issues in recent years, and the emergence of macrolide-resistant strains. It is a major public health problem worldwide.

Syphilis is a sexually or vertically (mother to fetus) transmitted disease caused by the infection of *Treponema pallidum* subspecies pallidum (TPA). The incidence of syphilis has increased over the past years despite the

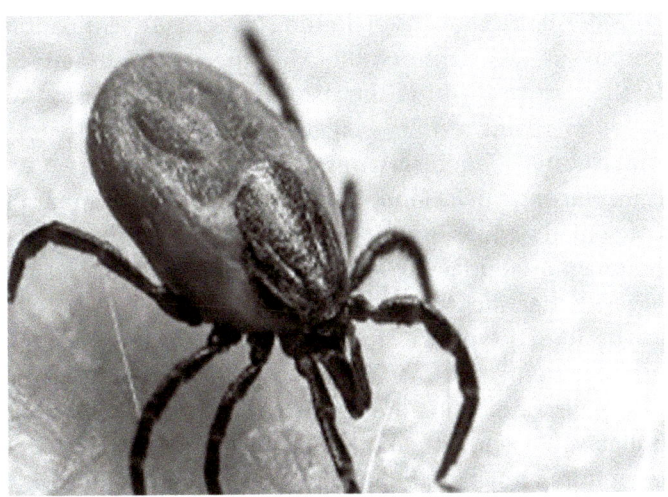

Fig. 1: Scrub typhus is spread by a bite of an 8-legged mite (also called a "chigger") infected with the bacteria that causes scrub typhus fever (mostly found in home backyard of Kerala and Tamil Nadu).

is spread to people by the bite of a mite (also called a "chigger") infected with the bacteria that causes scrub typhus fever. It is not spread from person to person. However, people residing in areas with active typhus outbreaks are at risk for the illness due to the presence of fleas, lice, or chiggers that spread the bacteria.

Mites do not have wings and cannot fly, but they are transported on their host and spread from host to host by direct contact. Most mites are very small, <1 mm in length, and have a very simple oblong-shaped body. The typical lesion of scrub typhus begins as a red, indurated lesion about 1 cm in diameter; it eventually vesiculates, ruptures, and becomes covered with a black scab. The capacity of different strains of *O. tsutsugamushi* to result in an eschar varies.

In 2019, data on scrub fever in Kerala state reported communicable diseases were around 570 and 14 deaths in that year (in 2021, reported cases were around 438 with the death of 6 patients due to scrub fever illness). Pediatric scrub typhus in Southern Kerala is now been an emerging public health problem *(Personal Communication with Dr Samitha Nayer, Laboratory Chief, KIMS Health, Trivandrum, India)*. Rise in scrub typhus cases in Tamil Nadu also worried in recent years. Health officials say, "45 scrub typhus cases were reported in Chennai and around 1,400 cases were reported across Tamil Nadu since January 2019"! The rise in scrub typhus cases in Tamil Nadu also worries in recent years; health officials say there were 1,400 cases reported across Tamil Nadu, India during the first 8 months in 2019.

fact that this bacterium is an obligate human pathogen, the infection route is well known, and the disease can be successfully treated with penicillin.

The US CDC warns that "cases of congenital syphilis are skyrocketing", recommends more testing and earlier treatment (November 7, 2023). More than 3,700 cases of congenital syphilis were reported in 2022, roughly 11 times the number recorded a decade ago. Having the disease during pregnancy can lead to miscarriage and stillbirth, and infants who survive may become blind or deaf or have severe developmental delays.

It is widely acknowledged that individuals who infect *T. pallidum* can be reinfected following treatment, and this cycle may recur multiple times. Human studies have demonstrated that individuals with late latent syphilis exhibit resistance to symptomatic reinfection with a heterologous strain of *T. pallidum*, whereas those in earlier stages display evidence of infection upon challenge.

The development of a syphilis vaccine may be crucial for controlling disease spread and/or severity, particularly in countries where the effectiveness of the preventive measures is limited. In the last century, several vaccine prototypes have been tested in preclinical studies, mainly in rabbits. While none of them provided protection against infection, some prototypes prevented bacteria from disseminating to distal organs, attenuated lesion development, and accelerated their healing.

The main limitation of syphilis research has been an inability to grow the delicate bacteria that causes it in the laboratory.

Humans are the only natural hosts, although in research studies, scientists have been able to infect other animals with *T. pallidum*. Despite these promising results, there is still some controversy regarding the identification of vaccine candidates and the characteristics of a syphilis-protective immune response. Vaccines represent the most cost-effective strategy to prevent and control the syphilis epidemic.

In light of the ongoing global COVID-19 pandemic, nucleic acid vaccines have gained prominence in the field of vaccine research and development, owing to their superior efficiency compared to traditional vaccines. A variety of strategies have been tested, including inactivated bacteria and subunit recombinant proteins, even though with limited success.

The ideal syphilis vaccine should protect against TPA infection. However, even if the vaccine is unable to completely prevent infection, it could still be worth considering as a means of limiting bacteria dissemination and tissue invasiveness, blocking the establishment of latency, or preventing the disease from progressing to secondary and tertiary stages. Additionally, a vaccine that reduces bacterial persistence or prevents TPA transplacental invasion might also reduce the number of congenital syphilis in endemic areas, where the number of nondiagnosed infected individuals might be high, and the access to healthcare may be limited.

Besides, a syphilis vaccine has to be effective against possible reinfections with similar or different TPA strains or isolates, indicating the importance of using conserved antigens. Recently, there has been evidence that TPA can be cultured in vitro, and that genetic manipulation of this pathogen can be accomplished. These scientific advances are likely to open the gateway to new research lines that can shed light on the current controversies.

It is well known that infection with *T. pallidum* reduces the body's autoimmunity and is complicated by the occurrence of many autoimmune diseases. The importance of *T. pallidum* vaccines is in addressing cross-infection or coinfection problems such as syphilis and HIV by reducing the risk associated with coinfection and improving the overall management of sexually transmitted infections.

Gonococcus Vaccines

Neisseria gonorrhoeae has presented challenges to researchers for decades. This sexually transmitted disease (STD) pathogen rapidly acquires AMR and does not confer protective immunity from natural exposure as a consequence of infection. There are no approved vaccines for gonorrhea anywhere in the world.

Attempts to generate an effective vaccine for gonorrhea have thus far been unsuccessful. Gonococcus (GC) causes illness in millions of humans and utilizes an arsenal of AMR strategies and highly variable surface structures to make treatment and prevention an enormous challenge. Despite these difficulties, bioinformatic tools and computational methods now make antigen identification and characterization easier than ever.

Recent data suggest vaccines for gonorrhea are biologically feasible; in particular, epidemiological evidence shows that vaccines against a closely related pathogen, serogroup B *Neisseria meningitidis* outer membrane vesicle (OMV) vaccines, may reduce gonorrhea incidence. There is evidence to suggest the Bexsero vaccine (GlaxoSmithKline, Kundl, Austria), developed and licensed to prevent group B meningococcal infections, provides some protection against gonorrhea. MenB given to children and young adults was associated with an approximately 30% reduction in gonorrhea diagnoses.

Two large clinical trials are underway to investigate the efficacy of Bexsero against *N. gonorrhoeae*; however, phase 3 trial results have been delayed by the COVID-19 pandemic. Another model in men who have sex with men (MSM) suggested that a vaccine would need a minimum efficacy of 90% and a fixed uptake of 40% to completely prevent AMR development.

The trial has received US FDA fast track designation (June 27, 2023), paving the way for their phase 2 trial of around 750 people including men and women considered at risk of infection with the GC in eight countries: the USA, the United Kingdom, France, Germany, Spain, Brazil, the Philippines, and South Africa. Participants are split into three groups; those who received the highest tolerated dose in the phase 1 trial; those receiving a dose below the highest tolerated dose; and those who received a placebo.

The primary outcome is local and systemic adverse events and hematological and biochemical abnormalities. Gonorrhea cases up to 13 months after vaccination will be a closely watched secondary endpoint.

Chlamydia

Chlamydia trachomatis is a gram-negative obligate intracellular bacterium. It is the leading cause of bacterial sexual transmitted infections (STIs). Infections often go undiagnosed, as they remain asymptomatic in 75% of women and 50% of men. *Chlamydia* is primarily a disease in young adults after their sexual debut with >131 million people infected each year.

The WHO figures estimated that over 90 million new cases of genital *C. trachomatis* infections occur worldwide each year. A vaccination program is considered to be the best approach to reduce the prevalence of *C. trachomatis* infections, as it would be much cheaper and have a greater impact on controlling *C. trachomatis* infections worldwide rather than a screening program or treating infections with antibiotics. Untreated infections in women increase the risk of developing severe complications, leading to pelvic inflammatory disease (PID) and long-term sequelae such as infertility and ectopic pregnancy. Thus, there is a great need to develop a vaccine against chlamydia.

Chlamydia is very much like a virus, meaning it relies totally on its host to survive and replicate. It has two developmental forms; a small (0.3 μm) nonreplicating infectious form which, after attachment, is internalized into the host cell and instantly reorganized into a metabolically active and replicating form of almost triple the size. After completion of a replicative cycle, it reorganizes into the infectious form again and is released from the host cell. If the bacteria are not controlled by the immune system, it may ascend to infect the fallopian tubes and can cause major damage leading to PID, scarring, and occlusion.

The development of a vaccine against chlamydia is an international priority, but the complex lifestyle of the pathogen makes vaccine development challenging. Currently, there are no vaccines available that effectively protect against a *C. trachomatis* genital infection despite the many efforts that have been made throughout the years.

Vaccination could be substantially more effective than other biomedical interventions in controlling epidemics of chlamydia infection. Administrating a protective vaccine to adolescents before their first sexual experience could induce a significant reduction in prevalence which could not be obtained by screening teenagers, even with a coverage of 100%. Unfortunately, no protective vaccines, either fully or partially, are available although there have been many attempts to develop one.

The clinical development of vaccines against urogenital *C. trachomatis* infection and disease is complicated for several reasons. The first difficulty relates to the choice of an ideal study population for late-stage efficacy trials. Another difficulty relates to the lack of reliable and well-validated biomarkers for ascension of infection and disease in the female upper genital tract.

The most advanced vaccine against infection with *C. trachomatis* is the CTH522 vaccine. The vaccine antigen CTH522 is a recombinant, engineered version of the *C. trachomatis* major outer membrane protein (MOMP), comprising heterologous immunorepeats from four genital *C. trachomatis* serovars (D, E, F, and G).

Preclinical research on the CTH522 vaccine led to selection of the liposome-based cationic adjuvant formulation CAF®01, which has been designed for the induction of a strong cell-mediated immune response combined with antibody induction.

The chlamydia field is coming of age and the first phase 1 clinical trial of a *C. trachomatis* vaccine has been successfully completed. Experts expect and hope that this will motivate various stakeholders to support further development of chlamydia vaccines in humans.

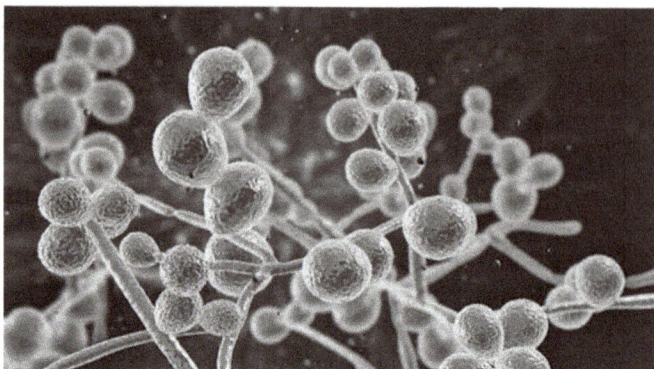

Fig. 2: A deadly fungus, *Candida auris*, emerges in the US and worldwide.

Vaccines Against Funguses

Antifungal Vaccines

In the context of viral and bacterial and viral diseases, there are currently no FDA-approved fungal vaccines available for clinical use.

Candida auris, a formidable yeast infection, has been escalating its presence, globally across the United States with a concerning rapidity **(Fig. 2)**. This emerging fungus, first identified in 2009, poses a significant global health threat due to its severe impact on hospitalized patients and its resistance to multiple antifungal treatments.

C. auris is notorious for its ability to cause a range of infections, from superficial skin conditions to invasive diseases such as bloodstream infections, which can be life-threatening. The fungus is most dangerous when it enters the bloodstream, with more than one-third of patients with invasive *C. auris* infections succumbing to the disease.

Transmission occurs in healthcare settings through contact with contaminated surfaces or equipment, or physical contact with an infected person. The fungus can survive on surfaces for several weeks, making stringent hygiene practices and thorough cleaning in healthcare facilities crucial for controlling its spread. Hand hygiene, using alcohol-based hand sanitizer or soap and water, is emphasized as a primary defense against *C. auris*.

C. auris's resistance to antifungal medications is a critical concern. While most infections can be treated with echinocandins, some strains have shown resistance to all three major classes of antifungals. In such cases, alternative or multiple antifungal medications may be necessary.

Candida Vaccines

Recently, preclinical and clinical studies of potential vaccine candidates have been published, which report good immunogenicity and a functional response against *Candida* spp.

Despite continuing efforts, there is currently no commercially available anti-*Candida* vaccine that has been approved for human use. Recently, preclinical and clinical studies of potential vaccine candidates have been published, which report good immunogenicity and a functional response against *Candida* spp. With this in mind, the development of an effective and successful vaccine against *Candida* infections could be a crucial step in preventing and controlling these potentially life-threatening fungal diseases.

While there is certainly a requirement for safe and efficient vaccines, the obstacles are significant in terms of both conceptual understanding and technical aspects in developing successful vaccines against conditions such as candidiasis and other fungal infections. Collaborations are warranted between researchers, healthcare providers, regulatory bodies, and industries to pave the way to the successful development of a novel anti-*Candida* vaccine.

Vaccines Against Parasites

There are no vaccines currently available to control the major human parasitic diseases, although there is evidence of acquired immunity and resistance to reinfection in most of the parasitic infections.

Commercially provided antiparasitic drugs with broad-spectrum action have successfully been used to control parasitic diseases in livestock and other domestic animals. However, frequent emergence of drug resistance in the target parasites has become a challenge. Boosting interest in alternative control methods and renewed the appeal of vaccines. Despite long-term work on vaccine development, notably in the fields of hookworm infection, leishmaniasis, malaria, onchocerciasis, and schistosomiasis, we have yet to see an effective vaccine being implemented against a human parasitic disease.

Malarial Vaccines

Malaria is a potentially life-threatening ID caused by parasites of the *Plasmodium* genus. It is transmitted to humans through the bites of infected female *Anopheles* mosquitoes and remains one of the biggest causes of fatalities across the world including in India.

The latest world malaria report states that in 2022, there were an estimated 249 million malaria cases and over 600,000 malaria deaths across the globe. India accounted for 66% of incidences in Southeast Asia regions. Changes in temperature, humidity, and rainfall can influence the behavior of the malaria-carrying anopheles' mosquito.

Developing vaccines with a high level of protective immunity against malaria has been challenging. The malaria parasite has >5,000 genes, which makes identifying the disease-causing gene or protein very difficult.

Researchers have been trying to develop a malaria vaccine for over 100 years, but "it is been pretty tough". "You need exceptionally high titers of antibodies to protect against any stage of the parasite's life cycle", which is hard to achieve. Stalled progress in reducing the global malaria burden since 2015 highlights the need for new interventions to interrupt malaria transmission and enable malaria elimination. A vaccine that prevents malaria transmission and can be implemented at scale and it could be a game-changer!

Earlier, the WHO formally recommended a recombinant protein-based malaria vaccine, e.g., *"RTS, S/AS01"* vaccine (the trade name *Mosquirix*) for wider clinical use. This malaria vaccine was found to be 77% effective in children.

The WHO (October 2023) has prequalified a *malaria vaccine (R21/Matrix-M)*, developed by the Oxford University and Serum Institute of India (SII), which is expected to rein in the disease that is not just a global problem but also affects India every season. This is the second malaria vaccine to be approved; it is meant for children under the age of 5 years and has three primary doses and a booster shot after a year. Since this vaccine is specific to *Plasmodium falciparum*, it cannot be used to prevent infections caused by other malaria parasites like P vivax, which is known to persist in the liver and trigger repeated infections.

Vivax is fairly widespread in India and there is no vaccine yet to tackle it.

At present, the R21/Matrix vaccine is meant for high-burden countries in Africa, where most of the cases are caused by *P. falciparum*. The burden of *P. falciparum* in India is already on the decline, the main concern being vivax. That's why many experts believe that a wide use of vaccines against *P. falciparum* might not be cost-effective.

Ghana and Nigeria have both approved the vaccine for use in children aged 5 months to 3 years, and in 2021 the WHO recommended RTS, S to all children under two in sub-Saharan Africa.

An alternative approach is to develop vaccines that are specifically designed to prevent malaria transmission to mosquitoes, known as transmission-blocking vaccines (TBVs). Only a limited number of TBVs have reached preclinical or clinical development with several major challenges impeding their development, including low immunogenicity in humans. TBV development efforts against *P. vivax*, the second major cause of malaria morbidity, lag far behind those for *P. falciparum* **(Fig. 3)**.

The WHO says, "We are at the crossroads of opportunities and challenges", and Medicine for Malaria Venture (MMV) research and development team is responsible for the full spectrum of the drug, vaccine discovery, and development. The MMVs claim that "almost 50 million young children received malaria prevention last year. If used in combination with the RTS,S vaccine, it could protect the lives of millions more, as shown in recent trials in Burkina Faso and Mali".

- Roll-out of the world's first malaria vaccine, RTS,S/AS01 in 2022 and a WHO recommendation for a second, cheaper vaccine, R21/Matrix-M, in 2023
- Both vaccines have the potential to make huge inroads against an ancient mosquito-borne disease that still kills more than half a million people, mainly young children in sub-Saharan Africa, every year.
- RTS,S has demonstrated a similar effectiveness to the R21 vaccine in similar settings, according to PATH.
- Cameroon launches world's first malaria vaccination program, January 2024 is set to expand beyond Cameroon to 19 other countries.
- Despite the vaccine's monumental role in combating malaria, it will not be the sole defense mechanism. It is planned to complement existing preventative measures, such as mosquito nets, to further minimize the risk of mosquito bites.
- For children younger than 5 years living in the African Sahel and sub-Sahel, the WHO recommends that seasonal malaria chemoprevention (SMC) with sulfadoxine, pyrimethamine, and amodiaquine be administered monthly during the rainy season when malaria transmission peaks.
- The recombinant circumsporozoite protein-based RTS,S/AS01$_E$ vaccine (*GlaxoSmithKline, Belgium*) is licensed for the control of malaria in Africa. In phase 3 trials, children were vaccinated with RTS,S/AS01$_E$ at months 0, 1, and 2, followed by a booster dose at month 20.
- Data from seven countries showed that RTS,S/AS01$_E$ had site-specific efficacy ranging between 22 and 74.6% and it waned rapidly after the last vaccination. Studies that modeled the decay of efficacy elicited by RTS,S/

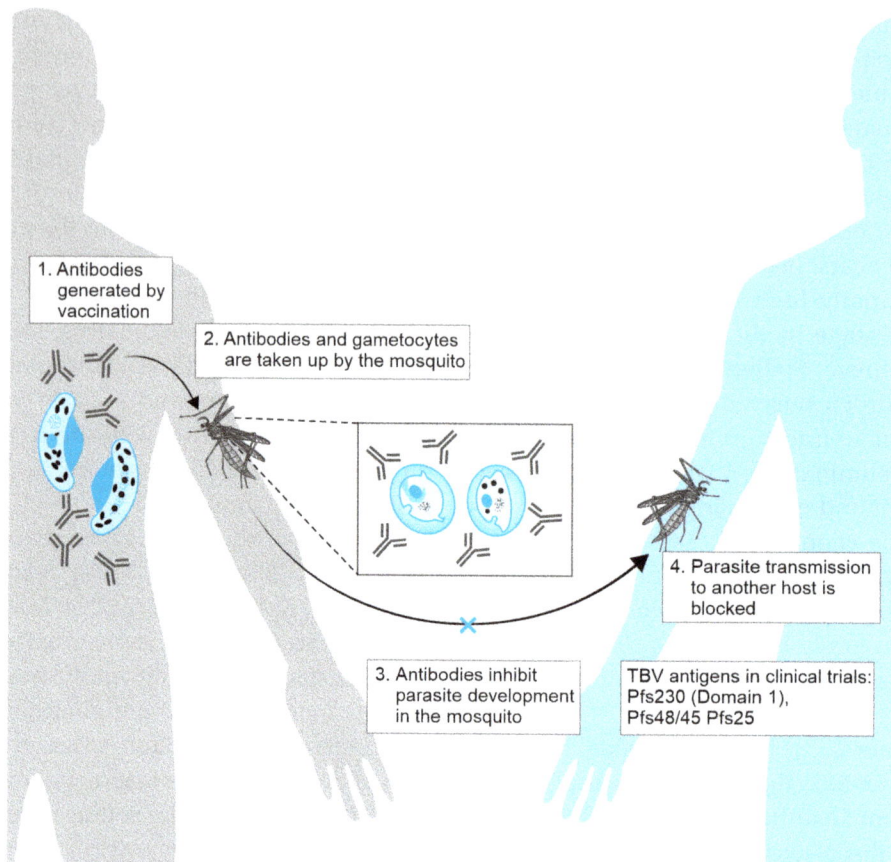

Fig. 3: Transmission-blocking vaccine (TBV).
Source: Dutta S, Thera MA. Seasonal RTS,S/AS01E vaccination with or without seasonal malaria chemoprevention. Lancet Infect Dis. 2024;24(1):9-11.

AS01, and SMC suggest that seasonal administration with RTS,S/AS01$_E$, in addition to SMC, might improve efficacy, in areas of high transmission.

- The introduction of R21/Matrix-M aims to address the urgent need for malaria vaccines, particularly among young children who face severe risks once maternal antibody protection wanes. With malaria mortality peaking around the first birthday, this age group is a crucial target for vaccination efforts.
- *To conclude*, vaccination is not a silver bullet. The wide range of nonvaccine interventions deployed since 2000 have helped reduce deaths by a third and their importance cannot be overstated.
- It must be used alongside existing malaria interventions such as insecticide-treated nets, indoor residual spraying, intermittent preventive treatment in pregnant women, use of antimalarials, plus effective case management and treatment.

Toxoplasmosis Vaccine

There is currently no licensed vaccine available for humans. A range of different veterinary vaccines are required to help control *Toxoplasma gondii* infection which includes vaccines to prevent congenital toxoplasmosis, reduce or eliminate tissue cysts in meat-producing animals, and to prevent oocyst shedding in cats.

Toxovax®, the only licensed vaccine for toxoplasmosis, administered to avoid abortion in sheep, is a live-attenuated vaccine, using the strain S48 tachyzoites, originally isolated from an aborted lamb in New Zealand.

The *Toxoplasma* parasite can live in the bodies of humans and other animals for long periods, possibly even for a lifetime. However, very few people who are infected have symptoms because a healthy person's immune system usually keeps the parasite from causing illness.

Congenital toxoplasmosis has a high impact on human disease worldwide, inducing serious consequences from fetus to adulthood. Over the past few years, various experimental approaches have shown that developing an effective vaccine against *T. gondii* is achievable. However, more remains unknown due to its complicated life cycle, difficulties in clinical translation, and lack of a standardized platform.

Patients with hematological malignancies might develop life-threatening toxoplasmosis, especially after allogeneic hematopoietic stem-cell transplantation (HSCT). Reactivation of latent cysts is the primary mechanism of toxoplasmosis following HSCT; hence, patients at high risk are those who were seropositive before transplantation. The lack of trimethoprim–sulfamethoxazole prophylaxis and various immune status parameters of the patient are other associated risk factors. The mortality of toxoplasma disease, e.g., with organ involvement can be particularly high in this setting.

Despite recent major advances in developing effective vaccines against toxoplasmosis, finding new protective vaccination strategies remains a challenging and elusive goal as it is critical to prevent the disease. With the identification of neoantigens, adjuvants, and immunization strategies, significant progress has been made in developing *T. gondii* vaccines. Candidate vaccines include recombinant antigens, multi-epitope antigens, DNA or RNA, and microparticles. Although there are many challenges in evolving a *T. gondii* vaccine, developing an effective vaccine to prevent and treat toxoplasmosis remains possible, particularly for women of childbearing age and HIV-positive patients.

Vaccines for Leishmaniasis

Leishmaniasis is a serious parasitic disease caused by *Leishmania* spp. transmitted through sandfly bites. This disease is a major public health concern worldwide.

It can occur in three different clinical forms, i.e., cutaneous, mucocutaneous, and visceral leishmaniasis (CL, MCL, and VL, respectively), caused by different *Leishmania* spp. Currently, licensed vaccines are unavailable for the treatment of human leishmaniasis. There are no approved vaccines for leishmaniasis. The development of a vaccine for this disease presents numerous challenges due to the complexity of *Leishmania* parasites and the different forms of the disease.

Leishmania has been a national scourge for several years. The disease is found everywhere in the world except Australia and Antarctica. Two million new cases occur each year worldwide, with one-tenth of the world's population

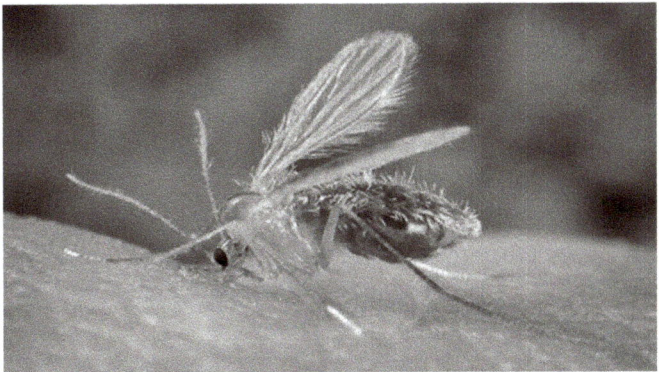

Fig. 4: Sand flies (*Phlebotomus* spp.) are more likely to bite people who are sleeping outdoors.

at risk of infection. In late 2023, numerous Israeli soldiers were under suspicion of having skin rashes attributed to the *Leishmania* parasite, characterized by ulcerative skin lesions. Sand flies (*Phlebotomus* spp.) are more likely to bite people who are sleeping outdoors in camps **(Fig. 4)**.

It is worth noting that in the absence of a vaccine, control measures for leishmaniasis currently rely on chemotherapy to alleviate the disease and on vector control to reduce transmission. The treatment relies mainly on chemotherapeutics, which are highly toxic and have an increasing resistance problem.

The development of a safe, effective, and affordable vaccine for all forms of vector-borne disease is urgently needed to block transmission of the parasite between the host and vector. Although cell-mediated immunity is known to play a crucial role in host protection, the immunological protective mechanism in the pathogenesis of leishmaniasis is complicated. As of February 2024, no vaccine for humans is available.

While there is currently no licensed vaccine for human leishmaniasis, extensive efforts are underway to develop a variety of vaccine modalities with promising results worldwide. Some of these modalities are in the clinical phase and successful results are obtained in terms of safety and immunogenicity. Meanwhile, it is considered that animal vaccines will play an important role in preventing the transmission of leishmaniasis to humans.

FUTURISTIC AND INNOVATIVE VIRAL VACCINES

Human Immunodeficiency Virus Disease Vaccine

In early 1980's, in US many were dying. But, it was not until 1984 that HIV was identified as the cause of acquired immunodeficiency syndrome (AIDS). HIV attacks the body's immune system, specifically targeting CD4 cells, weakening the immune system and making individuals vulnerable to opportunistic infections frequently. It can lead to AIDS if left untreated.

In March 1987, azidothymidine (AZT) became the first drug to gain approval from the U.S. FDA for treating AIDS. AZT was subsequently shown to markedly reduce the perinatal transmission of HIV.

HIV/AIDS Prevention Journeys

In 1995, a combination drug treatment known as the "AIDS cocktail" was introduced. This type of therapy was originally known as highly active antiretroviral therapy (HAART). It is also called combination antiretroviral therapy (cART) or simply antiretroviral therapy (ART).

- Taking *daily oral* *pill* called Truvada® or cabotegravir a new long-acting antiretroviral *injectable pre-exposure prophylaxis (PrEP)*, one shot every 2 months or an implant (a subcutaneous mall plastic rod) effective for about a year, similar technology to contraception implants.

*Truvada® contains two drugs in one pill; emtricitabine and tenofovir disoproxil fumarate. Both drugs are classified as nucleoside reverse transcriptase.

Toward Vaccine Preventions

As of March 2024, the US FDA and the EMA had not approved an HIV prevention vaccine. The National Institutes of Health (NIH) is investing in multiple approaches to prevent HIV, including a safe and effective preventive HIV vaccine. *"Developing safe, effective, and affordable vaccines that can prevent HIV infection in uninfected people is the NIH's highest HIV research priority given its game-changing potential for controlling and ultimately ending the HIV/AIDS pandemic".*

Therapeutic Vaccines against HIV

Human immunodeficiency virus has no vaccine up until now, but therapeutic vaccines could be the breakthrough for HIV. Such vaccines would enhance affected patients' immune systems to fight the disease. Many researchers are trying to develop and test therapeutic HIV vaccines to slow the HIV progression to AIDS. People affected with HIV normally have HIV at an undetectable level, which is detected by use of ART. If therapeutic vaccines for HIV work out, many lives will be saved. Many clinical trials are being conducted for HIV therapeutic vaccines, such as those conducted by AIDS.

Other prevention strategies such as PrEP and safe sexual practices are recommended to reduce the risk of HIV transmission. Developing an effective HIV vaccine has been a significant challenge due to the complex nature of the virus and its ability to mutate rapidly and evade the immune system. However, researchers and scientists have been working tirelessly to develop an HIV vaccine, and clinical trials are ongoing.

Nearly 40 years since HIV was identified as the cause of AIDS, and 36 years since the first HIV vaccine trial, the medical community still does not have a working vaccine. Although antiretroviral treatments are well established, (access varies). The Joint United Nations Program on HIV and AIDS (UNAIDS) estimates 630,000 people died from AIDS-related illness globally in 2022, while 39 million people are living with HIV, including 1.3 million people newly infected last year.

The Next Target for mRNA Vaccines: HIV?

Utilizing the same mRNA technology from their COVID vaccines, Moderna is now entering phase 1 clinical trials for their mRNA-based HIV vaccine. Earlier in 2021, this vaccine was shown to trigger the production of neutralizing antibodies against HIV-like viruses in monkeys, focusing on surface-bound glycoproteins, gp41 and gp120. Further research around these surface glycoprotein subunits has been shown to induce the production of antibodies that can neutralize over 80% of the virus **(Fig. 5)**.

The focal point of the investigation is the envelope glycoprotein, gp120, a tiny structure on the virus surface that plays a crucial role in its ability to dock and inject genetic material into human cells. Docking gp120 is a dynamic structure integral to the virus interaction with CD4 T-cell receptor. This receptor serves as the primary attachment point for the virus as it seeks the optimal site on a human T-cell. The binding triggers the opening of the envelope structure, revealing a co-receptor binding site, a pivotal event in the infection process. Researchers at the Duke Human Vaccine Institute (DHVI) have made a significant stride in understanding the intricate process of HIV infection (February 2, 2024). They believe attaching a specific antibody to this structure could prevent the virus from initiating infection.

Several approaches have been explored in HIV vaccine development:

- *Preventive vaccines:* Aim to stimulate the immune system to generate a protective response against HIV before exposure to the virus. Various vaccine strategies,

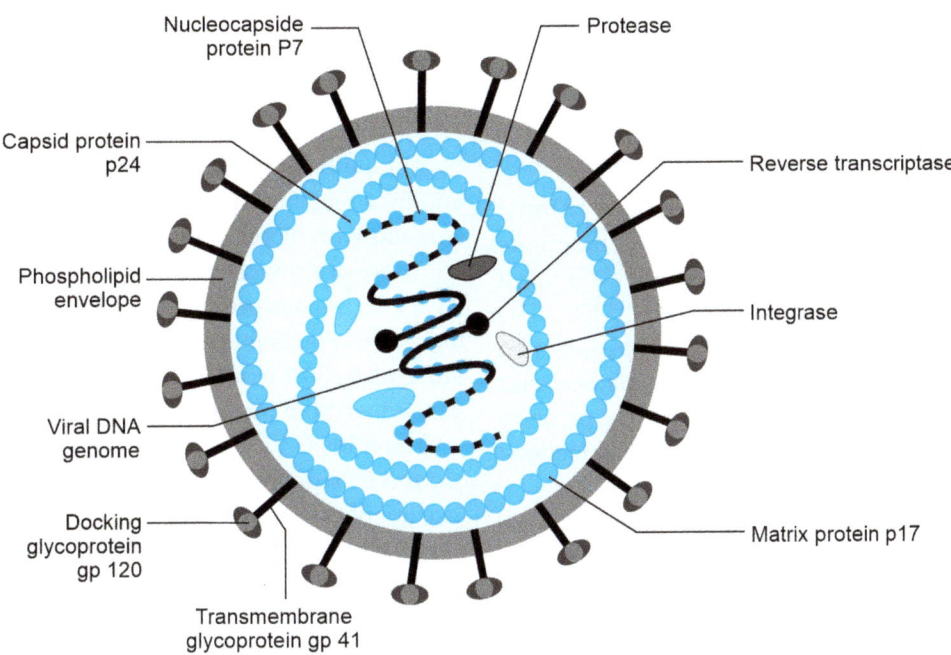

Fig. 5: Structure of human immunodeficiency virus (HIV) virus.

including viral vector-based vaccines, protein subunit vaccines, and DNA/RNA-based vaccines, have been tested in clinical trials. These vaccines typically aim to induce both antibody and cellular immune responses to prevent HIV infection.

- *Therapeutic vaccines:* These are designed to boost the immune response in individuals already infected with HIV. The goal is to control the virus, reduce viral load, and delay disease progression. Therapeutic vaccines are being studied in clinical trials to assess their ability to enhance immune responses and potentially improve long-term outcomes for people living with HIV.

Besides, HIV-infected individuals naturally produce antibodies that can neutralize a broad range of HIV strains. These "broadly neutralizing antibodies (bNAbs)" have provided insights into potential targets for vaccine development. Clinical trials are underway to evaluate the safety and efficacy of bNAbs as a preventive or therapeutic approach. The ultimate goal is to develop a vaccine that can provide durable protection against HIV infection or control the virus in individuals already infected.

A novel trial that has been described as "the last roll of the dice" for a generation of HIV vaccines called PrEPVacc, the trial is testing two vaccines alongside two forms of PrEP to test vaccine efficacy while offering protection to prevent the spread of HIV.

Even a partially effective vaccine could decrease the number of people who acquire HIV, further reducing the number of people who can pass the virus on to others. By substantially reducing the number of new infections, we can control the epidemic, especially for populations at high risk of getting HIV.

Recently Moderna announced it had begun another phase 1 of their experimental HIV trimer mRNA vaccine (mRNA-1574). The trial is expected to have a breakthrough in HIV vaccine discovery, hopefully.

Hepatitis C Virus Vaccines

Inquisitive Query on HCV Vaccine Answered

Authors have dealt with hepatitis C virus (HCV) vaccinations' role in recent years in Question and Answer format. These are our introductory messages for readers of this chapter.

Query from senior clinician cum medical school admin, NC, USA. Sayenna–I just heard the TV announced Noble Prizes for the year 2020 being shared by three scientists for their discovery on HCV. My question is many of us including children are being vaccinated regularly against hepatitis A and B viruses; why is not there a vaccine for hepatitis C?

Authors' responses: Though vaccines exist for hepatitis A virus (HAV) and hepatitis B virus (HBV), a vaccine capable of protecting against HCV, is not yet available. However, several candidate vaccines are currently under development despite many challenges.

Hepatitis C Virus Vaccines—Key Takeaways

Globally, an estimated 58 million people have chronic HCV infection, with about 1.5 million new infections occurring per year. There are an estimated 3.2 million adolescents and children with chronic HCV. The WHO estimated that in 2019, approximately 290,000 people died from hepatitis C, mostly from cirrhosis and hepatocellular carcinoma [hepatocellular carcinoma (HCC) = primary liver cancer]. "The annual number of new HCV infections has steadily increased over the past decade".

Direct-acting antiviral (DAAs) medicines can cure >95% of persons with HCV infection, but access to diagnosis and treatment is low. There is currently no effective vaccine against hepatitis C.

Worldwide, the prevalence of chronic HCV infection is highest in Eastern Europe, Central Asia, Northern Africa, and the Middle East. Therapeutic treatment of HCV has been vastly improved over the past decade due to the development of DAAs. Current treatments fail to prevent reinfection and remain expensive, limiting their use to developed countries.

The asymptomatic nature of acute infection can result in individuals not receiving treatment and unknowingly spreading HCV. A prophylactic vaccine is therefore needed to control this virus. Developing an HCV vaccine has been tough because the virus changes frequently, which makes it harder for our immune system to respond to it. In fact, we have currently identified seven main genotypes or virus strains, and 67 estimated subtypes.

In the 30 years since the discovery of HCV, it has been apparent that this virus is highly complex and presents a major public health challenge. Encouragingly, efforts toward a vaccine continue, and investigation into a range of approaches has yielded interesting results. Some vaccine candidates are still being designed or studied in animals, but few have progressed to human studies. It is a safe bet to assume that eventually, an HCV vaccine will be available.

Hepatitis C Virus Vaccine Perceptions

While vaccines exist for hepatitis A and B, the HCV has been more challenging to develop a vaccine for due to its high genetic variability and the way it evades the immune system. Several HCV vaccine candidates are currently being evaluated in clinical trials.

In addition to vaccination, other preventive measures for HCV include practicing safe injection practices, using barrier methods (such as condoms) during sexual activity, and avoiding sharing personal items that may come into contacts with blood, such as needles or razors.

There are several reasons why the development of an HCV vaccine has proven challenging. Genetically, HCV is highly diverse. Eight genotypes are currently known, each differing by 30% in nucleotide sequence (by contrast, HBV genotypes differ by only 8%).

Hepatitis C Virus genotypes are further classified into around 90 subtypes with 15% sequence variation. HCV is also adept at avoiding host immune responses. Beyond the peculiarities of the virus itself, research is hindered by a lack of in vitro and in vivo models of infection.

Conducting clinical trials for HCV vaccines can also be challenging, e.g., the relatively low incidence of HCV in many industrialized countries necessitates trials being run in the often-marginalized populations at high risk of HCV. The acute nature of COVID-19 has focused efforts to tackle SARS-CoV-2; by contrast, the chronic nature of HCV, often in marginalized communities, and in combination with the stigma associated with the disease, has left it neglected.

To Recap

- HCV vaccine development efforts were initiated after the discovery of HCV in 1989, but to date, no vaccine has been licensed protecting against chronic HCV infection.
- The HCV vaccine is urgently needed to address the ongoing public health crisis caused by this insidious pathogen—a major cause of liver cirrhosis and cancer.
- An increased understanding of HCV protective immunity and HCV envelope glycoprotein structure and function is paving the way toward rational vaccine design and evaluation.

Hepatitis E Virus Vaccines

Hepatitis E virus (HEV) is likely the most common cause of acute viral hepatic disease globally and has been the most common cause among adults in India. Pregnant women are at the highest risk for morbidity and mortality with HEV infection in most developing nations including India, Bangladesh, etc. Available evidence suggests that 20 million people are infected annually resulting in over 70,000 deaths. Considering the limited availability of diagnostics, insufficient surveillance, and investigation of hepatitis outbreaks, these are likely significant underestimates.

Yes, there is a vaccine that has been developed and is available in some countries. The vaccine is primarily used in regions where HEV is endemic and poses a significant public health threat.

One of the vaccines used to prevent HEV is called "Hecolin", and it was developed in China and was approved by the Chinese FDA in 2011. The HEV vaccine is an inactivated vaccine, typically administered in two or three doses to ensure optimal protection. Hecolin is currently licensed for use among individuals ≥16 years of age and there are no data regarding its safety, immunogenicity, or efficacy in younger age groups as they have not been included in any trial to date.

The need for vaccination depends on the prevalence of hepatitis E in a given region and individual risk factors. Not all countries have approved or widely distributed the hepatitis E vaccine, and its availability may vary. Because of this limited data, the WHO recommendations do not support the routine use of vaccines in pregnant women but do not preclude its use during an outbreak, relying on local risk-benefit judgment.

The availability and use of the HEV vaccine may vary depending on the country and specific healthcare guidelines. In some regions, the vaccine is recommended for individuals at high risk of HEV infection, such as travelers to endemic areas, individuals with chronic liver disease, and pregnant women in areas with high HEV prevalence.

In addition to vaccination, other preventive measures for HEV include practicing good hygiene, such as washing hands thoroughly with soap and water, avoiding consumption of contaminated water or food, and ensuring proper sanitation and hygiene practices in food preparation (similar to HAV precautions).

Although there are gaps in understanding the true burden of HEV globally, existing data are more than adequate to confirm that the prevalence and consequences of HEV infection are significant. The excess mortality and severe disease experienced by vulnerable groups, notably pregnant women, and displaced populations, are deserving of urgent global attention. Given the existence of a safe and highly effective vaccine, it is imperative that we identify and work to remove barriers and bottlenecks to its use in outbreaks and highly endemic settings.

Vaccines against Herpes Simplex Viruses Type 1 and Type 2

From our personal experiences, there have been ongoing efforts to develop vaccines against HSV-1 and HSV-2. Several vaccine candidates have been tested in clinical trials, with varying degrees of success. These vaccines aim to stimulate the immune system to produce a protective response against the herpes viruses, reducing the frequency and severity of outbreaks and potentially preventing transmission. The goal is to develop a vaccine that can provide long-lasting protection against HSV infection.

As of our knowledge update in February 2024, there was no approved vaccine for HSV types 1 and 2 available for general use. Although there are no currently available vaccines, there are various candidates in both the preclinical and the clinical phases currently in development. Vaccines are being developed with two broad focuses: preventative and therapeutic, some with dual use December 7, 2021.

Infections with the HSV are frequent and usually affect the skin and nervous system. These are brought on by two closely related but different viruses: type 1 (HSV-1), which affects up to 80–90% of older individuals and is more typically associated with oral infections, and type 2 (HSV-2), which affects 20–30% of adults and is more frequently associated with genital infections. Both types of herpes viruses can cause recurrent outbreaks and can be transmitted through close personal contact.

Although HSV can be more harmful to those with weakened immune systems, these viruses often do not pose a major risk to health because they often remain latent in the body. HSV may occasionally result in brain infections and corneal blindness. It may also be linked to neurodegeneration and Alzheimer's disease. One of the deadliest infections in babies is the HSV, which can spread to the brain and other organs. Severe infections can be extremely damaging.

The success of the VZV vaccine has resulted in more attention for an HSV vaccine due to the similarities between acute and latent infections. However, critical differences in immune response elicited by each virus and the evasion mechanisms used by HSV make development more difficult.

Preventive vaccines would be ideal to focus on primary infection prevention in a seronegative subject because it would prevent active disease and its sequelae and decrease transmission to others.

Therapeutic vaccines may be a more realistic focus to reduce disease severity and target a broader patient population, given the high number of seropositive individuals, especially at a young age. Therapeutic vaccines aim to prevent HSV reactivation, decrease the number of recurrences, or reduce the severity or duration of clinical symptoms.

Current HSV vaccine candidates in various stages of development use DNA, modified mRNA, protein subunit, and attenuated live virus vaccine technology to prevent the development of or mitigate symptoms and spread of HSV.

Protein subunit vaccines, such as the available VZV vaccine, are effective at eliciting an immune response against viral proteins. These vaccines are safer than live-attenuated vaccines but may not provide a long-lasting immune response.

GSK developed a glycoprotein D2 subunit vaccine consisting of the HSV-2 glycoprotein D (gD2-ASO4). In clinical trials, gD2-ASO4 induced protection against genital HSV-1 infection and disease but not disease or infection with HSV-2. Several other subunit HSV vaccines have been tested in animal models, with varying levels of success.

Nucleic acid vaccines include DNA plasmid vaccines and mRNA vaccines. These vaccines transfer genetic materials to cells to express and produce proteins that serve as immune system antigens. In a clinical trial of subjects infected with HSV-2, the vaccine demonstrated safety and reduced viral shedding after vaccine administration. A new formulation of a trivalent vaccine with HSV-2 glycoprotein C, D, and E as an mRNA vaccine was studied in animal models. Compared with a protein subunit vaccine, the mRNA vaccine provided a superior humoral response with higher titers of neutralizing antibodies, prevented HSV-2 infection of the dorsal root ganglia, and reduced viral shedding.

Live-attenuated vaccines for HSV are effective at generating an immune response but remain challenging in safety. HSV is an easily transmissible disease, with high levels throughout the world. Therefore, the highly prevalent disease is a target for developing preventive and therapeutic vaccines to curtail the pervasiveness and associated complications of HSV. Although an HSV vaccine is not currently available, advancements in vaccine technology and the development of an effective VZV vaccine provide hope that a safe and effective HSV vaccine is right around the corner.

In the absence of a vaccine, it is important to follow preventive measures to reduce the risk of HSV transmission, such as practicing safe sexual practices, using barrier methods (such as condoms), and avoiding close contact during active outbreaks.

Monoclonal Antibody against Respiratory Syncytial Virus

With prevention of RSV infection via palivizumab serving as a model of effective early life antibody therapy and several HSV-specific mAbs in clinical development for adult populations, the evidence reviewed here provides a strong scientific rationale to assess mAbs in human clinical trials for nHSV. Two out of three HSV-specific mAbs in human clinical trials have been tested and shown protection in a neonatal mouse model of HSV-1 and HSV-2 infection, further bolstering the promise of this approach.

HHV4 or Epstein Barr Virus (EBV) Vaccine

- First-ever vaccine against EBV shows promise, preventing the emergence of associated pluripotent cancers and potentially averting dangerous health complications like multiple sclerosis (MS).
- With human clinical trials on the horizon, there is more research to ensure comprehensive trials. These trials could commence as early as 2024 or 2025.

Challenges to developing an EBV vaccine include the virus's ability to establish lifelong, latent infection in the host, along with its complex interactions with the immune system. Despite these challenges, efforts in vaccine development remain strong, underpinned by the significance of EBV as a global health concern.

The EBV is a member of the herpes family of viruses; also known as human herpesvirus 4 (HHV4). Discovered in 1964 by Epstein and Barr, the EBV is widespread in all areas of the world, infecting over 95% of the adult population and earning it the informal name, *"Every Body's Virus"*.

In 1968, EBV was shown to be the causal agent of "kissing disease" or, infectious mononucleosis (IM). It is usually contracted during childhood and transmitted through saliva. Soon after contracting it, patients are typically asymptomatic or mildly symptomatic and lay dormant in B-cells over the lifespan, devoid of any significant symptoms. B-cells are immune cells key for producing antibody responses to other infections.

In 1970, the virus was shown to be able to immortalize B lymphocytes, which are one of its target cells. This oncogenic potential underlies the role of EBV in Burkitt's lymphoma, post-nasopharyngeal carcinoma, post-transplant lymphoproliferative disorders, and lymphoma in HIV-infected patients.

In India, the seroepidemiology of infection due to EBV has been limited or none. An earlier study on a limited people from Southern India shown that the age-specific prevalence of IgG antibodies to viral capsid antigen (VCA) rose rapidly to 90% by the age of 5 years. The prevalence of VCA-specific IgM and the geometric mean titer of VCA-specific IgG antibodies were highest between the ages of 6 months and 2 years, the median age of primary infection being 1.4 years. This pattern of other EBV viral markers and its prevalence suggests that the latent EBV infection that persists lifelong after primary infection may be reactivated in many individuals. These results are similar to data from areas where EBV-associated Burkitt's lymphoma is endemic and indicate a high EBV infection load early in life. Schematic representation of the evolution of antibodies to various EBV antigens in patients with IM is shown in **Figure 6**.

- The most commonly performed test is for antibody against the VCA of EBV. Because IgG antibodies against VCA occur in high titer early in infection and persist for life at modest levels.
- Testing of acute and convalescent serum specimens for IgG anti-VCA alone is not useful for establishing the presence of active infection. In contrast, testing for the presence of IgM anti-VCA antibody and the absence or very low titers of antibodies to EBV nuclear antigen (EBNA) is useful for identifying active and recent infections. Because serum antibody against EBNA is not present until several weeks to months after onset of infection and rises with convalescence, a very elevated anti-EBNA antibody concentration typically excludes active primary infection.
- Testing for antibodies against early antigen (EA) is not usually required to assess EBV-associated mononucleosis.
- Polymerase chain reaction (PCR) assay for detection of EBV DNA in serum, plasma, and tissue and reverse transcriptase-PCR assay for detection of EBV RNA in lymphoid cells, tissue, and/or body fluids are available and can be useful in evaluation of immunocompromised patients and in complex clinical situations.

There is no treatment or medical intervention for EBV available; however, virus-associated complications may be treated with various modes of immune modulation. Currently, radiotherapy and chemotherapy remain the

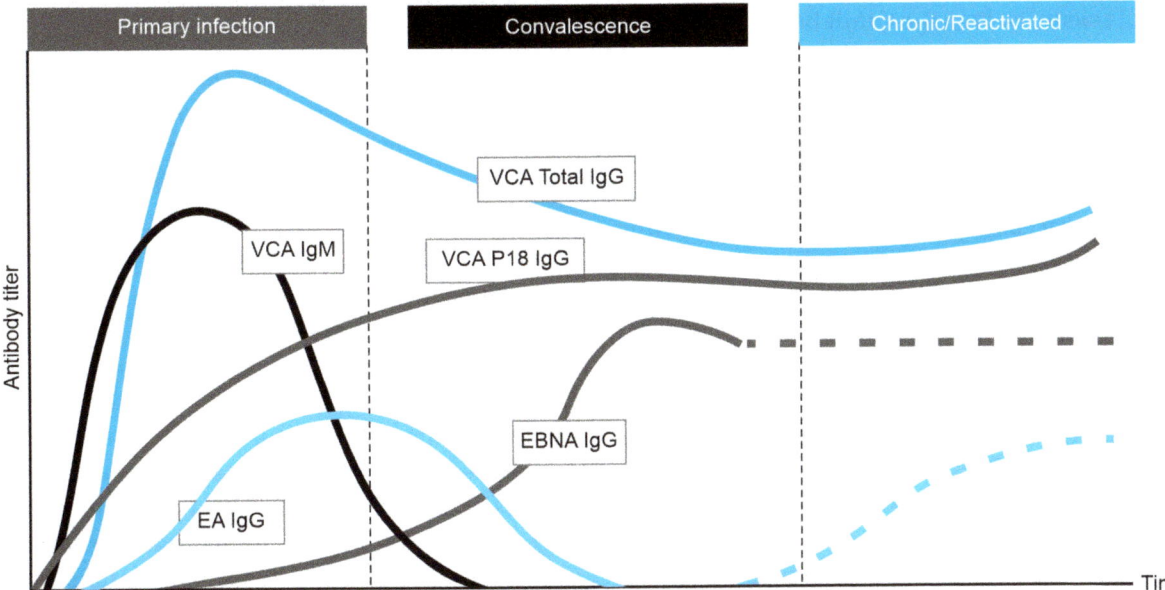

Fig. 6: Titers of neutralizing antibodies and antibodies to multiple EBV proteins increase over many months after primary infection with EBV. (EA: early antigen; EBNA: EBV nuclear antigen; EBV: Epstein–Barr virus; IgG: immunoglobulin G; IgM: immunoglobulin M; VCA: viral capsid antigen)

main treatments for EBV-associated malignancies. Recent evidence has suggested that adoptive therapy through infusions of human leukocyte-associated antigen-matched EBV cytotoxic T-cells may form a novel strategy for both prophylaxis and treatment of EBV-induced lymphoproliferative disorders. Additionally, a vaccine based on immunization with a structural antigen, gp350, is under evaluation.

Developing such interventions could reduce rates of EBV-related conditions, including MS, Hodgkin lymphoma, and various cancers especially gastric Ca. Recently, researchers developed a vaccine that can generate immunity against EBV in mice for seven months. Further tests are needed to know how these findings may apply to humans. A groundbreaking new vaccine for EBV may pave the way for better preventive and treatment options for conditions such as MS and various cancers.

Creating a vaccine for the EBV has historically been challenging as it changes over its life cycle. Moreover, as the virus itself can lead to the development of tumors, incorporating whole sections of its viral proteins into vaccines could increase cancer risk.

To overcome these issues, researchers incorporated 20 epitopes—small amino acid sequences that activate an immune response into their vaccine formula. Each epitope targets one of the proteins expressed by EBV at different stages of its life cycle. Also, have designed a novel adjuvant to accompany the vaccine to increase its efficacy.

A team of scientists, from the QIMR Berghofer Medical Research Institute in Australia, who have published their findings in the journal Nature Communications, have been able to design a vaccine targeting lymph nodes in mice, which are the key players in the functioning of the body's immune system.

- The new EBV vaccine targets multiple parts of the virus.
- It induces strong, long-lasting immunity in two vital arms of the immune system.
- The results in laboratory models support the progression to human clinical trials.

This vaccine not only elicited humoral antibodies and T-cells to combat EBV, but it also revealed the ability to induce a specific type of immunity that safeguards against the emergence of EBV-associated tumors. Given that EBV is a major risk factor for developing MS, an effective vaccine that prevents EBV infection in humans may also have an important role in preventing the onset of MS.

In the absence of a vaccine, it is important to follow preventive measures to reduce the risk of EBV transmission, such as practicing good hygiene, avoiding close contact with individuals who have active EBV infection (especially during episodes of IM), and refraining from sharing personal items that may come into contact with saliva.

HHV5 or Cytomegalovirus Vaccines

Cytomegalovirus is a common virus that infects people of all ages. Over half of adults have been infected with CMV by age of 40 years. Most people infected with CMV show no signs or symptoms. Pregnant people infected with CMV can give birth to a baby with congenital CMV (cCMV) which can cause hearing loss and developmental issues. CMV can cause serious complications in people who have a compromised immune system, such as transplant recipients.

In immunocompromised patients, CMV is a major cause of morbidity and mortality. Disease often results from reactivation of latent virus. The lungs, gastrointestinal tract, or central nervous system (CNS) may be involved. In the terminal phase of AIDS, CMV infection causes retinitis in up to 40% of patients and causes funduscopically visible retinal abnormalities. Ulcerative disease of the colon (with abdominal pain and gastrointestinal bleeding) or of the esophagus (with odynophagia) may occur.

A cCMV case scenario query answered by authors is as follows:

New query on Pediatric Oncall in your expertise category of "Infectious disease"—dated April 6, 2023.

"Is cCMV common in India? How often do obstetricians diagnose CMV infection in pregnant women? I had my child born full term normal delivery, but my doctor says my child was CMV infected before birth. Can you explain me, sir? I am worried. Is there a vaccine for CMV?"

Author's response: Certainly, the CMV maternal infection and the magnitude of the cCMV problem in India have major diagnostic issues. The various diagnostic modes used have not been adequately investigated in India. Consensus recommendations for prevention, diagnosis, and therapy are lacking.

In general, CMV infection causes few or no symptoms in most healthy individuals. Pregnant women can pass the virus on to the developing fetus, and this can have consequences for the fetus, neonate, and child. Maternofetal transmission of CMV can occur during pregnancy following primary or recurrent infections in mothers with different strains. For women who have a primary infection in pregnancy, there is around a 40% risk of transmission from mother to infant. If women have had CMV infection prior to becoming pregnant, the transmission risk is significantly less, around 1–2%.

In Western countries, around 50% of the women will have had CMV before, and this means they have got IgG antibodies for CMV (seropositive) *[CDC, USA data (2023)]*. About one out of every 200 infants is born with cCMV infection, and around one in five infected babies will have long-term health problems. In contrast, developing countries including India have a high maternal seropositivity prevalence of over 91%. However, we have a paucity of literature in India on cCMV infection-related neonatal clinical follow-up!.

In Pediatrics, cCMV infection is the leading nongenetic cause of sensorineural hearing loss (SNHL) in children. In the USA, approximately 20% of all hearing loss at birth and 25% of all hearing loss at 4 years of age is attributable to cCMV infection. But there are a number of other long-term health problems associated with cCMV. These include neurodevelopmental problems, including cognitive disabilities, gross motor impairment speech, and language delays, and there is a higher prevalence of autistic spectrum disorder (ASD) compared to the general population. Other problems include epilepsy and seizures and impaired vision as a result of chorioretinitis.

Development of preventive strategies is crucially important, with both risk and reduction to prevent CMV infection. Furthermore, currently, there are no approved vaccines to prevent CMV infection, no universal maternal or neonatal screening programs, and no consensus about treatment strategies in pregnancy for maternal or fetal CMV infection.

Cytomegalovirus Vaccine Needs and Challenges

An effective CMV vaccine could prevent the majority of birth defects caused by cCMV infections. Currently there is no licensed CMV vaccine. Challenges in developing a vaccine against CMV include adeptness of CMV in evading the immune system and limited animal models. However, scientists are making significant advances in their quest to develop a vaccine against this destructive virus **(Fig. 7)**.

Human CMV is probably one of the most common infections known to humans **(Fig. 8)**. Almost close to 90% of Indian adults by the age of 30 years have IgG antibodies

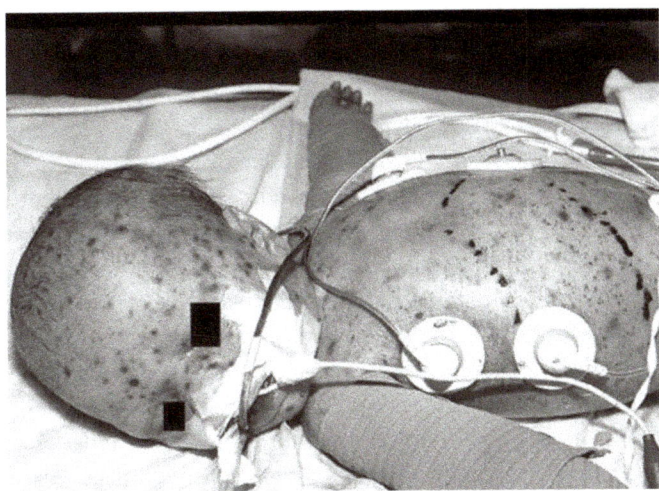

Fig. 7: Congenitally infected newborn (NB) with cytomegalovirus (CMV) disease with hepatospenomegally, jaundice, thrombocytopenic purpuric rashes, etc.
Source: CDC Redbook; 2022.

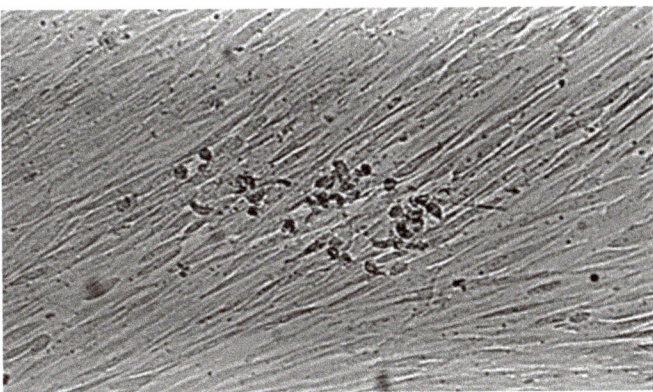

Fig. 8: Cytomegalovirus (CMV) isolated in human lung fibroblast (HLF) cell culture from affected body fluids. This shows the characteristic cytopathogenic effect (CPE) of CMV in a tissue cell culture.
Courtesy: Uduman et al.

against CMV suggestive of acquired CMV from early childhood onset asymptomatic infections.

Once CMV is in a person's body, it stays there for life and can reactivate. Healthy people who are infected with CMV usually do not require medical treatment.

Cytomegalovirus infection poses an important public health problem as it may cause serious morbidity and mortality in congenitally infected newborns and immunocompromised patients, most notably transplant recipients and HIV-infected persons. The magnitude of this problem in India and the various diagnostic modalities used have not been adequately investigated.

In the United States, nearly one in three children is already infected with CMV by the age of 5 years. Over half of adults have been infected with CMV by the age of 40 years. Once CMV is in a person's body, it stays there for life and can reactivate. A person can also be reinfected with a different strain (variety) of the virus. Most people with CMV infection have no symptoms and are not aware that they have been infected.

About 1 out of 200 babies in the United States are born with cCMV. But in India, it is much more frequent; one study reported that 19.4% of babies were congenitally infected resulting in various birth defects, including SNHL! The ultimate goal of the prevention program is to develop a vaccine that can be administered to seronegative women of childbearing age to prevent primary infection during pregnancy.

The development of a CMV vaccine has been an area of active research, but as of this time, no vaccine has received regulatory approval for general use. However, progress toward this goal has been made in recent clinical trials. CMV vaccine development started in the 1970s with attenuated strains. In the 1980s, one of the strains was shown to be safe and effective in renal transplant patients.

Currently, there is no vaccine available to prevent cCMV and to prevent the consequences of CMV disease in recipients of transplanted organs and hematopoietic cells. Numerous candidate vaccines are moving forward, and some are in clinical trials.

The diversity of novel strategies under development engenders optimism that a successful candidate will emerge **(Table 1)**. More, attention switched to the glycoprotein B (gB) vaccine, which was shown to give moderate protection against the acquisition of the virus in young women and adolescents. This has also provided benefits to CMV-seronegative SOT recipients. The identification of the pp65 tegument protein as the principal target of cellular immune responses resulted in new approaches, particularly DNA, and plasmids to protect hematogenous stem cell recipients.

On October 2023, ID Week (USA) presented an investigational mRNA-1647 vaccine that shows great promise in the fight against CMV infection. Developed using mRNA technology, it incorporates essential CMV antigens and has demonstrated safety and effectiveness in clinical evaluations. This vaccine incorporates six mRNA sequences, encoding two critical CMV antigens—gB and the pentameric glycoprotein complex—encapsulated in lipid NPs in a lyophilized presentation.

The clinical evaluation of mRNA-1647 demonstrated its overall safety, tolerability, and ability to induce antigen-specific immune responses across various dosage levels. This comprehensive assessment encompassed both CMV-seronegative and -seropositive participants. Based on these findings, the 100 μg dose of mRNA-1647 was selected for advancement to the phase 3 trial.

While the path to an effective COVID-19 vaccine can be described as a race, the long journey to develop a vaccine against CMV can be more seen as a quest, with innumerable obstacles and changes of direction. This journey presents us now with another promising vaccine candidate failing to provide the desired protective efficacy in a large phase 2b clinical trial. The V160 was generally well tolerated and immunogenic; however, three doses of the vaccine did not reduce the incidence of primary CMV infection in CMV-seronegative women compared with placebo. This study provides insights into the design of future CMV vaccine efficacy trials, particularly for the identification of CMV infection using molecular assays.

Compared with a previously moderately successful vaccine candidate called gB/MF59, the mRNA vaccine-elicited responses that were better at preventing the CMV virus from infecting epithelial cells that line the mouth

TABLE 1: Experimental cytomegalovirus vaccines in or approaching clinical evaluation.

Type	Vaccine	Developer	Components	Status
Live attenuated	Towne	Wistar	Whole virus	Phase 2
	Towne-Toledo 1, 2, 3, 4	Aviron/MedImmune	Whole virus	Phase 1
Subunit protein	gB/MF59	Chiron/Sanofi	gB/MF59	Phase 2
	GSK1492903A	GlaxoSmithKline	gB/ASO1	Phase 1
Subunit DNA vectored	TransVax	Vical	gB, pp65	Phase 2
	CyMVectin	Vical	gB, pp65	Late preclinical
Subunit viral vectored	AVX601	AlphaVax/Novartis	gB/pp65-IE1	Phase 1

and nose and provide the first line of defense against viral infection. The mRNA vaccine was also more effective at triggering the immune system to destroy CMV-infected cells.

After >50 years of research, we are closer than ever to having a licensed CMV vaccine. The Moderna mRNA vaccine has moved on to the first ever phase 3 clinical study to fight for a CMV vaccine, will lead ever to having a licensed CMV vaccine, which will help to stronger protection against CMV.

Vaccines for other Human Herpesviruses, HHV6, HHV7, and HHV8

Human Herpesviruses are among the most successful viruses found in human populations. They establish lifelong latent infections, which are punctuated by recurrent reactivations.

- *HHV6:* Causing roseola infantum (exanthema subitum). Antibodies to this virus are present in almost everyone by the age of 5.
- *HHV7:* Causing roseola like HHV6 and 7 are associated with rejection of transplanted kidneys; the pathogenesis is poorly understood.
- *HHV8:* Kaposi's sarcoma virus has been found associated with Kaposi's sarcoma in AIDS patients as well as intra-abdominal solid tumors.

Virtually nothing is known about the pathogenesis and epidemiology of this newly described HHV6 and 7. All HHVs can establish latent infection within specific tissues, which are characteristic of each virus. Reactivated viruses can cause disseminated disease in immune-compromised individuals.

Roseoloviruses Vaccines

Human herpesvirus 6 and HHV7 are roseoloviruses, which infect almost all babies and persist for their lifetime. Also, these viruses can be serious hazards during primary or reactivated infections, particularly in immunodeficient settings. Fortunately, despite their widespread nature, these T lymphotropic and neurotropic viruses are generally regarded as benign infections.

HHV8 or Kaposi's Sarcoma-associated Herpesvirus Vaccines

Kaposi's sarcoma-associated herpesvirus (KSHV) is the eighth HHV. This virus causes Kaposi's sarcoma, a cancer commonly occurring in AIDS patients, as well as primary effusion lymphoma, some types of multicentric Castleman's disease, and KSHV inflammatory cytokine syndrome. Despite the high prevalence and heavy disease burdens associated with HHVs, vaccines against these pathogens are still lacking, except for VZV.

Vaccine is the most effective method to prevent viral diseases, but there is no report describing a vaccine against HHV8 at present. No vaccine against HHV8 is commercially available now. KSHV vaccines designed to prevent a naïve host from infection and to boost the immune control of KSHV in persistently infected people will have a major impact on individuals who are at a high risk of developing KSHV-associated diseases.

Viral Hemorrhagic Fever Vaccines

The term viral hemorrhagic fever (VHF) refers to a condition that affects many organ systems of the body and reduces the human ability to function on its own. Clinical symptoms can vary but often include bleeding or hemorrhaging. Some VHFs cause relatively mild illness, while others can cause severe life-threatening disease. Management is largely supportive; most VHFs have no known cure or vaccine.

Although COVID-19 is very contagious, its fatality rate is relatively low in comparison with these 10 VHF causing viruses. From the Marburg to dengue, these viruses are not mere names but potent adversaries causing fear worldwide.

Viral hemorrhagic fevers are caused by several families of viruses and these viruses share some clinical commonalities **(Table 2)**:
- They are RNA viruses, as their genetic material.

TABLE 2: Viral hemorrhagic fever (VHF) diseases by virus family.

VHF virus family	VHF virus diseases
Arenavirus (order *Bunyavirales*)	Lassa fever, Lujo hemorrhagic fever (LUHF), Chapare HF (CHHF)
Flavivirus	Severe dengue, yellow fever, Kyasanur Forest disease (KFD), Alkhurma HF (AHF), Omsk HS (OHF)
Filovirus	Ebola disease, Marburg virus disease (MVD)
Hantavirus (order *Bunyavirales*)	Hantaviruses (HVs) with cardiopulmonary syndrome (HCPS) and with renal syndrome [hemorrhagic fever renal syndrome (HFRS)]
Nairovirus (order *Bunyavirales*)	Crimean-Congo HF (CCHF)
Phenuivirus (order *Bunyavirales*)	Rift Valley fever (RVF)

- VHF viruses exist in animal or insect populations and are generally restricted to the geographical areas where the host species live. After the initial spread into the human population, some VHF viruses can continue to spread from person to person [exceptions are dengue and Japanese encephalitis virus (JEV)].
- Most common cause of emerging disease in people because RNA viruses change over time at a high rate.
- They are covered, or enveloped, in a lipoprotein outer layer, making it easier to destroy these viruses with physical (heat, sunlight, and gamma rays) and chemical (bleach, detergents, and solvents) methods.
- Outbreaks of VHFs in people can be difficult to prevent since they can occur sporadically and cannot be easily predicted.

Viral Hemorrhagic Fever Challenges

- More of the world's population is at risk for VHFs. Spread is likely to shift due to globalization, climate changes, and international travel.
- Fast and accurate diagnostics are vital during outbreaks to confirm VHF cases. Improving VHF diagnostic techniques to make them faster, and easier to produce and use is an essential component of controlling these diseases.
- Person-to-person transmission of some VHFs can occur when people come in contact with infected animals or insects. For many VHFs, person-to-person transmission can then continue, often through direct contact or in healthcare facilities without adequate infection control procedures.
- Outbreak prevention is difficult. Because of VHF occurs sporadically and irregularly, and their unpredictable occurrence.
- The availability of vaccines and treatments are limited.

Crimean-Congo Hemorrhagic Fever Vaccine

The Crimean-Congo hemorrhagic fever (CCHF) is transmitted by ticks. It is similar to the Ebola and Marburg viruses in the way it progresses. During the first days of infection, sufferers present with pin-sized bleedings in the face, mouth, and the pharynx.

The CCHF outbreaks are an ongoing threat to public health. The disease is fatal in up to 40% of hospital-admitted cases, and it is difficult to prevent and treat as there are currently no approved treatments or vaccines. CCHF is found in Eastern and Southern Europe, throughout the Mediterranean, in Northwestern China, Central Asia, Africa, the Middle East, and the Indian subcontinent.

Risk of Exposure

Animal herders, livestock workers, and slaughterhouse workers in endemic areas are at risk of CCHF. Healthcare workers in endemic areas are at risk of infection through unprotected contact with infectious blood and body fluids. Individuals and international travelers with contact with livestock in endemic regions may also be exposed.

Transmission

Ixodid (hard) ticks, especially those of the genus *Hyalomma*, are both a reservoir and a vector for the CCHF virus. Numerous wild and domestic animals, such as cattle, goats, sheep, and hares, serve as amplifying hosts for the virus. Transmission to humans occurs through contact with infected ticks or animal blood. CCHF can be transmitted from one infected human to another by contact with infectious blood or body fluids. Documented spread of CCHF has also occurred in hospitals due to improper sterilization of medical equipment, reuse of injection needles, and contamination of medical supplies.

Treatment is primarily supportive. The virus is sensitive in vitro to the antiviral drug ribavirin. It has been used in the treatment of CCHF patients reportedly with some benefit.

Recovery

The long-term effects of CCHF infection have not been studied well enough in survivors to determine whether or not specific complications exist.

Prevention

Agricultural workers and others working with animals should use insect repellent on exposed skin and clothing. Insect repellants containing N, N-diethyl-m-toluamide (DEET) are the most effective in warding off ticks. Wearing gloves and other protective clothing is recommended. Individuals should also avoid contact with the blood and body fluids of livestock or humans who show symptoms of infection.

Currently, there are no licensed vaccines against CCHFV for widespread usage. However, a new vaccine against CCHF is being trialed in humans for the first time. The University of Oxford study aims to confirm the safety of the ChAdOx2 CCHF vaccine and investigate the development of immunity following vaccination.

Lassa Virus Fever Vaccine

A nurse in Nigeria was the first person to be infected with the Lassa virus fever (LASV). The virus is transmitted by rodents. LASV is an acute VHF endemic to West Africa. Confirmed outbreaks and sporadic cases have been reported in some other regions such as Mali, Ghana, Liberia, Sierra Leone, and Nigeria.

There is no licensed LASV vaccine approved for use in both humans and animals to reduce zoonotic transmission.

Kyasanur Forest Disease Virus

Kyasanur forest disease virus (KFDV), commonly known as "monkey fever" was identified in 1957 when it was isolated from a sick monkey from the Kyasanur forest in Karnataka (formerly Mysore) State, India. Since then, between 400 and 500 humans' cases per year have been reported. Hard ticks (*Haemaphysalis spinigera*) are the reservoir of KFDV and once infected, remain so for life.

A highly pathogenic KFDV is a rare, tick-borne, zoonotic disease that causes acute febrile hemorrhagic illness in humans and monkeys, especially in the southern part of India.

In January-February 2024, this tick-borne VHF claimed the lives of two of the 49 positive reported people. Most cases have been reported in Uttara Kannada district, followed by Shivamogga and Chikkamagaluru districts. State health department officials are actively reviewing preparedness to tackle the spread of the infection.

The only existing licensed vaccine is a formalin-inactivated tissue culture vaccine. The Institute of Animal Health and Veterinary Biologicals (IAH and VB) Bengaluru is producing the cell culture-based KFD vaccine and is supplying it to susceptible people in KFD disease-endemic regions of India for the past 23 years.

Vaccination regimes include two doses of vaccine administered at an interval of 1 month, by s/c route to persons aged from 7 to 65 years, since the immunity conferred by the vaccine is short-lived. Booster doses are recommended within 6–9 months of the primary vaccination. To combat the spread of KFD, the Indian Council of Medical Research (ICMR) has announced plans to develop a new vaccine in 2024. Previous vaccines developed for KFD have proven ineffective; however, a Hyderabad-based firm has stepped up to the challenge and is actively engaged in development.

Rift Valley Fever

Rift Valley fever (RVF) is a growing viral threat with emerging potential for global spread that has been largely neglected by major public health entities. Because of this lack of diagnostic and surveillance tools, the true prevalence of RVF is unknown. It is a zoonotic viral disease transmitted by mosquitoes and causes abortion storms, fetal malformations, and newborn animal deaths in livestock ruminants. In humans, RVF can manifest as hemorrhagic fever, encephalitis, or retinitis.

Since it was discovered in 1930, RVF virus has multiple outbreaks in Africa and the Middle East. People can be infected from the bite of a mosquito or through direct contact with the blood and tissues of infected animals. RVF is difficult to control because infected mosquito eggs can survive for years in the soil. Infected animals develop high levels of virus in their blood, making it easy for mosquitoes that bite these animals to then become infected with the virus. This chain of transmission must be broken to prevent disease in people and animals.

This disease outbreak is part of a growing problem; 39 countries in Africa and the Arabian Peninsula have reported RVF outbreaks, involving about 1000 total confirmed deaths since 1999. The WHO has identified RVF as one of nine priority diseases because of its potential to cause outbreaks, and healthcare practitioners remain without vaccines licensed for use in humans.

The development of RVF vaccines is crucial in preventing mortality and morbidity and reducing the spread of the virus. While several veterinary vaccines have been licensed in endemic countries, there are currently no licensed RVF vaccines for human use.

The CDC researchers have developed a vaccine. During early testing, all vaccinated animals were protected against the RVF virus. There were no negative side effects. The vaccine is also inexpensive to produce, and this makes it an affordable option for developing countries.

To reduce the likelihood of future devastating RVF outbreaks, effective RVF vaccination programs using appropriate vaccines for susceptible livestock animals are crucial. Promising RVF candidate vaccines require further safety and immunogenicity studies to reduce future RVF threats.

Ebola Vaccine

Ebola virus disease (EVD) is a severe and often fatal illness in humans. It is transmitted to people from wild animals and spreads through human-to-human transmission via direct contact with bodily fluids.

Ebola virus disease or Ebola is a rare but severe illness in humans and is often fatal. First appeared in 1976 in two simultaneous outbreaks, one in what is now Nzara, South Sudan, and the other in Yambuku, Democratic Republic of the Congo. The latter occurred in a village near the Ebola river, from which the disease takes its name.

There are five strains of the Ebola virus, each named after countries and regions in Africa: Zaire, Sudan, Tai Forest, Bundibugyo, and Reston. The Zaire Ebola virus is the deadliest, with a mortality rate of 90%. It is the strain currently spreading through Guinea, Sierra Leone, Liberia, and beyond. Scientists say flying foxes probably brought the Zaire Ebola virus into cities.

Ebola is a hemorrhagic fever virus that causes severe inflammation and tissue damage throughout the body. EVD outbreaks cause mortality ranging from 50 to 90%; however, no specified antiviral drugs are required for the treatment, which indicates the control of an outbreak by earlier identification through symptoms with early medical care. The current Ebola outbreak indicates an urgent requirement for a vaccine against EVD.

There are two EVD vaccines were approved for use: rVSV-ZEBOV-GP (trade name Ervebo) and Ad26.ZEBOV/MVA-BN-Filo (trade name Janssen). It was first used in a "ring vaccination" approach during the 2014–2016 outbreak in West Africa, where it was given to contacts of those infected with the disease.

The WHO has also prequalified this vaccine, which means that it meets WHO standards for quality, safety, and efficacy, and can be procured by international donors for use in emergencies. It is crucial for clinicians, especially those working in regions where EVD is endemic, to stay updated on vaccination guidelines, availability, and administration logistics.

Marburg Virus Disease Vaccine

Marburg virus disease (MVD), the most dangerous, is named after a small and idyllic town on the river Lahn, but that has nothing to do with the disease itself. As with Ebola, the Marburg is a hemorrhagic fever virus. It causes convulsions and bleeding of mucous membranes, skin, and organs. It has a fatality rate of 90%.

Marburg virus disease was first identified in Marburg, Germany in 1967; a severe, often fatal illness caused by the Marburg virus. Since then, there have been a limited number of outbreaks reported in Angola, the Democratic Republic of the Congo, Kenya, South Africa, and Uganda.

While rare, MVD remains a severe public health threat due to its high mortality rate and the lack of an effective antiviral treatment or vaccine. In 2023, two separate MVD outbreaks have been reported in two countries, Equatorial Guinea and the United Republic of Tanzania.

There are no approved vaccines; however, some experimental vaccines have shown promising results in first-in-human studies. The Sabin Vaccine Institute began a phase 2 clinical trial for a single-dose vaccine in Uganda.

Preventive measures against MVD are not well defined. However, avoiding fruit bats, and sick nonhuman primates in central Africa, is one way to protect against infection.

Hantaviruses Pulmonary Syndrome

Several types of Hantaviruses (HVs) can cause hantavirus pulmonary syndrome (HPS) and hemorrhagic fever with renal syndrome (HFRS). These are transmitted to humans through contact with rodent urine, droppings, or saliva. Symptoms include fever, muscle aches, and respiratory distress.

Hantaviruses are rodent-transmitted viruses that can cause HPS in the Americas and HFRS in Eurasia. Together, these viruses have annually caused approximately 200,000 human infections worldwide in recent years, with a case fatality rate of 5–15% for HFRS and up to 40% for HPS.

There is currently no effective treatment available for either HFRS or HPS. Only whole virus inactivated vaccines against HTNV or SEOV are licensed for use in the Republic of Korea and China, but the protective efficacies of these vaccines are uncertain. To a large extent, the immune correlates of protection against hantavirus are not known.

Dengue Hemorrhagic Fever

The dengue viruses (DENVs) are transmitted in tropical and subtropical regions by infected *Aedes* mosquito species as they take a blood meal from a susceptible host. Hundreds of millions of people are infected every year and an estimated 96 million infections are clinically apparent.

In India and Southeast Asia, 1.3 billion people live in dengue-endemic areas, with Thailand, India, and Indonesia among some of the most highly endemic countries. DENVs cause flu-like symptoms, including high fever, severe headache, pain behind the eyes, joint and muscle pain, rash, and mild bleeding. Severe cases can lead to dengue hemorrhagic fever (DHF) or dengue shock syndrome (DSS).

Individuals are at greatest risk for severe dengue when they experience two sequential DENV infections with two different DENV types separated in time by more than 18 months. The exact immunopathogenic mechanisms of sequential heterotypic DENV infections are incompletely understood, but considerable evidence points to humoral and cellular adaptive immune responses occurring in response to the first infection facilitating increased DENV replication during the second infection which, in turn, drives pro-inflammatory cytokine secretion.

Vaccination has long been recognized as the required foundation of a multipronged approach to reducing the global dengue burden. Sanofi Pasteur licensed the first dengue vaccine (Dengvaxia®). As expected, every dengue vaccine candidate following Dengvaxia® is being stringently reviewed for safety and efficacy in dengue immunes and nonimmunes, across a broad age range of recipients, and for their ability to protect against the full spectrum of disease outcomes caused by infection with any DENV type. There is also a requirement for demonstrating safety and efficacy across more than one dengue season.

■ OTHER MISCELLANEOUS VIRUSES

Other miscellaneous viruses include adenoviruses, chikungunya virus (CHIKv), RSV, non-polio enteroviruses, hand, foot, and mouth disease (HFMD) vaccine, Nipah vaccine, West Nile virus (WNV), and Zika virus (ZIKV).

Vaccine against Human Adenoviruses

Most human adenoviruses (AdHu) infections are mild and require only symptom relief for treatment. Adenoviruses viruses are common that can cause a range of illnesses, are associated primarily with respiratory tract disease, epidemic keratoconjunctivitis (EKC), "Madras eye", or gastroenteritis.

In healthy people, infection with one adenovirus type should confer type-specific immunity or at least lessen symptoms associated with reinfection, which forms the basis of adenovirus vaccines used in new military recruits. Human adenoviruses are an important cause of infections in both immunocompetent and immunocompromised individuals, and they continue to provide clinical challenges in diagnostics and treatment.

There is currently an adenovirus vaccine available, but it is not for general use. The adenovirus vaccine (live and oral) is a vaccine used to control disease caused by adenovirus types 4 and 7 and is currently approved for military personnel aged 17 through 50.

Immunocompromised persons are more likely to get seriously ill from an adenovirus infection. This includes people who have had stem cell transplants or organ transplants. It also includes people who have cancer or HIV/AIDS. If one has cardiac or respiratory disease, the chances of severe infection increase as well.

Transplant patients with severe hypogammaglobulinemia at the time of active adenovirus infection might benefit from immunoglobulin administration. Adoptive transfer of adenovirus-specific T-lymphocytes is under investigation for the treatment of severe adenovirus diseases in hematopoietic stem cell transplant recipients, but there is limited data in solid organ transplant recipients or other populations.

Adenovirus-based Influenza Vaccine

Replication deficient human adenovirus serotype 5 (AdHu5) vector expressing hemagglutinin antigen of avian influenza virus and a TLR-3 ligands has been found to induce antigen-specific immune responses in humans. Another novel approach is to use a chimpanzee adenovirus (AdC68)-based vector expressing artificial microRNAs to target matrix proteins or nucleoproteins of the influenza virus. Such vaccines have the potential to provide full protection from influenza infection by inhibiting viral replication.

Adenovirus-based Human Immunodeficiency Virus Vaccine

Trivalent AdHu5 vector expressing three HIV antigens, gag, pol, and nef, is the most widely studied HIV vaccine worldwide. However, this vaccine fails to reduce viral load clinically and increases the risk of HIV in AdHu5 seropositive males.

Another potential HIV vaccine candidate is the AdHu5 vector (replication-deficient) expressing simian immunodeficiency virus gag protein, and this vaccine has been shown to reduce viral load preclinically. Chimpanzee adenovirus (serotypes 3 and 63)-based vectors expressing gag, pol, and nef antigens have shown promising results in the murine model.

Adenovirus-based Tuberculosis Vaccine

There is only one clinically approved TB vaccine namely BCG; however, this vaccine cannot protect against pulmonary TB. AdHu5 is the most commonly used adenovirus serotype for the development of the TB vaccine. One of the major drawbacks of this type of vaccine is that having preexisting immunity against AdHu5 can drastically reduce vaccine efficacy. This drawback can be subsided by using less prevalent serotypes, such as Hu35. One such vaccine is rAd35-TBS, which is developed using the AdHu35 vector expressing three different antigens of Mtb under the control of the CMV promoter.

Chikungunya Virus Vaccine

There is a need for the CHIKv vaccine as the burden of disease is tremendous and infection rates are significant in developing countries. As of now, no commercial vaccines are available to prevent the occurrence of infection. Many vaccines have been tried in preclinical and phase 1 and 2 trials; like inactivated live-attenuated genetically engineered DNA, VLP vaccines are under trial.

The CHIKv is an old virus, but now it has become a global disease. The name "chikungunya" is derived from the "Kimakonde" language, meaning "to become contorted", which aptly describes the painful joint deformities characterized by a sudden onset of high fever, severe joint pain, and a range of other influenza-like symptoms, making it challenging to diagnose accurately. While it is not typically fatal, the acute phase of the illness can be extremely distressing and incapacitating, often leaving individuals bedridden for weeks.

Chikungunya disease has now been identified in over 110 countries in Asia, Africa, Europe, and the Americas. Over 2 million cases have been reported since 2005. This leads to socioeconomic impact, so there is an urgent need for a safe and effective CHIKv vaccine. A phase 3 clinical trial on a single-shot live-attenuated chikungunya vaccine (VLA1553) candidate for active immunization and prevention of disease caused by the CHIKv reports the safety and immunogenicity up to day 180 after vaccination with VLA1553.

First chikungunya vaccine, Ixchiq, approved by US FDA. The US FDA has authorized Ixchiq, the first chikungunya vaccine, for individuals 18 years of age and older who are at increased risk of exposure to mosquito-borne virus. Containing a live, weakened version of the chikungunya, it is administered as a single dose by injection into the muscle and may cause symptoms of a self-limiting nature.

Addendum, French drugmaker Valneva said that the application for its vaccine candidate against mosquito-borne viral disease chikungunya was accepted by the EMA which would now examine the drug in a fast-track procedure.

Dengue Vaccine

A single dose of Butantan–Dengue Vaccine (Butantan-DV) prevented symptomatic DENV-1 and DENV-2, regardless of dengue serostatus at baseline, through 2 years of follow-up.

A phase 3 trial, a single administration of Butantan-DV was shown to have a favorable safety profile and be efficacious in preventing symptomatic, virologically confirmed dengue caused by DENV-1 and DENV-2, irrespective of previous dengue exposure, throughout a 2-year follow-up. These data support the continued development of Butantan-DV for the prevention of dengue disease in adults and children. Butantan-DV is an investigational, single-dose, live, attenuated, tetravalent vaccine against dengue disease, but data on its overall efficacy are needed.

Respiratory Syncytial Virus Vaccine

- "2023 is the year of RSV", in terms of licensure, US FDA approval and, hopefully, deployment of new products.
- RSV vaccine research has only recently increased in intensity over the past decade after a long delay in activity following a deadly vaccine trial in the 1960s.

Past winters, RSV poses a significant threat to very young children and elderly adults in every country in the world, but the majority of hospitalizations and deaths occur in LMICs where care options may be limited at best and first come, first served at worst.

There are currently three strategies to mitigate RSV: (1) Live attenuated or mRNA vaccines for infants, toddlers, and older adults, (2) "immunization" of infants with a single dose of mAbs, and (3) passive immunization, which involves vaccinating pregnant women so they can pass on antibodies to the fetus.

There has been tremendous progress and advancements across all these above three RSV prevention strategies for infants, adults, and pregnant mothers. RSV vaccine prevention for people aged 50–59 years, including those with underlying comorbidities, and is expecting results from that trial later this year.

The maternal RSVpreF vaccine from Pfizer, which was given to pregnant women at 24–36 weeks of gestation during phase 3 clinical trials, saw 70–80% protection against severe disease for infants up to 6 months after birth.

Future RSV Vaccine Pipeline

Developing preventive therapies for RSV for all ages including newborns continues to be an active area of continued clinical investigation. Meanwhile, the FDA approved *nirsevimab* in July 2024 for the prevention of RSV in newborns and infants born during or entering their first RSV season and for children up to age 24 months who remain vulnerable to severe illness from the virus through their second RSV season.

Hand, Foot, and Mouth Disease Vaccine (Non-Polio Enteroviruses)

There is no specific medical or antiviral treatment for HFMD and most people get better on their own in 7–10 days. You can take steps to relieve symptoms and prevent dehydration while any adults or children are sick of HFMD. Antivirals such as pleconaril and pocapavir are not commercially available but may be accessible under a compassionate use mechanism. Fluoxetine has in vitro activity against group B and D enteroviruses (including EV-D68), but studies have not proven clinical benefit.

A HFMD typically affects young children in childcare and kindergarten settings, but anyone including adults can get it. That is because young children need frequent diaper changes and help using the toilet. They also tend to put their hands in their mouths. Older children and adults are thought to have immunity against this annoying disease.

It is different from foot-and-mouth disease (FMD) sometimes called hoof-and-mouth disease, which is an infectious viral disease found in farm animals. Humans cannot get FMD disease from pets or other animals, and HEMD cannot spread it to them.

There are seven different types and 70 subtypes of FMD. Thus, no single vaccine can be used to control this disease.

Thus, no single vaccine can be used to control this disease. About 15 different FMD vaccines manufactured throughout the world require the production and use of whole live viruses. Enterovirus A71 inactivated vaccines have been licensed in China and Thailand and are being evaluated in other Asian countries. Vaccines for other enterovirus serotypes associated with more severe diseases also are under investigation.

A HFMD vaccine that is available in Thailand is an inactivated enterovirus type 71 (EV71) vaccine. A randomized controlled trial study showed that the vaccine efficacy against EV71-associated disease was 97.3% after primary immunization in 1 year, and 93.77% during the second year after the primary immunization (*August 31, 2023*). This vaccine can induce immunity against EV71 only with no cross protectivity against other enteroviruses which is caused by infection of EV71 only. It cannot be used for the prevention of HFMD caused by other enteroviruses (including Coxsackievirus A16 etc.).

Nipah Virus Vaccine

Nipah virus (NiV) was first identified in 1998, and despite the first outbreaks of NiV, a zoonotic virus, occurring 25 years ago in Malaysia and Singapore, there are currently no approved vaccines or treatments.

The deadly NiV kills nearly 75% of the people it infects, but the circumstance under which the bat species, known as the Indian flying fox **(Fig. 9)**, transmits the virus to humans has remained a mystery. To prevent outbreaks in humans, we need to know when bats may transmit the virus, there is a "theoretical possibility of human infections any time of the year, wherever these bats and humans make contact". The NiV virus can also be transmitted through food contaminated with saliva, urine, and excreta of infected animals, or directly between people.

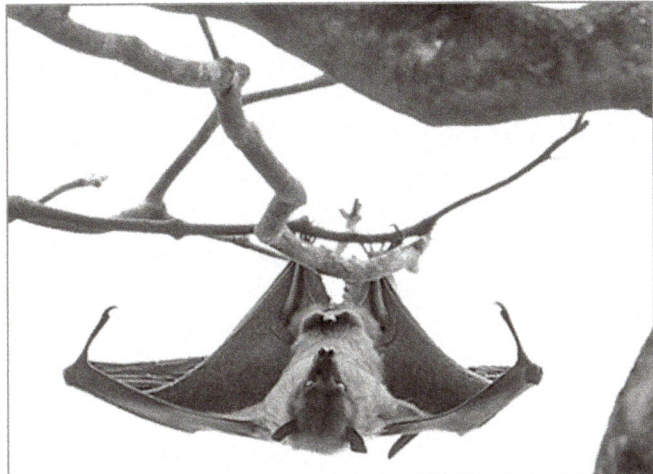

Fig. 9: The deadly Nipah virus (NiV) spreading the Indian bat species known as the Indian flying fox, transmits the NiV to humans has remained a mystery.

The NiV infection is a zoonotic disease, meaning that it is spread between animals and people. Fruit bats are the natural host for the virus. The first known Nipah outbreak occurred in 1998 in Malaysia and Singapore resulted in 265 human cases and 105 deaths, and caused significant economic damage to the swine industry there. It is endemic to Southeast Asia and the Western Pacific, with outbreaks occurring in Malaysia, Singapore, Philippines, India (Kerala), and Bangladesh. According to the WHO, the outbreak in Kerala in 2023 was the sixth outbreak of NiV in India since 2001.

The NiV is a highly lethal disease in humans who present with acute respiratory or neurological signs. No specific antiviral therapies or vaccines against NiV have been approved to date. Several candidate vaccines are at this time in clinical trials, including an mRNA-based vaccine. A single-dose ChAdOx1-vectored vaccine provides complete protection against Nipah Bangladesh and Malaysia in Syrian golden hamsters.

The National Institute of Allergy and Infectious Diseases (NIAID), part of the NIH, has launched an early-stage clinical trial evaluating an investigational vaccine to prevent infection with NiV. The experimental vaccine is manufactured by Moderna, Inc., Cambridge, Massachusetts, and was developed in collaboration with NIAID's Vaccine Research Center. It is based on a mRNA platform—a technology used in several approved COVID-19 vaccines, based on a protein from the closely related Hendra virus and another that uses a harmless vesicular stomatitis virus to deliver a NiV protein.

This virus replicon particle system provides a vital tool to the field and demonstrates utility as a highly efficacious and safe vaccine candidate that can be administered parenterally or mucosally to protect against lethal Nipah disease.

Also, a live, attenuated, recombinant vesicular stomatitis virus (rVSV-NiV vaccine) vector vaccine candidate (PHV02) has been licensed to Public Health Vaccines by the NIAID.

Noroviruses

Human norovirus (NoV) diarrhea and vomiting due to acute gastroenteritis (AGE) outbreaks are typically more common in cooler winter months, also called the "winter vomiting bug". Outbreaks with high attack rates tend to occur in semiclosed populations, such as schools, childcare centers, and long-term care facilities. Transmission is via the fecal-oral or vomitus-oral routes, either directly from person to person or indirectly by ingesting contaminated food or water or by touching surfaces contaminated with the virus and then touching the mouth. Common-source outbreaks have been described after ingestion of ice, shellfish, and a variety of ready-to-eat foods, including salads, berries, and bakery products.

Asymptomatic shedding of NoV is common across all age groups, with the highest prevalence in children. The infective NoVs and sapovirus are genera in the family Caliciviridae and are genetically diverse, with viruses from genogroups (G) I and GII causing most of the infections in humans. GII genotype 4 viruses have been causing >50% of all outbreaks globally over the past 15 years. Sapovirus GI, II, IV, and V cause acute gastroenteritis with symptoms indistinguishable from NoV in humans.

Several human NoVs vaccine candidates are being tested in clinical trials. However, the development of a broadly effective NoV vaccine remains difficult, owing to the wide genetic and antigenic diversity of viruses with multiple co-circulated variants of various genotypes.

On addition, the absence of a robust cell culture system, an efficient animal model, and reliable immune markers of NoV protection for vaccine evaluation further hinders the developmental process. Among the vaccine candidates that are currently under clinical studies, recombinant VP1-based VLPs that mimic major antigenic features of NoVs. This vaccine with proven safety, immunogenicity, and protective efficacy, supporting a high success likelihood of a useful NoV vaccine, hopefully.

While there is currently no approved NoV vaccine, recent human clinical efficacy trials with VLP-based vaccines have shown promise. Several additional NoV vaccine platforms are also currently under development and will likely improve the vaccines of the future. Vaxart's VP1-based oral tablet vaccine was developed to target the NoV GI. Norwalk and GII.4 Sydney strains, which are the predominant strains affecting humans. Vaxart's oral tablet vaccine candidate is designed to produce antibodies against NoV locally in the intestine.

Vaxart's development programs currently include pill vaccines designed to protect against coronavirus, NoV, seasonal influenza, and RSV, as well as a therapeutic vaccine for human papillomavirus (HPV).

West Nile Virus

In the last two decades, the WNV fever has emerged as a significant burden to public health worldwide, raising its threat as an emerging global pathogen. This virus is a neurotropic pathogen maintained through a mosquito–bird–mosquito (enzootic) transmission cycle. It primarily involves mosquitoes belonging to *Culex* spp. as vectors and birds as natural reservoirs (amplifying) hosts. Sometimes, due to spill-over from the enzootic cycle; horses and humans get infected. Neither horses nor humans develop sufficient viremia to transmit the virus, thus acting as "dead-end" hosts.

Although WNV fever-associated encephalitis is not well known in India, there have been serologically confirmed cases in Southern, Central, and Western India. In March 2019, a 7-year-old boy from the Malappuram District of Kerala was suffering from West Nile fever (WNF). WNV is commonly found in Africa, Europe, the Middle East, North America, and West Asia. WNV is maintained in nature in a cycle involving transmission between birds and mosquitoes. Humans, horses, and other mammals can be infected.

Physicians should consider arboviral infections in the differential diagnosis of aseptic meningitis and encephalitis, obtain appropriate specimens for laboratory testing, and promptly report cases to public health authorities.

In the absence of a vaccine or treatment the only way to reduce infection in people is by raising awareness of the risk factors and educating people about the measures they can take to reduce exposure to the virus. Four equine vaccines are licensed in the market; three are whole-inactivated virus (WN Innovator™, Vetera WNV, and Prestige® WNV) and one live chimeric virus expressing *prM/E* gene in canarypox virus (Recombitek™ Equine WNV). All the vaccines demonstrate a protective immune response in horses that lasts for 1 year. Several human vaccines have undergone preclinical studies and a few are in phase 2 trials. These vaccines have shown promising results in terms of safety and elicitation of antiviral immunity.

Future vaccine development against WNV is imminent due to an increase in the incidence of cases, mortality recorded, and the emergence of the virus in new geographical areas.

Zika Virus Vaccine Candidate

Zika virus is primarily transmitted to humans through the bite of infected *Aedes* mosquitoes, but it can also be sexually transmitted. Infection during pregnancy can lead to birth defects such as microcephaly and other neurological complications in infants. ZIKV infection can also cause pregnancy complications, including stillbirth or premature delivery.

Zika virus was originally isolated in 1947 in Uganda and has emerged within the last decade, causing significant outbreaks worldwide with an enormous impact on public health. Despite its importance, no vaccines are approved for use in humans. Insect-specific flaviviruses (ISFVs) have garnered increasing scientific interest in vaccine development and diagnostic applications, although several ZIKV vaccines are presently in clinical trials.

In immune-competent and immune-compromised mouse models, a single dosage of Aripo-Zika virus protected completely against viremia, loss of weight, and death. ARPV/ZIKV vaccination protects pregnant women and inhibits transmission to newborns in utero. Further research is required to identify the appropriate dosage, the effect of booster vaccinations on vaccine-elicited immunity, and the role of vertebrate-infectious flaviviruses (VIFs) during ARPV/ZIKV coinfection among vertebrate cells.

Vaccines against Variant Creutzfeldt–Jakob Disease or Bovine Spongiform Encephalopathy, or Mad Cow Disease

Bovine spongiform encephalopathy (BSE) or variant Creutzfeldt–Jakob disease (vCJD) is a progressive neurological disorder of cattle [mad cow disease (MCD)] that results from infection by an unusual transmissible *agent called a prion* (proteinaceous infectious particle). The nature of the transmissible agent is not well understood.

Currently, the most accepted theory is that the agent is a modified form of a normal protein known as prion protein. For reasons that are not yet understood, the normal prion protein changes into a pathogenic (harmful) form that then damages the CNS of cattle and human.

Prions are found in the brains of cows with "MCD" and in the brains of humans with vCJD. Prions can also be found in the spinal cord and in the back of the eye (retina). However, blood from infected animals or blood from infected people has never been shown to be a source of infection to humans. Researchers finding it difficult to explain; if prions are only found in the brain and spinal cord, why did people in England get vCJD after eating meat from cows?

What causes progressive neurological diseases like MCD disease or vCJD?

It was first reported from the United Kingdom in 1996, a progressive disease of the nervous system of cattle. Strong epidemiologic and laboratory evidence exists for a causal association between a new human prion disease called vCJD that was first reported from the United Kingdom in 1996 and the BSE outbreak in cattle.

This sporadic disease occurs worldwide, including the United States, at a rate of roughly one to two cases per 1 million population per year. The interval between the most likely period for the initial extended exposure of the population to potentially BSE-contaminated food (1984–1986) and the onset of initial vCJD cases (1994–1996) is consistent with known incubation periods for the human forms of prion disease.

Strong evidence indicates that classic BSE has been transmitted to people primarily in the United Kingdom, causing a vCJD. In the United Kingdom, where over 1 million cattle may have been infected with classic BSE, it is estimated that 232 people have died from vCJD which was likely a result of eating cows with BSE. Most of those lived in the UK and the risk to human health from BSE in the United States is extremely low. Indian neuropathologist Susarla Shankar says, "Officially, only 85 Indian CJD cases have been registered in the last 37 years". If our cattle would have had MCD, there would have been a major epidemic in Northern India long ago.

No effective treatment exists for CJD or any of its variants. Many medicines have been tested and have not shown benefits. Healthcare providers focus on relieving pain and other symptoms and on making people with these diseases as comfortable as possible.

In 2014, researchers at NYU Langone Medical Center and elsewhere say that a vaccination they have developed to protect US livestock from contracting the disease and preventing similar brain infections in humans.

Although "antiprion vaccine" experiments have so far been successful on mice and deer, and the concept could become a widespread technique for not only preventing, but potentially treating many prion diseases, hopefully. Vaccines may contain trace amounts of animal products used during the manufacturing process.

In July 2000, the FDA convened a meeting to discuss "the possibility that some vaccines were made using serum or gelatin derived from cows in countries that had MCD, including England". The risk of transmission of vCJD to humans from such vaccines was considered theoretical and remote. The recommendation was made that vaccines use bovine materials originating from countries without endogenous MCD. Mathematical models suggest that the agent of MCD first entered cattle feed in the United Kingdom around 1980; since the vast majority of initial cases of vCJD were born well before then, childhood vaccines were not likely to be the cause.

Experts' final reassurance comes from the fact that transmission of prions occurs from eating the brains of infected animals or from directly inoculating preparations of brains of infected animals into the brains of experimental animals. Transmission of prions has not been documented after inoculation into the muscles or under the skin, which are the routes used for vaccination. Taken together, the chances that currently licensed vaccines contain prions and represent a risk to humans is essentially zero.

FINAL WORD ON FUTURISTIC VACCINES

The development of vaccines is an ongoing, dynamic field of research and evolving new technologies are helping to develop future vaccines. Advances in our understanding of disease and leaps forward in science and technology are helping us design more effective vaccines, ones with a better immune response or vaccines that can be easier or quicker to manufacture.

Scientists and researchers continually work on creating vaccines for a wide range of bacterial and viral diseases. It is important to note that vaccine development is a complex and time-consuming process. The timeline for the availability of these vaccines may vary, and some may still be in the early stages of development.

Emerging New Infectious Diseases

The rapid development of COVID-19 vaccines in response to the SARS-CoV-2 virus is a recent example of this. Advances in mRNA vaccine technology may lead to the development of more effective and rapidly deployable vaccines for a variety of diseases.

The development of multipurpose vaccine platforms that can be adapted to different diseases, like the adenovirus vector platform used in some COVID-19 vaccines, may be applied to other diseases. Advances in our understanding of the immune system and disease mechanisms may reveal new targets for vaccine development, such as cancer vaccines and treatments for NCDs and chronic conditions.

The rise of antibiotic-resistant bacteria has renewed interest in developing vaccines against bacterial infections, particularly those caused by drug-resistant strains. Tackling AMR requires the development of new drugs and vaccines. AI-assisted computational approaches offer an alternative to the traditionally empirical drug and vaccine discovery pipelines. Increased antibiotic resistance in microorganisms, specifically among bacteria, has stimulated the development of novel antimicrobials and vaccines using AI and ML.

Bottom Line

Vaccine innovations save lives. Immunization has been a great public health success story. Vaccination saves lives at every stage of life.

■ CONCLUSION

With the Hi-Tech innovations, the future of vaccines is optimistic; poised to tackle existing and emerging infectious diseases more effectively. Universal vaccines provide broad protection against multiple strains of a virus, and new delivery methods will revolutionize disease prevention and control. Advances in our understanding of disease and leaps forward in science are helping us design more effective vaccines, ones with a better immune response or vaccines that can be easier or quicker to manufacture.

Throughout history, vaccines have led to the eradication of life-threatening or life-debilitating diseases. By saving millions of lives from contagious, serious diseases, vaccine innovations, and widespread vaccination efforts have a monumental impact on public health. One of the newest and most exciting areas in vaccine technology is the use of mRNA vaccines. Unlike conventional vaccines which can take many months or even years to cultivate mRNA vaccines can be developed quickly using the pathogen's genetic code.

Advancements in genomics and bioinformatics are paving the way for personalized vaccines. By analyzing an individual's genetic makeup, vaccines can be tailored to improve efficacy and minimize adverse effects. Personalized vaccines will be particularly important in managing diseases with high mutation rates, such as influenza and HIV.

Vaccines play a critical role in combating antimicrobial resistance (AMR), by preventing infections that would otherwise require antibiotic treatment. A vaccine directly blocks the transmission of pathogens that cause infections. Addressing these AMR challenges and ensuring global vaccine equity will be essential for maximizing the impact of these developments. Innovative vaccines targeting bacterial pathogens associated with high antibiotic resistance, such as Klebsiella pneumoniae and Pseudomonas aeruginosa, etc are under development.

As we look ahead, the continued evolution of vaccines will play a vital role in safeguarding public health and advancing medical science. Ensuring equitable access to vaccines is crucial for global health. Future strategies will focus on. improving vaccine distribution, affordability, and acceptance in low- and middle-income countries. Innovations in vaccine storage and transportation, such as thermostable vaccines, will also enhance global vaccine coverage.

■ SUGGESTED READING

1. Ávila-Nieto C, Pedreño-López N, Mitjà O, Clotet B, Blanco J, Carrillo J. Syphilis vaccine: challenges, controversies and opportunities. Front Immunol. 2023;14:1126170.
2. Al Hakeem WG, Fathima S, Shanmugasundaram R, Selvaraj RK. Campylobacter jejuni in Poultry: Pathogenesis and Control Strategies. Microorganisms. 2022;10(11):2134.
3. Alkan C, Jurado-Cobena E, Ikegami T. Advancements in Rift Valley fever vaccines: a historical overview and prospects for next generation candidates. NPJ Vaccines. 2023;8:171.
4. Association of the British Pharmaceutical Industry. (2023). The future of vaccines. Available from: https://www.abpi.org.uk/value-and-access/vaccines/the-future-of-vaccines/. [Last accessed Mat, 2024].
5. Baker CJ, Anderson AS. Plotkin's Vaccines, 8th edition. Amsterdam: Elsevier; 2023.
6. Beeson JG, Chan JA. A step forward for Plasmodium falciparum malaria transmission-blocking vaccines. Lancet Infect Dis. 2023;23(11):1210-2.
7. Boppana SB, Ross SA, Fowler KB. Congenital cytomegalovirus infection: clinical outcome. Clin Infect Dis. 2013;57(Suppl 4):S178-81.
8. Borges AH, Follmann F, Dietrich J. Chlamydia trachomatis vaccine development—a view on the current challenges and how to move forward. Expert Rev Vaccines. 2022;21(11): 1555-67.
9. Brisse M, Vrba SM, Kirk N, Liang Y, Ly H. Emerging Concepts and Technologies in Vaccine Development. Front Immunol. 2020;11:583077.
10. Carroll D, Daszak P, Wolfe ND, Gao GF, Morel CM, Morzaria S, et al. The Global Virome Project. Science. 2018;359: 872-4.
11. Dinc R. Leishmania Vaccines: the Current Situation with Its Promising Aspect for the Future. Korean J Parasitol. 2022; 60(6):379-91.
12. Dudhane RA, Bankar NJ, Shelke YP, Badge AK. (2023). The Rise of Non-typhoidal Salmonella Infections in India: Causes, Symptoms, and Prevention. Available from: https://www.cureus.com/articles/180658-the-rise-of-non-typhoidal-salmonella-infections-in-india-causes-symptoms-and-prevention#!/. [Last accessed May, 2024].

13. Duncan JD, Urbanowicz RA, Tarr AW, Ball JK. Hepatitis C Virus Vaccine: Challenges and Prospects. Vaccines (Basel). 2020;8(1):90.
14. Duthie MS, Machado BAS, Badaró R, Kaye PM, Reed SG. Leishmaniasis Vaccines: Applications of RNA Technology and Targeted Clinical Trial Designs. Pathogens. 2022;11:1259.
15. Dutta S, Thera MA. Seasonal RTS,S/AS01E vaccination with or without seasonal malaria chemoprevention. Lancet Infect Dis. 2024;24(1):9-11.
16. Dutta SS. What are Adenovirus-Based Vaccines? Available from: https://www.news-medical.net/health/What-are-Adenovirus-Based-Vaccines.aspx. [Last accessed May, 2005].
17. Finsterer J. Triggers of Guillain-Barré Syndrome: Campylobacter jejuni Predominates. Int J Mol Sci. 2022;23(22):14222.
18. Frost I, Sati H, Garcia-Vello P, Hasso-Agopsowicz M, Lienhardt C, Gigante V, et al. The role of bacterial vaccines in the fight against antimicrobial resistance: an analysis of the preclinical and clinical development pipeline. Lancet Microbe. 2023;4(2):e113-25.
19. HIV.gov. (2023). HIV Vaccines. Available from: https://www.hiv.gov/hiv-basics/hiv-prevention/potential-future-options/hiv-vaccines/. [Last accessed May, 2024].
20. In fact this source of information is from Pfizer's Vaccine Research and Development in Pearl River, New York, USA
21. Johnson B. GSK's gonorrhea vaccine receives fast-track designation to expedite clinical trials. Nat Med. 2023;29(9):2146-7.
22. Kallás EG, Cintra MAT, Moreira JA, Patiño EG, Braga PE, Tenório JCV, et al. Live, Attenuated, Tetravalent Butantan-Dengue Vaccine in Children and Adults. N Engl J Med. 2024;390:397-408.
23. Kaur G, Chawla S, Kumar P, Singh R. Advancing Vaccine Strategies against Candida Infections: Exploring New Frontiers. Vaccines (Basel). 2023;11(11):1658.
24. Khalil I, Walker R, Porter CK, Muhib F, Chilengi R, Cravioto A, et al. Enterotoxigenic Escherichia coli (ETEC) vaccines: Priority activities to enable product development, licensure, and global access. Vaccine. 2021;39(31):4266-77.
25. Laufer MK. (2021). WHO approved a malaria vaccine for children—a global health expert explains why that is a big deal. Available from: https://theconversation.com/who-approved-a-malaria-vaccine-for-children-a-global-health-expert-explains-why-that-is-a-big-deal-169501. [Last accessed May, 2024].
26. Li S, Li W, Jin Y, Wu B, Wu Y. Advancements in the development of nucleic acid vaccines for syphilis prevention and control. Hum Vaccin Immunother. 2023;19(2):2234790.
27. Marne Azarias Da Silva, Pierre Nioche, Calaiselvy Soudaramourty, et al. Repetitive mRNA vaccination is required to improve the quality of broad-spectrum anti-SARS–CoV-2 antibodies in the absence of CXCL13. Sci Adv. 2023; 9(31):2122. Published online 2023 Aug 4. doi: 10.1126/sciadv.adg2122
28. Marshall GS. (2010). Can Vaccines Transmit Mad Cow Disease? Available from: https://www.empr.com/home/features/can-vaccines-transmit-mad-cow-disease/. [Last accessed May, 2024].
29. NewsHub. (2014). First Successful Vaccination Against 'Mad Cow'-like Wasting Disease in Deer. Available from: https://nyulangone.org/news/first-successful-vaccination-against-mad-cow-wasting-disease-deer. [Last accessed May, 2024].
30. Fowler A, Van Rompay KKA, Sampson M, Leo J, Watanabe JK, Usachenko JL, et al. A virus-like particle-based bivalent PCSK9 vaccine lowers LDL-cholesterol levels in non-human primates. NPJ Vaccines. 2023;8(1):142
31. Permar S. Vaccine Shows Promise Against CMV, a Virus that Causes Birth Defects. https://news.weill.cornell.edu/news/2024/02/vaccine-shows-promise-against-cmv-a-virus-that-causes-birth-defects#:~:text=The%20study%2C%20published%20in%20the,to%20their%20babies%20during%20pregnancy. [Last accessed May, 2024].
32. Plotkin S. The history of vaccination against cytomegalovirus. Med Microbiol Immunol. 2015;204:247-54.
33. Poolman JT, Wacker M. Extraintestinal Pathogenic Escherichia coli, a Common Human Pathogen: Challenges for Vaccine Development and Progress in the Field. Infect Dis. 2016;213(1):6-13.
34. Sahadulla MI, Uduman S. Compendium of the Pandemic Era, 1st edition. Kottayam, Kerala: DC Folio (An Imprint of DC Books); 2022.
35. Sahadulla MI, Uduman S. Infectious disease of the head and neck. Comprehensive Textbook of Infectious Diseases, 2nd edition. New Delhi: Jaypee Brothers Medical Publishers (P) Ltd.; 2020. pp. 147-59.
36. Sahadulla MIS, Sayenna Uduman: KIMS Hospital, Thiruvananthapuram, India Comprehensive Text Book of Infectious Diseases-2019. Jaypee Medical Publishers, India.
37. Schautteet K, Clercq ED, Vanrompay D. Chlamydia trachomatis Vaccine Research through the Years. Infect Dis Obstet Gynecol. 2011;2011:963513.
38. Schneider M, Narciso-Abraham M, Hadl S, McMahon R, Toepfer S, Fuchs U, et al. Safety and immunogenicity of a single-shot live-attenuated chikungunya vaccine: a double-blind, multicentre, randomised, placebo-controlled, phase 3 trial. Lancet. 2023;401(10394):2138-47.
39. Slein MD, Backes IM, Garland CR, Kelkar NS, Leib DA, Ackerman ME. Effector functions are required for broad and potent protection of neonatal mice with antibodies targeting HSV glycoprotein D. Cell Rep Med. 2024;5(2):101417.
40. Tanelus M, López K, Smith S, Muller JA, Porier DL, Auguste DI, et al. Exploring the immunogenicity of an

insect-specific virus vectored Zika vaccine candidate. Sci Rep. 2023;13:19948.
41. The Lancet Infectious Diseases. A New Agenda to control tuberculosis. Lancet Infect Dis. 2023;23(11):1207.
42. Tilak R, Karade S, Yadav AK, Singh PMP, Shahbabu B, Gupte MD, et al. Lyme Borreliosis, a public health concern in India: Findings of Borrelia burgdorferi serosurvey from two states. Med J Armed Forces India. 2022.
43. Varadé J, Magadán S, González-Fernández A. Human immunology and immunotherapy: main achievements and challenges. Cell Mol Immunol. 2021;18(4):805-28.
44. Venkitaraman AR, Lenoir GM, John TJ. The seroepidemiology of infection due to Epstein-Barr virus in southern India. J Med Virol. 1985;15(1):11-6.
45. Wandera N, Olds P, Muhindo R, Ivers L. Rift Valley Fever—The Need for an Integrated Response. N Engl J Med. 2023;389:1829-32.
46. Wang H. (2023). Leprosy vaccines: developments for prevention and treatment. In: Christodoulides M (Eds). Vaccines for Neglected Pathogens: Strategies, Achievements and Challenges. Berlin: Springer, Cham; 2023. pp. 44-69.
47. WHO. Global Vaccination Strategy for COVID-19. Geneva; 2022.

SECTION 3

Vaccines for Travelers, School Children, and Healthcare Staff: Dispelling Myths with Medical AI and Ensuring Vaccine Safety

Sahadulla MIS, Zuhara PM, Reshmi Aysha, Uduman SA

14. Travel Vaccine (Travel Immunizations)
15. Vaccine Safety and Efficacy
16. Artificial Intelligence and Machine Learning in Vaccinology
17. Catch-up Vaccinations in Childhood Immunizations
18. Combination Vaccines (Combos)
19. School Health Immunization
20. Healthcare Personnel Vaccine Needs
21. Vaccine Hesitancy and Providing Confidence in Vaccinations
22. Some Facts, Myths, and Misconceptions

CHAPTER 14

Travel Vaccine (Travel Immunizations)

■ INTRODUCTION

With globalization and increased travel, the importance of travel vaccinations cannot be overstated. Adult vaccinations can help prevent the transmission of various infectious diseases. International travel plans require individuals to adhere to specific vaccine guidelines for the destination country, which may sometimes lead to confusion among travelers.

Travel vaccines, also called travel immunizations, are shots that travelers can get before visiting certain areas of the world. They are recommended to protect against diseases endemic to the country of origin or destination that may be prevalent in those areas. The specific vaccines recommended will depend on various factors, including the destination, duration of travel, purpose of travel, and individual's health status.

Travel vaccines are intended essentially to prevent the spread of diseases and ensure the health and safety of both travelers and the local population. It is best to get them at least four to six weeks before you travel to allow time to build up immunity and get the best protection, particularly from those that may require multiple doses.

Some travel vaccines include diphtheria, hepatitis A, tetanus, typhoid, hepatitis B, rabies, cholera, and Japanese encephalitis. The Centers for Disease Control and Prevention (CDC) and World Health Organization (WHO) recommend the following vaccinations for India—hepatitis A, hepatitis B, typhoid, cholera, yellow fever, Japanese encephalitis, rabies, meningitis, polio, measles, mumps, rubella (MMR), Tdap (tetanus, diphtheria, and pertussis), chickenpox, shingles, pneumonia, and influenza. These vaccines are recommended to protect against diseases endemic to the country of origin or destination. They are intended to protect travelers and to prevent disease spread within and between countries.

■ CDC YELLOW BOOK

It is a resource for health professionals providing care to international travelers. It compiles the US government's most current travel health guidelines, including pretravel vaccine recommendations, destination-specific health advice, and easy-to-reference maps, tables, and charts.

In India, travelers should visit their doctor at least a month before a planned trip to get vaccines or medicines they may need as they may be able to get some travel vaccines from local healthcare hospitals or health departments and travel medicine clinics. Make sure you are up-to-date on all routine vaccines before every trip and should receive personalized advice based on their specific circumstances. Vaccination recommendations for travelers can vary depending on various factors, including the destination, the duration of the trip, and the traveler's health status.

As of December 2023, common vaccines recommended for travelers from India may include routine vaccinations, such as MMR, diphtheria, tetanus, and pertussis (DTP), which are to be up-to-date. It is crucial to note that recommendations can change, and new vaccines may become available.

- *Travel-specific vaccinations:* Hepatitis A and B—recommended for many destinations
- *Typhoid:* Especially if traveling to areas with poor sanitation and hygiene
- *Polio:* Depending on the destination and individual vaccination history
- COVID-19 vaccine has become an essential consideration for international travel. Travelers should check for the latest updates and recommendations from health authorities, such as the WHO or the CDC, and consult with healthcare professionals.
- *Vector-Borne diseases:* Japanese encephalitis—for certain rural areas or during outbreaks. Yellow fever—required for travel to certain countries with a risk of yellow fever transmission.
- Respiratory Infections: Influenza (Flu)—advisable, especially during flu season or in crowded places. Meningococcal disease—for travel to areas with a high risk of meningococcal disease.

- *Rabies:* For travelers involved in outdoor activities, working with animals, or visiting areas with a high risk of rabies.
- *Malaria:* Prophylaxis may be recommended for certain regions.

The three most commonly recommended travel vaccines are:
- Typhoid vaccine for travel to countries where it is circulating.
- Hepatitis A vaccine for travel to most other countries in the world.
- Yellow fever vaccine (YFV) for travel to some parts of Africa and South America.

Here are some commonly recommended travel vaccines and the diseases they protect against.

Typhoid Vaccine

Recommended for travelers going to regions with poor sanitation and food hygiene, which is usually contracted by consuming contaminated food or water or where typhoid fever is endemic. The vaccine can help protect travelers from this potentially serious illness. Here are some key points to consider regarding typhoid vaccines for travelers.

High-risk areas include parts of South Asia, Southeast Asia, Africa, and Central and South America. Be sure to check with your family physician or travel clinic to determine if typhoid vaccination is recommended for your specific travel destination.

There are oral and parenteral types of typhoid vaccines:
- *Typhoid conjugate vaccine (TCV):* This is the preferred vaccine for travelers, as it provides longer-lasting protection and is suitable for individuals aged 2 years and older.
- *Typhoid polysaccharide vaccine (TYPV):* This vaccine is an older option and is typically recommended for travelers who are unable to receive the TCV or who are traveling to an area with a high level of drug-resistant typhoid.
- *Live typhoid vaccine* is administered orally (by mouth). It may be given to people 6 years and older. One capsule is taken every other day, for a total of four capsules. The last dose should be taken at least 1 week before travel.

Timing of vaccination: It is recommended to get the typhoid vaccine at least 2 weeks before traveling to allow your body to develop immunity. However, if you are short on time, you can opt for an accelerated schedule for some vaccines.

Booster doses: The duration of protection provided by the typhoid vaccine varies depending on the type of vaccine. TCV generally protects for several years, while TYPV may require a booster every 2 years if you remain at risk.

Other traveling precautions: While vaccination is an important preventive measure, travelers should also take precautions with food and water hygiene. This includes consuming only safe, cooked food, and drinking bottled or purified water. Good hand hygiene is also essential.

Before getting any vaccine, including the typhoid vaccine, it is important to consult with your family physician or travel medicine specialist. They can assess individual risk factors and health status to provide personalized recommendations.

Hepatitis A Virus Vaccine

Recommended for travelers visiting areas with poor sanitation to protect against hepatitis A virus (HAV), which is often transmitted through contaminated food and water; making it a concern for travelers visiting regions with poor sanitation and hygiene standards. The vaccine is also recommended for those engaging in high-risk activities, such as consuming street food or having close contact with the local population.

Hepatitis A virus vaccine is commonly known by several brand names, including *Havrix, Vaqta, and Avaxim*, among others.

It is important to plan because the vaccine takes some time to become fully effective. Ideally, you should start the vaccine series at least 2 weeks before traveling to a high-risk area.

Vaccination Schedule

The HAV vaccine is typically administered as a series of two doses. The second dose is usually given 6–12 months after the first dose. The vaccine is highly effective at preventing infection when administered according to the recommended schedule. A booster shot is not usually required for long-term immunity. The vaccine can provide protection for up to 20 years or more.

Common side effects of the HAV vaccines are generally mild and include pain or swelling at the injection site, fever, and fatigue. Serious side effects are rare.

Combo Vaccines

Like *Twinrix*, combine both HAV and hepatitis B virus (HBV) into one shot. This can be useful for travelers who need protection against both types HAV and HBV.

To determine the need for the HAV vaccine for your travel plans, consult with your family physician or travel medicine specialist to assess your specific risk factors and recommend the appropriate vaccinations. Additionally, practicing good hygiene, such as frequent handwashing and safe food and water consumption, is also important to minimize the risk of infection while traveling.

Yellow Fever Vaccine

Certain countries in Africa and South America where yellow fever is endemic require travelers to show proof of yellow fever vaccination when entering or leaving their borders. This is done to prevent the spread of the disease. YFV protects against this viral disease transmitted by mosquitoes. Here are some important points to know about the yellow fever travel vaccine:

- *Vaccine availability:* The YFV is a LAV and is typically administered as a single dose. It provides long-lasting immunity against the virus.
- *International Certificate of Vaccination or Prophylaxis (ICVP):* After receiving the YFV, travelers will be issued an ICVP, often referred to as a "yellow card". This card serves as proof of vaccination and may be requested by immigration authorities when entering certain countries.
- The YFV should ideally be administered at least 10 days before traveling to a yellow fever-endemic area to ensure immunity is developed. However, if you have limited time before your trip, it is still recommended to get the vaccine, as it may offer some protection.
- *Booster shots:* In the past, a booster dose of the YFV was recommended every 10 years. However, WHO revised its guidelines, stating that a single dose of the vaccine is likely to provide lifelong protection.
- The YFV is generally safe for most people. However, it may not be recommended for certain individuals, such as those with severe allergies to vaccine components, immunodeficiency disorders, or pregnant women. It is essential to consult your family doctor or travel clinic to assess whether the vaccine is suitable for you. It is advisable to schedule an appointment well in advance of your trip to ensure vaccine availability and the doctor can provide you the tips for preventing mosquito bites.
- Like any other vaccine, the YFV can have side effects, including mild ones like fever, headache, and soreness at the injection site. Serious adverse reactions are rare.

Hepatitis B Virus Vaccine

Recommended for travelers who may be at risk of contracting HBV during their travels. It is transmitted through intimate contact with local populations or requires medical treatment abroad via infected blood or bodily fluids including sexual contact, sharing needles, or exposure to contaminated medical instruments.

The risk is highest for travelers to regions with a high prevalence of hepatitis B surface antigen (HBsAg) carrier prevalence rates exceeding 8% and up to 20% in countries including sub-Saharan Africa, Far East Asia including India, and Mid-East countries. The longer you plan to stay in an area with a high HBsAg rate prevalence, the greater your risk of exposure. *Extended travelers may benefit from vaccination.* Healthcare professionals traveling to areas with a high prevalence of HBV should definitely get vaccinated, as they may be at increased risk through their work.

- *Routine vaccination:* In many countries, HBV vaccination is part of the routine childhood immunization schedule. If you were not vaccinated as a child and plan to travel to an area with a higher risk of HBV transmission, it is a good idea to get vaccinated.
- *Pre-exposure vaccination:* The HBV vaccine is given as a series of three shots. Ideally, you should start the vaccination series at least 6 months before your trip. However, if you do not have that much time, getting the first two shots before your trip and completing the series after you return is also an option.
- *Booster shots are generally not needed* for healthy individuals who have completed the HBV vaccination series. However, healthcare workers and those with weakened immune systems may need periodic testing to ensure ongoing protection. Additionally, it is important to practice good hygiene and take precautions to avoid exposure to the virus, even if you are vaccinated.

Polio Vaccine

The polio vaccine may be recommended for travelers to areas where polio is still a concern. Some countries may require proof of polio vaccination for entry. Travelers to regions with active polio outbreaks may also be advised to receive this vaccine. In some cases, a booster shot may be required.

- *Travelers should make sure they are properly vaccinated against polio before traveling to these countries:* Afghanistan, Democratic Republic of the Congo, Nigeria, Pakistan, Somalia, and Syria.

    There are two kinds of polio vaccines:
    1. *Inactivated polio vaccine (IPV):* This is the most common form of polio vaccine used in many countries. It is usually given as part of routine childhood vaccinations.
    2. *Oral polio vaccine (OPV):* Some travelers may need to take the attenuated virus, and it can provide a stronger immune response than IPV. However, it may be recommended only for specific situations.

- If one has completed the minimum of five doses of polio-containing vaccine, one should have a booster dose of polio-containing vaccine if >10 years since any previous doses. If you have not completed the minimum of five doses of polio-containing vaccine, you may need additional doses before you travel.
- Ideally, international travelers from all polio-infected countries should receive a dose of polio vaccine between 4 weeks and 12 months before departure.
- Travelers to countries where there is an increased risk of exposure to poliovirus may receive a one-time booster dose of IPV before traveling (CDC USA). The vaccine should be given between 4 weeks and 12 months before departure.

World Health Organization and the Center for Disease Control and Prevention, USA provide guidelines and recommendations for travelers regarding polio vaccination. These recommendations can change, so it is essential to check for the most up-to-date information before your trip. Be sure to get the recommended polio vaccine well in advance of your travel, as it may take time to build immunity.

Meningococcal Vaccines

Meningococcal disease is caused by the bacterium *Neisseria meningitidis* and can lead to severe illness, including meningitis and bloodstream infections. Meningococcal vaccines are important for travelers, especially those planning to visit regions where meningococcal disease is more common or where outbreaks have occurred.

Certain factors may increase the risk of contracting meningococcal disease. These include traveling to regions with known outbreaks, participating in crowded or close-contact settings (e.g., dormitories and military barracks), and having certain medical conditions that affect your immune system.

There are several types of meningococcal vaccines, and the choice of vaccine depends on various factors, including your age, destination, and specific risk factors. Types of meningococcal vaccines available, including:

- *Meningococcal conjugate vaccines:* These are typically recommended for travelers and provide protection against multiple serogroups (A, C, W, and Y).
- *Meningococcal B vaccines:* These vaccines protect against serogroup B, which is less common but can still cause disease.

The choice of a vaccine depends on your destination. Health authorities and travel clinics will provide specific recommendations based on the risk of meningococcal disease in the area you plan to visit. Common recommendations include the quadrivalent (A, C, W, Y) meningococcal vaccine. Should receive the meningococcal vaccine at least a few weeks before your trip to ensure that you are adequately protected. Check with your family physician or travel clinic for the recommended schedule.

Depending on the type of vaccine and your specific circumstances, you may need booster shots to maintain protection over time. One can often receive the meningococcal vaccine alongside other recommended travel vaccinations, such as hepatitis A, typhoid, or yellow fever, to minimize the number of shots you need.

Precautions

Like any vaccine, meningococcal vaccines can have side effects, but serious side effects are rare. It is essential to discuss any allergies or medical conditions you have with your healthcare provider before receiving the vaccine.

International Certificate of Vaccination

Some countries may require proof of meningococcal vaccination for entry, especially if you are traveling from or through an area with a high risk of meningococcal disease.

Dengue Fever Vaccines for Travelers

Dengue fever is the leading cause of febrile illness among travelers returning from the Caribbean, Latin America, and South Asia. Dengue occurs in people of all ages but occurs at higher rates in healthy adolescents and young adults and is most likely to cause severe disease in infants, pregnant women, and patients with chronic diseases (e.g., asthma, sickle cell anemia, and diabetes mellitus). Approximately 390 million dengue infections occur annually worldwide, of which 96 million have clinical manifestations, including 500,000 hospitalizations and 20,000 deaths every year.

Dengue fever (DF) vaccine called Dengvaxia (CYD-TDV) is approved for use in several countries for individuals aged 9–45 who live in or travel to areas with a high prevalence of dengue virus. However, the recommendations for its use varied by country and were often limited to specific age groups and regions where dengue was endemic. Therefore stay informed and consult with your family doctor or with those who are knowledgeable about the current status of DF and vaccinations in your specific travel destination.

Japanese Encephalitis Virus Vaccine

Japanese encephalitis virus (JEF) is a mosquito-borne virus that can cause serious encephalitis in humans. Travelers who are planning to visit areas where JEV is endemic, especially in parts of Asia, may consider getting vaccinated to protect themselves from the virus. Here is some information about the JEV vaccine for travelers:

There are several vaccines available for JEF. Two common vaccines are:

1. *Inactivated Vero cell-derived vaccine (JE-VC):* Administered in two doses, with the second dose given 7–28 days after the first. It provides long-lasting immunity and is suitable for travelers.
2. *Live attenuated SA 14-14-2 vaccine:* It is administered in a single dose and is often used in areas where JEF is endemic.

   Should start the vaccination series at least a month before your trip because the vaccines require multiple doses and take some time to become effective. Some individuals may not be suitable candidates for the vaccine due to contraindications or precautions, such as pregnancy, certain underlying medical conditions, or allergies to vaccine components. Discuss your medical history with your family physician. While vaccination is an effective measure, it is also crucial to take steps to prevent mosquito bites when traveling in areas with JEF risk. This includes using insect repellent, wearing long-sleeved clothing, and using bed nets if necessary.

Other Vaccines

Depending on your travel plans, you may also need other vaccinations, such as those for hepatitis A and B, typhoid, or rabies. Consult your family doctor for a comprehensive travel vaccination plan or with a medical center that specializes in travel medicine to create a personalized vaccination and health plan for your trip.

Cholera Vaccines

These are typically recommended for travelers going to areas with ongoing cholera outbreaks or poor sanitation conditions. Not all travelers will need this vaccine and is recommended for travelers to areas with ongoing cholera outbreaks. It is typically administered orally.

There are several cholera vaccines available for travelers. It is most commonly transmitted through contaminated water and food. Travelers to areas with known cholera outbreaks or poor sanitation may consider getting vaccinated to reduce their risk of infection.

Two cholera vaccines were widely used for travelers:

1. *Oral cholera vaccine (OCV):* Taken orally in two doses, typically at least 1 week apart. The two most common OCVs are *Dukoral and Vaxchora*. Dukoral provides some protection against enterotoxigenic *E. coli* (ETEC), a bacterium that can cause travelers' diarrhea. Cholera vaccines can have side effects, which are usually mild and temporary. Common side effects may include nausea, vomiting, and abdominal pain.
2. *Inactivated injectable cholera vaccine: Shanchol and Euvichol* are examples of inactivated injectable cholera vaccines. These vaccines require two doses given about 1–6 weeks apart.

   One should plan ahead because cholera vaccines require time for administration and for the body to develop immunity. Cholera vaccines are not 100% effective but can significantly reduce the risk of infection. They are often recommended alongside other preventive measures, such as practicing good hygiene, drinking safe water, and eating safe food.

Rabies Vaccine

Rabies infection is transmitted through the bite or scratch of an infected animal. The vaccine is recommended for travelers who are planning to visit regions where rabies is prevalent, especially if they will be engaging in close contact with animals, such as wildlife workers or adventure travelers. The vaccine can be administered in two ways—(1) preexposure prophylaxis (before potential exposure) and (2) postexposure prophylaxis (after potential exposure).

1. Preexposure prophylaxis involves a series of vaccinations before traveling to a high-risk area, followed by booster shots as needed. This can provide some level of protection in case of exposure.
2. *Postexposure prophylaxis:* It involves a different regimen of rabies vaccinations and, in some cases, rabies immune globulin (RIG). It is essential to start treatment as soon as possible after potential exposure.

Remember that the rabies vaccine is not a guarantee that you won't get rabies if exposed to the virus, but it significantly reduces the risk and buys you more time to seek medical treatment if bitten or scratched by a potentially rabid animal. Travelers should also take precautions to avoid close contact with animals, especially wild or stray ones, in rabies-endemic areas.

Tdap Vaccine

Tdap vaccine, which includes Tdap components, is recommended for travelers who have not had a dose in the past 10 years.

It is particularly important for travelers who may be in contact with infants or pregnant women, as pertussis can be life threatening for babies.

Before traveling, consult with your family doctor or a travel medicine specialist to review your vaccination history and assess any specific risks associated with your destination.

Measles, Mumps, Rubella, and Varicella Vaccine

The MMR and varicella vaccines are important vaccinations recommended for travelers, especially if they are traveling to regions or countries where these diseases are still prevalent or if they are at risk of exposure in outbreak situations.

Travelers should ensure they are up-to-date on their MMR vaccinations, especially if they were born after 1957 and have not received two doses of the vaccine, as measles outbreaks can occur in some areas.

- Infants 6–11 months old traveling internationally should get 1 dose of MMR vaccine before travel. This dose does not count as part of the routine immunization against MMR.
- Rubella can be particularly dangerous for pregnant women, as it can lead to birth defects. Travelers who are not immune to rubella should get vaccinated.
- For individuals who have not had chickenpox or the vaccine in childhood, it is advisable to get vaccinated before traveling to areas where the virus is still common.

Influenza Vaccine

Influenza vaccines are recommended for travelers in certain situations. Vaccination requirements and recommendations can vary, depending on factors such as destination, time of year, and individual health considerations.

Influenza is more common during the fall and winter months in the Northern Hemisphere (October through March months) and during the Southern Hemisphere's winter months (stars June month). If one plans to travel during these periods, getting a flu vaccine before your trip is a good idea.

The longer one plans to stay in an area with ongoing influenza transmission, the greater the risk of exposure. If you are planning an extended stay, getting vaccinated may be more important. It is advisable to get vaccinated at least 2 weeks before your trip so that your body has time to build immunity. However, getting vaccinated later is still beneficial, as it can protect the remainder of the flu season.

In addition to getting the vaccine, travelers should practice good hygiene, such as frequent handwashing, and avoid close contact with sick individuals. These measures can help reduce the risk of influenza transmission.

SARS-CoV-2 (COVID-19) Travel Vaccine

- Individuals who are fully vaccinated with updated booster doses can safely travel internationally.
- It is important to review the criteria of the countries you are traveling to or through before travel.
- WHO does not support using proof of vaccination as a requirement for international travel.
- It is not mandatory to be fully vaccinated to travel to India, but it is highly recommended for international travel.

Malaria Medications

- *While not a vaccine*, malaria prophylaxis involves taking prescription medications before, during, and after your trip to regions where malaria is prevalent.

- Malarial parasite, *Plasmodium* species transmitted to humans through the bite of infected Anopheles mosquitoes. Travelers to regions where malaria is prevalent should take preventive measures to reduce their risk of infection.
- Medications for malaria prevention, also known as malaria prophylaxis, are available and should be discussed with a healthcare professional before travel. The choice of medication depends on the destination, the type of *Plasmodium* species prevalent in that area, and individual factors such as medical history and allergies.
- Common medications used for malaria prophylaxis for travelers:
  - *Chloroquine:* Chloroquine used to be a widely used antimalarial drug, but its effectiveness has declined in many parts of the world due to drug-resistant strains of malaria. It is still effective in some regions with low levels of chloroquine resistance.
  - *Mefloquine:* Sold under the brand name Lariam, is an option for travelers but is associated with potential side effects such as neuropsychiatric symptoms. It is typically prescribed when other antimalarials are not suitable.
  - *Doxycycline:* It is an antibiotic that also has anti-malarial properties. It is often used for malaria prophylaxis, especially in areas with chloroquine-resistant malaria. It is taken daily and can have side effects such as sun sensitivity and gastrointestinal upset.
  - *Atovaquone/proguanil:* Sold under the brand name Malarone, this combination medication is highly effective and well-tolerated by most travelers. It is taken daily and is often recommended for travelers going to regions with chloroquine-resistant malaria.
  - *Dihydroartemisinin-piperaquine:* This medication is used in some areas where the malaria parasite has developed resistance to other drugs. It is taken as a single-dose treatment, typically once a week.
  - *Primaquine:* Primaquine is used to prevent relapse of *Plasmodium vivax* and *Plasmodium ovale* malaria. It is not effective against the initial infection and should be used in combination with another prophylactic medication. Additionally, primaquine requires testing for glucose-6-phosphate dehydrogenase (G6PD) deficiency, as it can cause hemolysis in individuals with this condition.

Additionally, travelers should continue to use mosquito bite prevention methods, such as using insect repellent, wearing long-sleeved clothing, and sleeping under insecticide-treated bed nets, to further reduce the risk of malaria infection.

CONCLUSION

Individual health conditions and travel plans vary, so it is essential to consult with a healthcare professional or a travel medicine specialist, ideally 4–6 weeks before travel for personalized advice. They can provide the most accurate information about necessary vaccines and other health precautions based on individual specific needs and circumstances.

SUGGESTED READING

1. Centers for Disease Control and Prevention.(2014). CDC Yellow Book. Available from: https://wwwnc.cdc.gov/travel/page/yellowbook-home [Last accessed April, 2024].
2. Schnyder JL, de Jong HK, Bache BE, Schaumburg F, Grobusch MP. Long-term immunity following yellow fever vaccination: a systematic review and meta-analysis. Lancet Publ Health. 2024;12:E445-56.

CHAPTER 15

Vaccine Safety and Efficacy

■ INTRODUCTION

Vaccine side effects can appear large in our minds as we consider the risks and benefits of vaccination. Today's side effects are generally few and mild, but severe side effects still crop up, especially when hundreds of millions of vaccinations allow even the rarest of cases to accumulate. Here is what to know about vaccine safety and side effects.

Vaccine safety is a critical aspect of public health, and vaccines undergo rigorous testing and monitoring to ensure they are safe and effective before they are approved for routine immunization use.

Vaccine effectiveness is the measure of how well vaccination protects people against infection, symptomatic illness, hospitalization, and death. In general, vaccines are safe, effective, and powerful weapons in the fight against IDs, while recognizing that many parents and patients may have concerns about vaccines.

Vaccines and vaccinations have a strong track record of safety and are one of the most effective tools for preventing and controlling infectious diseases. The safety of vaccines is rigorously monitored through a combination of preclinical testing, clinical trials, postmarketing surveillance, and ongoing research. Here are some key points about vaccine safety:

- Before a vaccine is tested in humans, it undergoes extensive preclinical testing, including laboratory and animal studies, to assess its safety and effectiveness.
- Human clinical trials involve testing in increasingly larger groups of people to evaluate their safety, efficacy, and appropriate dosing.
- Regulatory approval agencies, such as the United States Food and Drug Administration (US FDA), the European Medicines Agency (EMA), the National Regulatory Authority of India (NRA), and the WHO carefully review all the data from clinical trials before approving a vaccine for public use. These agencies have strict safety and efficacy standards that vaccines must meet.
- Vaccine safety is continually monitored through postmarketing surveillance systems, and regulatory agencies collaborate to ensure that vaccines are safe and effective. This helps ensure that rare or unexpected side effects are identified and addressed promptly.
- It is important to note that while vaccines, like any medical intervention, may have side effects, the vast majority of individuals experience no or mild side effects. The benefits of vaccination in preventing diseases and protecting public health generally far outweigh the risks. If you have concerns about vaccine safety, it is recommended to consult with healthcare professionals who can provide accurate information based on the latest scientific evidence.

VACCINE ADVERSE EVENT REPORTING SYSTEM

In many countries, there are systems for healthcare providers and the public to report any adverse events or side effects following vaccination. This data is critical for monitoring vaccine safety and researching vaccine safety.

In evaluating vaccine safety, it is important to consider the risks associated with vaccines relative to the benefits of disease prevention. Vaccines undergo rigorous safety assessments, and the vast majority of people experience only mild and temporary side effects, such as soreness at the injection site or a mild fever.

The risk of severe adverse events from vaccines is extremely low compared to the risk of contracting and suffering from the diseases they prevent. Vaccines have been instrumental in reducing the incidence of many serious diseases and their complications. The benefits of vaccination often outweigh the risks.

Vaccine ingredients are carefully evaluated for safety, and any potential risks are thoroughly assessed. The quantities of these ingredients in vaccines are typically very low and unlikely to cause harm.

Vaccine adverse event reporting system (VAERS) has successfully identified several rare adverse events related to vaccination. Among them are:
- An intestinal problem after the first vaccine for rotavirus was introduced (the vaccine was withdrawn in 1999)
- Neurologic and gastrointestinal diseases related to yellow fever vaccine
- According to Plotkin et al., VAERS identified a need for further investigation of measles, mumps, rubella (MMR) association with a blood clotting disorder, encephalopathy after MMR, and syncope after immunization.

Misinformation and myths about vaccines can contribute to safety concerns. It is important to rely on credible sources of information, such as public health agencies and healthcare professionals, for accurate and evidence-based information about vaccine safety.

Overall, vaccines have a strong safety record and are a crucial tool in public health for preventing infectious diseases.

As with any medical intervention, there may be safety concerns associated with vaccines or vaccinations. It is important to address these concerns and provide accurate information to help individuals make informed decisions.

ADVERSE EVENTS OF VACCINES

While vaccines are generally safe and effective, like any medical intervention, they can have side effects, and occasionally, adverse events can occur.

Vaccine adverse events refer to any undesirable or unexpected health effects that occur after vaccination. Adverse events can range from mild, such as soreness at the injection site, to more severe, although severe adverse events are relatively rare. However, many adverse events may be coincidental events that occur in temporal association after vaccination but are unrelated to vaccination. Observing the rate of an adverse event in the vaccinated population and comparing it with the rate of this event among the unvaccinated population can help to distinguish genuine vaccine reactions. Centers for Disease Control and Prevention (CDC) report asserts that "Just 33 people from 25 million immunized were affected" (August 2018).

It is important to note that vaccines undergo rigorous testing in clinical trials to ensure their safety and efficacy before they are approved for use. However, like any medical intervention, vaccines can have side effects, and some individuals may experience adverse events. Adverse events can range from mild and temporary, such as soreness at the injection site or a mild fever, to more severe and rare reactions. Serious adverse events are usually uncommon, and the benefits of vaccination in preventing diseases generally outweigh the risks.

Common vaccine adverse reactions usually are self-limited, i.e., mild-to-moderate in severity, e.g., low-grade fever or injection site swelling, pain, and redness, and have no permanent sequela. These include local inflammation after administration of DTwP, Td, or Tdap vaccines, and fever and rash 1-2 weeks after administration of MMR or MMRV vaccines.

As with all aspects of medicine, the benefits and risks from vaccines must be weighed against each other, and vaccine recommendations are based on this assessment. Recommendations are made to maximize protection and minimize risk by providing specific advice on dose, route, and timing and by identifying precautions or contraindications to vaccination.

It is important to remember that the overall benefits of vaccination in preventing serious and potentially life-threatening diseases often outweigh the risks of potential adverse events. Public health authorities and regulatory agencies work to strike a balance between ensuring vaccine safety and promoting disease prevention through vaccination.

A new systematic review of adverse events linked to routine childhood vaccines has found that vaccines associated with serious adverse events are "extremely rare and must be weighed against the protective benefits that vaccines provide".

MEASLES, MUMPS, RUBELLA VACCINATION, AND AUTISM

A recent Nationwide Cohort Study found again that the MMR "vaccine is not associated with an increased risk of autism even among kids who are at high risk because they have a sibling with the disorder". The researchers found that children who received "the MMR vaccine were 7% less likely to develop autism than children who didn't get vaccinated".

- *Autism Spectrum Disorders (ASD):* The US Kaiser Permanent researchers found that the prenatal Tdap vaccine was not associated with ASD after studying some 80,000 youngsters over 4 years.

Among children "whose mothers received prenatal Tdap, 3.78/1,000 person-years were diagnosed with autism compared to 4.05 per 1,000 person-years in children whose mothers were not vaccinated". The study authors concluded, "we provide evidence supporting the ACIP's recommendation to vaccinate pregnant women to protect vulnerable infants, who are at highest risk of hospitalization and death after pertussis infection".

- *Leukemia:* There was no association with leukemia among the following vaccines—MMR, diphtheria-tetanus-pertussis (DTaP), *Haemophilus influenzae* type B (Hib), and hepatitis B (high strength evidence). Literature provides no support for a link between the most common childhood vaccinations and childhood ALL development.

  Intussusception: Rotavirus vaccines (RV) were linked to intussusception (moderate evidence), but the occurrence was extremely rare. RV-associated intussusception is a rare (moderate evidence), but serious adverse event that has been associated with certain RV. Two RVs that were previously associated with an increased risk of intussusception are RotaShield and a previous version of the RotaTeq vaccine. RotaShield was withdrawn from the market in 1999 due to concerns about intussusception, while the RotaTeq, which was initially associated with a slightly increased risk, underwent additional safety evaluations and remains available as of my knowledge now childhood prevention use.

  A study conducted by the CDC Vaccine Safety Datalink (VSD) between May 2006 and February 2010 found no increased risk of intussusception following vaccination with RotaTeq. However, the study indicated an increased risk of intussusception following dose 1 and dose 2 of Rotarix. CDC estimates that there is a small increased risk of intussusception, usually within the first week after dose 1 or dose 2 of RV, resulting in one additional case for every 20,000–100,000 US infants who receive the vaccine.

- *Type 1 diabetes (T1D) and RV:* There is no association between rotavirus vaccination in children and the incidence or clinical manifestation of T1D.
- *Multiple sclerosis (MS):* HBV vaccine and risk of developing MS—a systematic review and the result of meta-regression and meta-analysis performed on 414 scientific papers showed that hepatitis B vaccination is not associated with an increased risk of developing MS.

  Hundreds of millions of people worldwide have received the hepatitis B vaccine without developing MS or any other autoimmune disease.

ADVERSE REACTIONS OF COVID-19 VACCINES

According to the findings of the voluminous kinds of literature available, the COVID-19 vaccine is safe to administer and induces protection against disease severity and deaths. It is critical to give the public accurate information on vaccine side effects, probable adverse reactions, and the safety level of the vaccines provided. Future research could look into the impact of the vaccine on patients of various ages and medical conditions.

Severe acute respiratory syndrome coronavirus-2 (SARS-CoV-2) vaccines-related adverse events were classified into three types—local side effects, systemic side effects, and other side effects such as allergies.

The adverse reactions to COVID-19 vaccines are mild-to-moderate in severity, which are typically short-lived with no significant influence or interference in individual daily activities and no unique patterns in cause of death among vaccine-related deaths. *These side effects are often a sign that the body is building protection against the virus.*

Allergic Reactions

Although rare, some individuals may experience severe allergic reactions (anaphylaxis) to COVID-19 vaccines. This is why individuals are monitored for 15–30 minutes after vaccination.

- *Blood clots and low platelets (Johnson & Johnson Vaccine):* There have been rare cases of blood clots with low platelets after vaccination with the Johnson & Johnson vaccine.
- *Myocarditis and pericarditis (mRNA vaccines):* In rare cases, there have been reports of myocarditis and pericarditis following mRNA COVID-19 vaccination, such as Pfizer and Moderna. These side effects are rare and occur more often in younger males. The risk of these side effects is still relatively low, and the benefits of vaccination generally outweigh the risks.
- *mRNA vaccine cuts COVID-related Guillain-Barré (GB) risk in practice:* While GB is extremely rare, people should be aware that having a COVID infection can increase their risk of developing the disorder, and receiving an mRNA vaccine can decrease their risk. People who received the COVID-19 vaccine were 59% less likely to develop GBS than those who did not get the vaccine

Multiple case reports describe Kikuchi–Fujimoto disease (KFD) following COVID-19 vaccination, but the true nature of this phenomenon is unknown, findings indicate that KFD is observed in association with COVID-19 vaccination and suggests that mechanistic studies are warranted.

If individuals experience adverse effects that are severe or persistent, it is important to contact ID experts. History of severe allergic reactions to any vaccine or its components, discuss your vaccination options with a healthcare provider. The decision to get vaccinated should be made after weighing the potential risks and benefits based on your circumstances.

It is essential to remember that these adverse effects are typically short-lived and mild, and they are far less severe than the potential complications of a COVID-19 infection, which can lead to hospitalization, long-term health issues, or death.

The claims that vaccines are unsafe when administered according to expert recommendations have been disproven by a robust body of medical literature, including a thorough review by the National Academy of Medicine (formerly known as the Institute of Medicine).

Put simply: Vaccines are safe. Vaccines are effective. Vaccines save millions of lives.

CONCLUSION

The safety and efficacy of vaccines are rigorously evaluated through extensive clinical trials before they are approved for public use. These trials are conducted in multiple phases to assess the vaccine's safety, efficacy, and potential side effects in different populations. After a vaccine is approved, its safety and efficacy continue to be monitored through post-marketing surveillance. This ongoing evaluation helps to ensure that any rare adverse effects or long-term side effects are identified and managed appropriately.

Vaccines have led to the eradication of smallpox, near elimination of wild polio, and significant reductions in the incidence of diseases such as measles, diphtheria, and pertussis. The COVID-19 vaccines, for example, are highly effective in preventing COVID-19 and reducing the severity of illness in those who get infected after vaccination.

Receiving several vaccines or combination vaccines in one visit is important to protect children from various diseases as early as possible. This also makes it easier to complete the recommended doses on time. Receiving multiple doses also does not overwhelm the immune system. The antigens present in vaccines are a small fraction compared to what our bodies naturally encounter every day.

Serious safety problems with vaccines are rare, and the benefits of vaccination in preventing illness and death from infectious diseases far outweigh the risks. Vaccination not only protects the individual who receives the vaccine but also helps protect the community by reducing the spread of infectious diseases.

SUGGESTED READING

1. Byington CL. Vaccines: Can transparency increase confidence and reduce hesitance. Pediatrics. 2014;134(2):377-9.
2. Craig JW, Farinha P, Jiang A, Lytle A, Skinnider B, Slack GW. Kikuchi-fujimoto disease following COVID-19 vaccination: experience at a population-based referral center. Am J Clin Pathol. 2023;160(2):114-8.
3. Dhamanti I, Suwantika AA, Adlia A, Yamani LN, Yakub F. Adverse reactions of COVID-19 vaccines: a scoping review of observational studies. Int J Gen Med. 2023;16:609-18.
4. Front Immunol. 2023 Oct 13:14:1243233
5. Hviid A, Hansen JV, Frisch M, Melbye M. Measles, mumps, rubella vaccination and autism: A nationwide cohort study. Ann Intern Med. 2019;170(8):513-20.
6. Plotkin SA. Vaccines, 5th ed. Philadelphia: Saunders; 2008.
7. Søegaard SH, Rostgaard K, Schmiegelow K, Kamper-Jørgensen M, Hargreave M, Hjalgrim H, et al. Childhood vaccinations and risk of acute lymphoblastic leukaemia in children. Int J Epidemiol. 2017;46(3):905-13.

CHAPTER 16

Artificial Intelligence and Machine Learning in Vaccinology

THE ARTIFICIAL INTELLIGENCE'S ROLE IN VACCINES

Artificial intelligence (AI) plays a crucial role in the development and optimization of vaccines through various approaches and applications. It helps in identifying target proteins or epitopes that stimulate the immune system, which are central to generating effective vaccines.

AI systems ensure that a vaccine remains effective over time by studying immunogenic viral antigens, such as the SARS-2 spike protein (S), which is one of the roles and functions of AI in developing COVID-19 vaccine development.

AI significantly contributes to vaccine development by enhancing the efficiency of research, aiding in the identification of effective vaccine components, estimating vaccine efficacy, and supporting public health efforts to combat misinformation and vaccine hesitancy.

Machine Learning and Deep Learning

Machine learning (ML) and Deep Learning (DL) are two subsets of AI that involve teaching computers to learn and make decisions from any sort of data. Sometimes, they are even used interchangeably. In broad terms, DL is a subset of ML which is a subset of AI.

They are interconnected fields that work together to analyze and make sense of large amounts of data. Some advantages of AI and ML include improved insight, enabling better decision-making, and increased efficiencies. Certainly, AI and ML are enhancing vaccine development processes. These technologies assist in predicting how a virus may mutate, enabling faster adjustments to existing vaccines or the creation of new ones. AI and ML also aid in vaccine trial optimization, accelerating the evaluation and approval phases.

NEW TECH USED TO CREATE VACCINES

The newest and most exciting area in vaccine technology is the use of messenger RNA (mRNA) vaccines. Unlike conventional vaccines—which can take many months or even years to cultivate—mRNA vaccines can be developed quickly using the pathogen's genetic code. Should a new pathogen emerge in the future, vaccine developers could quickly respond by selecting AI-identified antigenic determinants that would have already been validated in preclinical tests, thereby enabling vaccine candidates to be moved quickly into clinical testing.

The AI tools, such as ChatGPT, Ai Apple, and AI Google are the subject of intense debate regarding their possible applications in contexts such as vaccinations and healthcare.

Applications of AI in disease progression in hospitalized patients. Similarly, AI applications in the disease progression are also critical, helping medical staff find and treat high-risk patients early, estimate ICU events, formulate treatment plans, allocate medical resources, and reduce mortality (the COVID-19 Pandemic experiences)

In this chapter, we provide an overview of AI which has the potential to revolutionize various aspects of medicine, including drug discovery, vaccine development, and healthcare delivery. There are ways and means in which AI could be utilized in the field of vaccines, e.g., in various aspects of the vaccination process, from research and development to vaccine distribution and monitoring.

Historically, vaccine development is a long expensive process. As AI continues to advance, it is expected to contribute significantly to the field of vaccinations, designing clinical trials for vaccines identifying suitable trial participants, predicting patient recruitment rates, and even helping in monitoring and analyzing trial data.

- By analyzing large datasets, AI algorithms can identify patterns and potential correlations between vaccines and adverse events, aiding in early detection and enabling timely interventions.
- For safer and more effective vaccines, AI can assist in adjusting vaccine formulations, ensuring stability, and predicting potential side effects or adverse reactions.
- AI can aid in managing vaccine inventories, ensuring that vaccines are stored at the correct temperature, and tracking expiration dates

- AI algorithms can enhance vaccine distribution logistics, i.e., vaccine demand prediction. identifying the most efficient routes for distribution and ensuring that vaccines are delivered to the right locations at the right time.

AI can monitor disease trends and outbreaks which can help public health agencies respond quickly to potential vaccine-preventable disease outbreaks. By analyzing the biological pathways, AI can suggest existing medications that might have the potential to act as vaccines or vaccine adjuvants.

AI-based systems can be used to develop secure and verifiable vaccine passports, allowing individuals to prove their vaccination status for travel or access to certain facilities. Evolving AI systems can be utilized to identify and understand vaccine hesitancy trends and sentiments. This information can be used to develop targeted public health campaigns to address concerns and promote vaccination. It is expected to help healthcare providers create personalized vaccination plans based on an individual's medical history, allergies, and other factors.

AI can be a valuable tool and should be used in conjunction with rigorous scientific and ethical standards to ensure the safety, efficacy, and equitable distribution of vaccines.

The CDC in the United States adopted AI-based epidemiological surveillance to monitor the spread of infectious diseases. Their AI-based software utilizes various data sources as represented in **Figure 1** for various techniques to analyze, process, and issue early alerts as mentioned in **Figure 2**.

■ AI SYSTEM IN MEDICINE

A new study published in Frontiers in Immunology on March 9, 2023, and led by scientists at MIT reports successful experiments to inoculate mice with a new vaccine designed to protect against all COVID variants even ones that have not emerged yet. The vaccine was developed thanks to discoveries made using AI algorithms, and the new experiments demonstrate the vaccine's ability to prevent death from COVID-19 infection.

AI-based epidemiological surveillance can ensure more equitable vaccine access **(Figure 2)**. Techniques used by AI-based healthcare software to issue early alerts and improve public health.

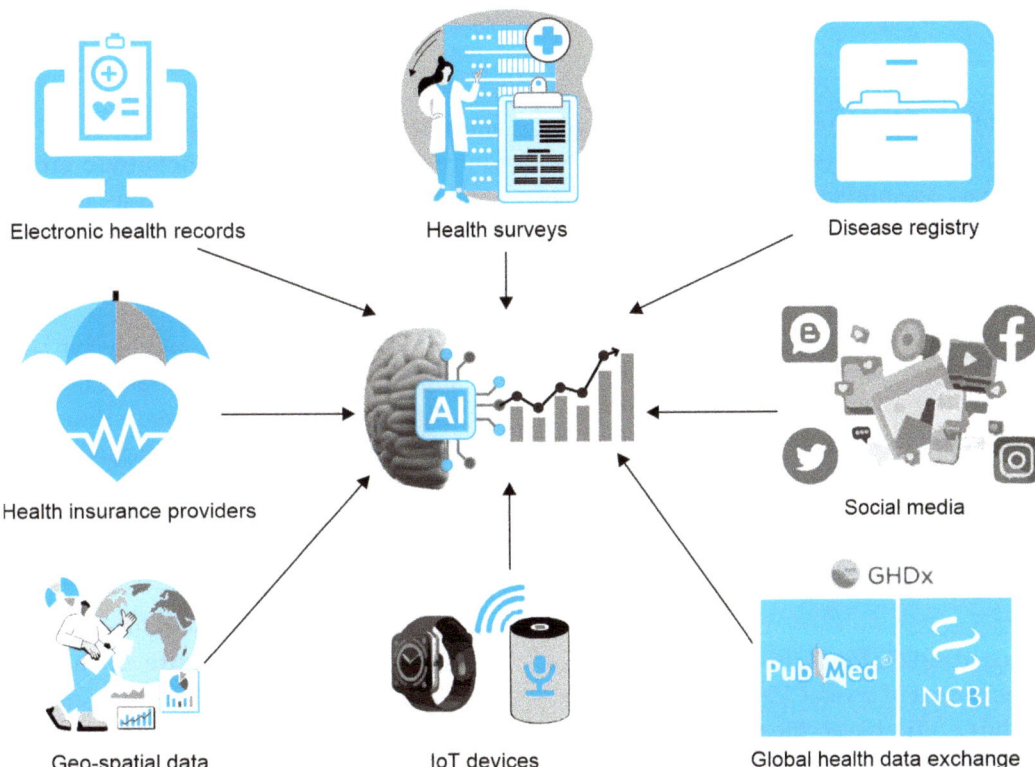

Fig. 1: Diverse sources that provide data to AI-powered health systems.

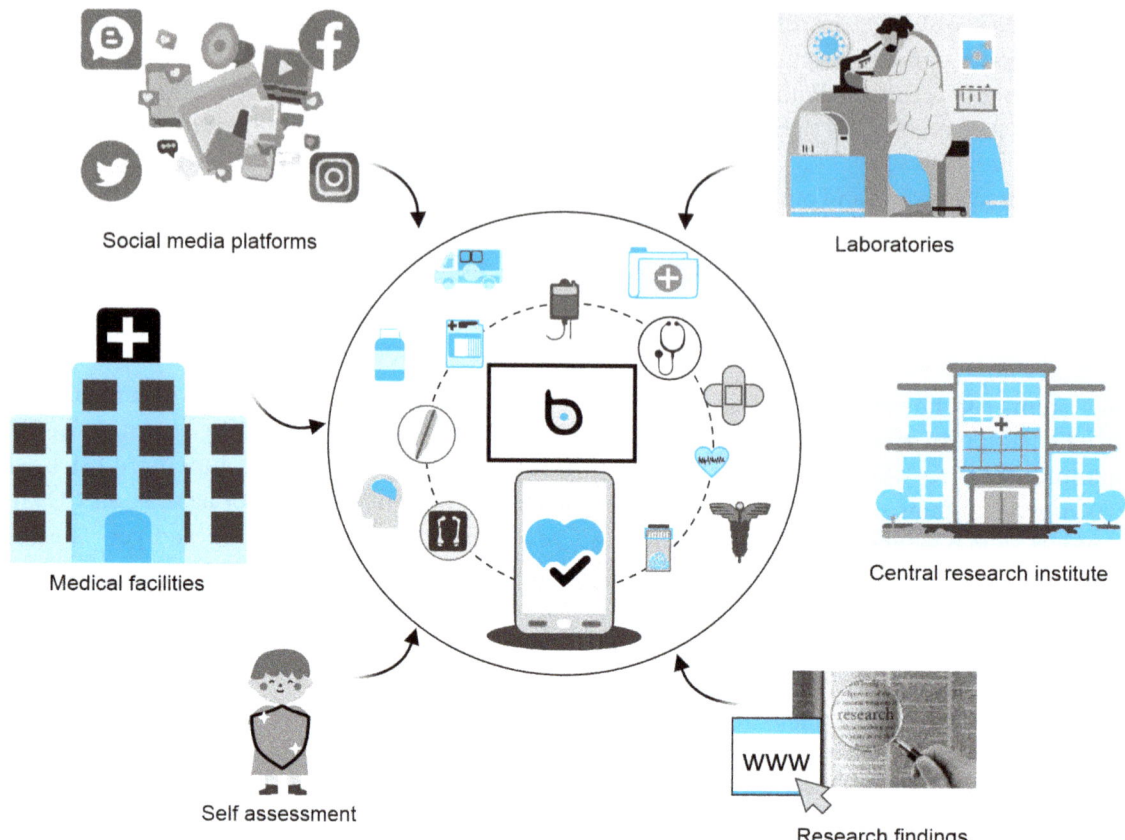

Fig. 2: AI-based epidemiological surveillance.

AI model could mitigate the inadequacies of imaging and the diagnostic errors in interpretation, which often contribute to delayed diagnosis of cancers. AI technology in combination with emerging blood-based biomarkers could speed up the development of future vaccines against novel viral threats.

AI-based approaches offer new opportunities for developing vaccine development. These approaches can quicken the process, improve accuracy, and reduce costs. Future research should concentrate on maximizing the application of AI-based techniques and combining them with conventional vaccine development methodologies.

AI/ML-BASED APPROACHES FOR DEVELOPING COVID-19 VACCINE

AI is being researched rapidly for use in the COVID-19 vaccination. The development of several AI/ML-based methods has accelerated the COVID-19 vaccine research process.

These approaches can accelerate the process, improve accuracy, and reduce costs. To guarantee the security and effectiveness of vaccines, and other infectious diseases, future research should concentrate on maximizing the application of AI-based techniques and combining them with conventional vaccine development methodologies.

CONCLUSION

The combination of AI should always complement and not substitute, rigorous "wet" laboratory testing research and clinical trials, which remain indispensable steps in ensuring vaccine safety, and efficacy that are essential for regulatory approval. However, continue to harness the power of AI-driven tools, the future holds great promise for the rapid creation of effective vaccines, particularly for emerging biological threats.

The ever-demanding workload of doctors will soon make AI an essential feature of medical care in the future. This will further enable medical personnel to focus more on human emotional components like care and compassion, which helps to build the doctor-patient relationship in medical care.

■ A NOTE OF CAUTION

Artificial intelligence technology cannot replace medical professionals, but it will indeed change their roles. AI has great potential in the field of vaccines but is not a substitute for rigorous scientific research and clinical trials. AI should be used as a tool to augment and support the work of researchers and clinicians in vaccine development and distribution. Collaboration between AI experts, vaccine researchers, and public health authorities is crucial to harness the full potential of AI in advancing vaccine science.

One potential disadvantage is the risk of software generating false positive or false negative test results. This limitation underscores the need for ongoing monitoring and evaluation to ensure the lasting effectiveness of AI-based epidemiological surveillance. Another challenge is protecting personal health information data which must be securely stored and protected.

Looking at medicine today, there are essentially two places, where we are at a fundamental turning point. One is AI, which gets so much attention and hype; this will change things in our clinical practices. The other is a bit more incomprehensible but may have a powerful impact on the RNA therapeutics medicines of the future.

■ SUGGESTED READING

1. Anjaria P, Asediya V, Bhavsar P, Pathak A, Desai D, Patil V. Artificial Intelligence in Public Health: Revolutionizing Epidemiological Surveillance for Pandemic Preparedness and Equitable Vaccine Access. Vaccines (Basel). 2023; 11(7):1154.
2. Sharma A, Virmani T, Pathak V, Sharma A, Pathak K, Kumar G, Pathak D. Kamla Pathak, Girish Kumar, and Devender Pathak. Artificial Intelligence-Based Data-Driven Strategy to Accelerate Research, Development, and Clinical Trials of COVID Vaccine. Biomed Res Int. 2022:7205241. https://www.ncbi.nlm.nih.gov/pmc/articles/PMC9279074/
3. Beam AL, Drazen JM, Kohane IS, Leong TY, Manrai AK, Rubin EJ. Artificial Intelligence in Medicine. N Engl J Med. 2023;388:1220-1.
4. Yu KH, Healey E, Leong TY, Kohane IS, Manrai AK. Medical Artificial Intelligence and Human Values. N Engl J Med. 2024;390(20):1895-1904.

CHAPTER 17

Catch-up Vaccinations in Childhood Immunizations

INTRODUCTION

"Catch-up vaccinations" are designed to ensure that individuals who have missed their scheduled vaccines can still receive those vaccines at a later date. This is particularly important for children and adolescents who may have missed one or more scheduled vaccines, but it can also apply to adults who have not been fully vaccinated. It is typically done to ensure that individuals are adequately protected against preventable diseases.

Catch-up vaccination programs are especially important for children and adolescents who may have missed scheduled vaccinations due to various reasons, such as missed doctor appointments, travel, or parental decisions. However, catch-up vaccination may also be necessary for adults who missed vaccinations in childhood or who require additional vaccines due to changing recommendations or travel plans.

Catch-up vaccination schedules are designed based on factors such as the individual's age, health status, previous vaccination history, and current recommendations from health authorities. The aim is to bring the individual up-to-date with their vaccinations as quickly and safely as possible.

The decline in vaccination coverage during the COVID-19 pandemic led directly to the current situation of rising diseases and child deaths. This pandemic has left >60 million children without a single dose of standard childhood vaccines. These, 60 million plus "zero-dose children" have not received any vaccines and have aged out of routine immunization. Many of these children who missed their shots have now aged out of routine immunization programs.

One of the biggest challenges is that the children who missed their first shots between 2020 and 2022 are now older than the age group typically seen routinely at primary healthcare centers and in normal vaccination programs. This is an example and challenge to all pediatricians and there is an urgency and need to move fast now to catch up with the children that were missed during the

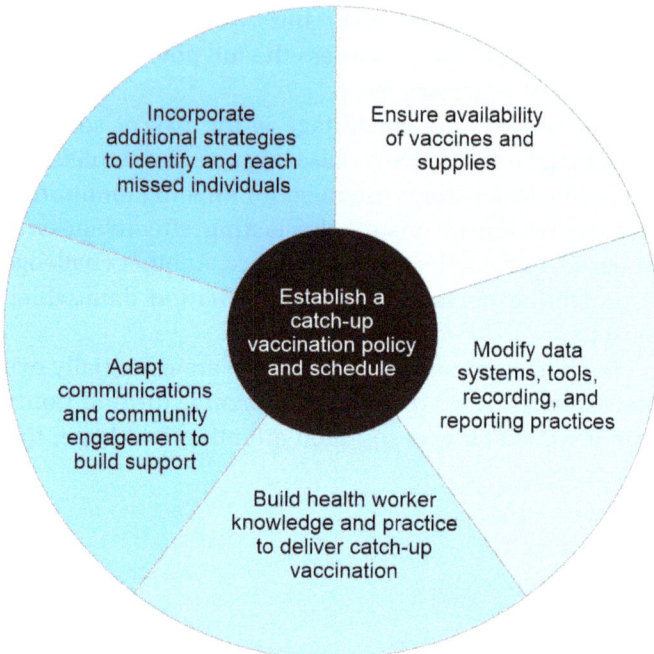

Fig. 1: Elements of a strong catch-up vaccination strategy: Leave no one behind guidance for planning and implementing catch-up vaccination.
Courtesy: WHO April 2021.

pandemic. *These aspects are dealt with in this section as follows*:
- *Background case scenario* Q and A format
- *Catchup Guidance* as per Centers for Disease Control and Prevention (CDC) USA, World Health Organization (WHO) catch-up vaccination strategy (2021 WHO **Fig. 1**).

BACKGROUND

The conundrum model queries with a conjectural answer by authors "on catch-up vaccination for an 11-month-old Indian child who received Bacillus Calmette–Guérin (BCG) at birth, one dose of diphtheria, tetanus, pertussis (DTP), pneumococcus, *Haemophilus influenzae* type B (Hib), and hepatitis."

■ AUTHORS RESPONSE

Catch-up guidance for the quoted a 11-month-old child, our suggestions are as follows:

Give dose # 2 now, DTP, Pneumo vax, Hib, and hepatitis B virus (HBV), preferably in combination vaccines, i.e., pentavalent shot and a separate conjugated Pneumo shot at a separate, distance site.

- The DTP, Hib, and HBV combo's shot in one site
- Another Pneumo shot separately [either pneumococcal conjugate vaccine-13 (PCV13) or PCV15] in another site (preferably into the anterolateral aspect of the thigh or the deltoid muscle of the upper arm, depending on the age of the child.)

Remember: This 11-month-old child has also missed polio, rotavirus dose, and also the 9-month MMR shot # 1. Should add to the varicella and hepatitis A virus (HAV) shots as recommended, subsequent visits.

■ VACCINE CATCH-UP GUIDANCE

The theme of the 2023 year's ("*the big catch-up*") World Immunization Week (April 24–30) is both a reference to the state of global immunizations following the acute phase of the COVID-19 pandemic and a call to action. The annual observance "comes at a critical time", because of COVID-19, "(immunization) levels decreased in >100 countries with millions of children missing out on lifesaving protection." It is critical that we mainly focus on accelerating speedy progress in nations to get back on track and protect more people, particularly children, from preventable diseases.

It is typically important for people who may have missed one or more doses of vaccines during their childhood or adolescence and need to "catch up" on their immunizations.

Catch-up vaccination refers to the action of vaccinating an individual who, for whatever reason, is missing or has not received doses of vaccines for which they are eligible, per the national immunization schedule. CDC has developed catch-up vaccine recommendations to assist and guide practicing pediatricians.

- When a vaccine is not administered at the recommended age, administer it at a subsequent visit.
- Children who start late or who are >1 month behind, administer recommended vaccines if immunization history is incomplete or unknown.
- Depending on the person's age and immunization history, their catch-up schedule may be different from the National Immunizations Program Schedule.
- Do not restart or add doses to the vaccine series for extended intervals between doses.

The catch-up schedule is designed to protect against vaccine-preventable diseases, including measles, mumps, rubella, polio, HBV, chickenpox (varicella), diphtheria, tetanus, whooping cough (pertussis), human papillomavirus (HPV), and more. Children, young people, and adults may miss a scheduled immunization for several reasons and need to start a catch-up immunization program.

Vaccination guidance for children and adolescents may vary by country and region. Therefore, it is important to consult with a local health department or pediatrics IDs expert in vaccinology for the most up-to-date and specific catch-up recommendations. Physicians or healthcare providers can contact 24/7 days with and/or ACIP for case-based catch-up vaccine recommendations

Catch-up vaccinations are essential for individuals who have missed one or more recommended vaccines or who may have fallen behind on their vaccination schedule. Catch-up schedules are designed to help bring individuals up-to-date on their vaccinations. Authors wish referring the attached website on: *4 Months–18 Years (July 25, 2023)"—a Medical Professionals References* as a guide to all healthcare-providing staff on individual cases with vaccination delay history.

The effectiveness of catch-up immunization in protecting vaccine efficacy depends on several factors:

- *Timing and the number of doses:* Catch-up immunizations are most effective when administered as soon as possible after the missed doses. Delaying catch-up immunization can increase the risk of exposure to vaccine-preventable diseases. The number of catch-up doses required may vary depending on the specific vaccine and how many doses were missed. Some vaccines require multiple doses to achieve full immunity, and catching up on all recommended doses is essential for protection.
- The effectiveness of vaccines can vary from person to person. Factors such as an individual's overall health, genetics, and underlying medical conditions can influence the strength of their immune response to vaccines. Different vaccines provide varying levels of protection, and some vaccines may be more effective than others in preventing specific diseases.

Some vaccines are more effective when given at specific ages. Catch-up immunizations may be less effective if administered too late in life. Therefore, it is important to follow the recommended age-specific vaccination schedules whenever possible.

In general, catch-up immunization is an effective way to help individuals become vaccinated and protected against vaccine-preventable diseases. The effectiveness of catch-up immunization also depends on the overall vaccination rates in the community. High vaccination rates contribute to herd immunity, which protects those who cannot be vaccinated, such as individuals with certain medical conditions.

Parents should consult with their family physician to ensure that the catch-up schedule is appropriate for the individual's specific circumstances. Vaccine efficacy is generally maintained when catch-up immunizations are administered according to the recommended schedule, and it is crucial to complete the full series of doses for each vaccine to maximize protection.

The CDC provides catch-up immunization schedules for children and adolescents who start late or are more than a month behind in their vaccinations. The schedules take into account the minimum ages and minimum intervals between doses for each vaccine.

For example, if a child has missed their first dose of the MMR vaccine normally given at 12–15 months, the catch-up schedule allows for the first dose to be given at any age, with a second dose at least 28 days later.

Similarly, for the HPV vaccine, if the vaccination series is started after the 15th birthday, three doses are recommended, with the second dose given 1–2 months after the first, and the third dose 6 months after the first.

It is important to note that catch-up vaccination schedules can be complex, as they need to take into account the vaccines already received, the ages at which they were received, and the current age of the individual. Therefore, Pediatricians often play a crucial role in determining the appropriate catch-up schedule for each individual.

■ CONCLUSION

Should always consult with an ID physician or vaccination clinic to determine the appropriate catch-up vaccination schedule based on individual circumstances and the specific vaccines needed for optimal protection.

The "World Immunization Day" is a momentous occasion commemorated every year and mainly educates people about the benefits of vaccination against several diseases and disorders. This day honors the advancements, breakthroughs, and tireless efforts dedicated to immunizing individuals across the globe. Immunization has transformed public health, significantly reduced the burden of diseases, and saved countless lives.

■ SUGGESTED READING

1. CDC. (2024). Children and adolescents age 7 through 18 years. Available from: https://www.cdc.gov/vaccines/schedules/hcp/imz/catchup.html#table-2 [Last accessed April, 2024].
2. CDC. (2024). Recommended Catch-up Immunization Schedule for Children and Adolescents Who Start Late or Who Are More than 1 Month Behind. Available from: https://www.cdc.gov/vaccines/schedules/hcp/imz/catchup.html [Last accessed April, 2024].
3. Medical Professionals References. (2024). 2024 Catch-Up Vaccination Schedule: 4 Months-18 Years. Available from: https://www.empr.com/charts/https-www-empr-com-charts-child-adolescent-catch-up-vaccine-schedule-vaccines/ [Last accessed April, 2024].
4. New Pediatric Oncall query dated Feb 3rd, 2023 on expertise category of 'Vaccines'.

CHAPTER 18: Combination Vaccines (Combos)

INTRODUCTION

Combination vaccinations, also known as combos or multivalent vaccines, are vaccines that protect against multiple diseases with a single injection. These vaccines combine antigens from different pathogens into a single formulation, allowing them to build up immunity against multiple diseases simultaneously.

At present, combination vaccines are being advised for many children. Combination vaccines can be beneficial for children as they can help them to prevent various diseases. Instead of receiving separate vaccinations for each disease, combination vaccines offer the convenience of fewer injections, potentially reducing the number of healthcare visits needed and improving overall vaccine coverage rates.

The Combos offer the advantage of reducing the number of injections required for immunization. This can improve convenience for patients and healthcare providers, as well as increase adherence to the recommended vaccination schedule. By reducing the number of clinic visits and injections, combination vaccines can help ensure that individuals receive all the necessary vaccinations.

SAFETY AND EFFECTIVENESS OF THE COMBOS

Combination vaccines are carefully developed and undergo rigorous testing to ensure their safety and efficacy. Before a combo vaccine is approved for use, they follow the same regulatory processes as single vaccines and are recommended by health authorities like the Centers for Disease Control and Prevention (CDC) and the World Health Organization (WHO) based on their demonstrated effectiveness in preventing diseases.

During the past two decades, the number of injections that are required per clinic visit to fulfill the recommended childhood immunization schedule has been increasing dramatically. This has created problems for patients and practitioners, sometimes risking a missed opportunity for vaccination. The use of combo vaccines can simplify vaccination schedules and reduce the number of injections required by combining multiple vaccines into a single syringe to improve vaccination coverage rates. The combo shots are particularly useful and welcome in populations where access to healthcare services is limited. However, healthcare physicians must consider factors such as individual vaccine components, timing of doses, and potential interactions with other vaccines when administering combination vaccines.

The administration schedule for combination vaccines is determined based on the recommended immunization schedule for each included disease. The timing and number of doses may vary depending on the specific combination vaccine and the target population. Healthcare providers follow national immunization guidelines to determine the appropriate schedule for administering combination vaccines.

Combos that have been available for many years include diphtheria, tetanus toxoid and pertussis vaccines (DTP); and measles, mumps, rubella (MMR). Also, the vaccines containing immunizing antigens against more than one serogroup or serotype of the same disease, i.e., the pneumococcal, quadrivalent meningococcal, and human papillomavirus (HPV) vaccines are symbolic. Improved vaccines are evolving continually and are expected to be marketed for immunization purposes **(Table 1)**.

- The Health Ministry in each country has its combo preference and there have been no universally acceptable schedules in use.

As many countries begin to include inactivated polio vaccine (IPV) in routine vaccination programs, the use of high-valency combination vaccines is increasing [including hexavalent diphtheria, tetanus, and acellular pertussis–hepatitis B virus–IPV/*Haemophilus influenzae* type b disease vaccine [DTPa-HBV-IPV/Hib)]. Combination vaccines are generally licensed on the basis of immunogenicity data, but these data can be inconclusive,

TABLE 1: Combination vaccines licensed by the US Food and Drug Administration (FDA).

S. No.	Combo vaccines	Trade name (Year licensed)	Age group	Use in the immunization schedule
	DTP	1949	Early infancy	The development of numerous effective DTP vaccines quickly stimulated efforts to combine DTP with other routine vaccines for infants
	MMR	1971	Over 12 months	The measles vaccine was developed in 1963, mumps by 1967, and rubella (1969). Combined into the MMR vaccine by Dr Maurice Hilleman in 1971. Administered as a single shot
	MMR-V	2005	Over 12 months	
1.	HepA-rHepB	Twinrix (2001) GSK	≥18 years	Three doses on a 0-, 1-, and 6-month schedule
2.	DTaP-rHepB-IPV	Pediarix (2002) Five diseases	6 weeks through 6 years	Three-dose series at 2, 4, and 6 months of age
3.	MMRV	ProQuad (2005). Merck Four diseases	>12 months	12 months through 12 years, two doses
4.	DTaP-IPV	Kinrix (2008) or Quadracel	4 years through 6 years	Booster for fifth dose of DTaP and fourth dose of IPV
5.	DTaP-IPV/Hib	Pentacel (2008) Five diseases	6 weeks through 4 years	Four-dose series administered at 2, 4, 6, and 15 through 18 months of age
6.	Hib-MenCY	MenHibrix (2013) GSK	6 weeks through 18 months	Four-dose series administered at 2, 4, 6, and 12 through 15 months of age
7.	DTaP-IPV-Hib-HepB	Vaxelis (2018) Six diseases	6 weeks through 4 years	Three-dose series administered at 2, 4, and 6 months of age@
8.	B + A, C, W-135, and Y conjugate meningococcal vaccine	Penbraya (2023) (meningococcal groups A, B, C, W, and Y) Five most common serogroups	Children and adult	Combines components from those two vaccines and is approved for use in individuals 10 through 25 years of age

@A fourth dose of acellular pertussis vaccine is needed to complete the pertussis primary series in infants who receive three doses of Vaxelis.
(DTaP: diphtheria–tetanus-acellular pertussis; Hib: Haemophilus influenzae type b; HepA: hepatitis A; IPV: inactivated poliovirus; MMRV: measles-mumps-rubella-varicella; MenCY: meningococcal conjugate vaccine Serogroup C and Y; rHepB: recombinant hepatitis B)
Courtesy: Redbook, 2018.

and the interpretation of differing antibody titer responses to different products can be challenging.

Penbraya Vaccine against Five Meningococcal Serogroups Together

In October 2023, The FDA approved a new meningococcal vaccine, clearing Pfizer's shot Penbraya in teenagers and young adults for protection *against the five most common disease-causing serogroups*. Penbraya is the first vaccine available that can provide such broad protection, which may make it more convenient than current options. While meningococcal disease is rare, it can be serious and even deadly.

The Future of the combo vaccines; other combination vaccines that are being studied include:
- Now, the Advisory Committee on Immunization Practices (ACIP) recommending Hexavac (DTaP-rHepB-IPV/Hib) vaccine is especially exciting, might be just two shots for your child during infancy [Hexavac and pneumococcal conjugate vaccine 13 (PCV13)].
- Other good combinations might include putting PCV and Hexavac together. That would mean just one shot at 2, 4, and 6 months!

Fewer shots are good, but even more exciting would be the development of edible vaccines. Early research showed that producing edible vaccines is theoretically possible, but the production of the first edible vaccines is likely way off.

When patients have received the recommended series of immunizations for a particular antigen, administering an extra dose of this antigen as part of a combination vaccine is permissible as long as the vaccines are age-appropriate and there are no contraindications.

Side effects from combination vaccines are usually mild. They are similar to those of the individual vaccines given separately. Sometimes combo vaccines cause slightly more pain or swelling where the shot was given. But if a child got the shots individually, he or she might have pain or swelling in two or three spots, instead of just one.

NOVEL COMBINATION FUTURE—VACCINATION APPROACH

- Pfizer's combination vaccine candidate for influenza and COVID-19, for children and adults
- Moderna's mRNA combination vaccine generated immune responses similar to existing flu and COVID-19 vaccines. It will start the phase 3 trial of the vaccine, will start later this year.
- Respiratory syncytial virus (RSV), flu, and COVID-19 Combos are awaiting Emergency Use Authorization (EUA)
- Investigational mRNA influenza vaccine expanding its mRNA program to develop vaccines against human immunodeficiency virus (HIV) and Nipah virus, with a good primary endpoint in phase 3 clinical trials.

To mitigate confusing ambiguities, regulatory authorities and vaccine manufacturers should adhere to established guidelines for vaccine naming. Unambiguous vaccine naming is a critical aspect of public health efforts to combat infectious diseases and protect populations from preventable illnesses.

SUMMARY

In summary, the recommended vaccines are as effective in combination as they are individually. Serious safety problems with vaccines are rare, and the benefits of vaccination in preventing illness and death from infectious diseases far outweigh the risks. Rarely, certain combinations of vaccines given together can cause fever and febrile seizures; these are temporary and do not cause any lasting damage.

SUGGESTED READING

1. Monge S, Hahné SJ, de Melker HE, Sanders EA, van der Ende A, Knol MJ. Effectiveness of the hexavalent diphtheria, tetanus, and acellular pertussis-hepatitis B virus-inactivated polio virus/Hib vaccine (DTaP-HBV-IPV/Hib) against invasive Haemophilus influenzae type b disease in the Netherlands (2003–16): a case-control study. Lancet Infect Dis. 2018;18(7):749-57.

CHAPTER 19

School Health Immunization

INTRODUCTION

A school health immunization program is a coordinated effort by schools, healthcare providers, and public health agencies to ensure that students are up-to-date on their vaccinations. These programs are crucial for preventing the spread of communicable diseases within the school setting and the wider community.

School health settings provide good opportunities to integrate vaccine delivery with other health interventions aimed at reducing vaccine-preventable diseases (VPDs). The primary objectives are to protect the health and well-being of students and the broader community by preventing the spread of VPDs in a school setting.

School health immunization is important in India, just as it is in many other countries. Immunization plays a crucial role in protecting children and the broader population from preventable diseases.

SCHOOL-BASED DELIVERY OF VACCINES PROVIDES AN OPPORTUNITY TO ACCESS YOUNG ADOLESCENT POPULATIONS WHO MAY NOT ATTEND REGULAR HEALTH SERVICES

Yes, the Government of India launched the School Health Program (SHP) in 2018. The SHP is a joint program between the Ministry of Health and Family Welfare and the Ministry of Human Resource Development. The SHP would benefit 22 Crore students in 12,88,750 schools all over India. The program's goal is to strengthen health promotion and disease prevention.

Shots for School Immunization

School health immunizations, also known as school immunization requirements, are policies implemented by schools, school districts, and educational authorities to ensure that students are up-to-date on their vaccinations before they can attend school.

School entry booster vaccination is the link between infant vaccination and adolescent vaccination. It boosts the immune response in these children and helps to restore the immunity gap. The impact of the introduction of pertussis-containing diphtheria, tetanus, pertussis (DTaP or Tdap) vaccine at school entry in Norway was seen with 65% reduction in pertussis cases. In India, schools are the perfect touch-point for monitoring immunization status improving coverage, and catching up on the immunization schedule. Checking the vaccination status of each child during school admission allows an opportunity to identify children that have missed their first dose of BCG or DPT or any other routine vaccine, especially amongst those born at home, or from hard-to-reach geographic.

Providing human papillomavirus (HPV) vaccine in the school setting has led to high HPV vaccination rates in Australia, Canada, and Great Britain. Even in the absence of a national school immunization program in the United States, there are opportunities in the school setting that can be leveraged to improve vaccination rates. These include school-located vaccination clinics, school mandates for HPV vaccination, and utilizing school-based health centers (SBHCs). Parents report a willingness to have their adolescents receive the HPV vaccine in schools and some school-located programs have been successful.

Meningitis, measles, hepatitis B, tetanus toxoid (TT), and HPV, COVID-19 etc., are examples of vaccines offered in schools, either as routine primary or booster vaccinations or through campaigns for catch-up strategies or disease control.

The Ministry of Health and Family Welfare, Government of India has an ongoing scheme to provide vaccines for the prevention of cervical cancer to girls aged between 9 and 14 years through their schools. Certain Indian States also initiated school-based COVID-19 administrations, at free of cost.

KEY POINTS ABOUT SCHOOL HEALTH IMMUNIZATIONS

These immunizations are typically required or recommended for school-aged children and often obligatory for school entry.

- Common vaccines that are typically required for school entry include those for diseases such as polio measles, mumps, rubella (MMR), DTaP or Tdap, hepatitis A, B, chickenpox (varicella), and more. The specific vaccines required for school entry can vary by location and may change over time based on recommendations from health authorities.
- The updated school health immunization requirements should conform with current national recommendations including COVID-19 vaccinations from KG classes to grade Plus 2 students.
- With the conjugated quadrivalent vaccine (MenACWY) available, World Health Organization (WHO) and Centers for Disease Control and Prevention (CDC) now routinely recommend all school-attending 11–12-year-olds should get meningococcus preventive vaccines with a booster dose at 16 years old. Teens and young adults (16 through 23 years old) also may get a meningococcal group B (MenB) vaccine. CDC also recommends meningococcal vaccination for other children and adults who are at increased risk for certain vaccines may be required for students entering kindergarten, while additional vaccines may be required for students entering middle or high school.

In some places, individuals may be eligible for medical exemptions if they have a valid medical reason for not receiving vaccines (e.g., severe allergies to vaccine components). Some regions also allow for religious or philosophical exemptions, although these are becoming less common due to concerns about VPD outbreaks.

Respiratory virus infections are common in school-aged children, but not well documented even in most developed countries such as the UK and USA. The COVID-19 pandemic highlighted the gap in knowledge related to the prevalence and symptoms of respiratory viruses among children and in schools. These data are important to improve understanding of the epidemiology of respiratory infections in any school setting, including but not limited to severe acute respiratory syndrome coronavirus 2 (SARS-CoV-2).

To support healthy learning environments for all, it is important to implement strategies to prevent and reduce the spread of infectious diseases, including staying up to date with recommended vaccinations, including COVID-19 and influenza vaccines. Also, now with pandemic lessons, it is ideal, e.g., practicing good hand hygiene and respiratory etiquette, staying home when sick, and improving indoor ventilation. These approaches lessen respiratory-related illnesses among children in any educational setting and could direct guidance in primary and secondary schools.

Immunization efforts help prevent outbreaks of diseases, particularly in densely populated areas like schools, where infectious diseases can easily spread. By ensuring that a significant portion of the population is immunized, school health immunization programs contribute to the overall improvement of community health, reducing the burden of disease on healthcare systems.

With immense gains for child health, and school health immunity at large, it is a continuous process to step up the focus on vaccinations from birth till 18 years of age and make other VPDs a word of the past, much like we did with smallpox, Hib and polio. From 1990 to 2015, the annual number of deaths among children under the age of 5 years fell from 12.7 million to 5.9 million globally and from 3.4 million to 1.2 million in India.

If schoolchildren were vaccinated at higher rates, the estimated positive associations between the universal immunization program (UIP) could be complementary to provide herd protection to unvaccinated people. Children especially those living near vaccinated individuals, such as within the same school, household, or village fixed-effect models, as the control group may have received unobserved secondary immunity. These observations reemphasize the need for universal coverage of routine childhood vaccines among Indian school children.

HEALTH EDUCATION AND AWARENESS PROGRAM

It could provide information to parents, students, and school staff about the importance of immunizations in preventing diseases and protecting public health. This includes educating them about VPDs, the safety and efficacy of vaccines, and the importance of maintaining immunization records.

Overall, a well-designed school health immunization program plays a vital role in promoting the health and well-being of students, staff, and the broader community by preventing the spread of VPDs.

SUMMARY

School health vaccination programs are vital initiatives aimed at protecting students and the broader community from preventable diseases. It provides critical access to vaccines for children and adolescents. This is particularly important in communities where healthcare access might be limited. By offering vaccines in schools, these programs ensure that more children receive necessary immunizations.

Overall, school health vaccination programs play a vital role in public health by facilitating widespread immunization, promoting equity, and supporting educational outcomes. School health vaccination programs are integral to public health strategies, particularly in preventing disease outbreaks and promoting community health.

SUGGESTED READING

1. Aase A, Herstad TK, Jørgensen SB, Leegaard TM, Berbers G, Steinbakk M, et al. Anti-pertussis antibody kinetics following DTaP-IPV booster vaccination in Norwegian children 7-8 years of age. Vaccine. 2014;32:5931-6.
2. Goldman JL, Lee BR, Porter J, Deliu A, Tilsworth S, Almendares OM, et al. Notes from the Field: Multi-pathogen Respiratory Virus Testing Among Primary and Secondary School Students and Staff Members in a Large Metropolitan School District - Missouri, November 2, 2022-April 19, 2023. MMWR Morb Mortal Wkly Rep. 2023;72(28):772-4.
3. Oliver K, McCorkell C, Pister I, Majid N, Benkel DH, Zucker JR. Improving HPV vaccine delivery at school-based health centers. Hum Vaccin Immunother. 2019; 15(7-8):1870-77.
4. To have logistic school Health vaccinations are a rarity. Therefore the appropriate reference is as follows: Operational Guidelines on School Health Programme under Ayushman Bharat, April 2018. A Joint initiative of Ministry of Health & Family Welfare and Ministry of Human Resource & Development, Government of India.

CHAPTER 20

Healthcare Personnel Vaccine Needs

INTRODUCTION

Patients harboring vaccine-preventable diseases (VPDs) are treated regularly by healthcare workers (HCWs), who may or may not have received all the recommended childhood immunizations. Therefore, healthcare professionals (HCPs) across all levels, have an "ethical responsibility" to protect patients from communicable diseases and vaccinations for healthcare staff are crucial to protect both the HCWs and the patients they serve. Vaccination is a simple, safe, and effective way of protecting HCPs against harmful diseases before they come into contact with IDs in any hospital setting. Vaccination as a primary prevention strategy is a well-established public health policy for preventing highly contagious diseases, in the modern era.

Despite strong recommendations, vaccination coverage among health workers is still not satisfying.

The specific vaccinations required or recommended for healthcare staff can vary depending on the country, healthcare facility, and the nature of the work. There is also, a risk that infected health workers could contribute to nosocomial transmission of disease to vulnerable patients at higher risk for severe illness, complications, and death. The protection of HCPs through vaccination is, therefore, an important part of patient safety and infection prevention and control programs in all hospital care settings, as well as a cornerstone of job-related health and safety.

Vaccination of HCPs and personnel—from doctors and nurses to admissions clerks and ambulance drivers—protects from potentially dangerous diseases like flu and COVID-19, and protects patients and the community at large as well.

MANDATORY VACCINATION POLICIES FOR HEALTHCARE EMPLOYEES AT THE GLOBAL LEVEL OR IN INDIA

Basically, there have been no stipulated/mandatory vaccination policies for healthcare employees at the global level nor in India!

- *In general, unions representing hospital* and nursing care staff have been vocal in opposing vaccine mandates. However, they normally support voluntary vaccination and strongly encourage their members to comply, they believe that each HCW should be entitled to make his or her own decision. Vaccination coverage among HCWs is still at an unsatisfactory level. This is despite the majority of the HCPs accepting that the vaccine is safe and preventive against influenza. Efforts are still needed to improve the coverage.
- *The swift development of effective vaccines against COVID-19* was an unprecedented scientific achievement. Close to three years after COVID-19 emerged, nearly one-third of the global population is yet to receive a vaccine dose. As the number of cases, hospitalizations, and deaths continue to rise, so do the number of hospitals, health systems, and other healthcare institutions across the country mandating vaccination for employees. In a major recent judgment, the Delhi High Court (24-Jan 2023) ruled that employers cannot insist on their employees getting the COVID-19 vaccine and disposed of all pending applications concerning the matter, directing that vaccines cannot be 'insisted upon by the employer'.
- *Although hospital admin requirements* differ between states and institutions, HCWs have routinely been required to obtain vaccination against infectious diseases including COVID-19.
  - Beyond COVID-19 shots, healthcare employers may require their staff to be vaccinated against other diseases including periodic TB screening, vaccine completion against Influenza, hepatitis B (HepB), measles, varicella, tetanus, diphtheria, pertussis (Tdap), etc.
  - Depending on the specific healthcare setting and potential exposures, additional vaccines may be recommended, such as the hepatitis A vaccine, pneumococcal vaccine, and other travel-related vaccines.

- *There are WHO-issued specific recommendations* for vaccines of particular importance to health workers, against VPDs for which there is a higher risk of transmission within healthcare settings. These recommendations include vaccines that are part of the routine immunization schedule that all health workers should receive ideally before entering the workforce, as well as annual vaccinations and, in some circumstances, emergency, or outbreak response vaccinations.

■ VACCINATIONS FOR HEALTH WORKERS

Broadly speaking, vaccinations for health workers fall into three general categories:

1. Routine immunizations which all HCWs should receive, ideally before entering the health workforce or beginning clinical contact **(Table 1)**.
2. Annual or periodic vaccinations (e.g., seasonal influenza vaccine); and
3. Exceptional or emergency vaccinations for which HCWs are a priority group (e.g., pandemic influenza and Ebola vaccine)

When establishing a health worker vaccination platform, policymakers should recognize that each of these categories will require different planning and implementation considerations.

Preservice screening and vaccination, vaccination of current health workers, and vaccination of health workers during emergencies or outbreaks.

The requirement for tuberculosis (TB) testing for HCWs may vary depending on the country, healthcare facility, and specific job responsibilities. However, in many healthcare settings, TB testing is recommended or required for HCWs due to the increased risk of exposure to TB patients. Here are some key points regarding TB testing for HCW:

- Tuberculin skin test (TST), also known as the Mantoux test or purified protein derivative (PPD), is a common method used for TB screening. The interferon-gamma release assays (IGRAs), such as the QuantiFERON-TB Gold test, are blood tests that detect the release of interferon-gamma in response to TB antigens. These tests are an alternative to the TST and may be used for TB screening in HCWs.

TABLE 1: WHO recommendations for healthcare vaccination need and screening for IDs National and International perspective.

Vaccine/immunization	WHO recommendations for all Health Workers
TB screening [tuberculin skin testing (TST)]	For BCG unvaccinated, TST- or IGRA-negative persons are at risk of occupational exposure in low and high TB incidence areas (e.g., health workers, laboratory workers, medical students, and other individuals with occupational exposure)
HepB immunization	It is suggested for groups at risk of acquiring infection who have not been vaccinated previously (e.g., health workers who may be exposed to blood and blood products at work)
Influenza	Health workers are an important group for influenza vaccination. Annual immunization with a single dose is recommended
Measles	All health workers should have immunity or be vaccinated against measles
Meningococcal	One booster dose 3–5 years after the primary dose may be given to persons considered to be at continued risk of exposure, including health workers
Pertussis	Health workers should be prioritized as a group to receive pertussis vaccine
Polio	All health workers should have completed a full course of primary vaccination against polio
Respiratory syncytial virus (RSV)	Two RSV vaccines (Arexvy by GSK and Abrysvo by Pfizer) have been licensed and recommended by CDC for adults ages 60 and older (2023–24 season onward)
Rubella	All health workers should have immunity or be vaccinated against rubella
SARS-CoV-2	Health workers should be included in (the highest priority group for vaccination) against COVID-19
Varicella	Should consider vaccination of potentially susceptible health workers (i.e., unvaccinated and with no history of varicella) with two doses of varicella vaccine

(BCG: bacillus Calmette–Guérin; CDC: Centers for Disease Control and Prevention; IGRA: interferon-gamma release assay; TB: tuberculosis; TST: tuberculin skin test; SARS-CoV-2: severe acute respiratory syndrome coronavirus-2; WHO: World Health Organization)
Source: WHO. BCG vaccines: WHO position paper–February 2018–Vaccines BCG: Note de synthèse de l'OMS – Février 2018. Weekly Epidemiol Rec. 2018;93:73-96.

- *Screening frequency:* HCWs may vary depending on the local guidelines and risk assessment. In some settings, initial baseline testing is performed, followed by periodic retesting at regular intervals (e.g., annually) or as per specific risk factors.
- *Latent TB infection (LTBI) treatment:* If an HCW tests positive for LTBI, which indicates exposure to TB bacteria without active disease, treatment may be recommended to prevent the development of active TB disease. The decision to initiate treatment is based on individual factors and local guidelines.
- *Active TB disease:* If an HCW is suspected or diagnosed with active TB disease, appropriate diagnostic evaluation, treatment, and infection control measures should be implemented to protect both the HCW and patients.

Regular TB screening helps identify and manage TB infection or disease among HCWs, reducing the risk of transmission in healthcare settings.

Hepatitis B

Screening typically involves testing for hepatitis B surface antigen (HBsAg) and hepatitis B surface antibody (anti-HBs). Additional tests, such as HepB core antibody (anti-HBc), may be performed to assess previous exposure. Vaccination is highly recommended for those who have not been previously vaccinated or who do not have evidence of immunity.

Unvaccinated HCPs and/or those who cannot document previous vaccination should receive either a two-dose series of Heplisav-B at 0 and 1 month or a three-dose series of either Engerix-B or Recombivax HB at 0, 1, and 6 months.

After completing the HepB vaccine series, HCW may undergo postvaccination testing to ensure an adequate immune response. This typically involves testing for anti-HB antibody levels.

If adequate anti-HBs (at least 10 mIU/mL) is present, no further antibody testing should be done, and no further HepB vaccine doses are recommended, even if subsequent antibody tests showed a titer of <10 mIU/mL.

If an HCW tests positive for HBsAg, indicating current infection, appropriate management, and follow-up are necessary. This may involve referral to a specialist, initiation of antiviral therapy, and implementation of infection control measures to prevent transmission to others.

Flu Vaccination

It is highly recommended for all HCWs to protect both themselves and the patients they care for. All HCWs should receive the flu vaccine every year, as the flu virus strains can change from season to season. Vaccination is the most important way to prevent the spread of the flu.

Annual vaccination ensures that HCWs are protected against the most prevalent flu strains and should aim to receive the flu vaccine before the start of the flu season. Getting vaccinated early helps to ensure optimal protection throughout the flu season. The specific vaccine type may depend on factors such as age, health status, and availability. By getting vaccinated against the flu, HCWs play a vital role in protecting themselves, their patients, and the community from the flu virus.

Measles Vaccination

Those without evidence of immunity should get two doses of the measles, mumps, rubella (MMR) vaccine, separated by at least 28 days. The Centers for Disease Control and Prevention (CDC) recommends that most adults born in 1957 or later who cannot show that they have had all three diseases get an MMR vaccine. Those born before 1957 should be considered for MMR vaccination in the absence of an outbreak. During an outbreak of measles, healthcare facilities should recommend two doses of the MMR vaccine for unvaccinated personnel born before 1957. If a measles case or an outbreak occurs within or in the areas served by a hospital, clinic, or other medical or nursing facility, all personnel regardless of birth year, should receive two doses of MMR vaccine, unless they have other documentation of measles immunity.

Meningococcal Vaccine

It is not common for HCW to become infected with meningococcal disease from patients, but it can occur if there is direct exposure to saliva or respiratory secretions (whether from contact with patients or saliva or sputum samples obtained for the laboratory). This is especially true during outbreaks at universities or colleges where the disease can spread rapidly through residence halls. Two doses of MenACWY, given ≥8 weeks apart and followed by a booster every 5 years, are required for adults who have anatomic or functional asplenia, HIV infection, or persistent complement component deficiencies or who take eculizumab or eculizumab.

Pertussis

After exposure to pertussis, HCW requires antibiotic postexposure prophylaxis (PPE). If not receiving PPE, restrict from contact (e.g., furlough, duty restriction, or reassignment) with patients and other persons at increased risk for severe pertussis for 21 days after the last exposure may consider a single dose of Tdap.

Polio

Unvaccinated HCWs (rare) should be given three doses of IPV at the recommended intervals.

Respiratory Syncytial Virus

New respiratory syncytial virus (RSV) vaccines are available for adults 60 and older. Healthcare providers should be aware of underlying conditions that may increase the risk of severe RSV illness, and who might be most likely to benefit from these new vaccines.

Currently, the RSV vaccine series consists of a single dose. Studies are ongoing to determine whether older adults might benefit from receiving additional RSV vaccines in the future. Healthcare providers should consider the RSV vaccine especially adults ages 60 and older—two RSV vaccines (Arexvy by GSK and Abrysvo by Pfizer) have been licensed by FDA and recommended by CDC for adults ages 60 and older, using shared clinical decision-making.

Healthcare pregnant women: One RSV vaccine (Abrysvo by Pfizer) has been licensed and recommended during weeks 32 through 36 of pregnancy to protect both them and their infants.

So far, RSV vaccines appear to provide some protection for at least two RSV seasons.

Rubella

In many healthcare settings, HCWs are strongly recommended or required to provide documentation of their immunization status or undergo serologic testing to confirm their immunity to rubella if they have not been previously vaccinated. This is done to ensure that HCW is adequately protected and not at risk of transmitting the disease to patients.

SARS-CoV-2

The requirements for severe acute respiratory syndrome coronavirus-2 (SARS-CoV-2) (COVID-19) vaccination for HCW may vary depending on the country, healthcare facility, and local guidelines. However, COVID-19 vaccination is strongly recommended for HCWs due to their increased risk of exposure to the virus and the potential for transmission to vulnerable patients.

- Healthcare staff were among the first to be prioritized for vaccination in many countries to protect against the spread of the virus.
- National and international health authorities recommend COVID-19 vaccination for all eligible individuals, including HCWs. The specific vaccine(s) authorized for use may vary by country. HCWs are typically considered a priority group for COVID-19 vaccination due to their frontline role in patient care.
- HCWs may be required to provide documentation of COVID-19 vaccination to their employers or regulatory bodies. This documentation may include proof of vaccination dates, vaccine type, and any booster doses.
- HCWs should be informed about the potential side effects of COVID-19 vaccines and the importance of reporting any adverse events. Monitoring systems should be in place to track and manage any vaccine-related concerns among HCWs.

Varicella (Chickenpox)

In many countries, including the United States, HCWs are strongly recommended to receive the varicella vaccine, to protect themselves and their patients from the disease. However, specific requirements may differ depending on the healthcare facility, local regulations, and individual circumstances.

- The CDC in the United States recommends that all healthcare personnel without evidence of immunity to varicella should receive two doses of the varicella vaccine.
- HCWs may require employees to undergo immunity testing (serologic testing) to determine if they are already immune to varicella.
- Facilities may require HCWs to provide documentation of their vaccination or immunity status. Those who are not immune may be recommended to receive the vaccine.
- Check with your specific healthcare facility's occupational health policies and guidelines for the most accurate information on varicella vaccination requirements.

CHECKING FOR IMMUNITY OR HISTORY OF PREVIOUS VACCINATION (SCREENING)

In countries with established and high-performing immunization programs, younger HCWs may have already received the recommended vaccinations in their childhood or before entering the workforce, or through health worker vaccination programs offered at previous places of employment.

In some settings (e.g., where measles is still endemic or where HepB is known to be highly prevalent) a substantial portion of adults may already have acquired natural immunity through prior infection or exposure. Policies may therefore specify that serological testing for confirmation of immunity, where available and reliable, be accepted instead of requiring revaccination.

Healthcare workers have a responsibility to know their immune status and share the obligation to protect themselves and their patients. Unvaccinated/nonimmune may be temporarily (or permanently) reassigned to areas where they are less likely to encounter high-risk patients or be required to wear personal protective equipment such as face masks while caring for patients. For health workers who refuse or opt out of vaccination for nonmedical reasons, some policies include repercussions such as mandatory unpaid leave during an outbreak or periods of peak transmission, or even requirements to appear before a committee to explain reasons for not following the policy.

ETHICAL ISSUES ASSOCIATED WITH HCWs VACCINATION

The main issues at which ethical decisions must be made are individual, institutional, and governmental policies. The role of institutions in terms of promoting or mandating vaccination is the subject of ongoing ethics debates.

All frameworks could accommodate a mandatory vaccination policy with termination of employment for offenders, but it should be preceded by a successful educational campaign for most of them, and a consensus should be reached before the implementation of a mandate. This is especially true when considering that a mandate without a consensus can lead to a serious backlash against vaccines in general.

CONCLUSION

Vaccination of HCWs is an important aspect of comprehensive programs such as infection, prevention and control (IPC) and occupational health and safety (OHS). Direct protection for health workers will maintain the function and resilience of the health system. Indirectly, it will also contribute to the protection of vulnerable patients and increase the likelihood of health workers recommending vaccination to their patients.

Healthcare professionals must recognize that vaccines have benefits and risks, which misunderstand current global recommendations and programmatic considerations for establishing and/or strengthening platforms for the vaccination of health workers.

Improving vaccine coverage among HCWs is challenging, but benefits patients getting contagious diseases from attending HCWs. Education and academic leadership play a role here, but other interventions can be useful and must continue to be tried and implemented. In addition to vaccination, traditional infection control measures also have a role to play.

Nosocomial transmission of VPDs can be avoided thanks to immunization. The ideal coverage is dynamic for each disease, depending on the effective reproductive rate, which itself varies with the level of herd immunity in the population (from vaccination and infection), and the density of contacts.

SUGGESTED READING

1. Arjun P, Abraham SV, Koul PA. Knowledge, attitude and practices toward seasonal influenza vaccination among healthcare workers. Lung India. 2022;39(5):437-42.
2. https://www.cdc.gov/vaccines/adults/rec-vac/index.html

21 Vaccine Hesitancy and Providing Confidence in Vaccinations

■ INTRODUCTION

The World Health Organization (WHO) defines "vaccine hesitancy" as the "delay in accepting or refusing immunization" due to the perception of low disease risk, reduced accessibility, and lack of confidence in safety and efficacy. It is a complicated phenomenon that is closely related to social contexts and has various elements such as historical events, confidence in vaccines, geographical setting, and political background.

Vaccine hesitancy or uncertainty is a significant barrier to vaccination coverage increasing the risk of vaccine preventable disease (VPD) outbreaks and epidemics.

Vaccine hesitancy is an important health threat to communities and has been since the first smallpox vaccine became available >200 years ago. The extent of vaccine hesitancy varies by community and type of immunization. In recent years, antivaccinationists have been known as "antivaxxers" or "antivax" and "antivaccinationism" refers to total opposition to vaccination. *Vaccine hesitancy is nothing new. Pockets of people have criticized vaccines for ages.* This may have increased in the face of widespread misinformation and disinformation, political polarization, and the Covid-19 pandemic.

In the 20th century, several vaccines have drawn praise and anger. The US entered a golden age of vaccine development from the 1920s through the 1970s with the arrival of vaccines for diphtheria, pertussis, polio, measles, mumps, and rubella (MMR). Opposition diminished as infection rates, particularly for polio, fell. As vaccines to protect people from COVID-19 started becoming available in late 2020, the rhetoric of antivaccine groups intensified. Efforts to keep vaccines out of arms reinforce misinformation about the safety and effectiveness of the vaccines and spread disinformation—deliberately misleading people for political, ideological, or other reasons.

Vaccine hesitancy, also known as immunization hesitancy, refers to the reluctance or refusal of individuals or communities, to accept vaccines despite the availability of vaccination services. The antivaccine movement has gained traction in many countries since the COVID-19 pandemic began. The plethora of literature about the vaccine hesitation phenomenon is becoming more common during the severe acute respiratory syndrome coronavirus 2 (SARS-CoV-2) pandemic and following the marketing of the various types of COVID-19 vaccines. Exploratory analysis reveals that COVID-19 vaccine hesitancy has a negative and statistically significant impact on COVID-19 vaccinations.

- Vaccine hesitancy can stem from a variety of factors, including individual and religious beliefs, societal attitudes, and misinformation.

In India, COVID-19 is yet not completely over; however, many people are hesitant to take COVID-19 vaccines despite their availability. It is now well recognized that vaccine hesitancy is not a monolithic issue, and it varies by region and population. Addressing it effectively requires a "nuanced and adaptable" approach that takes into account the unique factors influencing each community or individual.

The vaccination schedule in India is designed to ensure timely and comprehensive immunity against various diseases. According to NFHS-5 (National Family Health Survey) 2019-21, the country's full immunization coverage is 76.1 percent. Despite the availability of vaccines, many parents in India remain hesitant and uninformed of the serious diseases that can harm their children if they do not receive proper vaccinations at the right time.

Vaccine hesitancy can have significant public health implications, as it can lead to lower vaccination rates. Addressing vaccine hesitancy is crucial for achieving herd immunity and preventing the spread of vaccine-preventable diseases. Here are some approaches to provide confidence in vaccinations and to provide overviews to combat the phenomenon of vaccine hesitancy.

■ SAFETY CONCERNS

Vaccine-hesitant individuals may worry about potential side effects or long-term risks associated with vaccines.

Rare adverse events can receive significant media attention and fuel concerns. However, it is important to note that vaccines undergo rigorous testing for safety and efficacy before they are approved for use.

Spikes in vaccine hesitancy often coincide with new information, new policies, or newly reported vaccine risks. These aspects use the examples of hesitancy regarding pertussis, MMR, human papillomavirus (HPV), and COVID-19 vaccines to look at the multifaceted issues that fuel vaccine hesitancy. Each of these examples is part of a larger, complex story.

However, the pertussis component of the diphtheria, tetanus, and pertussis (DPT/DTP) vaccine was responsible for severe postvaccine reactions, such as febrile seizures and encephalopathy, or nonfocal diseases of the brain, that occurred infrequently post-DTP vaccination. During the late 1970s and early 1980s, there was significant controversy concerning the safety of the pertussis component. One large study conducted in England between 1976 and 1979 suggested that encephalopathy was more common following DTP vaccination, but still rare (1 in 110,000 vaccinations) with long-term effects being seen in 1 in 310,000 vaccinations.

Likewise, claims of a link between the MMR vaccine and autism have been extensively investigated and found to be false. The link was first suggested in the early 1990s and came to public notice largely as a result of the 1998 Lancet MMR autism fraud, characterized as "perhaps the most damaging medical hoax of the last 100 years". The fraudulent research paper authored by Andrew Wakefield and published in The Lancet falsely claimed the vaccine was linked to colitis and autism spectrum disorders.

Vaccines are notable scientific achievements that have significantly reduced rates of death and disease around the world, underpinning public confidence in today's vaccines. Together, the accumulated scientific evidence explains the far-sightedness of routine immunization are the safest of all medications. Before FDA licensing, vaccines were studied in larger populations than other drugs. Once licensed and put to use, multiple layers of safety surveillance continue as long as the vaccines are distributed.

Every scientific authority, including WHO, the Centers for Disease Control and Prevention, globally, Academic Medical Associations, the National Academy of Medicine, and every Nation's health department, recommends routine vaccinations. To improve vaccination uptake, it is crucial to address the systemic and personal needs of each individual.

Parents can be reassured to know that there have been hundreds of large-scale studies around the world on vaccine safety during the past few decades. They demonstrate that recommended vaccines are safe for children and teens. Vaccines are not associated with conditions such as diabetes, problems with fertility, autism, or developmental delay. Vaccine ingredients are safe. Measles-containing vaccines are safe.

Research continues to confirm that vaccines are safe and effective, and they protect children and teens from serious diseases.

Adult immunization has recently emerged as an area of great emphasis in research and policy. Increasing life expectancy, outbreaks like COVID-19, and the endemic nature of diseases such as dengue, and malaria have underscored its importance.

- Yes, vaccines are generally safe and effective for adults, just as they are for pediatric populations, and have a long history of safety and effectiveness in both pediatric and adult populations.
- Vaccine safety monitoring systems allow for the ongoing assessment of vaccine safety in real-world conditions and the prompt identification of any rare or unexpected side effects.
- Vaccines undergo extensive clinical trials involving adults to assess their safety and effectiveness.

While vaccines are generally safe for adults, it is important to consider individual factors such as underlying health conditions, allergies, or specific contraindications. Healthcare providers assess these factors and make recommendations based on an individual's medical history and risk-benefit valuation.

- *Lack of trust:* Some people may not trust the pharmaceutical companies that produce vaccines, government health agencies, or healthcare providers. Mistrust in healthcare systems or pharmaceutical companies can also contribute to vaccine hesitancy.
  - Convincing individuals with vaccine hesitancy or mistrust requires a thoughtful and empathetic approach. Should offer them support and resources to help individuals make informed decisions. Include providing educational materials, connecting them with healthcare professionals for further discussions, or addressing any logistical barriers to vaccination.

- *Cultural beliefs, religious, or philosophical principles including peer pressure* can influence vaccine hesitancy. For example, some communities may stigmatize vaccination or prioritize alternative medicine. Understanding and addressing these factors are important when providing support to individuals who are hesitant about vaccines.
  - Building trust and establishing open lines of communication are key components of community engagement to promote accurate information and positive attitudes toward vaccination. It is important to approach counseling with cultural humility, respect, and a willingness to listen and understand the perspectives of individuals and communities.
  - Certain religious groups may oppose vaccines that contain animal-derived components or those that go against their beliefs. which can impact their decision to vaccinate. Religious reasons are distinct from other factors in that they are generally linked to core principles, which makes it extremely difficult to convince individuals to change their opinions on immunization.
- *Misinformation and disinformation:* The spread of false or misleading information about vaccines on social media and other platforms can contribute to vaccine hesitancy. This misinformation can include claims about vaccines causing autism, containing harmful ingredients, or being part of a government conspiracy.
  - Antivaccination activism has existed as long as there have been vaccines. But the movement picked up steam in 1998 when British physician Andrew Wakefield published a now-discredited study that falsely claimed a link between childhood vaccines and autism.
  - Handling vaccine misinformation and disinformation requires a multifaceted approach that involves addressing false claims, promoting accurate information, and building trust in reliable sources. This can involve debunking myths and engaging with social media platforms to limit the spread of false information.
- *Vaccine mandates and government policies:* Related to vaccination can sometimes lead to resistance and hesitancy. Some individuals may perceive these mandates as infringing on personal freedoms or distrust the motivations behind them.
  - *Legislation and policies:* Implementing vaccine mandates or strengthening vaccine requirements for certain activities, such as attending school or traveling, can increase vaccine uptake through legislation and health guidelines.
- Despite evidence of the vaccine's safety profile, closing the gap on the remaining unvaccinated adolescents and adults; "will likely require a mix of current and newer approaches to address vaccine hesitancy".
- *Ongoing research and surveillance:* Continuously monitoring vaccine safety and efficacy and promptly addressing any concerns is crucial to maintaining public confidence in vaccines. In this way, should work toward achieving higher vaccination rates and protecting individuals and communities from vaccine-preventable diseases.

ENCAPSULATE

- It is essential to double down on efforts to increase confidence and trust in vaccines Because of the complexity of this issue, addressing parental vaccine hesitancy requires partnerships among academic experts in various disciplines, community leaders, policymakers, public health professionals, and parents.
- Addressing this breadth of concerns requires a multifaceted approach that addresses individual and social concerns as these are often interlinked.
- Vaccine-hesitant parents who are on the fence far outnumber vaccine refusers; therefore, counseling this group might be more effective. The reasons behind vaccine hesitancy are complex and encompass more than just a knowledge deficit. As a trusted source of information on vaccines, pediatricians and family physicians play a key role in driving vaccine acceptance.
- Importantly, healthcare providers, public health agencies, and trusted sources should communicate and discuss the benefits, safety, and importance of vaccines in a clear and accessible manner. Rather than labeling individuals as "anti-vaxxers". It is more beneficial to engage in open and respectful conversations to address their concerns.
- Some individuals may have been exposed to misinformation or myths about vaccines through social media, websites, or word of mouth. Addressing these misconceptions with accurate information can be helpful. Engaging with people, understanding their concerns, and involving them in decision-making

processes can help address vaccine hesitancy effectively.
- For those who may have religious or philosophical objections to vaccines, it is essential to approach discussions with understanding and respect for diverse perspectives while providing the right useful information on how vaccines align with public health goals. It is important to explain the risks and potential complications associated with natural infection compared to the safety and efficacy of vaccines. And ensuring equitable access to vaccines and addressing barriers to vaccination, such as cost or availability, in reducing vaccine hesitancy.
- Education about the importance of maintaining high vaccination rates for community immunity can be helpful. It is crucial to approach these conversations with empathy, respect, and a willingness to listen. Public health efforts often focus on providing accurate information, debunking myths, and addressing concerns to promote vaccine acceptance and protect community health.

■ SUGGESTED READING

1. Dubé E, Laberge C, Guay M, Bramadat P, Roy R, Bettinger J. Vaccine hesitancy: an overview. Hum Vaccin Immunother. 2013;9(8):1763-73.
2. Gidengil C, Goetz MB, Maglione M, Newberry SJ, Chen P, O'Hollaren K, et al. Agency Healthc Rese Qual. 2021:21-EHC024.
3. Higgins DM, O'Leary ST. The risks of normalizing parental vaccine hesitancy. N Engl J Med. 2024;390:485-7.
4. Larson HJ, Gakidou E, Murray CJL. The vaccine-hesitant moment. N Engl J Med. 2022;387(1):58-65.
5. Science & Society. (2021). Vaccine hesitancy is nothing new. Here's the damage it's done over centuries. Available from: https://www.sciencenews.org/article/vaccine-hesitancy-history-damage-anti-vaccination [Last accessed April, 2024].

22 Some Facts, Myths, and Misconceptions

■ INTRODUCTION

Myths and misinformation about vaccines can spread quickly and have a detrimental impact on public health. Sahadulla et al. (2018–2022) have answered many such commonly encountered parental doubts on "vaccines-related misinformation and immunization in their earlier publications".

During these coronavirus disease 2019 (COVID-19) pandemic years, they have continually reemphasized vaccine's importance and its human values. Parental and public concerns and misconceptions about immunization are dealt with factual information beyond what they have already dealt with on this subject. Here are some common myths circulating about the vaccine and clear up confusion with reliable facts about vaccines and immunizations.

Again, the facts are that vaccines and vaccinations have been repeatedly demonstrated to be one of the most effective interventions to prevent many life-threatening diseases. Most of the arguments against vaccination appeal to the public and parents are understandably derived from speculative fears and worries. Groundless allegations regarding adverse effects from vaccines including autism, sudden infant death syndrome (SIDS), multiple sclerosis, etc. and in some instances, concerns about the safety of certain vaccines have led to declines in vaccination rates and outbreaks of disease. Potential immunologic overload resulting from concomitant vaccination with too many antigens as a result of infant immunization is a parental and societal concern that may limit confidence in and thus affect immunization programs.

It is crucial to rely on accurate information from reputable sources, such as health organizations and medical professionals, when making decisions about vaccinations. Here are some common myths and the corresponding facts.

▌ LET US BUST MYTHS AND LEARN THE FACTS ABOUT COVID-19 VACCINES

Further, there are concise pieces of information on a range of vaccine-related topics ("*Fast facts*"), to some of the common "Myths and Misconceptions" that are frequently come across by healthcare professionals:

Myth: Vaccinations only matter for children.
Fast facts:
- Childhood vaccines are important, but that is not the only time you may need a vaccine. Vaccines are crucial for individuals of all ages.
- Vaccines for adults are recommended based on various factors such as age, prior vaccinations, health conditions, lifestyle, occupation, and travel.
- Certain vaccines, such as influenza and pneumonia vaccines, are recommended for adults, especially those with underlying health conditions.
- The various vaccines for adults recommended by the Centers for Disease Control and Prevention (CDC), United States and Advisory Committee on Immunization Practices (ACIP), United States.

Myth: I received all the childhood vaccines as a child, so I did not need vaccines anymore any longer.
Fast fact: While childhood vaccinations provide initial protection against many diseases, immunity can wane over time. It is essential to receive booster shots or additional vaccines to maintain optimal protection.

The vaccines recommended for adults over the age 19 years vary from those for children. The recommended vaccination schedule for adults may vary based on factors such as age, health condition, occupation, and travel plans. Additionally, new vaccines have been introduced in recent years that target-specific diseases prevalent in adulthood.

Adult vaccination is a crucial aspect of maintaining good health and preventing the spread of diseases.

Myth: Some parents believe in "not to vaccinate their children" because all the other children around them are already immune.
Fast facts: Herd immunity occurs when a large portion of a community is immunized against a contagious disease, reducing the chance of an outbreak. Infants, pregnant women, and immunocompromised people who cannot

receive vaccines depend on this type of protection. However, if enough people rely on herd immunity as the method of preventing infection from vaccine-preventable diseases, herd immunity will soon disappear.

Myths: Vaccines cause autism and SIDS.

Fast facts:
- Extensive research has found no credible evidence linking vaccines to the development of autism or SIDS. Science has not yet determined the cause of autism and SIDS. These diagnoses are made though, during the same age range that children are receiving their routine immunizations.
- The 1998 study that raised concerns about a possible link between the measles–mumps–rubella (MMR) vaccine and autism was retracted by the journal that published it because it was significantly flawed by bad science.
- One of the most definitive findings of no causal link between the MMR vaccine and autism was by a Danish group and published in the New England Journal of Medicine (NEJM) in 2002. The authors reviewed the records of more than half a million children born in Denmark during the study period (1991–1998) and found no association between age at vaccination, receipt of vaccination, or time passed since vaccination and the development of autism spectrum disorders.
- Large epidemiological studies clearly refuted the postulated link and have substantively affirmed that vaccination, and the MMR vaccine in particular, have neither a correlative nor causative link to autism spectrum disorders.

The benefits of vaccination greatly outweigh the risks and without vaccines, many more injuries and deaths would have occurred.

Myths: Vaccines can overload the immune system.

Fast facts:
- Vaccines contain only a small fraction of the antigens that the immune system naturally encounters.
- The immune system is capable of handling the antigens present in vaccines along with the numerous other challenges it encounters daily.
- "Most vaccines contain weakened or killed germs, which are not strong enough to overwhelm the immune system".

Myth: Vaccines weaken our immune system.

Fast facts:
- Vaccines and immunizations do not weaken overall immune systems, instead vaccines can strengthen our immune system by training it to recognize and fight specific pathogens.
- Vaccines stimulate the immune system without causing the disease, strengthening the body's ability to fight off the actual infection.
- Although there are slight differences in the ways that the various COVID-19 vaccines work, they all follow the same principle. They help the body create immunity or resistance to severe acute respiratory syndrome coronavirus 2 (SARS-CoV-2), the virus that causes COVID-19 by mimicking an infection. The immune system then remembers how to fight that infection in the future.
- COVID-19 vaccines strengthen and prime the body's immune response and help prevent serious COVID-19 disease and hospitalization.
- It is essential to rely on credible sources of information, such as public health agencies and healthcare professionals, to get accurate and up-to-date information about vaccines.

Myth: Natural immunity is better than vaccine-induced immunity.

Fast facts: While natural infection can provide immunity, it also carries risks of severe illness, complications, and death. Vaccination is a safer way to achieve immunity without the same risks.

Myth: The COVID-19 vaccines can give you COVID-19 disease!

Fast facts:
- No vaccine is 100% effective. All of the current COVID-19 vaccines approved for use in the United States do not contain the live virus, which means you cannot contract COVID-19 from these vaccines.
- The COVID-19 vaccine is a safer and more dependable way to build immunity to SARS-CoV-2, the virus that causes COVID-19 than getting sick with COVID-19.
- Vaccination causes a more predictable immune response than an infection with the virus that causes it. Vaccines do not create or cause variants of the virus that causes COVID-19.
- Some people may experience mild side effects such as fever or fatigue after vaccination, but these are signs that the body is building immunity and not getting sick with the virus.

Myth: The COVID-19 vaccines were rushed and are not safe.

Fast facts:
- Yes, there was an unprecedented, incredible amount of work that went into the COVID-19 vaccine discovery and distribution.
- In a sense of worldwide urgency with great scientific attention and an incredible amount of teamwork to help make the vaccine possible and to save lives.
- The COVID-19 vaccines went through rigorous testing in clinical trials to ensure their safety and efficacy.
- The speed of development was due to first-time global collaboration and investment not because safety was compromised.
- The vaccines authorized for emergency use or full approval by health authorities such as the Food and Drug Administration (FDA) and the World Health Organization (WHO) have undergone thorough repeated and ongoing review processes.

Myth: Vaccines contain many harmful ingredients, so the vaccines are not safe.

Fast facts:
- Vaccine ingredients are carefully selected and monitored for safety. Common ingredients such as thimerosal, formaldehyde, and aluminum are present in tiny amounts and is a widely used preservatives for vaccines that are manufactured in multidose vials.
- Vaccines contain ingredients at a dose that is even lower than the dose we are naturally exposed to in our environment. Thimerosal, a mercury-containing compound, is naturally exposed to mercury in milk, seafood, and contact lens solutions. There is no evidence to suggest that the amount of thimerosal used in vaccines poses a health risk. Many vaccines are now produced in single-dose vials, which have greatly decreased the use of thimerosal in vaccine production.
- Formaldehyde, another vaccine ingredient, is in automobile exhaust, household products, and furnishings, such as carpets, upholstery, cosmetics, paint and felt-tip markers, and in health products, such as antihistamines, cough drops, and mouthwash. The dose of vaccines is much lower than the amount we are exposed to in our daily lives.
- Another example of an ingredient in vaccines is aluminum which is added in order to boost and build a stronger immunity to the vaccine. Not all vaccines contain aluminum, but those that do typically contain aluminum in amounts that are much less than what the average person consumes in a day from foods, drinking water, and medicines.

Myth: A child can get the disease from a vaccine.

Fast facts:
- A vaccine causing complete disease would be extremely unlikely.
- Most vaccines are inactivated (killed) vaccines, which makes it impossible to contract the disease from them.
- A few vaccines contain live organisms and when vaccinated with live vaccines, it may lead to a mild case of the disease. Chickenpox vaccine, for example, can cause a child to develop a mild rash. This is not harmful and can actually show that the vaccine is working.
- One exception was the live oral polio vaccine which could very rarely mutate and actually cause a case of polio. However, the oral polio vaccine is no longer administered in many developed nations including the United States.

Myth: Vaccines are not necessary because the diseases they prevent are "no longer a threat".

Fast facts:
- Vaccine-preventable diseases still exist and can cause outbreaks if vaccination rates decline.
- Globally, studies suggest past suboptimal vaccine coverage has contributed to infectious disease outbreaks in vulnerable populations.
- Vaccines have been successful in reducing the incidence of many diseases, but they are still necessary to maintain herd immunity and protect vulnerable populations.

Myth: Vaccines are not effective and do not work.

Fast facts:
- Vaccines trigger our immune response to recognize and fight disease-causing organisms.
- Vaccines have been proven to be highly effective in preventing diseases and have significantly reduced the incidence of many infectious diseases and saved countless lives.
- Vaccine effectiveness is continuously monitored through ongoing research and surveillance.

Myth: There are microchips in the COVID-19 vaccine.

Fast facts: There are no microchips in the COVID-19 vaccines currently on the market or currently being investigated. The vaccines are not tracking people or gathering their information in any way, shape, or form.

Myth: Those already had COVID-19 and recovered do not need to be vaccinated.

Fast facts:
- There is not enough information available to determine how long immunity against the SARS-CoV-2 virus will last after recovering from the infection.
- Studies are ongoing to determine how long natural immunity lasts; however, there is some evidence that immunity may not last long.
- The CDC currently recommends that you receive a COVID-19 vaccine when you are eligible regardless of whether you already had COVID-19 disease.
- One should schedule his/her vaccine after quarantine or isolation time is complete. For patients who received monoclonal antibodies or convalescent plasma to treat COVID-19 disease, they should wait 90 days before getting the vaccine.

Myth: There are new COVID-19 vaccines that have come up. Do we need the extra protection?

Fast facts:
- Yes, there are a few updated COVID-19 booster shots that have been approved for all people aged 6 months and older.
- The new shot is formulated specifically to target the XBB.1.5 subvariant, which made up a considerable percentage of COVID cases through July 2023 (CDC, WHO).
- Even for those who were vaccinated or got the booster in the past, their COVID-19 immunity has likely waned. The new shot is a chance to strengthen it.

Myth: Which immunity is better: Disease-induced natural immunity or vaccination-induced immunity?

Fast facts:
- Yes, natural immunity can occur after recovering from an infection; it comes with the risk of severe complications and even death.
- Studies now show that both types of immunity are beneficial and do a pretty good job of protecting from severe COVID-19 illness and death.
- "Recent data analyses indicate that disease-induced immunity can be as long-lasting or even longer-lasting in some instances than vaccine-induced immunity".
- Vaccines provide a safer way to develop immunity without the risks associated with the actual disease.
- It is not an either-or situation. Limitations exist with gaining immunity either way.
- According to an analysis published in The Lancet Infectious Diseases, a recent, robust study shows that hybrid immunity is longer lasting and more effective than disease-induced immunity or vaccination alone. *(Hybrid immunity = Natural immunity + vaccination)*

Myth: Individuals who have comorbidities such as diabetes and heart disease cannot take the COVID vaccines.

Fast facts:
- A comorbid person should get vaccinated as soon as possible because COVID complications are more common in people with such comorbidities.
- It is recommended to consult the doctor before getting vaccinated.

Myth: COVID-19 vaccines can alter human deoxyribonucleic acid (DNA).

Fast facts:
- The genetic material delivered by messenger ribonucleic acid (mRNA) vaccines never enters the nucleus of our cells, which is where our DNA is kept, so the vaccine does not alter the DNA.
- Both mRNA and protein subunit COVID-19 vaccines work by delivering instructions (genetic material) to our cells to start building protection against the virus that causes COVID-19.
- None of the authorized COVID-19 vaccines in the United States, Europe, or most other countries can alter our DNA. They use different mechanisms like mRNA or viral vector technology to stimulate an immune response. These mechanisms do not change our genetic code. After the body produces an immune response, it gets rid of all the vaccine ingredients just as it would get rid of.

Myth: Vaccination and the risk of childhood cancer

Fast facts: Literature-reported results are consistent with the hypothesis that vaccinations reduce the risk of childhood leukemia.
- Literature evidences an inverse association between Bacillus Calmette–Guérin (BCG) vaccination and leukemia death, Hemophilus influenzae type b (Hib) vaccination and acute lymphoblastic leukemia (ALL), and a high number of unspecified vaccinations and ALL as well as leukemia.
- Large cohort studies are needed to assess the association between different types of vaccinations and specific childhood cancers.

Myth: Can I have the second or subsequent dose with a different vaccine than the previous dose?

Fast facts:
- It is safe for you to receive a second primary, first booster, or any additional booster dose with a different COVID-19 vaccine than the one used for the previous dose(s), according to your country's recommendations.
- Depending on the type of vaccine, using a different type of vaccine may even provide better protection than using the same type of vaccine.
- *Mixing and matching COVID-19 vaccine booster doses:* Mixing vaccines may enhance the immune response and it increases flexibility for when people need a booster dose but doses of the vaccine they first received are not available.

Myth: The COVID-19 vaccines contain microchips that can track you and can make people magnetic.

Fast facts:
- There is no evidence to support this claim. COVID-19 vaccines do not contain microchips or tracking devices. Such claims are baseless conspiracy theories.
- COVID-19 vaccines are free from metals such as iron, nickel, cobalt, lithium, and rare earth alloys.
- They do not contain ingredients that can produce an electromagnetic field at the site of your injection.
- In fact, vaccines work by stimulating the immune system to produce antibodies. After getting vaccinated, people develop immunity to that disease, without having to get the disease first.

Myth: COVID-19 vaccines and people with cancer

Fast facts:
- The CDC recommends that everyone aged 6 months and older stay up to date with COVID-19 vaccination. That includes most people with underlying medical conditions, including cancer.
- A number of research groups are studying COVID-19 vaccine efficacy in people with cancer, from those with solid tumors to those receiving bone marrow transplants.
- For example, there are researchers looking at people who have blood cancers, like chronic lymphocytic leukemia (CLL) or chronic myeloid leukemia (CML) because they are more likely to have immunodeficiency over a long period of time.
- Data from immunosuppressed patient populations have indicated that additional COVID-19 vaccine doses in the primary series and boosters can help improve immune responses in some people with cancer.

Myth: You do not need to wear masks or practice social distancing after getting vaccinated.

Fast facts:
- While vaccines are highly effective at preventing illness, they are not 100% foolproof.
- It is important to follow public health guidelines, which may include mask wearing and social distancing until a sufficient portion of the population is vaccinated and the spread of the virus is controlled.
- The question of whether to drop or to continue wearing face masks especially after being vaccinated is controversial.
- Studies show that the increased extent of wearing of face masks by vaccinated individuals at increasing levels of vaccine and face mask average protection results in a highly accelerated decrease in COVID-19 infections.

Myth: COVID-19 vaccines can affect fertility.

Fast facts:
- Currently, no evidence shows that any vaccines, including COVID-19 vaccines, cause fertility problems (problems trying to get pregnant) in women or men.
- COVID-19 vaccination is recommended for people who are pregnant, trying to get pregnant now, or might become pregnant in the future, as well as their partners.
- As of this date and time, there is no scientific evidence to suggest that COVID-19 vaccines can affect fertility. Extensive clinical trials and ongoing monitoring of vaccine safety have not shown any conclusive evidence linking COVID-19 vaccines to fertility problems.

Rumors and misinformation about COVID-19 vaccines and fertility have circulated on social media and other platforms, causing unnecessary concern. It is important to rely on credible sources of information, such as health authorities and medical experts, for accurate and up-to-date information regarding COVID-19 vaccines and their safety.

Myth: Pregnant women should avoid vaccines.

Fast fact: Vaccination during pregnancy helps protect both the mother and the developing baby. Certain vaccines, such as the flu shot and tetanus–diphtheria–acellular pertussis (Tdap), are recommended for pregnant women to reduce the risk of complications and protect newborns through passive immunity.

In general, the CDC recommends pregnant people receiving influenza vaccine be given in any trimester of pregnancy. One dose of Tdap is recommended during each pregnancy, preferably between the 27th and 36th week of gestation to protect the newborn against whooping cough.

Likewise, pregnant people should receive the respiratory syncytial virus (RSV) vaccine between the 32nd and 36th week of gestation to protect the newborn. COVID-19 can be more severe in pregnancy. Ensure you are up-to-date with the recommended updated COVID-19 vaccine.

Myth: COVID-19 vaccines can cause long-term health problems.

Fast facts:
- Extensive monitoring and research have found that the authorized COVID-19 vaccines are safe and do not cause long-term health problems.
- The benefits of vaccination in preventing severe illness and death far outweigh any potential risks.

The available COVID-19 vaccines, including Pfizer-BioNTech, Moderna, Johnson & Johnson, AstraZeneca, and others have been administered to hundreds of millions of people worldwide. These vaccines went through extensive clinical trials involving tens of thousands of participants before receiving emergency use authorization or full approval from regulatory agencies in various countries.

It is important to note that vaccine safety is continuously monitored through various systems, such as the Vaccine Adverse Event Reporting System (VAERS) in the United States and similar programs in other countries. These systems allow for the identification and investigation of any potential adverse events associated with vaccines, including rare ones.

Myth: COVID-19 vaccines cause new variants.

Fast facts:
- The development of new variants is a natural occurrence in viruses, including the SARS-CoV-2 virus that causes COVID-19. New variants of the COVID-19 virus (SARS-CoV-2) happen because the virus constantly changes through a natural ongoing process of mutation (change).
- COVID-19 vaccines do not create or cause variants of the virus. As the COVID-19 virus spreads, it has more opportunities to change.
- There is currently no scientific evidence to support the claim that SARS-CoV-2 vaccines cause the emergence of new variants. Vaccines are designed to target-specific viral proteins and stimulate an immune response against those proteins.
- While some variants may exhibit reduced susceptibility to certain vaccines, authorized COVID-19 vaccines have shown effectiveness against multiple variants, including the Delta variant. Vaccination remains a crucial tool in reducing the severity of illness, hospitalizations, and deaths caused by COVID-19, including variants.

Vaccination plays a critical role in controlling the spread of the virus and reducing the likelihood of new variants emerging. By reducing the number of infections and transmission, vaccines help limit the opportunities for the virus to mutate and generate new variants. Monitoring and research—ongoing surveillance and research are conducted to monitor the emergence of new variants and assess their impact on vaccine effectiveness. This allows for the identification of any potential changes in the virus and the development of strategies to address them, such as updating vaccine formulations if necessary (WHO, CDC).

Myth: Administering the MMR vaccine may diminish septic inflammation associated with the COVID-19 infection.

Fast facts:
- Although a little scientifically weird, it is worth pursuing to find out cross-protective effects of the MMR vaccine; after all, these are all RNA viruses!
- Researchers' intent is needed to have a clinical trial to test the efficacy of MMR vaccine in protecting COVID-19 and, in the meantime, suggest that all adults, healthcare workers, and individuals in nursing homes, in particular, get the vaccine.

Myth: Giving combination (combos) vaccinations, i.e., multiple vaccines in a single visit may overwhelm or weaken the children's immune systems.

Fast fact: It is recommended to vaccinate young children early in life as this is when they are most susceptible to dangerous infectious diseases. Many vaccines are given as combination vaccines. This reduces the number of shots a child receives at each vaccination visit and provides protection early on.

Many studies show that vaccines are as effective when given as a combination, as they are when given individually. More importantly, getting multiple vaccinations does not weaken the child's immune system, which is capable of responding to multiple vaccine antigens at the same time.

MYTHS AND FACTS ABOUT IMMUNOTHERAPY FOR CANCER

Myth: All cancers are curable by immunotherapies.

Fast facts: There is not enough research to say that immunotherapy can help with all types of cancer.

However, evidence suggests that immunotherapy is an effective treatment for lung, kidney, skin, and bladder cancers.

Myth: Immunotherapy makes cancer worse.

Fast facts: With most medical treatments, one can expect to experience side effects. Immunotherapy is no different. The potential side effects individuals may experience can vary based on their cancer stage, overall health, the type of immunotherapy they receive, and other factors.

Myth: Immunotherapy can cure stage 4 cancer.

Fast facts: While immunotherapy does not cure stage 4 cancer, it can improve the quality and longevity of your life. Because immunotherapy is a relatively newer cancer treatment, receiving FDA's approval in 1986, more research is needed to learn about its ability to reduce or eliminate cancer symptoms across all stages.

Myth: Immunotherapy helps with cancer pain management?

Fast facts: Immunotherapy, like other treatments, may help with cancer pain management in people with advanced-stage cancers. One 2022 study involving 356 people with hepatopancreatic biliary cancer found that immunotherapy reduced the need for opioids and helped with pain management.

QUASHING MYTHS ASSOCIATED WITH BRAIN TUMORS

Myth: Brain tumors are always accompanied by severe headaches.

Fast fact: While headaches can be a symptom of brain tumors, they are not always present.

Myth: Cell phone use is dangerous to human health and causes brain tumors.

Fast facts: To date, no conclusive evidence suggests a direct causal relationship between the potential link between cell phone use and brain tumors. Studies published in the Journal of the Neurological Sciences (2017) concluded that in the higher-quality studies, long-term use of mobile phones was linked to an increase in the risk of brain tumors. Long-term use was defined as >10 years or more than 1,640 hours.

The good news is that between 2008 and 2017 in the United States, the overall trend in brain and central nervous system cancer incidence decreased by 0.8% annually.

Myth: Brain tumors are almost always cancerous.

Fast facts: Many brain tumors are noncancerous, while some brain tumors are cancerous and can be effectively treated or managed.

Myth: Brain tumors are always fatal.

Fast fact: Brain tumors can be life-threatening and prognosis/outcomes depend on the tumor type, location, size, and the individual's overall health.

Brain tumors can also be fast growing (high grade) and can recur despite treatment. Early detection, appropriate treatment, and ongoing care can significantly improve the prognosis.

Myth: Does immunotherapy cure brain tumors?

Fast facts: There has been less success in immunotherapy for brain tumors than in other cancer types. When it comes to the brain, immune-based treatments face several obstacles before they can even reach the tumor.

CONCLUSION

It is important to rely on accurate and evidence-based information from reputable sources, such as healthcare professionals, public health organizations, and scientific research, to understand the facts about immunotherapies. Vaccines are a crucial tool in preventing the spread of infectious diseases and protecting individual and public health.

SUGGESTED READING

1. Atmar RL, Lyke KE, Deming ME, Jackson LA, Branche AR, El Sahly HM, et al. Homologous and Heterologous Covid-19 Booster Vaccinations. N Engl J Med. 2022;386: 1046-57.
2. CDC. National Center for Immunization and Respiratory Diseases (NCIRD). (2023). Division of Viral Diseases (DVD). Available from: https://www.cdc.gov/ncird/dvd.html [Last accessed April, 2024].
3. Marron M, Brackmann LK, Kuhse P, Christianson L, Langner I, Haug U, et al. Vaccination and the Risk of Childhood Cancer-A Systematic Review and Meta-Analysis. Front Oncol. 2021;10:610843.
4. Notarte KI, Catahay JA, Velasco JV, Pastrana A, Therese Ver A, Pangilinan FC, et al. Impact of COVID-19 vaccination on

the risk of developing long-COVID and on existing long-COVID symptoms: a systematic review. EClinicalMedicine. 2022;53:101624.
5. Sahadulla MI, Uduman SA (Eds). Vaccinology (Principles and practices: an essential guide). Comprehensive Textbook of Infectious Diseases, 2nd edition. New Delhi: Jaypee Brothers Medical Publishers (P) Ltd.; 2019. pp. 450-89.
6. Sahadulla MIS and Sayenna Uduman. Compendium of the Pandemic Era; SARS-2 CoV 19 Virology Timelines; in Questions & Answers format. KIMS Health, Thiruvananthapuram. DC India Publishers, 2022.
7. Taylor B, Miller E, Farrington CP, Petropoulos MC, Favot-Mayaud I, Li J, et al. Autism and measles, mumps, and rubella vaccine: no epidemiological evidence for a causal association. Lancet. 1999;353(9169):2026-9.
8. Zaçe D, La Gatta E, Petrella L, Di Pietro ML. The impact of COVID-19 vaccines on fertility—a systematic review and meta-analysis. Vaccine. 2022;40(42):6023-34.

Index

Page numbers followed by *f* refer to figure and *t* refer to table.

A

Abciximab 145, 166, 170
Abemaciclib 197
Acellular pertussis 89
Acinetobacter baumannii 260, 264
    infections 265
Acquired immunodeficiency
        syndrome 20, 34, 111
Acyclovir, intravenous 175*f*
Adalimumab 135, 166, 170, 171, 250
Addiction, vaccine against 252
Adenovirus 39, 155, 220, 244, 289
    vaccine 36, 39, 40, 289
        basis of 289
Adipose tissue 236
Adoptive cell therapy 137
Adriamycin 210
Aducanumab 166
Advisory Committee on Immunization
        Practices 173, 320
Aedes
    aegypti 46, 93
    albopictus 46, 93
    mosquito 288, 293
        vectors 65
Alanine aminotransferase 121
Alcohol abuse, chronic 184
Aldesleukin 206
Alemtuzumab 166, 187
Alirocumab 166
Allergens 247
Allergic diseases 247
Allergic reaction 70, 247
Allergies 174, 313
Allogeneic hematopoietic stem-cell
        transplantation 275
Allogenic chimeric antigen receptor
        T-cell therapy 150
Allograft 173
Alpha-beta T-cells 139
Alzheimer's disease 5, 147, 154, 225, 227,
        228, 234
    vaccines 227, 228, 228*t*
American Cancer Society 196, 198
American College of Obstetricians and
        Gynecologists 198
American Society for Colposcopy and
        Cervical Pathology 198

American Society of Transplantations 178
Amivantamab 166
Anakinra 135
Anaphylactic reaction 70
Anaphylaxis 71, 72, 75-82
Angioedema, hereditary 164
Angiotensin 244
Anicteric hepatitis, mild 48
Aniridia 218
Annual flu 84
    vaccine 87
Anopheles mosquitoes 272
Anthrax 92
    vaccine 40, 93
Anti-acetylcholine receptor 232
Anti-allergen monoclonal
        antibodies 247
Antibiotic postexposure prophylaxis 328
Antibody 181
    against early antigen, testing for 281
    cytokine fusion proteins 133
    dependent cell-mediated
        cytotoxicity 140, 147*f*
    directed enzyme prodrug therapy 147*f*
    neutralizing 20, 277
    producing lymphocyte 146
    titer, protective cut-off 49
Anticancer therapy 221
Anti-candida vaccine 272
Anticytotoxic T lymphocyte antigen 194
Antidrug antibodies 146
Antigen
    early 281*f*
    multiple 53
    presentation 39
    presenting cells 191, 258
    selection 192
    single 50
    specific immunity 56
    types of 192
    vaccines 192
Antigenic drift 57
Anti-hemoglobin antibody levels 327
Anti-inflammatory cytokines 251
Antimicrobial prophylaxis 40
Antimicrobial resistance 32, 103, 257,
        259, 295
    bacteria 259

Anti-myasthenia gravis 232
Antiretroviral therapy 113
Antisense oligonucleotide 234
Antivaccinationism 330
Antiviral medicines, direct-acting 278
Applied behavioral analysis 235
Arenavirus 285
Aripo virus 109
Aromatic-L-amino-acid deficiency 163
Arthritis 166, 168, 178
    juvenile idiopathic 170
Artificial intelligence 7, 21, 22, 258, 312
    based epidemiological surveillance
        313, 314*f*
    role of 21
    system 197, 313
    technology 315
Artificial neural networks 22
Aspartate aminotransferase 121
Asplenia 60
    functional 76, 77
Asthma 81, 245, 305
    allergic 5, 38
    severe 147
Astrazeneca's nirsevimab 104
Atezolizumab 166
Atherosclerosis 5, 225
Atovaquone 307
Attenuated live poliovirus strain 9
Atypical hemolytic uremic syndrome 188
    management of 167
Autism 334
    spectrum disorders 162, 309, 235
        development of 335
        higher prevalence of 283
        immunotherapy for 235
Autograft 173
Autoimmune
    diseases 38, 138, 145, 149, 175, 225, 230
    disorder 147, 168, 232
    therapeutics 135
Autologous hematopoietic stem cell
        transplantation 231
Avaxim 302
Avelumab 166, 199, 206
Axalimogene filolisbac 134
Axicabtagene ciloleucel 150, 209
Azidothymidine 276

B

Baby's brain 109*f*
Bacillus anthracis 40
Bacillus Calmette-Guérin 7, 8, 24, 26, 36,
    41, 68, 69, 134, 191, 193, 259,
    316, 326
  history 8
  vaccination 41, 69, 337
  vaccine 40, 41
Bacteremia 60
Bacteria 146, 245
  antibiotic-resistant 294
  based delivery systems 157
  dissemination 270
  extracellular 259
Bacterial cellular vaccines 259
Bacterial diseases 146
Bacterial sexual transmitted infections
  cause of 271
  vaccine against 269
Bacterial vaccines
  preventive 257
  role of 259
Bacterium 265
Bad cells 38
Basiliximab 166, 187
B-cell
  depleting agents 250
  driven 180
  lymphatic leukemia 166
  lymphoma 168
  maturation antigen 209
Beckwith–Wiedemann syndrome 218
Belagenpumatucel-L vaccine 212
Belatacept 188
Belimumab 166
Beneficial monoclonal antibody
    therapies 233
Benralizumab 166, 245
Beta-amino esters 159
Beta-amyloid vaccines 226, 228
Beta-thalassemia 247, 248
Bevacizumab 166, 171, 199, 201, 205
Bezlotoxumab 167
Bharat Biotech's covaxin 33, 43
Biliary cholangitis, primary 184
Bioconjugation technology 258
Bispecific antibodies 133
Black-legged ticks 268
Bladder cancer 193, 340
Blinatumomab 167, 168
Blood
  brain barrier 163, 164*f*, 194
  cerebrospinal fluid barrier 163
  clots 310
  meal 288
  retina barrier 163
Bococizumab 167

Body's immune
  response 37
  system 276
Body's nerve cells 230*f*
Bone
  cancer 216
    primary 216
  marrow 232
Bordetella pertussis 30, 47
Borrelia burgdorferi 268
Bovine spongiform encephalopathy 293
Brain tumor 194, 340
  primary malignant 194
Breakthrough varicella disease 64
Breast cancer 189, 196, 197
  female 189
  triple negative 197
  vaccines 196, 197
Breastfeeding 97, 106, 115
Brentuximab vedotin 167
Brexucabtagene autoleucel 150, 209
Brodalumab 167
Bronchial asthma vaccine 245
Bunyavirales 285
Burkholderia cepacia complex 267
Butantan-Dengue Vaccine 290

C

Campylobacter 264
  jejuni 237, 238, 259, 263
Cancer 5, 145, 148, 149*f*, 175, 190, 198, 225
  advanced urothelial 167
  cells 190*f*, 220
    killer uterine carcinoma 169
    killing 168
  colon 151, 189, 201, 202, 214
  curing, miracles of immunotherapy
      for 194
  esophageal 203
  hepatocellular 189
  immune system 5
  immunotherapy 5, 151
  microbiome research 222
  therapy 157, 190
  treatment 129, 202, 221, 222
  vaccines 148, 190, 192, 202, 219, 294
    background 190
    preventive 148, 189
    therapeutics 189
Cancerous cells 190*f*
Candida
  auris 272, 272*f*
  vaccines 272
Capromab pendetide 167
Capsular polysaccharide 103
Carcinoma, hepatocellular 48, 246, 278
Cardiac failure 80
Cardiovascular diseases 225
  vaccine 241

Casirivimab 169
Castleman's disease 169, 285
Cataracts 106*f*
Catch-up
  immunization 74, 174, 318
  vaccination 316
    programs 316
    schedules 316, 318
Cell
  based therapies 231, 237, 252
  nucleus 153*f*
  phone use 340
  therapy 209, 213, 235
Cellular immunotherapies 251, 266
Cellular therapies 187
  vaccination following 187
Cemiplimab 167
Centers for Disease Control and
    Prevention 191, 301, 319, 326,
    327, 334
Central nervous system 110, 152, 229
  disorders 241
  malignancies 219
  tumors 190
Cerebrospinal fluid 76, 81, 110, 233
Certolizumab pegol 135, 167
Cervarix 55
Cervical cancer 54, 198, 199
  screening 198
Cervix cancer 189
Cetuximab 167, 170
Chemokines 135
Chemotherapy 210, 213, 217
Chickenpox 14, 15, 68, 107, 122, 174, 301,
    323, 328
  vaccination 82
  vaccine 85, 91, 336
Chikungunya 46, 269, 290
  disease 290
  vaccine 46, 290
  virus 93, 146, 289
    vaccine 93, 290
Chimeric antigen receptor 129, 194, 209
  T-cell 209
    therapy 136, 149*f*, 150*t*, 186, 207,
      209*t*, 210
Chimeric yellow fever virus 17
Chimpanzee adenovirus 289
Chinese vaccines 18
Chlamydia 112, 269, 271
  trachomatis 271
  vaccine 112
Chloromycetin 269
Chloroquine 307
Cholera
  toxin, B-subunit of 240
  vaccine 46, 305
    several 305
Cholesterol, familial 166

Chondrosarcoma 216
Chordoma 216
Chorioretinitis 110
Chronic inflammatory demyelinating
   polyneuropathy 143
   polyradiculoneuropathy 237, 238
Chronic obstructive pulmonary
      disease 87, 225
Ciltacabtagene autoleucel 150, 209
Cinpanemab 167, 169
Cirrhosis 121, 278
Clostridium
   botulinum 143
   difficile 259
      infection 262
      toxin 167
Cochlear implants 90
Combination vaccines, side effects from 321
Combo vaccines 303, 320
Conjugate vaccines 36, 59, 64, 245
Conventional messenger ribonucleic
      acid vaccines 257
Conventional vaccine development
      methodologies 314
Coronary artery
   abnormalities 242
   preventions 241
   atherosclerosis 266
Coronavac 179
Coronavirus disease-2019 (COVID-19) 3,
      5, 7, 8, 17, 41, 46, 68, 99, 111, 135,
      143, 148, 178, 180, 182, 190, 230,
      245, 323, 325, 334, 335, 337
   booster shots 337
   catastrophic effects of 33
   combos 321
   infection 120, 146, 190, 243, 339, 338
   pandemic 4, 6, 42, 63, 131, 132, 226,
      256, 270, 330
   severe 182
   vaccination 70, 98, 121, 176, 178, 243,
      310, 311, 328
      documentation of 328
      schedule 182t
   vaccine 19, 24, 32, 33, 42-44, 84, 99,
      100, 115, 116, 120, 123, 178-180,
      182, 231, 292, 301, 310, 325, 331,
      334-339
      booster doses 338
      development 312
      discovery 336
      doses 338
      effective 284
      hesitancy 330
      rapid development of 294
      research process 314
      side effects of 45
      types of 330
      work 335
   variants 313

Corticobasal ganglionic
      degeneration 233
Covaxin 33, 179
Covishield 179
Cowpox 25
   virus 25
Crimean-congo hemorrhagic fever
      vaccine 286
Crizanlizumab 167, 249
Crohn's disease 5, 38, 147, 166, 169, 170,
      226, 249, 250
   vaccine 249
Culex tritaeniorhynchus 94
Cyclophosphamide 210
Cystic fibrosis 156, 162, 167, 168, 245,
      246, 265
   immunotherapy 245
Cytokine 135, 137, 196, 266
   release syndrome 186
   storm 135, 243f
Cytomegalovirus 97, 109, 110, 143, 257, 283f
   disease 283f
      prophylaxis of 143
   infection 110, 110t, 283
   vaccine 109, 282, 283, 284t
Cytotoxic T cells 199, 282
Cytotoxicity, complement-dependent 147f

D

Daclizumab 167
Daratumumab 167
Deer ticks 268
Delivery system, targeted 258
Dementia 227, 233
Demyelinating acute
      inflammatory demyelinating
      polyneuropathy 263
Dendritic cells 137, 190
Dengue 92
   fever 132
      vaccine 25, 304, 305
   hemorrhagic fever 288, 289
   infection 17
   serotype of 47
   severe 285
   shock syndrome 289
   vaccine 7, 47, 289, 290
      candidates 17
      development 17
      second 47
      tetravalent 17
   virus 16, 39, 71, 93, 288
      fever 46
      vaccination 71
      vaccine 16, 17, 46
Dengvaxia 17, 305
Denosumab 167, 171
Denys–Drash syndrome 218

Deoxyribonucleic acid 4, 110
   platforms, recombinant 257
   vaccine 37, 192, 280
Depemokimab 167
Dexamethasone 210
Diabetes mellitus 119, 173, 225, 240, 305
   type 1 5, 38, 240, 310
   type 2 240
   vaccines 239
Diarrhea 82
Dihydroartemisinin 307
Dinutuximab 167
Diphtheria 30, 181, 245, 325
   component of 331
   pertussis 3, 330
   tetanus 69
      acellular pertussis 69, 320
      pertussis 7, 10, 25, 47, 68, 71, 76, 85,
         259, 316, 319, 322
      toxoid 181
   toxoids 89, 119
   vaccine 30
Disease-modifying antirheumatic drugs 250
Disinformation 330
Donepezil 227
Dostarlimab 167, 206
Down syndrome 162
Doxorubicin hydrochloride 210
Doxycycline 269, 307
Drives pro-inflammatory cytokine
      secretion 289
Drug addictions, prevent 253
Duchenne's muscular dystrophy 158, 161
   gene therapy 161
Ductal carcinoma in situ 196
Duke human vaccine institute 276
Dukoral cholera vaccine 263
Dupilumab 167, 245
Durvalumab 167, 170, 199

E

Ebola
   vaccine 288
   virus 39, 146
      disease 288
      strains of 288
Ectopic pregnancy 271
Eculizumab 78, 167, 187, 238
Edmonston-Ender's strain 14
Edrecolomab 145
Effusion lymphoma, primary 285
Electroporation 157
Elotuzumab 167
Emerging new infectious diseases 294
Emicizumab 167
Emphasis 265
Enbrel 135
Encapsulate antigens 36

Encephalitis syndrome, acute 269
Endometrial cancer 200
Enfortumab vedotin 167
Enlimomab 145
Enteric multicenter study 264
Enterobacter cloacae 265
Enterococcus faecium 260, 264
Enterotoxigenic *Escherichia coli*
    vaccines 263
Enterovirus 244
Epcoritamab 167
Epidermal growth factor receptor 166
Epigenetic therapy 159, 160
Epiglottitis 259
Epstein–Barr virus 196, 204, 226, 229, 257, 281*f*
    infection 19
    nuclear antigen 281*f*
    part of 230*f*
    role 229
    vaccine 280
Erenumab 167
Erythema infectiosum 107
Esophageal cancer 203
    treatment 203
Esophagus 173
Estimated glomerular filtration rate 183
Etanercept 135
European Medicines Agency 268, 308
    Regulatory Committee 154
Evolocumab 168
Ewing sarcoma 216
Ex vivo gene therapy 154, 155*f*, 163
Exanthema subitum 285
Eyes, clouding of 106*f*

F

Fatigue 120
Fatty liver disease 121
    nonalcoholic 184, 246
Febrile illness 304
Fetal hemoglobin 158
Fever 82, 120
    low-grade 309
Flavivirus 65, 76, 108, 285
Fleas, presence of 269
Flu 321
    strains, prevalent 327
    vaccination 327
    vaccine 37, 85, 88, 98, 100, 114, 119, 120, 182
        adjuvanted inactivated 120
        higher-dose 120
        side effects of 100
        updated 57
    virus antigen 120
Fluzone 120
Follicular lymphoma 169

Food and Drug Administration 190, 209, 336
Foot-and-mouth disease 291
Formaldehyde 336
Formic acid excretion 226
Formidable yeast infection 272
Fragile X
    messenger ribonucleoprotein 1 162
    syndrome 162
Frexalimab 168, 231
Fungal diseases, potentially life-threatening 272
Fusion proteins 133

G

Galantamine 227
Gamma delta T-cells 139
Gardasil 9V vaccine 55
Gastric cancer 204, 267
Gastroenteritis 289
    acquired acute 29
Gastroesophageal reflux disease 203
Gastrointestinal oncology 202
Gastrointestinal tract 102, 173
Gelatin 123
Gelsinger's death shocked gene therapy community 156
Gemtuzumab 168
Gene
    addition 141, 163
    editing 141, 163, 165
    inhibition 141
    replacement 141
    silencing 163
        targeted 157
    therapy 129, 141, 152, 153, 153*f*, 154, 155, 155*f*, 156, 163, 237
        background 248
        delivery system 164*f*
Genetic metabolic disorder 154, 156
    historical background of 161
Genital tracts 102
Genitourinary abnormalities 218
Germ cell tumors 217
Germline gene therapy 153
Gestational age 110
Glaxosmithkline 273
Glioblastoma 194
Global cancer burden 189
Global vaccine action plan 8
Glycogen storage diseases 154, 156
Golimumab 168
Gonococcus 269
    vaccines 270
Gonorrhea 112
Good hand hygiene 302
Graft versus host disease 138, 168
Granular lymphocytes, large 140

Granulocyte-macrophage colony-stimulating factor 191
Granulomatosis, eosinophilic 168
Granulomatous disease, chronic 82
Group A *streptococcus* 241, 266
    vaccines 241
Group B *streptococcus* 7, 21, 102, 267
    vaccine 21, 85, 267
Guillain–Barré syndrome 72, 90, 97, 99, 102, 103*f*, 232, 237, 263
Gut microbiota, role of 221

H

H1N1 232
Haemaphysalis spinigera 287
Haemophilus influenzae 7, 24, 53, 60, 68, 72, 86, 187, 310, 319
    B 3, 69, 87, 142, 176, 245, 261, 316, 320, 337
        disease 26
        immunization 11
        vaccine 11, 53, 85
Hand-foot-mouth disease 37
    antiviral treatment for 291
    vaccine 291
Hantavirus 285
    pulmonary syndrome 288
Harboring vaccine-preventable diseases 325
Hard ticks 286
Headache 82
    migraine 167
Health Education and Awareness Program 323
Healthcare 328
    professionals, vaccination of 325
    setting, specific 325
    worker 325
        vaccination programs 326, 329
Heart 180
    disease 119, 173, 225
        acquired 241, 242, 266
        chronic 80
        congenital 80
        coronary 241
Hecolin 53, 279
Helicobacter pylori 204, 260, 267
Hematopoietic stem cell transplantation 54, 110, 174, 207
Hemihypertrophy 218
Hemodialysis 50
    disease 181
Hemoglobin 158, 247
Hemoglobinopathies 145
    vaccine against 247
Hemophilia 167
Hemorrhagic fever
    renal syndrome 285
    virus 288

Hepatitis 31, 110, 316
  A 86, 87, 115, 143, 176, 181, 320, 323
    vaccine 16, 49, 85, 87, 302
  A virus 24, 48, 49, 68, 99
    control 31
    infection 104
    vaccine 16, 104
  autoimmune 121
  B 3, 32, 68, 69, 73, 86, 119, 143, 176, 181, 322, 323, 325, 327
    birth dose 69
    immunization 326
    immunoglobulin 50, 105, 142, 143
    infection 51
    recombinant 320
    special situations 121
    surface antibody 181, 327
    vaccination 50, 73
    vaccine 49, 50-52, 69, 74, 85, 87, 121
  B virus 7, 48, 49, 68, 99, 105, 148, 206, 303
    vaccination success story 31
    vaccine 8, 37, 49, 104, 105, 183, 189
  C 111, 121
    virus 48, 49, 52, 146, 277, 278
  D virus 49
    vaccines 52
  E virus 48, 49, 278
    infection, chronic 48, 178
    vaccine 53, 105, 278
  vaccines 104
  viral 32
  viruses, multiple 16
Hepatotropic viruses 48, 49
Herceptin 194
Herd immunity 49, 175, 334
  level of 329
Herpes simplex virus 257
  vaccines against 279
Herpes zoster 91, 174
  subunit vaccine 65
  vaccine 15, 85, 285
Heterologous flavivirus vaccination 109
Hexavalent vaccine 53
High tumor mutational burden 201
Histocompatibility complex, major 139
Hodgkin's disease 175f
Hodgkin's lymphoma 167, 207
Host immune responses 278
Human adenovirus 39, 289
  serotype, replication deficient 289
  vaccine 92
    against 289
Human anthrax 40
Human body cells 43
Human diploid cell vaccine 62
Human epidermal growth factor receptor 145
Human herpesvirus 280
  vaccines for 285

Human immunodeficiency virus 7, 39, 71, 87, 111, 132, 191, 256, 276, 321
  antigens 289
  disease vaccine 275
  infection 20, 71, 77, 92, 121, 175
  maternal 115
  structure of 277f
  transmission of 115
  vaccine 25, 289
    developments 20
Human infections, theoretical possibility of 291
Human insulin, B-chain of 240
Human lung fibroblast cell culture 283f
Human malignancies 148
Human norovirus diarrhea 292
Human papillomavirus 7, 24, 37, 54, 68, 99 129, 176, 189, 317, 331
  infection 19
  serotypes 191
  vaccine 19, 32, 54-56, 84, 85, 87, 105, 106, 115, 173, 292, 319
    doses of 55
    providing 322
    therapeutic 198
Human prostatic acid phosphatase 191
Human rabies immunoglobulin 62
Humoral immunodeficiency, primary 143
Huntington's disease 154, 234
Hyalomma 286
Hyaluronidase 169
Hybridomas 146
Hypercholesterolemia 168, 244
  familial 148
  heterozygous familial 244
  vaccine for 244
Hypertension 5, 244
  controlled 119f

I

Ibalizumab 168
Ibritumomab tiuxetan 168
Idarucizumab 168
Idecabtagene vicleucel 150, 209
Illness, risk for 269
Imatinib 168
Imdevimab 167
Immune
  cells, interaction of 190f
  checkpoint 132, 152
    blockade 196
    inhibitor 132, 132f, 152, 166-168, 199, 200, 211
  deficiencies 77
  effector cell 151
  globulin subcutaneous 143
  memory 39
  response, strong 268

  stimulating antibodies 208
  suppressed, vaccine second booster for 182
  system 15, 124, 190f, 211, 230f, 271, 276, 335
    childhood 339
  tolerance 19
Immunity 29, 329
  acquired 272
  community herd 95
  confirmation of 329
  herd 49, 175, 334
  hybrid 337
  induction of 142
  preservation of 187
  tetravalent 94
  vaccine-induced 337
  waning 30, 84
Immunization 3, 4, 24, 38, 85, 173, 290, 323, 326
  active 62, 141
  adult 3, 84, 95
  childhood 68, 316
  hesitancy 330
  passive 142
  pediatric 68
  practices 124
  routine 55
    childhood 60
  strategic principles 68
  timing of maternal 98
  travel 301
Immunocompromise, severe 182t
Immunodeficiency
  severe 71, 77, 82
  syndrome 276
Immunogenic cell death 136
Immunoglobulin
  deficiency 73
  G 42, 235, 267, 281f
  intravenous 143, 232, 238, 243
  M 281f
Immunomodulators 206
Immunomodulatory drugs 237
Immunopathogenesis, perspective of 241
Immunotherapy 4, 115, 129, 149f, 163, 165, 189, 190, 193, 196, 199, 200-202, 204, 205, 211, 216, 217, 219, 239, 241, 246, 265, 340
  advantages of 129
  bacteria-based 134
  biomarkers 211
  checkpoint 201
  compilation of 6
  marks 129
  passive-mediated 131
  perspective of 243f
  types of 202, 266

Inactivated influenza vaccine 88
Inactivated pertussis toxin 47
Inactivated polio
   vaccine 304, 319
   virus 181, 320
Inactivated vero cell-derived vaccine 305
Inactivated virus vaccines 71
Inclacumab 168
Indian Council of Medical
       Research 205, 287
Indian flying fox 291*f*
Indian typhus fever 269
Induced pluripotent stem cells 236
Infections 291, 337
   asymptomatic nature of 278
   bacterial 265
   blocking vaccine 5
   hospital-acquired 262, 264
   natural 47
   primary source of 263
   vaccine-preventable 175
   viral 146
Infectious disease 11, 14, 129, 145, 175,
       221, 225, 256
   spread of 83
Infertility 271
Inflammatory neuropathies 237
Infliximab 135, 145, 168, 170, 188, 250
Influenza 36, 37, 68, 76, 84, 119, 120, 181,
       245, 301, 306, 325, 326
   pandemic 57
   vaccination 75, 243
   vaccine 15, 16, 25, 57, 58, 75, 76, 85,
       87, 98, 100, 114, 180, 182, 306,
       323, 339
      adenovirus-based 289
      types of 15
   virus 15, 25, 39, 89, 146, 244
Inhalation anthrax 169
   treatment of 143
Inherited genetic disorders,
       prevalence of 162
Inherited neuromuscular disorders 162
Innate immune system 140, 264
Innate lymphoid cells 190, 193
Innovative viral vaccines 266, 275
Inotuzumab ozogamicin 167, 168
Intensive care unit 71
Interferons 135
   gamma release assay 326
Interleukin 135, 250
International Certificate of
       Vaccination 303, 304
International Diabetes Federation 239
Intestinal problem 309
Intestines 180
   large 173
Intramuscular injections 5
Intranasal flu vaccines 44

Intranasal vaccines 5
Intrapartum antibiotic prophylaxis 103
Intrauterine infection 111
Intravenous immunoglobulin 143, 232,
       238, 243
   immune regulations 238
Intussusception 310
Invasive pneumococcal disease 122
Inverse vaccine 38, 230
Ipilimumab 133, 168, 201, 206
Isograft 173
Ixekizumab 168
Ixodid ticks 286

J

Janus kinase inhibitors 250
Japanese encephalitis 68, 269, 301
   virus 76, 108, 286
      vaccine 76, 94, 109, 113, 114, 305
Jaundice 283*f*
Joints
   inflammation of 170
   pain 289

K

Kaposi's sarcoma 285
   virus 285
Kawasaki disease 241, 243, 243*f*, 266
Kawasaki syndrome 143
Keratoconjunctivitis, epidemic 39, 289
Kidney 180
   cancer 205
      therapeutic treatment 205
   disease, chronic 181, 181*t*, 185, 225
   solid organ transplantation of 173
   transplant 180, 181
      recipients 167
   tumors, childhood 218
Kikuchi–Fujimoto disease 310
Kissing disease 280
Klebsiella pneumoniae 259
   vaccine 265
Kyasanur forest disease 285
   virus 287

L

Lactation, vaccination during 114
Lassa virus fever 285, 287
   vaccine 287
Latent tuberculosis infection
       treatment 327
Leishmania 275
   parasite 275
Leishmaniasis, vaccines for 275
Lentivirus 155
Leprosy vaccine 260

Leukemia 137, 190, 310
   acute
      lymphoblastic 209, 337
      myeloid 207
   childhood 218
   chronic
      lymphocytic 168-170, 338
      myeloid 338
   death 337
   vaccines for 207
Lewy bodies 233
Limb-girdle muscular dystrophy 161
Lipo-oligosaccharides, pathogenic 264
Lipopolysaccharide 237
Lisocabtagene maraleucel 150, 209
Listeria monocytogenes 134
Live typhoid vaccine 302
Live vaccine 15, 177, 245
Live-attenuated vaccine 36, 57, 71, 88, 91,
       97, 141, 175-177, 280
Liver 180
   cancer 184, 206
      treatment 207
   cirrhosis 48
   disease
      alcoholic 121
      chronic 121, 184
   failure, acute 105
Loncastuximab 168
Lou Gehrig disease 162
Low birth weight 69
Low-density lipoprotein
   cholesterol 148
   high levels of 244
Lower respiratory tract disease 38, 103
   severe 123
   prevention of 21
Lujo hemorrhagic fever 285
Lung 180
   cancer 189, 210
      treatment 211
Lyme disease 268
   post-treatment 268
   vaccination against 268
   vaccine 268
Lymphadenopathy 41
Lymphoblastic leukemia, treatment of
       acute 133
Lymphocyte-activated killer cells 139
Lymphocytic lymphoma, small 208
Lymphoid cells, innate 140
Lymphokine 135
Lymphoma 137, 167, 168, 190, 208, 218
   vaccine 207, 208

M

Machine learning 22, 258, 312
Macular degeneration 169
Maculopapular skin eruption 269

Mad cow disease 293
Madras eye 289
Malaria 20, 132, 269, 302
    medications 306
    prevention, medications for 307
    prophylaxis 307
    vaccine 7, 21, 25, 95, 256, 272
    venture research, medicine for 273
Malarial parasite 92, 146, 307
Malignant melanoma 212
Mantle cell lymphoma 209
Mantoux test 326
Maraba virus 220
Marburg virus disease vaccine 288
Margetuximab 197
Maternal group B streptococcus 84
Maternal health 102
Maternal immunity 21
Maternal immunization 21, 98, 101
Maternal infections 111
Maternal pertussis 101
Maternal pneumococcal vaccination 102
Maternal respiratory syncytial virus 92, 103
Maternal vaccination 101, 102
Maternal vaccines, development of 103
Measles 3, 13, 14, 68, 143, 220, 245, 322, 325, 326
    antigen 58
    control 27
    elimination 27
    vaccination 327
    virus transmission 27
Measles, mumps, and rubella 25, 69, 86, 99, 174, 176, 181, 256, 301, 309, 319, 330, 335
    and varicella 320
        vaccinations 106
        vaccine 13, 306
    vaccination 77, 98, 309
    vaccine 58, 85, 87, 90
        doses of 327
Measles, rubella 58
    containing vaccine 14
Medicine, history of 9
Mefloquine 307
Melanoma 152, 212, 213
    associated antigen 3 212
Membrane attack complex 238
MenABCWY vaccine 79
Meningitis 13, 60, 259, 301, 322
    illnesses 259
Meningococcal 326
    B 176
        vaccines 304
    bacteria, types of 77
    conjugate 13, 99, 102
        vaccine 58, 176, 304, 320
    disease 59
    polysaccharide vaccine 59
    septicemia 259
    vaccine 13, 34, 77, 85, 90, 115, 304, 327
    types of 304
Meningococcus serogroup 86
Mepolizumab 168, 245
Mesenchymal stem cells 137, 236
Messenger ribonucleic acid 4, 5, 36, 70, 173, 182, 226, 257
    technology 4
    therapeutics 5
    therapy 246
Messenger ribonucleic acid vaccine 18, 36, 257, 276, 310
    against cystic fibrosis 246
    consideration of 173
    nasal 37
    oral 37
    self-amplifying 257
Metabolic dysfunction 246
Metastatic bladder cancer 193
Metastatic carcinoma breast 169
Metastatic colorectal cancer 169
Metastatic melanoma 168
Methyltransferase 196
Microarray patches 38
    administrations 37
Microbiome in immunotherapy, role of 152
Microorganisms, antibiotic resistance in 295
Midesophagus 203
Miller Fisher syndrome 238
Minimal residual disease 195
Mismatch repair gene 201
Mite-borne scrub-bush typhus diagnosis 269
Mites 269
Mitigate confusing ambiguities 321
Molecular mimicry 238
Monkeypox 26
    high risk for 63
    prevention of 26
    vaccine 63
    virus 25
Monoclonal antibiotics 142, 144
    major types of 144
Monoclonal antibody 62, 116, 131, 143, 145, 186, 187, 194, 199, 201, 202, 208, 211, 215, 231, 235, 240, 241, 244, 250, 253, 280
    therapeutic
        role 249
        utility 246
    therapy 187, 200, 228, 232
    use of 170
Monoclonal IG antibody therapy 144*t*
Monovalent hepatitis B vaccine 74
Monovalent specificity 144
Mosquirix 273
Mosquito 287
    bite spreading dengue fever 269
Mosquito-bird-mosquito transmission cycle 293
Motor axonal neuropathy, acute 238, 263
Mouth disease vaccine 289
Mpox vaccine 86, 90
Mucosal immunity 38
Mucosal vaccines 44
Multicomponent vaccines 21
Multidrug resistance, rise of 260
Multi-epitope antigens 275
Multi-epitope vaccine 268
    construction of 268
Multifocal motor neuropathy 143
Multipathogen vaccines 258
Multiple myeloma 167, 209
    vaccine for 208
Multiple sclerosis 5, 38, 168, 225, 229, 231, 280, 310, 334
    cell-based therapies for 231
    development, model for 229
    risk of 230*f*
    vaccine 229
Multiple system atrophy 233
Multiple vaccines 319
Mumps 14, 28, 68, 77, 106
Murine antibodies 144
Muromonab 147, 168, 187
Muscle
    aches 120
    disorders 239
    pain 289
Mutant huntingtin protein 234
Mutating bacteria 30
Myasthenia gravis 5, 232
    vaccines for 232
Mycobacterium 261
    avium 249
    leprae 261
    tuberculosis 8, 26, 39, 259
        vaccine for drug resistance 260
    bovis 8, 40, 134
Mycophenolate mofetil 180
Mycoplasma pneumoniae 245, 264
Myeloma, vaccines for 207
Myocarditis 310
Myxoma virus 220

N

Nairovirus 285
Nanoparticle vaccines 258
Nanotechnology, role of 36
Nasal vaccine 38, 44
    types of 38
Natalizumab 168, 231, 233
National Family Health Survey 330
National Immunization Programs 3, 12
National Institute of Allergy and Infectious Diseases 292

National Institutes of Health 17, 276
National Kidney Foundation 182
National Regulatory Authority 308
Natural immunity 335, 337
Natural killer cells 140
Natural products 268
Nausea 82, 120
Necitumumab 168
Necrotizing fasciitis 103
Neisseria
   gonorrhoeae 112, 259, 261
   meningitidis 12, 34, 58, 59, 79, 90, 304
      vaccines 12
   meningitis 7
Neoantigen 193, 195, 199
Neoantigen vaccines 211
Neomycin 123
Neurobiology 22
Neuroblastoma, high-risk 167
Neurodegenerative disorders, gene therapy for 163
Neurological diseases 293
Neurological disorder 145, 147, 293
Neurotoxicity syndrome 151
Neurotropic viruses 285
Neutralizing antibodies, titers of 281*f*
New pentavalent meningococcal vaccine 59
New tuberculosis vaccine 42
Newcastle disease virus 220
Next-generation sequencing 195
Nipah
   outbreak 292
   vaccine 289
   virus 291, 321
      vaccine 291
Nirsevimab 80, 104, 291
Nivolumab 133, 168, 171, 199, 193, 201, 206
   incorporation of 205
Nonalcoholic steatohepatitis, nomenclature of 246
Noncommunicable disease 5, 23, 96, 147, 225
   immunotherapy against 225
   vaccines for 226
Non-Hodgkin lymphoma 170, 207-209
Non-polio enteroviruses 289, 291
Nonreplicating viral vectors 257
Non-small cell lung cancer 152, 170, 210
   diagnosis 210
Non-typhoidal salmonella 263
Nonviral gene delivery systems 157
Norovirus 29, 292
Nose drop vaccine 227
Novavax 33
   unique 44
   vaccine 44, 70
Novel antimicrobials, development of 295

Nucleic acid 159
   amplification test 112
   vaccines 270, 280
Numerous enzyme deficiency disorders 156

O

O-antigen conjugates 263
Oat cell carcinoma 210
Obesity vaccine 252
Obiltoxaximab 168
Obinutuzumab 168, 208
Occupational exposures 174
Occupational health and safety 329
Occupational therapy 235
Ocrelizumab 168
Ofatumumab 168, 207, 208, 231
Off-the-shelf car t-cell therapies 150
Olaratumab 169
Olokizumab 251
Omalizumab 169, 170, 245, 247
Oncological drugs 115
Oncolytic virotherapy 219
Oncolytic virus 136, 136*f*, 154, 194, 205, 219, 220
   therapy 154, 220, 220*f*
Ophthalmic diseases 145
Opioid use disorder 252
Oral cholera vaccine 305
Oral human-attenuated monovalent rotavirus 79
Oral polio vaccine 61, 69, 304
Oral route administrations 37
Organ transplantation 143, 175
Orthopneumoviruses 46
Orthopoxviruses 63
Oseltamivir 76
Osteitis 41
Osteoarthritis 225
   pain vaccine 252
   vaccine for 251
Osteoporosis 225
Osteosarcoma 216
Otitis media, acute 80
Outer membrane vesicle vaccines 270
Ovarian cancer 189, 199
   immunotherapy 199
   vaccine targets 200

P

Pain, abdominal 82
Palbociclib 197
Palivizumab 145, 146
   med immune 169
Pancreas 180
Pancreatic cancer 202, 213, 214
   vaccine 213

Pancreatic ductal adenocarcinoma 213
Panitumumab 169
Paralytic poliomyelitis, vaccine-associated 28
Parasites 146
   vaccines against 272
Parasitic infections 272
Parkinson disease 154, 167
Parkinson plus syndrome 233
Parkinson's disease 163, 169, 225, 233, 234
Parkinsonism 233
Particle based vaccines, virus-like 257
Particle vaccines, virus-like 37, 198
Parvovirus 220
   B19 107
   infection 107
Pathogen-infected cells 96
Pediatric dose vaccine 73
Pediatric malignancy
   and immunotherapy, vaccines for 217
   vaccines against 190
Pelvic inflammatory disease 271
Pembrolizumab 133, 167, 169, 171, 193, 199, 200, 201, 204, 206, 213, 216
Pemphigus vulgaris 170
Penbraya vaccine 320
Penicillin G 112
Pentavalent vaccine 13
Peptide 198
   vaccines 37, 198, 207, 232, 257
Percutaneous coronary intervention 145, 166
Pericarditis 310
Perlman syndrome 218
Persistent asthma, moderate-to-severe 170
Personal communication 269
Personalized cancer vaccine 221
Personalized chimeric antigen receptor t-cell therapy process 209
Personalized messenger ribonucleic acid vaccines 214
Personalized neoantigen vaccine 201
Personalized vaccines 4, 190, 192
Pertussis 48, 245, 317, 326, 328
   vaccination 101
   vaccine 30
Pertuzumab 169, 170, 197
Pharmaceutical applications 22
Pharyngitis 256
Phenuivirus 285
Phlebotomus spp 275, 275*f*
Physical therapy 235
Picornavirus 220
Piperaquine 307
Plague psoriasis 167, 168, 169
Plasma kallikrein activity, inhibitors of 164
Plasmapheresis 238

Plasmodium
   Berghei sporozoites 20
   genus 272
   ovale malaria 307
   parasite 20
   species 20, 307
   vivax 307
      infections 21
   falciparum 21, 39, 273
Platelet
   disorder 70
   low 310
Platelet-rich plasma therapy 252
Pneumococcal 181
   conjugate 176
      vaccine 11, 60, 86, 121, 122, 176, 185, 242, 261
   disease 11, 32, 245
   polysaccharide vaccine 121, 185
   vaccination 242
   vaccine 32, 59, 85, 90, 101, 115, 119*f*, 121, 184, 259
      types of 101
Pneumococcus 121, 316
   bacteria 90
   vaccine 142
Pneumonia 11, 60, 119, 301
   bacteremic 60
   prevent 119
Pneumonitis 110, 175*f*
Polio 3, 9, 68, 245, 301, 326, 330
   toward eradication 28
Polio vaccine 9, 61, 69, 303, 304
   birth dose 69
   childhood 92
Polio virus 7, 79
   vaccination 79
   vaccine 9
   vaccine-derived 28
Political polarization 330
Polyangiitis 168
Polyclonal IG antibody therapy 144*t*
Polymerase chain reaction 110, 198, 281
Polysaccharide 245
   vaccine 11, 36, 59, 102
Positron emission tomography 226
Post-CA prostate 167
Postexposure prophylaxis 62, 143, 306
Postherpetic neuralgia 15, 91, 122
Post-liver transplant
   cases 143
   vaccination 184
Post-menopausal osteoporosis 167
Postpartum vaccination 102, 105
Post-transplant vaccinations 184
Postvaccination serologic testing 50
Potential disadvantage 315
Potential exposures 325

Potential immunologic overload resulting 334
Poxviruses 220
Prasinezumab 169
Pre-exposure vaccination 303
Pregnancy 174
   vaccination during 338
Pre-liver transplant vaccination 184
Preterm infant 69
Pretransplant vaccinations 184
Primaquine 307
Prime-boost vaccinations 19
Probiotics 268
Progressive multifocal leukoencephalopathy 208
Progressive supranuclear palsy 233
Proguanil 307
Prophy organ rejection 167
Prophylactic vaccines 191
Prophylaxis, pre-exposure 40, 93, 306
Prostate cancer 214, 215, 215*f*
   castration-resistant 191
   vaccines 214
Prostate health index 215
Prostate-specific antigen 215
Protective immune response 262, 293
Protein
   F 92, 124
   recombinant 266
   subunit vaccines 280
Proteinaceous infectious particle 293
Protein-based vaccine 200, 240
Pseudomonas aeruginosa 260, 264, 265
Psoriasis 166, 169
Psoriatic arthritis 168, 169
Public health 9, 334
   authorities 315
   campaigns 313
   efforts, critical aspect of 321
   guidelines 338
   protecting 323
   threat 34
Pyrazinamide 41

Q

Quadrivalent influenza vaccine 16, 87, 100

R

Rabies 37, 62, 301, 302
   immune globulin 62, 142
   immunoglobulin products 63*t*
   infection 305
   postexposure treatment of 143
   vaccination 62
   vaccine 143, 305
      intradermal use of 62
   virus 39
Racotumomab 212

Radiation 217
Ramucirumab 169
Ranibizumab 169
Rapid plasma reagin 112
Rash 82
Ravulizumab 78
Raxibacumab 169
Receptor-binding domain 18
Recombinant antigens 275
Rectal cancer 167
Remicade 135
Renal cell carcinoma 205
Renal disease
   advanced 182
   chronic 173
   end-stage 87, 180
Renal failure, chronic 181
Renal transplant 167
   rejects propyl 166
Reovirus 220
Residual disease 210
Reslizumab 169, 245
Respiratory diseases 245
   chronic 173
   vaccine 244
Respiratory infections 301
Respiratory infectious diseases 38
Respiratory related illnesses 323
Respiratory syncytial virus 7, 46, 62, 68, 99, 119, 132, 244, 245, 256, 280, 321, 326, 328
   infection 123
   vaccination 80
   vaccine 21, 84, 85, 103, 123, 124, 290, 339
Respiratory tract disease 39, 289
Respiratory virus infections 323
Retinoblastoma 190, 217
Rheumatic fever
   acute 241, 266
   prevention vaccines 266
Rheumatic heart disease 226, 256
Rheumatoid arthritis 135, 147, 169, 170
   vaccine 250
      roll of 251
Rhinovirus 244
Ribociclib 197
Ribonucleic acid 99, 243
   therapy 158, 159
   vaccine 37, 159
Rift valley fever 285, 287
Rindopepimut 195
Ring vaccination 288
Rituxan 208
Rituximab 145, 169, 170, 187, 207, 208, 231, 238, 251
Robust cell culture system 292
Roseola infantum 285
Roseoloviruses 285
   vaccines 285

Rota shield vaccine 29
Rotavirus 12, 36, 68, 178
    diarrhea 3
    gastroenteritis disease 12
    vaccination 79
    vaccine 61, 310
        development 12
Routine immunization programs 4
Routine vaccination 47, 58, 71, 122, 303
Rozanolixizumab 169
Rubella 3, 14, 106, 143, 245, 326, 328
    infection 110t
    syndrome, congenital 25, 106f, 110
    vaccine development 14
Russian vaccine 18

S

Saccharomyces cerevisiae 107
Safety during pregnancy 106
Salmonella
    serotype *paratyphi* 259
    typhi 64, 82, 261
    typhimurium 134, 135
Salmonella paratyphi 261, 262
    drug-resistant 262
Sand flies 275, 275f
Sarcomas 216
Sarilumab 169, 250
School entry booster vaccination 322
School health immunization 322, 323
    program 322, 323
School Health Program 322
School Health Vaccination Programs 324
School immunization, shots for 322
Sclerosing cholangitis, primary 184
Sclerosis, amyotrophic lateral 162, 239
Scrub typhus 269, 269f
    vaccine 268
Scrub, vaccination against 269
Seasonal influenza 292
Seasonal malaria chemoprevention 273
Secukinumab 169
Seizures
    febrile 321
    history of 77
Senior care vaccinations 119
Senior flu 58
Sensorineural hearing loss 110
Sepsis 11, 60
    bacterial cause of 261
Septicemia, invasive 259
Serogroup B
    meningococcal 59
    Neisseria meningitidis 270
    vaccines 102
Serologic testing 62, 98, 175

Severe acute respiratory
    syndrome 71, 328
Severe acute respiratory syndrome
    coronavirus 2 17, 18f, 37, 71, 143,
    176, 181, 230, 244, 257, 323, 326,
    328, 330
    travel vaccine 306
    vaccination 17, 114
    vaccine 32, 42, 85, 89, 310
    virus 339
Severe allergic reaction 71, 72, 75-82
    history of 75, 174
Sexual abuse, history of 75
Sexual assault, history of 75
Sexually transmitted
    disease 270
    infection 90, 111
        during pregnancy 111
        prevention 112
Shigella 256, 264
    flexneri 264
    spp. 259, 263
    vaccine 264
        development 264
Shigellosis vaccine prevention 264
Shingles 15, 119, 301
    vaccination 107
    vaccine 85, 91, 119, 123
Shingrix 123
Sibeprenlimab 169
Sickle cell 158
    anemia 162, 305
    crisis 167
    disease 54, 81, 90, 156, 168, 247, 249
Silent killer 213
Siltuximab 169
Single-dose vaccines 38
Sinopharm 33, 43
Small cell lung cancer 210
    diagnosis 210
Small intestine 173
Smallpox 26, 63, 90
    eradication 24
    high risk for 63
    prevention of 26
    success story 25
    vaccination 143
Soft tissue sarcoma 169
Solid organ cancers 190
Solid organ transplant 173, 176, 178, 186
    candidates and recipients,
        vaccination for 176
    recipients 187
    vaccines for 180
Somatic gene therapy 152
Sophisticated human systems 6
Sore throat 256

Spike glycoprotein 18
Spinal cord 230f
    injury 236
Spinal muscular atrophy 160
Spleen
    cancer 217
    tyrosine kinase 218
Splenectomy 217
Sporadic disease 294
Sputnik V 33, 43
Squamous cell carcinoma 203
Staphylococcus aureus 260, 265
Steatohepatitis 246
    nonalcoholic 246
Steatotic liver disease 246
Stem cell
    based therapies 237
    therapy 231, 236, 239
    types of 236
Stereotactic body radiotherapy 205
Stimulus-responsive nanocarriers 157
Stimuvax 212
Stomach 173
Strain specific vaccination 57
Strep throat 256
    fever illnesses 256
Streptococcus 256
    pneumococcal vaccinations 80
    pneumoniae 11, 68, 101, 121, 187, 245,
        259, 261
Strokes 225
Subcutaneous abscess 41
Sudden infant death syndrome 334
Sulfamethoxazole prophylaxis 275
Syphilis 111, 269
    congenital 270
    prevention 112
    vaccine, development of 270
Systematic vaccination 27

T

T cells 190f
T lymphotropic 285
Talimogene laherparepvec 136, 191
T-based immunotherapy 194
T-cell 149, 209
    based therapy 148
    costimulation blockers 250
    driven 180, 181
    engaging bispecific antibodies 209
    receptor vaccines 232
    regulatory 139
    targeting 251
    therapy 5, 129, 199, 202
Tecemotide 212
Temozolomide 194
Teplizumab 169

Testicular germ cell tumors 217
Tetanus 3, 29, 99, 119, 317, 325
    prophylactic treatment of 143
    therapeutic treatment of 143
    vaccine 30
Tetanus and diphtheria 31, 84, 176
    and acellular pertussis 101, 174, 176, 338
    and pertussis 301, 323
        vaccination, timing of 101
        vaccine 114, 119, 120, 306
    control 24
    vaccine 101
        role 29
Tetanus toxoid 89, 322
    conjugated vaccine 63
    containing vaccine 72
Tetravalent vaccine 53, 61
Thalassemia 162, 247
Therapeutic cancer vaccines 189
Therapeutic monoclonal antibodies 166
Therapeutic vaccination 197
Therapeutic vaccines 56, 191, 276, 277, 280
Thermostable vaccines 37
Thrombocytopenic purpura
    chronic idiopathic 143
    rashes 283*f*
Thrombosis 166
Thrombotic thrombocytopenia, vaccine-induced 179
Tildrakizumab 169
Tisagenlecleucel 150, 209
Tissue
    biopsies 210
    cell culture 283*f*
    invasiveness 270
Tocilizumab 135, 169, 170
Tolerance-inducing therapies 252
Tonsillitis 256
    causing pathogens 256
Toxoid vaccine 36, 245
Toxoplasma
    gondii infection 274
    parasite 274
Toxoplasmosis
    congenital 274
    vaccine 274
Transitional cell bladder 193
Transmission blocking vaccine 274*f*
Transparent public health 22
Transplant rejection 145
Trastuzumab 145, 169, 170, 197
Travel vaccine 113, 301
Travel-specific vaccinations 301
Treponema pallidum 111
    subspecies *pallidum* 269
Trimethoprim 275

Tuberculin skin test 40, 326
Tuberculosis 3, 25, 26, 69, 260, 326
    contagious pulmonary 26
    disease, active 327
    testing, requirement for 326
    vaccine, adenovirus-based 290
Tumor
    associated antigens 149, 190
    hematologic 71
    lysate 195
    microenvironment 194
    necrosis factor-alpha 135
    specific antigens 190
Tumor cell 136*f*
    immune mediated destruction of 132*f*
    surface of 132*f*
    vaccines 192
Tumor-infiltrating lymphocyte 199
    therapy 138
Typhoid 301
    conjugate vaccine 64, 82, 302
    fever 113, 245
        vaccine 113
    illnesses 259
    immunization 63, 82
    polysaccharide vaccine 302
    vaccine 64, 68, 82, 85, 89, 113, 302
Tyrosine kinase inhibitors 206

U

Ublituximab 169
Ulcerative colitis 166, 168, 169
Umbilical cord tissue 236
United Nations International Children's Emergency Fund 9
Universal flu vaccine 89
Universal immunization 50
    Program 3, 16, 69, 207, 323
Unvaccinated healthcare workers 328
Upper respiratory tracts 38
Urinary tract infections, majority of 261
Urticaria 82
Ustekinumab 169
Uterine
    cancer immunotherapies 200
    endometrial cancer 200, 201

V

Vaccination 31, 243
    adolescent 322
    bacterial 256
    benefits of 335
    childhood 25
    facilities, adequate 40
    guidance 317
    regimes 287
    saves lives 295

Vaccine 3, 7, 24, 219, 228, 237, 305, 311, 326, 331, 336, 337
    adjuvant action 68
    adjuvant-based 240
    adverse event 309
        reporting system 308, 309, 339
    antifungal 272
    availability 303
    bacterial 259, 260, 267
    catch-up guidance 317
    coadministration of 180
    delivery 36
    development 15, 37, 238, 263, 265
        progress of 36
    distribution 23
    dose 45
        primary 182
    effectiveness 44, 308, 317, 336
    efficacy 56, 308
    elicited antibodies 143
    evolution 7
    field of 315
    formulation 192
    hesitancy 3, 5, 30, 56, 330
        spikes in 331
    immunity, duration of 88
    innovation 256, 295
    mandates 332
    manufacturers 321
    nonresponders 50
    play 295
    policy decisions 22
    preventable disease, risk of 330
    preventing aspects 42
    preventive 19, 191, 198, 276, 279
    protection 63
    protein 268
    recombinant 268
    recommendations 175
    refusal 5
    related misinformation 334
    responses 180
        depends, nature of 142
    safety 45, 308
        concerns 14
        monitoring systems 331
    shelf life of 258
    targeting bacteria 259
    technology 312
    trigger 336
    type 70, 240, 328
        B 264
    virus 93
Vaccine-preventable diseases 3, 10, 25, 226, 336
Vaccinia virus 25, 220
Valent pneumococcal conjugate vaccine 60

Valent polysaccharide pneumococcal
    vaccine 60
Variant Creutzfeldt-Jakob disease 293
Varicella 14, 68, 107, 122, 143, 181,
    325, 328
  postexposure prophylaxis 143
  severe 175*f*
  syndrome, congenital 106, 107*f*, 110
  vaccination 82
  vaccine 15, 64, 85, 91, 123
Varicella-Zoster
  immunoglobulin 107, 143, 142
  virus 15, 122, 257
Vascular endothelial growth
    factor 199
Vascular parkinsonism 233
Vaso-occlusive crises 247
Vector-based vaccines 192
Vector-borne diseases 301
Vedolizumab 169
Vesicles, extracellular 160
Vesicular stomatitis virus 37, 220
  recombinant 292
Vincristine sulfate 210
Viral capsid antigen 281, 281*f*
Viral disease 93
Viral gene delivery systems 157
Viral hemorrhagic fever 285, 286
  diseases 285*t*
  vaccines 285
  virus
    diseases 285
    family 285

Viral hepatitis
  A 184
  B 32, 184
  C 32, 184
  D 184
  E 184
Viral infections, prevention of 41
Viral replication 289
Viral vaccines
  futuristic 275
  recombinant 200
Viral vector 257
  types of 39
  vaccine 18, 36, 245
Virus 244
  based therapy 136
  miscellaneous 289
Vivax 273
Vomiting 82

W

Wegener's granulomatosis 170
West-Nile
  fever 293
  virus 289, 292
Whole-cell pertussis 69
  vaccines 10
Whooping cough 3, 25, 245, 317
Wild poliovirus 29
Wilms tumor 190, 217, 218
Winter vomiting bug 292
Woman's rubella immunity 106
Wound management 72

X

Xenografts 173

Y

Yellow fever 94, 113, 285
  vaccine 65, 94, 95, 113, 302, 303
  virus 108

Z

Zaire Ebola virus 288
Zanamivir 76
Zika
  infection 110*t*
  purified inactivated virus 109
  vaccine candidates 109
Zika virus 108, 109*f*, 146, 289
  fever 269
  infection 109, 293
  range of 109*f*
  vaccine 95, 108, 293
Zilebesiran 244
Zinc finger protein therapies 234
Zolgensma 161
Zoonotic viral disease
    transmitted 287
Zostavax 15, 65, 123, 178
  single dose of 91
Zoster vaccination 15, 65, 107
Zoster vaccine 123
  recombinant 86, 122, 176, 178

EU GSPR Authorised Reprsentative
Logos Europe, 9 rue Nicolas Poussin
1700, La Rochelle, France
Phone: +33 (0) 6 67 93 73 78
E-mail: contact@logoseurope.eu

www.ingramcontent.com/pod-product-compliance
Ingram Content Group UK Ltd.
Pitfield, Milton Keynes, MK11 3LW, UK
UKHW051847210426
5322IPUK00019B/285